Essentials of

Radiodiagnosis

Essentials of **Radiodiagnosis**

As per the Revised Competency-based Medical Education Curriculum 2024 (NMC)

Rachna Chaurasia MD (Radiodiagnosis)
Professor and Academic Head
Department of Radiodiagnosis
Maharani Laxmi Bai Medical College
Jhansi, Uttar Pradesh, India

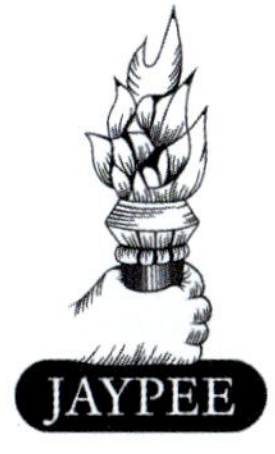

JAYPEE BROTHERS MEDICAL PUBLISHERS
The Health Sciences Publisher
New Delhi | London

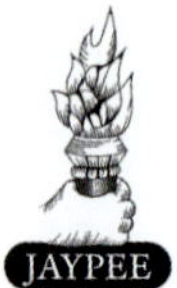

JAYPEE **Jaypee Brothers Medical Publishers (P) Ltd**

Headquarters
Jaypee Brothers Medical Publishers (P) Ltd.
EMCA House
23/23-B, Ansari Road, Daryaganj
New Delhi - 110 002, India
Landline: +91-11-23272143, +91-11-23272703
+91-11-23282021, +91-11-23245672
Email: jaypee@jaypeebrothers.com

Corporate Office
Jaypee Brothers Medical Publishers (P) Ltd.
4838/24, Ansari Road, Daryaganj
New Delhi 110 002, India
Phone: +91-11-43574357
Fax: +91-11-43574314
Email: jaypee@jaypeebrothers.com

Overseas Office
J.P. Medical Ltd.
83 Victoria Street, London
SW1H 0HW (UK)
Phone: +44 20 3170 8910
Fax: +44 (0)20 3008 6180
Email: info@jpmedpub.com

Website: www.jaypeebrothers.com
Website: www.jaypeedigital.com

Inquiries for bulk sales may be solicited at: jaypee@jaypeebrothers.com

Essentials of Radiodiagnosis

First Edition: **2025**

ISBN: 978-93-6616-175-4

Printed at Samrat Offset Pvt. Ltd.

Dedicated to

My late father Shri PC Chaurasia and brother Dr Vikas Chaurasia, whose dreams for me have shaped my path. Your belief in my potential to heal and help others guided me to the world of radiology. Every page of this book holds a piece of the legacy you envisioned. Thank you for inspiring me to see beyond the visible.

Contributors

Anil Kumar Singh
Additional Professor
Department of Radiodiagnosis
Sanjay Gandhi Post Graduate Institute
Lucknow, Uttar Pradesh, India
Gastrointestinal Tract Imaging, Ch-27

Ankur J Shah
Consultant Radiologist
Department of Radiodiagnosis
Sadbhav Imaging Centre
Ahmedabad, Gujarat, India
Musculoskeletal Imaging, Ch-14

Ashish Verma
Professor
Department of Radiodiagnosis
Banaras Hindu University
Varanasi, Uttar Pradesh, India
Pediatric Neuroimaging, Ch-21

Deb K Boruah
Additional Professor
Department of Diagnostic and
Interventional Radiodiagnosis
All India Institute of Medical Sciences
Guwahati, Assam, India
Radiology in Geriatric Patients, Ch-30

Dhruv Gehlot
Ananta Institute of Medical Sciences and
Research Centre
Rajsamand, Rajasthan, India
Hepatobiliary and Pancreatic Imaging, Ch-28

Digish Vaghela
Professor
Department of Radiodiagnosis
BJ Medical College
Ahmedabad, Gujarat, India
Neurological Imaging, Ch-11

Dinesh Patel
Senior Cardiac Imaging Radiologist
Department of Radiodiagnosis
UN Mehta Institute of Cardiology and
Research Centre
Ahmedabad, Gujarat, India
Cardiovascular Imaging, Ch-32

Gaurav Raj
Professor and Head
Department of Radiodiagnosis
RML Hospital, Lucknow, Uttar Pradesh, India
Oncological Imaging, Ch-31

Hit B Jivani
Ex-Assistant Professor
Department of Radiodiagnosis
UN Mehta Institute of Cardiology and
Research Centre
Ahmedabad, Gujarat, India
Cardiovascular Imaging, Ch-32

Ishan Kumar
Professor
Department of Radiodiagnosis
IMS, Banaras Hindu University
Varanasi, Uttar Pradesh, India

Kalyan Sarma
Associate Professor
Department of Diagnostic and Interventional
Radiodiagnosis
All India Institute of Medical Sciences
Guwahati, Assam, India
Radiology in Geriatric Patients, Ch-30

Kunal Gehlot
Radiologist
Department of Radiodiagnosis
RNT Government Medical College
Udaipur, Rajasthan, India
Hepatobiliary and Pancreatic Imaging, Ch-28

Kushal Gehlot
Professor
Department of Radiodiagnosis
RNT Government Medical College
Udaipur, Rajasthan, India
Hepatobiliary and Pancreatic Imaging, Ch-28

Malvika Gehani
Radiologist
Department of Radiodiagnosis
RNT Government Medical College
Udaipur, Rajasthan, India
Hepatobiliary and Pancreatic Imaging, Ch-28

Mansi Jain
Consultant, Fetal and Women Imaging Specialist
Department of Radiodiagnosis
IRIS Imaging Centre
Bhopal, Madhya Pradesh, India
Obstetric Emergencies, Ch-18

Mashoo Neil Dubey
Director, Neil Ultrasound and Diagnostic Solutions
Chief Consultant, Adi Shankar Hospital
Jabalpur, Madhya Pradesh, India
Fetal Imaging—Developmental Anomalies, Ch-16

Megha M Sheth
Cardiac Imaging Radiologist
Department of Radiodiagnosis
UN Mehta Institute of Cardiology and
Research Centre
Ahmedabad, Gujarat, India
Cardiovascular Imaging, Ch-32

Milin Garachh
Cardiac Imaging Radiologist
Department of Radiodiagnosis
UN Mehta Institute of Cardiology and
Research Centre
Ahmedabad, Gujarat, India
Cardiovascular Imaging, Ch-32

Neeraj Prajapati
Professor
Department of Radiodiagnosis
Shri Ram Murti Smarak Institute of
Medical Sciences
Bareilly, Uttar Pradesh, India
Spinal Imaging, Ch-13

Neha Singh
Additional Professor
Department of Radiodiagnosis
RML Hospital
Lucknow, Uttar Pradesh, India
Breast Imaging, Ch-25

Pankaj Sharma
Additional Professor
Department of Diagnostic and
Interventional Radiology
All India Institute of Medical Sciences
Rishikesh, Uttarakhand, India
Urinary Tract Imaging, Ch-29

Pooja Kundu
Ex-Senior Resident
Department of Radiodiagnosis
All India Institute of Medical Sciences
Rishikesh, Uttarakhand, India
Urinary Tract Imaging, Ch-29

Pranjal Phukan
Professor
Department of Diagnostic and
Interventional Radiodiagnosis
All India Institute of Medical Sciences
Guwahati, Assam, India
Radiology in Geriatric Patients, Ch-30

Pratyaksha Rana
Assistant Professor
Department of Radiodiagnosis
UN Mehta Institute of Cardiology and
Research Centre
Ahmedabad, Gujarat, India
Cardiovascular Imaging, Ch-32

Priscilla Joshi
Professor and Head
Department of Radiodiagnosis
Bharati (DU) Medical College and Hospital
Dhankawadi, Pune, Maharashtra, India
Pediatric Musculoskeletal Imaging, Ch-22

Rashmi Singh
Co-founder and Consultant Radiologist
Healthscan Diagnostic
Varanasi, Uttar Pradesh, India
Basics of Obstetric Imaging, Ch-15

Samir Patel
Cardiac Imaging Radiologist
Department of Radiodiagnosis
UN Mehta Institute of Cardiology and Research Centre
Ahmedabad, Gujarat, India

Sanket
Consultant Interventional Radiologist
Department of Radiodiagnosis
Yashoda Hospitals
Hyderabad, Telangana, India
Interventional Radiology, Ch-7

Saurabh Deshpande
Ex-Senior Resident
Department of Radiodiagnosis
UN Mehta Institute of Cardiology and Research Centre
Ahmedabad, Gujarat, India
Cardiovascular Imaging, Ch-32

Shamrendra Narayan
Professor
Department of Radiodiagnosis
RML Hospital
Lucknow, Uttar Pradesh, India
Imaging in Joint Disease, Ch-26

Shikha Khandelwal
Chief Consultant
CT and MRI Division
Gujarat Imaging Centre
Ahmedabad, Gujarat, India
Advanced Imaging Techniques, Ch-6

Shivam Angiras
MRI Technician
Department of Diagnostic and Interventional Radiodiagnosis
All India Institute of Medical Sciences
Guwahati, Assam, India
Imaging in Geriatrics, Ch-30

Shruti Mehta
Professor and Head
Department of Radiodiagnosis
Smt GR Doshi and Smt KM Mehta Institute of Kidney Diseases and Research Centre and
DR HL Trivedi Institute of Transplantation Sciences (IKDRC-ITS)
Gujarat University of Transplantation Sciences
Ahmedabad, Gujarat, India
Imaging in Transplant Medicine, Ch-36

Suvinay Saxena
Assistant Professor
Department of Radiodiagnosis
Chirayu Medical College and Hospital
Bhopal, Madhya Pradesh, India
Musculoskeletal Imaging, Ch-14

Vipul Solanki
Associate Professor
Department of Radiodiagnosis
Government Medical College
Bhavnagar, Gujarat, India
Neurological Imaging, Ch-11

Vishal Patel
Associate Professor
Radiation Safety Officer (High Dose)
Department of Nuclear Medicine
UN Mehta Institute of Cardiology and Research Centre
Ahmedabad, Gujarat, India
Nuclear Medicine in Radiology, Ch-35

Vivek Singh
Professor
Department of Radiodiagnosis
Sanjay Gandhi Postgraduate Institute of Medical Sciences
Lucknow, Uttar Pradesh, India
Interventional Radiology, Ch-7

Preface

Radiodiagnosis stands as a cornerstone in modern medical practice, bridging gaps across various specialties by providing crucial insights that guide diagnosis and treatment. With the evolving landscape of medical education and the heightened emphasis on competency-based assessments, there arises a need for a resource that not only simplifies this complex field but also aligns seamlessly with the current educational standards.

Essentials of Radiodiagnosis is crafted with the dual intent of serving as a foundational text for MBBS students and a comprehensive review guide for postgraduate (PG) students. This book is designed to cater to the academic requirements of students at different levels of their medical education, offering a thorough exploration of radiodiagnostic techniques from basic to advanced levels.

For MBBS students, this book covers all essential aspects of radiodiagnosis, ensuring alignment with the Competency-Based Medical Education (CBME) curriculum. It not only prepares them for their regular assessments but also equips them with the knowledge necessary for their exit exams, encapsulating key concepts in a manner that is both digestible and retainable.

Postgraduate students will find this text equally beneficial. The detailed exposition of advanced imaging techniques, interventional procedures, and latest advancements in the field makes it an invaluable tool for quick revision and deep dives into complex topics. The structured format of the book helps in reinforcing knowledge and preparing for Postgraduate Medical Entrance Examinations (PGMEE), with chapters logically organized to build on foundational concepts and advance to more intricate discussions.

In crafting this edition, we have integrated feedback from a wide array of radiology educators and students, ensuring that the content not only meets educational standards but also addresses the practical needs of learners. With contributions from experts across various subspecialties of radiology, the book offers diverse perspectives and insights, enhancing the learning experience.

Essentials of Radiodiagnosis also emphasizes radiation safety and protection, with dedicated chapters that are crucial in everyday clinical practice, especially for those handling radiological equipment and interpreting results.

It is our hope that this book will serve as a comprehensive resource, aiding students in mastering radiodiagnosis and ultimately fostering a deeper understanding of this pivotal field in medicine.

Rachna Chaurasia

Acknowledgments

The journey to compile "Essentials of Radiodiagnosis" has been both challenging and enlightening. This endeavor would not have been possible without the support and guidance from many who have contributed their expertise and time.

Foremost, I extend my heartfelt appreciation to my mentors, Dr Ganesh Kumar and Dr AK Gupta, whose profound teachings have not only enriched my understanding but also guided my approach to radiodiagnosis. Their mentorship has been invaluable.

I owe a deep gratitude to my husband, Professor Anshul Jain, whose unwavering support and insight have been crucial throughout this process. His encouragement and belief in my capabilities have been a constant source of motivation.

Special thanks go to my parents, Shree PC Chaurasia and Shakuntala Chaurasia; in-laws, Dr DB Jain and Smt Saroj Jain; uncles Shri Subhash Chandra Chaurasia and Dr Atish Sharma; brother and sister-in-law Mr Vishal Chaurasia and Smt Kavita Chaurasia for their blessings and the values they have instilled in me. Their support has been a cornerstone of my personal and professional life.

Gratitude is also due to my children, whose patience and love have lightened the burden of this comprehensive endeavor. Their presence brings joy and balance to my demanding schedule.

I am also thankful to my academic peers, including Drs Rajeev Sinha, Naveen Malhotra, Sanjaya Sharma, Pramodita Agarwal, Pushpendra Agarwal, Teena Sahu, SV Sahu, Manita Devariya, Rajkumar Rajpoot, and Kajal Kumari, whose collaborations and discussions have enriched this text significantly.

Additionally, I would like to acknowledge the support from colleagues and friends within the community, especially those who have provided feedback and constructive criticism that have greatly enhanced the quality of this work.

This book is a testament to the collaborative efforts of many dedicated individuals, especially my PG students Shivam and Shweta and all staff of Aashirvad Diagnostic Centre. To everyone who has been a part of this journey—your contributions are immensely appreciated and have been pivotal in the creation of this resource.

My sincere appreciation extends to the entire team of M/s Jaypee Brothers Medical Publishers (P) Ltd, New Delhi, for their tremendous effort and unwavering support, Shri Jitendar P Vij (Group Chairman), Mr Ankit Vij (Managing Director), Mr MS Mani (Group President), Dr Madhu Choudhary (Director-Educational Publishing), Ms Pooja Bhandari [Director—Production (Books and Journals)], Dr Upma Tomar (Senior Development Editor), Ms Sunita Katla (Executive Assistant to Group Chairman and Publishing Manager), Ms Samina Khan (Executive Assistant to Director—Educational Publishing), Mr Ajay Kumar Sharma [Deputy General Manager (Books and Journals)], Mr Vijay Kumar Bhatia (Production Manager), Ms Seema Dogra (Cover Visualizer), Ms Neha Verma (Graphic Designer—Cover), Mr Mithlesh Kumar Singh (Quality Analyst), Mr Jagvir Singh Tomar (Typesetter), and Mr Sumit Kumar (Team Lead-Graphic Designer). Without their cooperation, I could not have completed this project.

Contents

UNIT 3: Obstetric and Gynecological Imaging

UNIT 4: Pediatric Radiology

UNIT 5: Comprehensive Radiological Review

Competency Table

Competency number	*Competency name*	*Unit*	*Chapter*
RD1.1	Knowledgeable about the general principles of functioning of imaging modalities such as plain X-ray, fluoroscopy, CT, ultrasound, nuclear medicine modalities (bone scan, PET) and MRI, to the extent that they would be able to (a) exhibit mindful behavior regarding the potential hazards associated with each imaging modality (b) make rational choices about the appropriateness of the modality for a particular purpose, such as what will be seen better in which modality (e.g., air-containing structures would be imaged better in X-ray than in ultrasound)	1 2 7	1, 2, 5, 6, 8 9 35
RD2.1	Obtain relevant clinical history to select patients for imaging modalities, in order to determine suitability for radiation exposure/contrast administration/exposure to magnetic fields (including allergies, renal function, pregnancy, implanted devices)	1 7	3, 4, 5 36
RD2.2	Select the correct imaging modality and procedure for broad pathology type (infections, tumor, trauma, congenital), body part/system (CNS, head and neck, chest, abdomen and extremities) in adults, children and pregnant women, mindful of unique needs of pediatric patients with respect to radiation and sedation	2 3 4 5 Glossary, annexure	9 to 14 15 to 19 20 to 24 25 to 32
RD3.1	Awareness of different types of radiation and the stochastic and nonstochastic hazards of radiation in human beings (acute and long-term)	1	3, 4
RD3.2	Knowledgeable about best practices (time, distance and shielding) and provisions to keep X-ray exposure ALARA (as low as reasonably achievable) in clinical practice of radiology and general principles to be followed as per AERB regulatory guidelines	1	3, 4
RD3.3	Knowledgeable about monitoring radiation exposure in healthcare workers with dosimeter such as thermoluminescent dosimeter and awareness of the units to measure radiation exposure in human beings	1	3, 4

Competency number	*Competency name*	*Unit*	*Chapter*
RD3.4	Knowledgeable about the purpose and components of the PC-PNDT Act relevant to a primary care physician	7	37
RD4.1	Collaborate with imaging specialists for optimum patient care—provide relevant and clear clinical information in requisitions for imaging, convey appropriate clinical urgency to facilitate correct scheduling of patients for imaging, clarify from imaging specialists when in doubt about appropriateness of imaging procedure	1 Annexure	5
RD4.2	Apply appropriate safety measures when transporting critically ill patients for imaging competencies such as checking adequacy of oxygen cylinder, following correct precautions in MRI room	6	33, 34
RD4.3	For diseases that can be encountered by primary care physician such as osteoarthritis (X-ray), deep vein thrombosis, cholecystitis, apply anatomical-radiological-pathophysiology correlations as a basis of clinical reasoning and interdisciplinary communication	5 Annexure	25 to 32
RD5.1	Interpretation of normal X-ray images of the chest, abdomen, musculoskeletal system by identifying normal structures in chest X-ray, abdominal X-ray, musculoskeletal X-ray (upper limbs, lower limbs, spine), PNS – Water's view in adults; normal neonatal chest X-ray (thymic shadow identification); normal joint X-ray in children (epiphysis and growth plate identification)	2 3 4 5 Glossary, annexure	9 to 14 15 to 19 20 to 24 25 to 32
RD5.2	Age estimation from X-rays by selecting and using appropriate reference standards	Glossary	
RD5.3	Image interpretation of emergency conditions in chest X-ray, abdominal X-ray and skeletal X-rays such as pneumoperitoneum, acute fracture, differentiating acute from chronic fracture etc.	5 2	26 12
RD5.4	Image interpretation of normal/abnormal position of devices in the chest X-ray of adult and pediatric ICU patients	6	34
RD6.1	Ability to provide written and verbal instructions tailored to the patient and imaging procedure such as fasting requirement, medication adjustments, bowel preparation	1	5, 7
RD7.1	Integrate provided imaging findings and description of appearances in the management of PCOD, ectopic pregnancy, evaluation of infertility in the obstetrics and gynecology department	3	15 to 19

Competency number	*Competency name*	*Unit*	*Chapter*
RD7.2	Integrate provided imaging findings and description of appearances in the management of ASOM/CSOM, evaluation of sensorineural hearing loss in the ENT department	2	10
RD7.3	Integrate provided imaging findings and description of appearances in the management of stroke (CT brain), pulmonary embolism, findings associated with cardiac failure and liver parenchymal diseases in the internal medicine department	2 5	11 28, 32
RD7.4	Integrate provided imaging findings and description of appearances in the management of head injuries, hernia with strangulation, appendicitis and intestinal obstruction in the surgery department	5	27
RD7.5	Integrate provided imaging findings and description of appearances in the management chest infections, foreign body aspiration, urinary tract infection in the pediatrics department	4	20 to 24
RD7.6	Integrate provided imaging findings and description of appearances in the screening for breast cancer and management of breast cancer patients	5	25

UNIT 1

Fundamentals and Techniques in Radiodiagnosis

Unit Outline

CHAPTER

1 Introduction

"In a world of shadows, radiologists bring light to the truth hidden within."

Radiodiagnosis stands as a cornerstone in the realm of modern medicine, harnessing the power of advanced imaging techniques to unveil the mysteries within the human body. This medical specialty transcends traditional boundaries, offering a window into the intricate structures and functions that lie beneath the surface, all without a single incision. With the ability to visualize everything from the sprawling network of bones and vessels to the delicate nuances of soft tissue, radiodiagnosis provides clinicians with unprecedented insights into the nature and extent of diseases. It plays a critical and expanding role in patient care, empowering physicians with precise diagnostic information, guiding the trajectory of treatment plans, and offering a means to monitor the effectiveness of interventions over time. As technology advances, so too does the scope and accuracy of radiodiagnostic tools, continually pushing the limits of what is possible in medical imaging and diagnosis. This chapter embarks on a journey through the role of radiologist, exploring the transformative impact of imaging modalities on patient care, the intricate dance of radiological interpretation, and the profound influence of these technologies in shaping the future of healthcare.

ROLE OF THE RADIOLOGIST

Radiologists are highly trained medical doctors who specialize in interpreting medical images to diagnose and manage diseases. The role of the radiologist is multifaceted, extending far beyond the interpretation of medical images to encompass a broad spectrum of responsibilities that significantly impact patient care and treatment outcomes. Radiologists are medical doctors with specialized training in reading and interpreting a wide range of diagnostic images, including X-rays, CT scans, MRI scans, and ultrasounds. Their expertise is pivotal in diagnosing diseases, identifying injuries, and even guiding certain therapeutic procedures. Broadly radiologist plays important role in

Diagnostic Expertise

Radiologists play a critical role in the diagnostic process. They analyze images to identify abnormalities such as fractures, tumors, fetal anomaly or diseases in various body parts. Their interpretations help in confirming or diagnosing medical conditions, thereby informing the next steps in patient management. This diagnostic insight is crucial for developing effective treatment plans tailored to the specific needs of patients.

Interventional Procedures

A subset of radiologists, known as interventional radiologists, perform minimally invasive procedures under the guidance of imaging technologies. These procedures can include anything from biopsies, where small tissue samples are removed for analysis, to the treatment of blocked arteries or the delivery of targeted cancer therapies. Interventional radiology offers alternatives to open surgery for certain conditions, often resulting in shorter recovery times and less risk for patients.

Consultation and Collaboration

Radiologists consult with other healthcare professionals to ensure a comprehensive approach to patient care. They discuss their findings with physicians, surgeons, and other medical staff to develop or adjust treatment plans based on the diagnostic images. This collaborative approach ensures that treatment decisions are indirectly based on radiological findings.

Research and Education

Many radiologists are also involved in research, contributing to advancements in imaging techniques and technologies that continue to revolutionize patient diagnosis and treatment. They play a vital role in educating clinicians, residents, and other healthcare professionals about the latest developments in early diagnosis and their applications in clinical practice.

For example, IRIA Samrakshan develop protocol at national level for early screening of pre-eclampsia and fetal growth restriction.

Patient Advocacy and Communication

Although radiologists often work behind the scenes, their role in patient advocacy is significant. They ensure that imaging studies are performed safely, adhering to protocols that minimize exposure to radiation. Additionally, radiologists may communicate directly with patients to explain imaging procedures, discuss findings, and sometimes provide recommendations based on the imaging results.

IMAGING MODALITIES AND THEIR APPLICATIONS

In the realm of radiodiagnosis, a variety of imaging modalities stand as the cornerstone for diagnosing and managing patient care. These modalities, each with its unique capabilities and applications, form the backbone of medical imaging, offering unparalleled insights into the structure and function of the human body. The choice of imaging modality is dictated by the specific clinical question at hand, considering factors such as the area of the body being examined, the nature of the suspected condition, and the patient's overall health status. Each modality employs a different physical principle to create images, from the density-based contrast of X-rays to the intensity of magnetic properties of tissue utilized in MRI, upto the metabolic insights provided by PET scans **(Table 1.1)**.

As we proceed through the book, we will expand on this foundation, providing a comprehensive understanding of how these technologies work, their advancements, and their critical roles in patient care and treatment planning. The journey through the evolution and detailed exploration of each technique will equip you with the knowledge to appreciate the full spectrum of possibilities that modern radiodiagnosis offers to healthcare.

Table 1.1: Overview of imaging modalities.

Modality	*Principle*	*Primary Use*
X-ray	Electromagnetic radiation	Bone fractures, lung imaging
Ultrasound (US)	Sound waves	Soft tissues, pregnancy, vascular systems
Computed tomography (CT)	X-ray with computer processing	Detailed bone and lung pathology
Magnetic resonance imaging (MRI)	Magnetic fields and radio waves	Soft tissue, spine, brain, joints
Positron emission tomography (PET)	Radioactive tracers	Metabolic activity, cancer detection
Single-photon emission computed tomography (SPECT)	Gamma rays	Blood flow, functional imaging of organs

PRACTICAL ASPECTS OF RADIODIAGNOSIS

When a patient presents with symptoms that require further exploration, the clinician evaluates the clinical picture and decides on the necessary investigations. If imaging is deemed necessary, the patient is referred to a radiology center, marking the beginning of a critical journey in their care pathway. This journey, intricate and multifaceted, encompasses not just the technical execution of imaging studies but also the preparation of the patient, interpretation of the images, and effective communication of the results.

Patient Preparation and Safety

Upon arrival at the radiology center, the first step involves preparing the patient for the imaging procedure **(Table 1.2)**. This preparation varies significantly depending on the type of study being performed but generally includes a review of the patient's medical history, explanation of the procedure to alleviate any anxiety and instructions on how to prepare physically and mentally. For some procedures, this might mean fasting, while for others, it could involve drinking contrast media. Safety protocols are paramount, especially concerning the use of ionizing radiation and contrast agents, to minimize any potential risks and manage allergies.

Table 1.2: Pre-procedural patient preparation in various modalities.

Radiological test	*Patient preparation*
X-ray	No special preparation required in plain X-rays remove jewelery and metallic objects though bowel preparation fasting, etc., required in case of procedures
Ultrasound	Fast for 6–8 hours if abdominal ultrasound (especially for hepatobiliary system); drink water for pelvic and KUB scans to fill the bladder
CT scan	May need to fast for a few hours; possible administration of contrast material orally or intravenously
MRI	Remove all metallic objects, inform technician if there are any implants; fasting may be required for specific studies
PET scan	Fast for at least 4–6 hours before the test; avoid strenuous exercise for 24 hours prior to the test

Imaging Technique Execution

The technical execution of the imaging procedure is a delicate balance between acquiring the highest quality images and ensuring patient comfort and safety. Radiologists and technologists meticulously select imaging parameters and position the patient to capture the most diagnostic views of the area of interest. Protective measures are also employed to shield both patients and staff from unnecessary radiation exposure.

Image Interpretation

The interpretation of radiologic images is a nuanced process that requires extensive knowledge of anatomy, pathology, and the specific characteristics of various imaging modalities. Radiologists systematically analyze images to identify normal versus abnormal findings, utilizing their expertise to distinguish between benign conditions and those necessitating further investigation or immediate intervention. This interpretative process is critical in providing accurate diagnoses that guide patient management.

Communication of Results

Communicating the findings of radio diagnostic studies to referring clinicians is a crucial step in the diagnostic process. The radiologist's report must be clear, concise, and timely, providing actionable insights that can directly impact treatment decisions. This communication is often facilitated by standardized reporting system (e.g., BIRADS, ORADS, etc.) and digital platforms (e.g., PACS) that ensure the swift transmission of information.

Quality Control and Continuous Learning

Maintaining the highest quality standards in radiodiagnosis requires ongoing efforts in quality control and professional development. This encompasses everything from regular maintenance of imaging equipment to participation in continuing education and peer review activities. Such practices ensure that radiologists and technologists remain at the forefront of technological advancements and best practices in patient care. Every machine has to be managed by combined effects of radiologist, technician and engineer of concerned firm which provide latest upgradation of technologies. QA of machines has to be done yearly.

FUTURE DIRECTIONS IN RADIODIAGNOSIS

The field of radiodiagnosis is on the cusp of transformative changes, driven by advancements in technology, artificial intelligence (AI), and the increasing emphasis on personalized medicine. These innovations promise to enhance diagnostic accuracy, improve patient outcomes, and streamline workflow processes within radiology departments.

Integration of Artificial Intelligence

One of the most significant advancements is the integration of AI and machine learning algorithms into radiodiagnositc practices. AI has the potential to revolutionize how images are interpreted by assisting radiologists in detecting subtle abnormalities that may be overlooked by the human eye. Furthermore, AI can automate routine tasks, such as measuring lesions or identifying standard anatomical structures, thereby reducing the time radiologists spend on monotonous activities and allowing them to focus on more complex cases.

Advanced Imaging Techniques

The development of more sophisticated imaging techniques offers unprecedented detail and clarity, enabling earlier detection of diseases and more accurate assessments of treatment efficacy. Techniques such as 4D imaging, functional MRI (fMRI), and molecular imaging are pushing the boundaries of traditional radiodiagnosis, offering insights into the functional aspects of tissues and organs, in addition to their anatomical structure.

Radio Genomics

Radio genomics is the integration of genomic information with imaging data, is an emerging field that promises to link genetic mutations with specific imaging patterns, facilitating more personalized treatment strategies especially for tumors based on a patient's genetic profile.

Enhanced Patient Experience

Future developments in radiodiagnosis also focus on enhancing the patient experience. This includes reducing the time required for imaging procedures, minimizing the need for invasive contrast agents, and developing more comfortable and less claustrophobic imaging environments. Efforts are also being made to reduce radiation exposure, especially in modalities that rely on ionizing radiation, to ensure patient safety.

Teleradiology and Global Collaboration

Teleradiology continues to expand, breaking down geographical barriers and enabling the sharing of images with specialists around the world. This global collaboration enhances diagnostic accuracy through second opinions and facilitates access to expert consultations, particularly in underserved areas.

In conclusion, the journey through the world of radiodiagnosis is a testament to the dynamic interplay between technology, medicine, and patient care. It underscores the importance of radiodiagnosis in the healthcare continuum and sets the stage for its evolving role in shaping the future of medical diagnostics. As the field continues to grow and evolve, it remains a beacon of innovation, committed to improving the lives of patients through enhanced diagnostic precision and care.

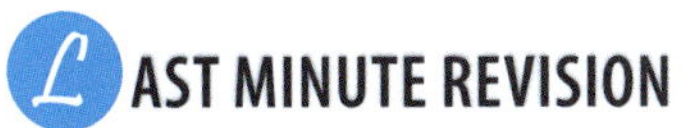

- Radiodiagnosis is a branch deals with diagnosis as well as management of patient (example guided procedures and therapeutic interventions like peripheral vessel angioplasty)
- Guided procedures like biopsy and abscess drainage can be performed with all modalities depending on type/origin of pathology, condition of patient and availability of modality
- Usage of X-rays related modalities are contraindicated in pregnancy
- USG and MRI are safer modality during pregnancy
- X-ray related modalities should be AERB approved and should be installed as per AERB guidelines
- USG and even cross-sectional modalities like CT and MRI should be registered under the PC-PNDT act.

REVIEW QUESTIONS

Multiple Choice Questions (MCQs)

1. **Which of the following imaging modalities uses sound waves to create images of the body?**
   a. X-ray
   b. MRI
   c. Ultrasound
   d. CT scan
2. **What is the significance of contrast agents in radiodiagnosis?**
   a. They help in reducing radiation exposure
   b. They are used to improve the visibility of internal structures
   c. They are used to treat the diseases being imaged
   d. They decrease the imaging time
3. **Which of the following is a key consideration when preparing a patient for an MRI scan?**
   a. Ensuring the patient has fasted for 12 hours
   b. Confirming the patient has no metal implants
   c. Applying a contrast agent topically
   d. Ensuring the patient is hydrated
4. **What future direction in radiodiagnosis involves enhancing image quality through artificial intelligence?**
   a. Reducing the need for contrast agents
   b. Decreasing imaging time
   c. Increasing radiation dose for clearer images
   d. Improving image analysis and interpretation

Answer Key

1. c 2. b 3. b 4. d

SUGGESTED READING

1. Barreiro-Ares A, Morales-Santiago A, Sendra-Portero F, Souto-Bayarri M. Impact of the Rise of Artificial Intelligence in Radiology: What Do Students Think? Int J Environ Res Public Health. 2023 Jan; 16;20(2):1589. doi: 10.3390/ijerp0021589. PMID: 36674348; PMCID: PMC9867061.
2. Zuhir Bodalal, Stefano Trebeschi. Radiogenomics: Bridging imaging and genomics. Abdom Radiol (NY). 2019 Jun;44(6):1960 -1984. doi: 10.1007/s00261 -019-02028-w.

CHAPTER

2 Evolution of Radiodiagnosis

"Radiodiagnosis has evolved, but its purpose endures—to decode the silent signals and lead the way."

INTRODUCTION

In the ever-evolving landscape of medical sciences, radiodiagnosis stands as a cornerstone, continually reshaping the way we understand, diagnose, and treat a myriad of health conditions. Radiodiagnosis has emerged as a highly sought-after field for MBBS graduates today, a shift driven largely by its remarkable technological advancements. This chapter offers an in-depth look at the evolution of radiodiagnosis, a field that has dramatically transformed in the previous 25–30 years. As mandated by the NMC competency-based curriculum, our exploration will encompass all pertinent aspects of radiodiagnosis, ensuring a thorough understanding of both its historical context and current applications. We embark on this journey with a recognition of how radiodiagnostic techniques have revolutionized medical diagnostics, offering unprecedented insights into the human body.

This chapter is designed to offer MBBS students a comprehensive insight into the field of radiodiagnosis. Starting from the initial discovery of X-ray imaging, it traces the path leading to advanced techniques such as MRI, CT scans, mammography, ultrasound, and PET. Timeline of radiodiagnosis evolution discussed in **Table 2.1**.

Table 2.1: Timeline of radiodiagnosis evolution.

Year	*Milestone*
1895	Discovery of X-rays by Wilhelm Conrad Röentgen
1896	First use of X-rays for medical diagnosis
1913	Invention of the Coolidge tube, improving X-ray tube design
1927	Introduction of contrast agents for X-ray imaging
1950s	Development of ultrasound for medical imaging
1960s	First commercial CT scanners developed by Godfrey Hounsfield
1970s	Introduction of MRI technology by Raymond Damadian
1980s	Digital radiography begins to replace traditional film
1990s	Advancements in 3D imaging and Doppler ultrasound
2000s	Integration of PET with CT for combined imaging (PET/CT)
2010s	Widespread use of AI and machine learning in image analysis
2020s	Emergence of advanced interventional radiology techniques

The chapter will provide MBBS students with a broad understanding of radiodiagnosis. It familiarizes you with the various diagnostic machines and the types of images they produce. Beyond this, it provides a brief overview of the wider aspects of the field, including ethical considerations and the impact of these technologies on patient treatment and overall healthcare.

RADIOLOGICAL DIVISIONS IN THE CURRENT ERA

Radiodiagnosis has evolved dramatically from its early days, beginning with conventional X-ray radiography. Today, it encompasses a range of technologically advanced modalities, each offering unique insights into the human body. As we journey through the timeline of innovations in this field, showcased in **Table 2.1**, we observe a rich diversity of advanced imaging techniques now at our disposal. These modalities can be utilized independently or in conjunction with others, enhancing diagnostic accuracy and patient care. In the current era, the key modalities include:

X-ray Radiography

X-ray radiography, the oldest form of medical imaging, remains a staple in diagnostic radiology. It operates on the principle of passing X-rays through the body to create images of internal structures. The varying densities of different tissues and organs—like bones, muscles, and organs—result in varying shades on the X-ray film, providing critical information about conditions like fractures, infections, and obstructions.

As you have read in the subsequent chapter, the journey of conventional X-ray radiography began with the discovery of X-rays by Wilhelm Conrad Röentgen. Following this ground-breaking discovery, the first conventional X-ray machines were developed and introduced to the market. However, it wasn't until after the second world war that X-ray machines became widely available and began to be commonly used in medical diagnostics, marking the start of a new era in medical imaging. Initially, conventional radiography was the norm, where images were captured directly on film. This process required a dark room (**Wet processing**) for developing the images, much like traditional photography. As technology progressed, computed radiography (**CR = Dry processing with cassette**) was developed. In this method, the exposure is carried out by a conventional X-ray machine, but instead of using film, a special imaging plate captures the image. This plate is then scanned by a dedicated reader, converting the captured image into a digital file. This advancement bridged the gap between traditional film-based radiography and the modern digital era, enhancing image processing efficiency and quality **(Fig. 2.1)**.

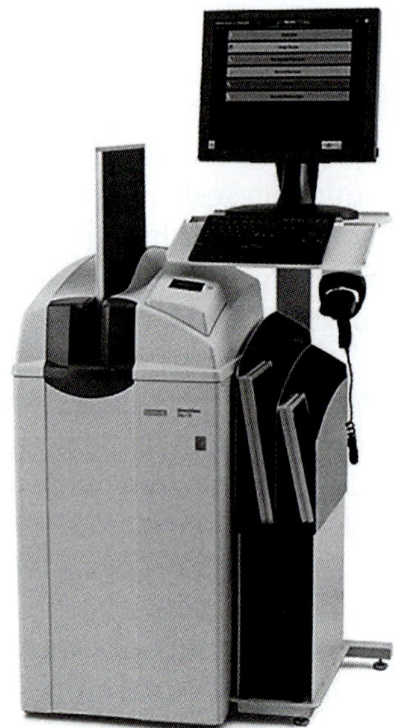
Fig. 2.1: Computed radiography system.

The latest advancement in this domain is digital radiography (**DR = cassette-less dry processing**), **(Fig. 2.2)** which bypasses the

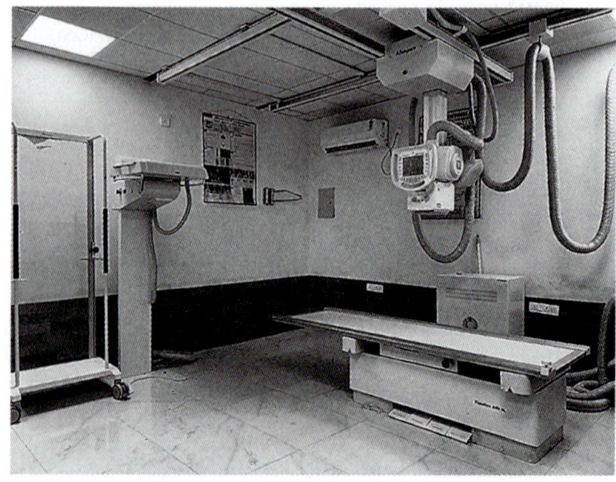
Fig. 2.2: Digital radiography system.

Table 2.2: Distinguishing features of conventional, computed, and digital radiography.

Feature	*Conventional radiography*	*Computed radiography (CR)*	*Digital radiography (DR)*
Image capture	Directly on film	On a special imaging plate	Direct digital capture (cassette-less x-ray)
Image processing	Requires dark room development (wet processing)	Scanner reads imaging plate (dry processing)	Instant digital processing (dry processing)
Image quality	Standard	Improved over conventional	Superior, with enhanced detail
Radiation exposure	Standard	Lower than conventional	Lowest among the three
Image storage	Physical storage of films	Digital file storage	Integrated with electronic medical records
Turnaround time	Longer due to manual processing	Faster than conventional	Immediate image availability

need for film or imaging plates altogether. In DR, the detectors directly capture the image and convert it to a digital format. This leap offers numerous advantages, including immediate image availability, better image quality and reduced radiation exposure to patients. The digital format also facilitates the integration of images with electronic medical records and teleradiology, allowing for easier sharing and consultation. Differentiation features between conventional, computed and digital radiography are discussed in **Table 2.2**.

Computed Tomography

Computed tomography (CT) **(Fig. 2.3)** has revolutionized diagnostic imaging by providing detailed cross-sectional views of the body. Unlike conventional X-rays, CT scans can differentiate between tissues with very similar densities, making them particularly useful for detecting diseases and injuries in complex organs like the brain. Modern CT scanners are faster and more precise with capable of generating 3D images. The development of spiral and multislice CT scan offers a critical advantage in diagnosing a wide range of diseases and injuries:

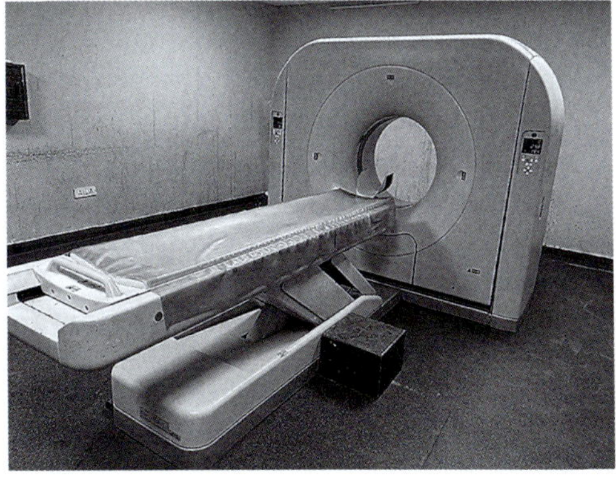

Fig. 2.3: Computed tomography machine.

- **Craniocerebral injuries:** Computed tomography (CT) stands as the definitive diagnostic tool in the wake of traumatic head injuries. Its swift imaging capabilities are essential for the evaluation of craniocerebral trauma, allowing for the quick identification of intracranial hemorrhages, fractures of the skull, and any signs of cerebral edema. CT imaging is the gold standard for diagnosing cervical spine injuries especially in bony structures for detecting fractures, and dislocations, or any other spinal abnormalities.
- **Neuroimaging for stroke:** CT's role in neuroimaging, especially in the setting of stroke, is pivotal. The swift differentiation between ischemic and hemorrhagic stroke by a CT scan directly informs the therapeutic approach. According to the American Heart Association 2020 guidelines, the CT scan should be completed within 10–25 minutes of the patient's arrival at

the emergency department and interpreted within 45 minutes to ensure rapid initiation of reperfusion therapy in suitable candidates.

- **Cardiac CT**, particularly the coronary CT angiography (CCTA), is a powerful noninvasive imaging tool that offers a clear view of the heart's anatomy. By using contrast material, it highlights the coronary arteries, enabling physicians to assess the presence and severity of plaque that may cause coronary artery disease. This advanced imaging is very helpful to determine whether a patient might be a candidate for angioplasty and stenting or if they may require coronary artery bypass surgery, depending on the extent and location of arterial blockages.
- **Thoracic CT:** Thoracic CT has become an indispensable tool in diagnosing a wide array of lung diseases. Its detailed cross-sectional images provide vital insights into various pathologies, from infections to malignancies. During the COVID-19 pandemic, thoracic CT scans have been integral in detecting characteristic patterns of pneumonia. Beyond infectious diseases, contrast-enhanced thoracic CT scans are essential in the diagnosis and staging of lung cancer, giving clarity on tumor size, location, and potential spread. Furthermore, CT pulmonary angiography has a definitive role in diagnosing pulmonary thromboembolism, allowing for timely therapeutic interventions. Beside this, abnormalities of thoracic cage are also best assessed by 3D-CT only.
- **CT abdomen:** CT imaging of the abdomen has become a cornerstone in diagnosing a range of acute and chronic conditions, offering detailed insights into abdominal and pelvic pathologies. CT is particularly valuable in the urgent assessment of the acute abdomen. The use of oral contrast, further enhances the visualization of gastrointestinal structures, aiding in the accurate localization and characterization of abdominal pathology. In cases of suspected renal colic, abdominal CT is the diagnostic standard, offering clear images of the urinary system. It efficiently detects urinary stones, revealing their size, location, and potential for spontaneous passage. Additionally, CT urography, which involves imaging the urinary tract with contrast, has significant utility. It is particularly effective in evaluating patients with hematuria and in detecting urothelial abnormalities. CT urography complements the diagnostic capabilities of standard abdominal CT, providing a more comprehensive assessment of the urinary system.
- **Contrast-enhanced CT scans:** The fundamental principle behind contrast-enhanced CT is that the iodinated contrast agent accumulates in areas of increased blood flow and perfusion. This property is particularly useful in highlighting regions of inflammation or tumor growth, as these areas typically have higher blood supply compared to normal tissues. The contrast agent enhances the density of these areas on the CT images, allowing for a more distinct delineation between normal and pathological tissues. Contrast-enhanced CT scans significantly enhance the diagnostic capabilities of standard CT imaging. The use of iodinated contrast agents pose additional risk, especially in patients with allergies to iodine or those with impaired kidney function. In such cases, the potential risks of contrast-induced nephropathy need to be weighed against the diagnostic benefits of the enhanced imaging.

Both X-ray and CT imaging use X-rays, a form of ionizing radiation that can lead to various effects at nuclear level. While occasional X-ray imaging poses minimal risk, repeated or high-dose exposure can lead to potential health risks, such as an increased chance of developing cancer later in life. Comparatively, the radiation dose from a standard X-ray is relatively low. For instance, a chest X-ray exposes a patient to a small amount of radiation, equivalent to a few days' worth of natural background radiation that everyone is exposed to from the environment. On the other hand, a CT scan, which involves multiple X-ray beams and a higher level of

Table 2.3: Comparative radiation doses in diagnostic imaging.

Imaging modality	*Approximate radiation dose (mSv)*	*Equivalent in natural background radiation*
X-Rays		
Chest X-ray	0.1 mSv	10 days
Limb X-ray	0.001 mSv	A few hours
Dental X-ray	0.005 mSv	1 day
OPG (Dental panoramic radiograph)	0.01 mSv	1–2 days
CT scans		
Head CT	2 mSv	8 months
Abdomen and pelvis CT	10 mSv	3 years
Chest CT	7 mSv	2 years
Cardiac CT for coronary evaluation	12 mSv	4 years
Other imaging modalities		
Mammography	0.4 mSv	7 weeks
DEXA scan	0.001–0.01 mSv	A few hours to 1 day

detail, typically results in a significantly higher radiation dose **(Table 2.3)**. This is especially a concern for sensitive groups like children and pregnant women. This risk necessitates careful consideration, especially in repeat imaging. Strategies to minimize exposure include protocol optimization and the use of newer, low-dose CT technology.

Magnetic Resonance Imaging

Magnetic resonance imaging (MRI) **(Fig. 2.4)** is distinguished by its ability to produce high-resolution images of soft tissues, such as the brain, muscles, and heart. This modality utilizes powerful magnetic fields and radiofrequency pulses to generate detailed images without the use of ionizing radiation. In upcoming chapters, you'll read in detail about the principle and physics behind the magnetic resonance imaging. One of MRI's most significant benefits is its use of nonionizing radiation, eliminating the radiation exposure risks associated with X-rays and CT scans. This makes it a safer option for repeated imaging and imaging of vulnerable populations like pregnant women and children. MRI is renowned for its exceptional ability to differentiate between various soft tissues, making it superior to CT scans for imaging muscles, ligaments, and the brain. Its detailed views are crucial for diagnosing soft tissue pathology, brain disorders, and musculoskeletal injuries.

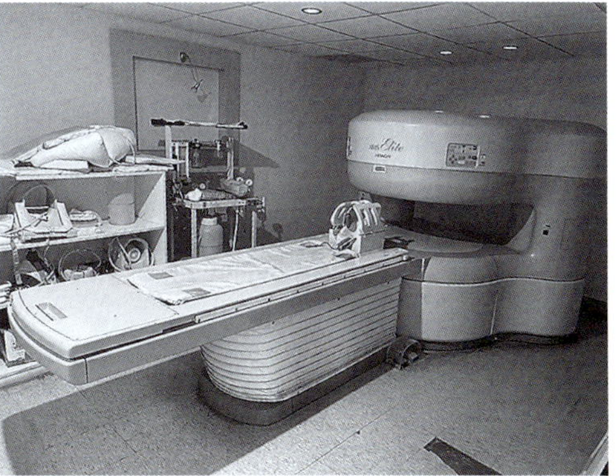

Fig. 2.4: Magnetic resonance imaging machine.

- **Neurological imaging:** For neurological assessments, MRI is indispensable. It can detect abnormalities such as tumors, inflammation, and demyelinating diseases with greater clarity than other imaging modalities. Its capability to visualize neural tissues in fine detail aids in the precise planning of neurosurgical procedures.

- **Musculoskeletal applications:** In orthopedics, MRI's sensitivity to detect changes in cartilage and bone marrow makes it the imaging choice for joint and spine pathologies. It is particularly beneficial for detecting subtle injuries such as meniscal tears, ligament sprains, and intervertebral disc herniation.
- **Cardiac assessments:** Cardiac MRI provides a comprehensive evaluation of the heart and great vessels, offering exquisite details on cardiac structure, function, and myocardial tissue characterization offering insights into congenital heart defects, cardiomyopathies, and myocardial infarction. It is an essential tool in the noninvasive assessment of cardiac diseases.
- **Abdominal and pelvic imaging:** MRI is advantageous for imaging the abdomen and pelvis because it provides clear visualization of organs and soft tissues, including the liver, kidneys, and reproductive organs, without the need for ionizing radiation. It is particularly useful for characterizing masses, identifying liver diseases, and staging pelvic cancers.
- **Oncology and breast imaging:** In oncology, MRI is a powerful tool for tumor detection and staging. It is especially valuable for breast imaging in high-risk patients due to its high sensitivity and specificity, often used in conjunction with mammography.
- **Vascular imaging:** With magnetic resonance angiography (MRA), MRI provides clear images of blood vessels without the need for contrast agents, though gadolinium-based contrasts can be used to enhance images. It's used to diagnose vascular abnormalities, aneurysms, and blockages.

The field of MRI continues to advance with innovations such as functional MRI (fMRI) for brain activity mapping (by detecting changes in blood flow) and diffusion tensor imaging (DTI) for visualizing white matter tracts. Despite its advantages, MRI is often more expensive than other imaging modality like CT scan, which can affect its accessibility. Additionally, the length of time required for scanning can be a challenge for patient comfort. Moreover, the presence of strong magnetic fields requires careful screening for contraindications, such as certain metal implants, pacemakers, or foreign bodies **(Table 2.4)**.

Table 2.4: Comparative overview of MRI and CT scan.

Aspect	*MRI*	*CT scan*
Principle	Utilizes magnetic fields and radio waves	Uses ionizing radiation (X-rays)
Imaging time	Slower, ranging from 15 minutes to over an hour	Quick, typically completed within a few minutes
Patient comfort	Can be challenging for claustrophobic patients	More open and often shorter duration, better for claustrophobic patients
Applications		
Bone imaging	Offers less detail for bones compared to CT	Superior for detailed bone imaging, such as fractures or bone pathology
Soft tissue imaging	Excellent contrast resolution, superior for soft tissue structures like the brain and muscles	Good for soft tissue, but with less contrast resolution compared to MRI
Neuroimaging	Gold standard for imaging the brain and spinal cord	Used when MRI is not available, or for rapid imaging in acute trauma
Organ imaging	Superior for organ systems due to better soft tissue contrast	Adequate for organ systems, but with potential contrast limitations

Contd...

Contd...

Aspect	*MRI*	*CT scan*
Trauma	Not typically used in acute trauma due to slower speed	Often used in emergency settings due to fast image acquisition
Functional imaging	Capable of functional and metabolic imaging (e.g., fMRI)	Limited functional imaging capabilities
Disadvantages		
Radiation exposure	No exposure, making it safe for repeated use	Exposure present; cumulative dose considered in repeat imaging
Contrast use	Uses gadolinium-based contrast, which is less likely to cause nephrogenic systemic fibrosis	Uses iodinated contrast, which can pose a risk for patients with kidney issues
	Can be challenging for claustrophobic patients, not suitable for patients with certain metal implants	Ionizing radiation exposure, potential allergic reactions to iodinated contrast material
Cost	Generally higher due to longer scan times and equipment costs	Comparatively lower

Mammography

Mammography **(Fig. 2.5)** is a specialized form of imaging used primarily for breast cancer screening and diagnosis. It employs low-dose X-rays to create detailed images of breast tissue. The technology has evolved to include digital mammography, which offers clearer images and easier storage and sharing. The advent of 3D mammography, or tomosynthesis, marks a significant advancement by providing layered images of the breast, improving the detection of small tumors in dense breast tissue. Mammography plays a crucial role in early cancer detection, significantly impacting treatment outcomes.

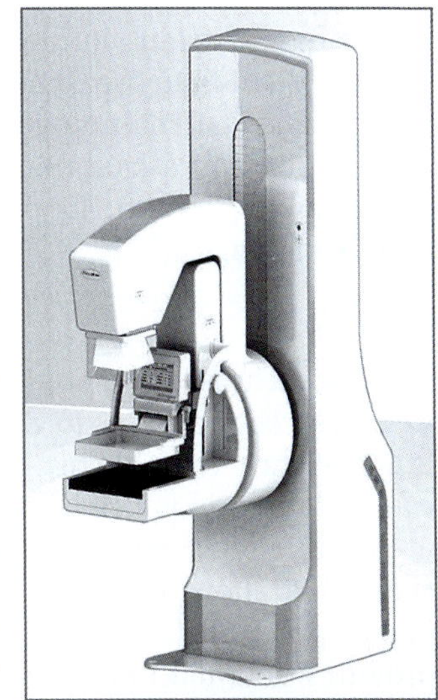

Fig. 2.5: Mammography machine.

- **Screening mammography:** Screening mammography is a preventive measure for women who do not have any symptoms of breast cancer. It plays a vital role in early detection, allowing for the discovery of breast tumors that may be too small to be felt. Regular screening mammograms can detect cancer early, often up to two years before a tumor can be physically felt, enhancing the chance for successful treatment and survival.
- **Diagnostic mammography (Fig. 2.5):** When a lump or other sign of breast cancer is present, diagnostic mammography is used. It focuses on obtaining more images to carefully evaluate an area of concern. Diagnostic mammography can also monitor changes in breast tissue found on a screening mammogram.
- **Mammosynthesis and breast cancer detection:** Mammosynthesis is particularly beneficial in detecting cancer early in women with dense breast tissue, where traditional mammograms may be less effective. Statistics indicate that 3D mammography may detect up to 40% more breast cancers than conventional mammography alone.

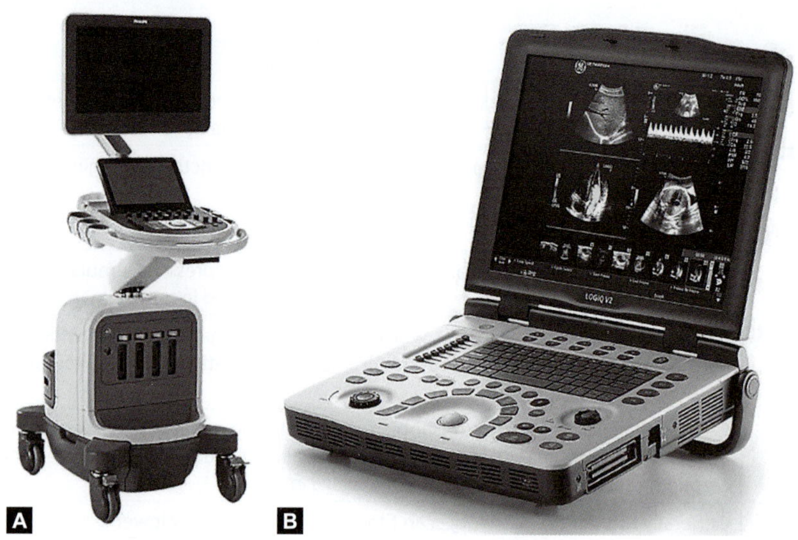

Figs. 2.6A and B: (A) Ultrasonography machine (fixed); (B) Portable Ultrasonography machine.

- **Mammographic-guided biopsy:** When mammography reveals a suspicious area, a mammographic-guided biopsy can be performed. This procedure uses mammography imaging to guide a needle to the area of concern, allowing for tissue sampling and subsequent pathological examination.

The effectiveness of mammography in reducing breast cancer mortality is significant. According to various studies, the use of mammography for screening has been associated with a reduction in breast cancer mortality by about 20–40% in women aged 40–74. One of the drawbacks of mammography is the discomfort or pain some women experience during the breast compression necessary for clear images. While the compression is brief, it can be distressing. Healthcare providers often work to minimize discomfort while ensuring the quality of images.

Ultrasound

Ultrasound imaging, or sonography, is a versatile and noninvasive technique that uses high-frequency sound waves to visualize internal organs, blood flow, and soft tissue structures. It is particularly valuable in obstetrics for monitoring fetal development, but its applications extend to cardiology, musculoskeletal imaging, and abdominal imaging. The development of portable ultrasound machines **(Figs. 2.6A and B)** has made this modality even more accessible, allowing for bedside examinations and use in remote locations. Advancements like Doppler ultrasound, which can visualize blood flow, and 3D/4D ultrasound, which provides detailed images of fetal anatomy, demonstrate the ongoing evolution of this technology. You will learn a lot about ultrasound in the upcoming chapters.

Positron Emission Tomography

Positron emission tomography (PET) scans represent a sophisticated combination of nuclear medicine and imaging technology. By using radioactive tracers, PET scans **(Fig. 2.7)** can visualize metabolic processes within the body, making them particularly useful in oncology for identifying cancerous tissues, as well as in neurology and cardiology. When combined

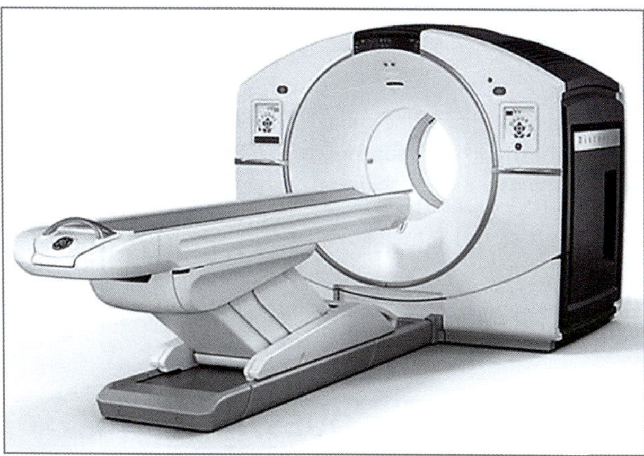

Fig. 2.7: Positron emission tomography machine.

with CT or MRI, PET provides comprehensive information about both the structure and function of tissues and organs. This dual capability makes PET scans invaluable in the diagnosis, staging, and monitoring of various diseases.

ADVANCES AND INNOVATIONS IN RADIODIAGNOSIS

The field of radiodiagnosis has witnessed significant advancements and innovations, enhancing diagnostic accuracy and patient care.

Digital Imaging and PACS

The transition to digital imaging has been transformative, allowing for immediate image processing, easier storage, and rapid sharing among healthcare providers. Picture archiving and communication systems (PACS) facilitate this by enabling the storage and convenient access to images from multiple modalities.

Interventional Radiology

Interventional radiology has burgeoned as a subspecialty, utilizing imaging techniques for guidance in minimally invasive procedures, such as angioplasty, stent placement, and tumor ablation.

3D Imaging

Three-dimensional imaging techniques have improved, aiding in complex surgeries and treatment planning. This includes 3D reconstructions from USG, CT and MRI scans, as well as advancements in 3D printing for surgical planning.

Artificial Intelligence and Machine Learning

AI and machine learning are increasingly being integrated into radiodiagnosis. They assist in teaching students, pattern recognition, predictive analysis, and improving diagnostic workflows (image analysis, measurement, reporting) leading to more personalized patient care.

These innovations collectively push the boundaries of traditional imaging, offering a glimpse into the future where radiodiagnosis is not just about detecting disease, but also about personalized and precision medicine.

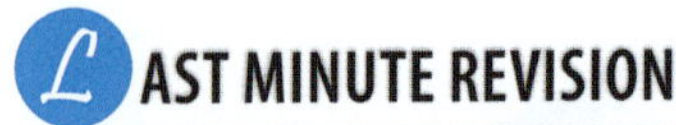

LAST MINUTE REVISION

- CT scans are the gold standard for diagnosing cranial and cervical bony injuries, especially after trauma.
- MRI excels in soft tissue contrast, making it superior for neurological and musculoskeletal imaging.
- Digital mammography and tomosynthesis significantly enhance breast cancer detection, especially in dense breast tissue.
- Use of contrast in CT scans is crucial for distinguishing between types of soft tissues and identifying vascular structures.
- AI in radiodiagnosis improves accuracy and efficiency but cannot replace the need for expert radiologists.

REVIEW QUESTIONS

Multiple Choice Questions (MCQs)

1. **What is the significance of using contrast material in CT imaging?**
   a. It helps in the visualization of digestive processes
   b. It increases the speed of the CT scan
   c. It enhances the differentiation between various types of pathologies
   d. It reduces the need for patient preparation before the scan
2. **What does PACS stand for in medical imaging?**
   a. Patient Archive Communication System
   b. Picture Archiving and Communication System
   c. Public Access to Computerized Services
   d. Picture Access and Communication Service
3. **Which of the following is not a typical use of interventional radiology?**
   a. Angioplasty
   b. Joint replacement
   c. Stent placement
   d. Tumor ablation
4. **How does artificial intelligence (AI) contribute to radiodiagnosis?**
   a. Replaces the need for radiologists
   b. Provides automated image interpretation
   c. Decreases image clarity and quality
   d. Increases the radiation dose to patients

Answer Key

1. c 2. b 3. b 4. b

SUGGESTED READING

1. Giaquinto AN, Sung H, Miller KD. Breast Cancer Statistics, 2022. CA Cancer J Clin. 2022 Nov;72(6):524-541. doi: 10.3322/caac.21754. Epub 2022 Oct 3.
2. Kessner R, Barnes S, Halpern P. CT for acute nontraumatic abdominal pain-is oral contrast really required? Acad Radiol. 2017 Jul;24(7):840-845. doi: 10.1016/j.acra.2017.01.013. Epub 2017 Feb 23.

CHAPTER

3 Radiation and its Effects

"Radiation, when guided with knowledge and care, transforms energy into healing—turning invisible waves into visible hope."

INTRODUCTION

Radiation, in its various forms, plays a pivotal role in the field of medicine, offering both diagnostic and therapeutic capabilities. At its core, "Radiation", refers to energy emitted as electromagnetic waves or particles. This encompasses a broad spectrum, from electromagnetic waves, such as light and radio waves, to particulate radiation, like alpha and beta particles. In the realm of radiodiagnosis, understanding the nature and effects of radiation is fundamental, as it directly impacts patient care and safety.

For medical professionals, especially those specializing in radiodiagnosis, a thorough understanding of the various types of radiation, their sources, and their interactions with biological tissues is essential. This knowledge is crucial not only for the effective application of diagnostic and therapeutic techniques but also for ensuring patient and healthcare worker safety in the face of potential radiation exposure.

This chapter aims to offer a thorough exploration of radiation's principles, its interactions with matter, biological impacts, and the clinical relevance of radiation-induced conditions. By equipping medical practitioners with this insight, we aim to enhance their ability to leverage radiation's benefits while minimizing risks in patient care.

FUNDAMENTALS OF RADIATION

Radiation is a form of energy that travels through space and matter, existing in various types that are broadly categorized into ionizing and non-ionizing radiation **(Table 3.1)** based on differences in mass, energy and depth of penetration. Ionizing radiation includes subatomic particles and the high energy, short-wavelength portion of the electromagnetic spectrum, whereas non-ionizing radiation includes the visible spectrum and the low energy, long-wavelength part of the spectrum beyond the visible light **(Fig. 3.1)**.

Ionizing Radiation

This type possesses enough energy to remove electrons from atoms, creating ions. It includes:

- **X-rays:** High-energy electromagnetic waves produced by the deceleration of fast moving electrons from cathode to target anode in vacuum tube. X-ray photon causes interaction with matter, commonly used in medical imaging.
- **Gamma rays:** Electromagnetic waves emitted from the nucleus of radioactive atoms, used in diagnostic imaging and cancer therapy.

Table 3.1: Comparison of ionizing and non-ionizing radiation.

Feature	*Ionizing radiation*	*Non-ionizing radiation*
Definition	Radiation with enough energy to remove tightly bound electrons from atoms, creating ions	Radiation that does not have enough energy to remove electrons from atoms
Types	• X-rays • Gamma rays • Alpha particles • Beta particles	• Ultraviolet (UV) light • Visible light • Infrared (IR) radiation • Microwaves • Radio waves
Sources	• Natural: Cosmic rays, terrestrial sources • Artificial: Medical imaging (X-rays, CT scans, PET scan), nuclear industry	• Natural: Sunlight (UV, visible light) • Artificial: Lasers, LED lights, radio transmitters, MRI, USG
Medical applications	• Diagnostic imaging (X-rays, CT scans) • Cancer treatment (radiotherapy) • Sterilization of medical equipment	• Diagnostic imaging (MRI, ultrasound) • Phototherapy (UV light therapy for skin conditions) • Infrared saunas (pain relief)
Health risks	• Increased risk of cancer • Genetic damage (at high doses)	• Skin burns (from UV exposure) • Cataracts (from prolonged IR exposure) • Generally considered safer than ionizing radiation at low to moderate levels
Safety precautions	• Lead shielding • Limiting exposure time • Maintaining safe distances	• Protective eyewear (for UV, IR radiation) • Regulation of exposure times • Use of non-ionizing radiation sources at safe power levels

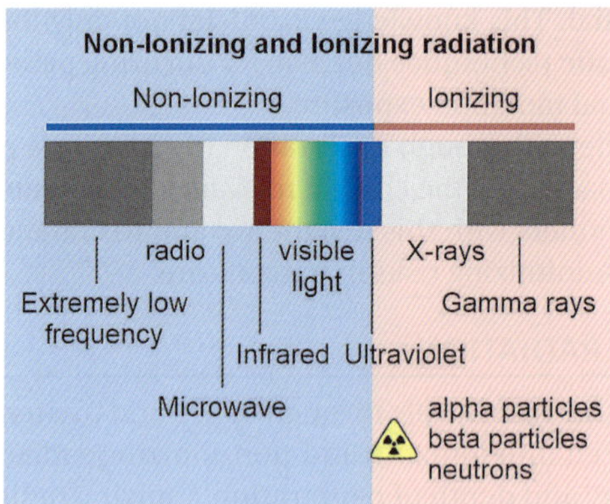

Fig. 3.1: Non-ionizing and ionizing radiation.

- **Alpha particles:** Heavily charged particles from the decay of radioactive materials, not typically used in diagnostics due to their inability to penetrate human skin but relevant in understanding radiation safety.
- **Beta particles:** High-energy, charged particles from radioactive decay, with limited penetration and more relevance in radiation therapy and safety.

Non-ionizing Radiation

Lacks the energy to ionize atoms but includes important modalities in medical diagnostics:

- **Ultraviolet light (UV):** Has roles in dermatological treatments but is not used for internal imaging due to its non-penetrative nature.
- **Microwaves and radio waves:** Utilized in MRI scans, these waves resonate with atoms in the body under magnetic fields to produce images.
- **Infrared radiation:** Used in some therapeutic and diagnostic applications for its heat-producing effects.

Note: Radiation is classified on the basis of source too, according to which radiation can be either natural or artificial.

- **Natural sources:** Include cosmic rays from outer space, terrestrial radiation from radioactive materials in the earth, and radon gas.
- **Artificial sources:** Primarily from medical applications (X-rays, CT scans), industrial uses, and nuclear power generation.

MECHANISMS OF RADIATION INTERACTION

Atomic makeup of biological tissues, not its molecular structure is the fundamental of interactions that forms the basis for both the diagnostic, therapeutic capabilities and potential risks of radiation in medical applications.

Interaction with Matter

Radiation interacts with matter through several mechanisms, which determine its penetration depth, energy deposition, and potential biological effects.

- **Photoelectric effect:** Predominant at lower energies, this effect involves the "absorption" of the entire energy of an X-ray photon by an electron in an atom, leading to the electron's ejection and ionization of the atom. It is maximum with elements like barium and iodine having high atomic number. This effect is crucial in diagnostic radiography, providing high-contrast images (Characteristic radiation) but also contributes to dose absorption in tissues.
- **Compton scattering:** Occurs when an X-ray or gamma ray photon collides with a loosely bound outer electron, imparting some of its energy to the electron and scattering at a changed angle. This interaction is more significant in therapeutic X-rays (Radiation therapy) than diagnostic imaging as it affects the distribution of radiation within the body and can lead to scattered radiation outside the intended treatment area.
- **Pair production:** Relevant at very high energies, this phenomenon occurs when a photon converts into an electron-positron pair near a nucleus. While not typically encountered in diagnostic radiology, it's important in the context of particle accelerators and some types of radiation therapy.

  Note: Two other interactions are coherent scattering and photodisintegration.

Absorption and Scatter

- Absorption of radiation in tissues is a critical concept, determining both the effectiveness of radiation in imaging and therapy and the potential for tissue damage. In the context of biological tissues, the degree of absorption is influenced by several factors:
  - *Type of radiation:* Different types of radiation are absorbed at different rates. For instance, X-rays and gamma rays can penetrate deeper into the body than alpha or beta particles.

  - *Tissue composition:* Tissues with higher atomic numbers (e.g., bone) absorb more radiation than those with lower atomic numbers (e.g., soft tissues), leading to the contrast seen in radiographic images.
  - *Energy of radiation:* Higher energy radiation penetrates further before being absorbed, affecting both its diagnostic utility and the potential for tissue damage.
- Scatter on the other hand refers to the deflection of radiation from its original path upon interacting with matter. In medical imaging, scatter can arise from interactions such as Compton(Incoherent) scattering, where photons are deflected by electrons. Scatter has significant implications:
  - *Image quality:* Scatter can degrade the quality of radiographic images by introducing noise and reducing contrast, complicating the interpretation of diagnostic images, e.g., coherent scattering forms film fog.
  - *Exposure to surrounding tissues:* Scattered radiation can expose surrounding tissues to unintended radiation, potentially increasing the risk of radiation-induced damage.
  - *Radiation protection:* Managing scatter is crucial for protecting both patients and healthcare workers from unnecessary radiation exposure. Techniques such as collimation, which narrows the beam of radiation, and the use of shielding materials, are employed to minimize scatter.

Dose-response Relationships

The biological effects of radiation depend on the dose absorbed by the tissues. This relationship helps in understanding the risk of radiation exposure and is fundamental in setting safety standards and protocols for radiation use in medicine.

BIOLOGICAL EFFECTS OF RADIATION

The interaction of radiation with biological tissues can lead to a range of effects, from benign to severely detrimental, depending on various factors such as the type and amount of radiation, the rate of exposure, and the sensitivity of the tissue **(Fig. 3.2)**. The biological interaction can be classified as:

Cellular Damage

Radiation can cause damage to cells in two primary ways: directly, by interacting with and damaging the DNA or other critical cellular components, and indirectly, through the generation of reactive oxygen species (ROS) that can damage DNA, proteins, and lipids.

1. **Direct damage:** Occurs when ionizing radiation directly interacts with DNA, leading to breaks in the DNA strands or other molecular injuries that can disrupt cellular function.
2. **Indirect damage:** Most cellular damage from radiation results from water radiolysis, where radiation interacts with water molecules within the cell to produce ROS. These reactive molecules can then damage various cellular components, including DNA.

The cell's ability to repair this damage is crucial in determining the outcome of radiation exposure, with ineffective repair processes potentially leading to mutations, cancer, or cell death.

Acute and Chronic Effects (Table 3.2)

The biological effects of radiation can be categorized as either acute, manifesting shortly after exposure, or chronic, developing over a longer period.

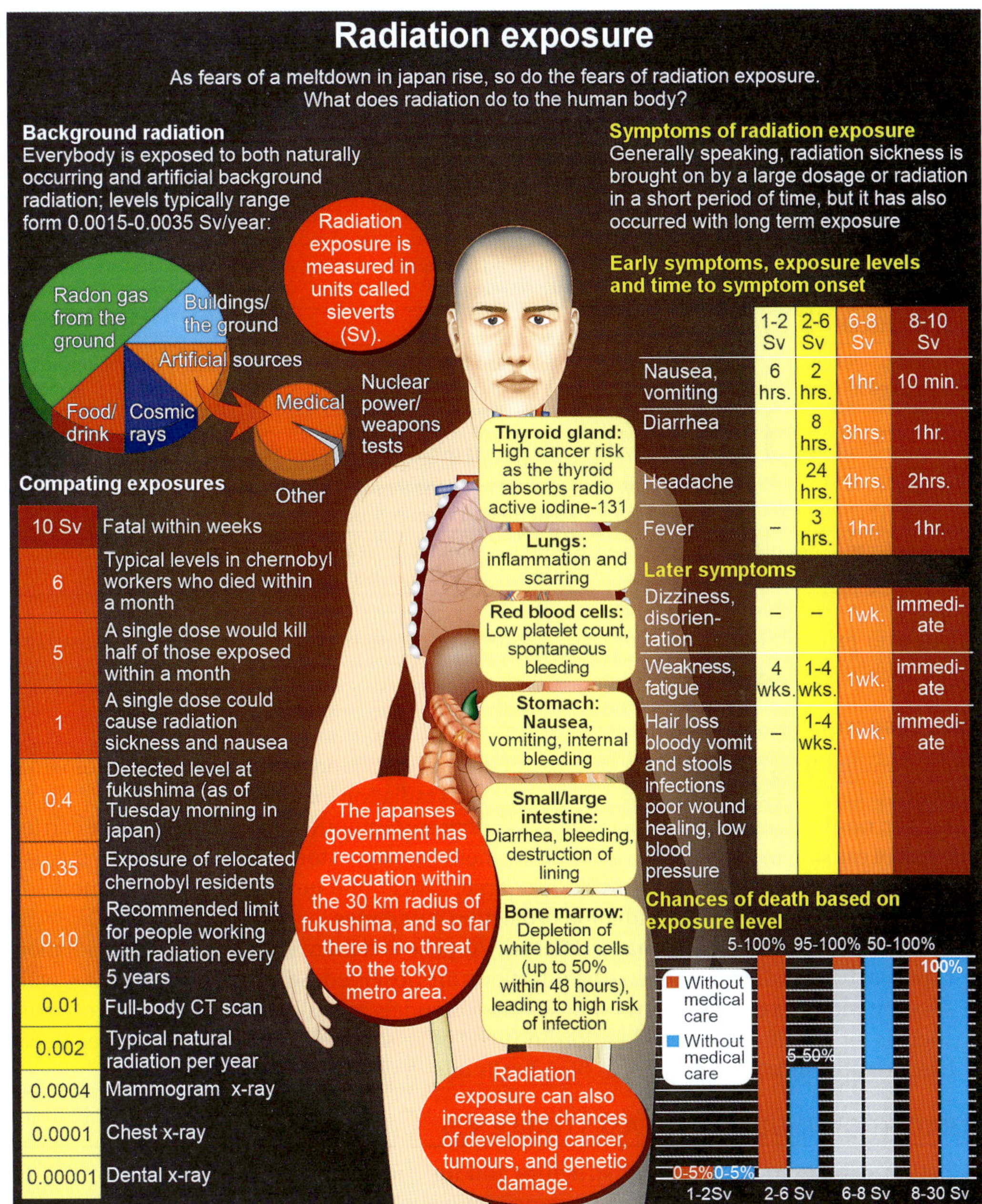

Fig. 3.2: Effect of radiation over various organ system.

- **Acute effects:** Include skin burns, acute radiation syndrome (ARS), and hematopoietic damage, typically occurring after exposure to high doses of radiation over a short period. Symptoms can range from nausea and fatigue to more severe consequences such as infection due to immune system damage.
- **Chronic effects:** Long-term effects of radiation exposure can include cancer, cardiovascular disease, and cataracts, among others. These effects often result from lower doses of radiation

Table 3.2: Summary of acute and chronic effects of radiation.

Effect type	*Dose range gray*	*Potential health outcomes*	*Time to onset*
Acute effects			
Skin erythema	2–5	Reddening or burning of the skin	1–24 hours
Acute radiation syndrome (ARS)	>1 (whole body)	Nausea, fatigue, hair loss, hemorrhage, infection due to immune suppression	Hours to weeks
Hematopoietic damage	0.5–1 (whole body)	Decreased production of blood cells, leading to anemia, infection, and hemorrhage	Weeks to months
Chronic effects			
Cancer (e.g., leukemia, thyroid, breast)	Variable; increased risk at doses >0.1 (cumulative)	Development of cancer in various organs	Years to decades
Cardiovascular disease	>0.5 (cumulative)	Increased risk of heart disease and stroke	Years to decades
Cataracts	>0.5 (cumulative)	Clouding of the lens of the eye, leading to decreased vision	Years to decades
Genetic effects	Variable; increased risk with higher doses	Heritable mutations leading to increased risk of genetic disorders in offspring	Generational

but over extended periods, emphasizing the importance of monitoring and minimizing cumulative radiation exposure.

Dose-response Relationships

Understanding the relationship between the dose of radiation received and the biological response is key to assessing the risks associated with radiation exposure.

- **Linear, no-threshold (LNT) model:** Suggests that any amount of radiation exposure carries a risk of causing health effects, (all or none phenomenon = stochastic effects), with the risk increasing linearly with the dose. For example, cancer and genetic effects. This model is widely used for establishing radiation protection guidelines.[1]
- **Threshold models (non-stochastic effects):** Propose that there is a certain level of radiation exposure below which no adverse health effects are observed. Somatic effect increases with severity with increasing absorbed dose. These models are considered in some contexts, such as for specific types of radiation-induced effects. For example, degenerative effects like lens opacification, changes in blood cells and decreased sperm production.

RADIATION-INDUCED DISEASES (TABLE 3.3)

Radiation's ability to alter cellular structure and function means it can lead to a variety of diseases, primarily cancers, but also non-cancerous conditions. Understanding these potential health impacts is critical for medical professionals, particularly those specializing in fields heavily reliant on radiation for diagnostics and treatment.

Cancer

Radiation exposure is a well-documented risk factor for several types of cancer. The mechanism typically involves DNA damage that either kills the cell, repairs it incorrectly, or leaves it in a mutated form that can proliferate uncontrollably. Key cancers associated with radiation include:

Table 3.3: Major radiation-induced diseases and associated radiation types.

Disease	*Associated radiation type(s)*	*Description*	*Latency period*
Leukemia	Ionizing (X-rays, Gamma rays)	Cancer of the body's blood-forming tissues, including the bone marrow and the lymphatic system	2–10 years
Thyroid cancer	Ionizing (I-131, X-rays)	A type of cancer that occurs in the thyroid gland, it's more likely to be caused by exposure to radioactive iodine	5–30 years
Breast cancer	Ionizing (X-rays, Gamma rays)	Cancer that forms in the cells of the breasts, possibly linked to cumulative exposure to ionizing radiation	10+ years
Lung cancer	Ionizing (Radon, X-rays, Gamma rays)	A malignant lung tumor characterized by uncontrolled cell growth in tissues of the lung. Exposure to radon gas is a significant risk factor	5–25 years
Skin cancer	Non-ionizing (UV light), ionizing (X-rays)	Cancer that forms in the skin cells. Non-ionizing UV radiation from the sun and tanning beds are primary causes, though ionizing radiation can also contribute	Variable
Cataracts	Ionizing (Gamma rays, X-rays), non-ionizing (UV light)	Clouding of the lens of the eye, leading to decreased vision. Both ionizing and non-ionizing radiation exposures are risk factors[2]	5–15 years
Cardiovascular diseases	Ionizing (X-rays, Gamma rays)	Diseases of the heart or blood vessels, including coronary artery disease, attributed to high doses of ionizing radiation	10–30 years

- **Leukemia:** Most strongly linked with radiation exposure, especially after high-dose exposure, with increased incidence observed after atomic bomb explosions and in medical therapeutic contexts.
- **Thyroid cancer:** Particularly associated with radiation exposure in childhood, often through medical treatments or environmental exposure.
- **Breast cancer:** Increased risk with higher doses of radiation, especially in medical diagnostic contexts or radiation therapy.
- **Lung cancer:** Associated with radon exposure, a naturally occurring radioactive gas, in addition to occupational or therapeutic exposures.

Non-cancer Effects

In addition to carcinogenesis, radiation can lead to various non-cancerous conditions, often resulting from its cumulative damage to tissues and organs over time.

- **Cardiovascular disease:** Long-term, high-dose radiation exposure can increase the risk of heart disease and stroke by damaging the cardiovascular system.
- **Cataracts:** Exposure to moderate doses of radiation can accelerate the development of cataracts, leading to impaired vision.
- **Skin conditions:** Chronic low-dose exposure can lead to dermatitis and other skin conditions, while high-dose exposure can cause burns and necrosis.

Genetic Effects

Radiation exposure can also have heritable effects, causing genetic mutations that are passed on to future generations. These effects are of particular concern in populations exposed to high levels of radiation, such as survivors of atomic bombings or nuclear accidents.

Prevention and Management

Understanding the link between radiation exposure and disease is crucial for preventing these conditions and managing them effectively when they occur. This involves adhering to safety protocols to minimize exposure, employing protective measures in medical and occupational settings, and monitoring individuals at higher risk due to previous exposure.

In summary, while radiation is a powerful tool in medicine, its potential to induce a wide range of diseases necessitates careful management and adherence to safety standards to protect both patients and healthcare professionals. Awareness and education on these risks are paramount in mitigating the adverse effects of radiation exposure.

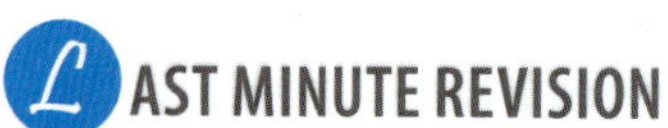

- Ionizing radiation, including X-rays and gamma rays, has enough energy to ionize atoms, while non-ionizing radiation, such as UV light and microwaves, does not.
- Radiation exposure can cause a range of biological effects, from immediate cellular damage to long-term chronic diseases like cancer.
- Photoelectric effect is the most useful type of radiation interaction with matter for diagnostic radiology

REVIEW QUESTIONS

Multiple Choice Questions (MCQs)

1. **What type of radiation is capable of ionizing atoms?**
   a. Ultraviolet light
   b. Radio waves
   c. X-rays
   d. Microwaves
2. **Which mechanism of radiation interaction involves a photon being converted into an electron-positron pair?**
   a. Photoelectric effect
   b. Compton scattering
   c. Pair production
   d. Coherent scattering
3. **Which of the following is a chronic effect of radiation exposure?**
   a. Skin erythema
   b. Acute radiation syndrome
   c. Leukemia
   d. Hematopoietic damage
4. **Which safety measure is effective in protecting against scatter radiation?**
   a. Using higher doses of radiation for clearer images
   b. Collimation
   c. Avoiding protective lead aprons
   d. Increasing the distance from the radiation source

5. **The linear no-threshold (LNT) model suggests that:**
   a. There is a safe level of radiation below which no effects are seen.
   b. Radiation effects do not increase linearly with dose.
   c. Any amount of radiation exposure has the potential to cause harm.
   d. Only high doses of radiation can cause cancer.

Answer Key

1. c 2. c 3. c 4. b 5. c

SUGGESTED READING

1. Chodick G, Bekiroglu N, Hauptmann M, et al. Risk of cataract after exposure to low doses of ionizing radiation: a 20-year prospective cohort study among US radiologic technologists. Am J Epidemiol. 2008 Sep 15;168(6):620-31. doi: 10.1093/aje/kwn171.
2. Tubiana M, Feinendegen LE, Yang C, Kaminski JM. The linear no-threshold relationship is inconsistent with radiation biologic and experimental data. Radiology. 2009 Apr;251(1):13-22. doi: 10.1148/radiol.2511080671.

CHAPTER

4 Radiation Safety and Protection

"Protection isn't a barrier—it's empowerment. Safe practices in radiation ensure precision, confidence, and care for every life we touch."

INTRODUCTION

In modern medicine, ionizing radiation plays a crucial role in both diagnostics and treatment, offering invaluable insights into the human body and disease management. However, as highlighted in the previous chapter, it also carries potential health risks. Radiation safety is a concern not only for patients, but for physicians, and staff as well. Radiation protection aims to reduce unnecessary radiation exposure with a goal to minimize the harmful effects of ionizing radiation This chapter aims to delve into radiation protection and safety, equipping students with essential knowledge and practices to minimize exposure risks. By emphasizing the principles of justification, optimization, and dose limitation, we foster a safety culture that balances well-being with diagnostic effectiveness, building on the foundational understanding of radiation's biological impacts.

FUNDAMENTAL PRINCIPLES OF RADIATION PROTECTION

The fundamental principles of radiation protection, designed to safeguard both healthcare professionals and patients from unnecessary exposure, are encapsulated in three key concepts:

1. **Justification:** Any use of radiation must have a net benefit. This principle requires that the advantages of radiation exposure (e.g., diagnostic clarity, treatment effectiveness) outweigh the potential risks (e.g., radiation-induced damage).
2. **Optimization (Follow "ALARA—as Low as Reasonably Achievable" Principle):** All exposures should be kept to the minimum necessary level, even applicable to USG Doppler studies. This involves using the least amount of radiation to achieve the desired outcome, employing various strategies to reduce dose without compromising diagnostic quality.
3. **Dose limitation:** Predefining the limits that can produce harmful effects. Dose limitation sets caps on the amount of radiation that individuals can be exposed to over specific periods. For healthcare workers and the public, these limits are designed to prevent excessive exposure and protect against the harmful effects of radiation.

DAMAGING EFFECT OF RADIATION

Understanding the harmful impacts of radiation plays a pivotal role in developing protective measures for healthcare workers and patients alike. As discussed n detail in previous chapter,

X-rays, are high-energy photons within the electromagnetic spectrum, stand out because of their ability to ionize atoms by breaking molecular bonds. This ionization process generates free radicals, which are chemically active and capable of causing indirect DNA damage through their interactions.

PROTECTION TECHNIQUES AND STRATEGIES

In clinical practice, minimizing radiation exposure is crucial and hinges on controlling exposure time, increasing distance from the source, and using effective shielding. Planning ahead to streamline the number and extent of radiographic images is a key strategy. The main modifiable factors are:

1. **Time of exposure:** Limiting the duration of radiation exposure to minimize risk.
2. **Increasing distance from the source:** The principle is simple: the farther is the recipient from the radiation source, the lower the exposure. Clinically in diagnostic radiology this is accomplished by maximizing the space between the radiation source and individuals to reduce exposure levels.
3. **Shielding:** Utilizing barriers or protective equipment to absorb or deflect radiation away from the body. Clinically shielding is the primary defense against unwanted radiation exposure, so would be discussed in detail.

   Note: Time, distance, shield (TDS) should be appropriate for radiation protection.
4. **Equipment:**
   - *Maintenance, optimization and inspection of protective gear:* Regular checks (yearly QA report) and updates to ensure radiation-emitting devices operate efficiently, minimizing unnecessary exposure.
   - *Installation:* All equipment's should be AERB and FDA approved. Room location, size, wall thickness and its design should be preapproved by AERB before installation of machine. After submission of installation report through ELORA system (e-licensing of radiation applications) on institutional AERB ID, only registered equipment is allowed to use for diagnosis and therapeutic purposes.
   - *Collimator:* It is the best x ray beam restrict or having dual function
     - Decreases patient exposure by accurate localization region of interest
     - Well collimated beam reduces scatter radiation
5. **Procedural protocol:** Adherence to best practices for patient positioning only by trained personnel and the optimization of imaging parameters to achieve the lowest possible dose for diagnostic efficacy. Using magnification cautiously is advised, as it elevates radiation dose. An alternative to continuous fluoroscopy is pulsed fluoroscopy, which lessens exposure without compromising image quality by reducing the number of images taken per second. Above all, limiting the time of radiation exposure remains a fundamental safety measure.

Shielding

Appropriate shielding is the most important factor in protecting individuals from radiation exposure. There are three types of shielding:

Structural Shielding

This type of shielding is integrated into the infrastructure of medical suites, offering defense against direct radiation **(always nine-inch brick wall thickness)**. Its effectiveness varies with the material used, such as mobile, transparent, and leaded acrylic shields, which provide lesser protection against scattered radiation.

Table 4.1: Room requirements of various types of machines.

Machine	*Room size*	*Door lining*	*Protective barrier*
X-ray machine	400 × 450 cm	2 mm lead	2 mm
Mammography/OPG/CBCT	300 × 350 cm	1 mm lead	1.5 mm
CT gantry	400 × 625 cm	2 mm lead	2 mm (100 × 80 cm)
CT console	400 × 200 cm	—	—
Dexa SCAN/BMD	350 × 400 cm	—	—
Interventional radiology (C-arm)	500 × 500 cm	2 mm lead	2 mm (120 × 100 cm)
Interventional console	500 × 200 cm	—	—

Equipment Mounted Shielding

Incorporating leaded drapes and acrylic barriers attached to medical devices, this shielding method helps protect medical staff during radiographic procedures.

Personal Protective Devices

PPE includes garments and accessories like lead aprons, thyroid shields, and protective eyewear, essential for personnel involved in fluoroscopic-guided procedures. These items are designed from lead or alternative lightweight materials to mitigate scatter radiation exposure. In clinical practice the application of PPE is indispensable in regard to radiation protection. Lead aprons, thyroid shields, and lead glasses serve as frontline defense for healthcare workers by providing targeted protection to vulnerable parts of the body that are most susceptible to radiation damage. These are also yearly inspect for wear and tear such as cracks, or holes. These protective items are designed to absorb or block the penetration of X-rays and gamma rays, thus reducing the dose of radiation received during medical procedures **(Table 4.1)**.

Regulatory Framework and Safety Culture

Various regulatory bodies like International Atomic Energy Agency (IAEA) and Atomic Energy Regulatory Board (AERB) have devised the upper limits of professional exposure and the technique to monitor them **(Table 4.2)**.

Thermoluminescence dosimetry (TLD) has been a key tool for nearly a century, used for measuring ionizing radiation doses (Personnel Dosimetry). TLDs, owing to their varied materials and forms, can assess a broad spectrum of radiation types across different dose levels. They are pivotal in both radiation safety, where they track minuscule dose levels, and in radiotherapy, for gauging doses that can reach several grays. TLDs are favored for their compact size and the convenience of not needing wires or additional devices during measurement. TLD is based on phosphorescence phenomenon. It commonly uses small chips of activated lithium fluoride as it has similar density to human tissues.

TLD batch in radiodiagnosis involves a cycle of calibration, distribution, usage, collection, analysis, reporting, and recordkeeping to ensure the safety of healthcare workers and compliance with radiation safety regulations. For analysis they are sent to different organizations like BARC, radiology safety division of AERB, etc., either monthly or quarterly or biannual or yearly as per TLD service providers or institution norms or level of radiation exposure.

The important step to optimizing safe radiation practice is educating hospital staff on radiation best practices. Regular radiation safety workshops and program should be conducted to educate both patients and professionals with the goal to minimize iatrogenic radiation exposure.

Table 4.2: Personal protective equipment (PPE) for radiation protection.

PPE type	*Description*	*Design variations*	*Key features*
Lead aprons	Primary protective garment used during fluoroscopy to shield the body from radiation	• Front coverage only • Wraparound • Vest and kilt combination	• Lead equivalent thickness typically 0.25–1 mm • A 0.5 mm thick apron can attenuate 90% of scatter radiation • Designs to fit various body types and procedural needs • Importance of proper fit to reduce exposure, particularly for breast tissue in female staff
Thyroid shields	Designed to protect the thyroid gland from scatter radiation, reducing the risk of thyroid cancer	Standard, adjustable for fit	• Recommended to have at least 0.5 mm lead equivalent thickness for effective protection • Proper adjustment enhances protection efficiency • Regular inspection and proper fit are crucial
Lead glasses	Eyewear providing protection against scatter radiation to reduce the risk to the lens of the eye, the most radiation-sensitive part of the body	• Various frame styles • Prescription and nonprescription options	• Lead equivalent thickness of 0.5–0.75 mm can reduce more than 95% of scatter radiation • Essential for all personnel performing or assisting in fluoroscopic procedures
Caps and gloves	Additional accessories offering protection for the head and hands, areas also susceptible to scatter radiation exposure	• **Gloves:** Available in different sizes and lead equivalent thicknesses • **Caps:** One-size-fits-most, with or without lead	• Gloves and caps made of lead composite or lighter lead-free materials • Designs vary to accommodate different procedural requirements and personal preferences • Aim to attenuate scatter radiation effectively, with gloves particularly focused on hand protection during close proximity to radiation sources
Special considerations	Considerations for long-term use, health implications, and ergonomic design to reduce physical strain and increase compliance among healthcare professionals	N/A	• Newer aprons made from lightweight materials like barium, tungsten, tin, and antimony to reduce musculoskeletal problems and fatigue • Regular inspection for damage such as cracks or holes • Proper handling and storage to maintain integrity and extend lifespan • The ergonomic design of vests and kilts reduces spine burden by distributing weight evenly

Table 4.3: Dose limits.

Type of dose limit	*Limit on dose from occupational exposure*	*Limit on dose from public exposure*
Effective dose	20 mSv/yr, averaged over defined five-year periods, with no single year exceeding 50 mSv	1 mSv/yr
Effective dose	Once employee declares pregnancy, the dose to embryo/fetus should not exceed 1 mSv during remainder of pregnancy	—
Equivalent dose: Lens of the eye	20 mSv/yr, averaged defined five-year periods, with no single year exceeding 50 mSv	15 mSv/yr
Equivalent dose: Skin	500 mSv	50 mSv/yr
Equivalent dose: Hands and feet	500 mSv/yr	—

RADIATION AND PREGNANCY

While selecting the most appropriate imaging modality for pregnant patients, the primary concern is balancing the need for accurate diagnosis with the safety of both the mother and the fetus. The ALARA (As Low As Reasonably Achievable) principle guides this balance by minimizing radiation exposure without compromising diagnostic efficacy.

During pregnancy, the unique challenge lies in minimizing fetal radiation exposure while still obtaining the necessary diagnostic information. Each imaging modality has different implications for fetal radiation exposure, and the choice must consider both the immediate clinical needs and the potential long-term effects on the fetus.

Imaging Modalities and Fetal Radiation Exposure

1. **Ultrasound (US):**
   - *Radiation exposure:* None
   - *Advantages:* Safe for both mother and fetus, making it the first-line imaging modality in pregnancy. It is widely used for evaluating fetal development, placental position, and maternal pelvic conditions.
   - *Limitations:* Operator-dependent, and certain maternal conditions may limit the effectiveness of ultrasound.
2. **Magnetic resonance imaging (MRI):**
   - *Radiation exposure:* None
   - *Advantages:* No ionizing radiation, providing excellent soft-tissue contrast. MRI is particularly useful for detailed evaluation of fetal anatomy and maternal conditions when ultrasound findings are inconclusive.
   - *Limitations:* Costly, less available in some settings, and may require sedation in claustrophobic patients.
3. **X-ray and computed tomography (CT):**
   - *Radiation exposure:* Varies depending on the study. Fetal exposure during a single abdominal CT scan is approximately 10–25 mGy.
   - *Advantages:* Rapid and widely available, providing critical information in emergencies, particularly in trauma or suspected pulmonary embolism.
   - *Techniques to reduce exposure:* Shielding the abdomen, using the lowest effective dose, and considering alternative imaging modalities when possible.

- *Limitations:* The potential for higher radiation doses compared to other modalities makes it less preferred unless absolutely necessary.

4. **Nuclear medicine studies:**
   - *Radiation exposure:* Depends on the radiopharmaceutical used. Typically, fetal doses are low but must be calculated on a case-by-case basis.
   - *Advantages:* Useful in specific scenarios, such as evaluating thyroid function or pulmonary embolism with V/Q scanning.
   - *Limitations:* Exposure to both ionizing radiation and radiopharmaceuticals; often avoided unless the benefit clearly outweighs the risk.

Radiation Protection in Pregnancy

- **Tailored imaging protocols:** Modifying imaging techniques to reduce dose, such as adjusting CT parameters or use ultrasound/MRI as first-line modalities.
- **Fetal shielding:** When appropriate, physical shielding can reduce fetal exposure during radiologic procedures.
- **Judicious use of imaging:** Limiting imaging studies to those that are clinically indicated, and considering alternative diagnostic methods when possible.
  - *Dose reduction techniques:* Use of pelvic lead aprons, PA projection over AP, optimal patient positioning, minimize repeat exams, limit radiographs to essential cases.
  - Use pulse fluoroscopy, last image hold, and appropriate collimation. Avoid unnecessary magnification in case of angiography.

Distribution of Effects of Radiation on Fetus (Table 4.4)

Table 4.4: Distribution of effects of radiation on fetus.

Gestational period	*Potential effects*	*Radiation sensitivity*	*Dose relationship*
Less than 2 weeks	Pregnancy loss	Very high sensitivity	Any exposure can lead to pregnancy loss ("all-or-none" effect)
2 to 8 weeks	Malformations and developmental delays	High sensitivity during organogenesis	**Below threshold:** Minimal disruption. **Above threshold:** Dose-dependent malformations
Throughout pregnancy	Carcinogenesis	Present throughout pregnancy	**Stochastic effect:** No safe threshold, but risk increases with dose

Guidelines of Radiation Dose in Pregnancy (Table 4.5)

Table 4.5: Guidelines of radiation dose in pregnancy.

Parameter	*Details*
USNRC recommended fetus exposure (total, pregnancy)	Less than 5.0 mSv (500 mrem)
Safe fetal radiation dose	Below 50 mGy
Inconclusive fetal radiation dose	50–100 mGy
Risk threshold for negative fetal consequences	Doses above 100 mGy (especially >150 mGy)

Contd...

Contd...

Parameter	*Details*
Fetal susceptibility (2nd and 3rd trimester)	More resistant as compared to first trimester; dose between 0.05 and 0.5 Gy generally considered safe, but high doses (>0.5 Gy) may result in adverse effects
Potential adverse effects of high radiation (>0.5 Gy)	Miscarriage, growth reduction, IQ reduction, severe mental retardation
Occupational exposure limit (total, pregnancy)	Should not exceed 500 mrem (NCRP recommendation)
Occupational exposure limit (monthly)	Should not exceed 50 mrem per month during pregnancy

Note: 1 Gy (unit of absorbed dose) = 100 rads
1 Sv (unit of equivalent dose) = 100 rems

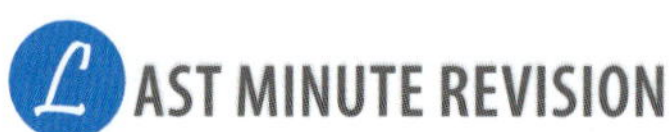

- All x-ray using radiological equipments and its room should be AERB approved.
- A lead apron typically has a lead equivalent thickness of 0.5 mm, which can attenuate 90% of scatter radiation.
- Lead glasses with a lead equivalent thickness of 0.5–0.75 mm can reduce over 95% of scatter radiation, essential for eye protection.

REVIEW QUESTIONS

Multiple Choice Questions (MCQs)

1. **What principle of radiation protection involves using the least amount of radiation necessary to achieve the desired outcome?**
   a. Justification
   b. Optimization
   c. Dose limitation
   d. Time reduction
2. **Which type of personal protective equipment (PPE) is NOT commonly used in radiation protection?**
   a. Lead aprons
   b. Thyroid shields
   c. Nitrile gloves
   d. Lead glasses
3. **Thermoluminescence dosimetry (TLD) is used to measure:**
   a. Only high doses of radiation, such as those in radiotherapy
   b. Only low doses of radiation, such as those monitored in radiation protection
   c. A wide range of absorbed doses, from microgray to several gray
   d. The temperature of the radiation source
4. **Which of the following is NOT a fundamental principle of radiation protection?**
   a. Justification
   b. ALARA (As Low As Reasonably Achievable)
   c. Cost-benefit analysis
   d. Dose limitation

5. **In diagnostic radiology, reducing the duration of radiation exposure can be achieved by:**
   a. Using continuous fluoroscopy at maximum intensity
   b. Increasing the number of images captured per second
   c. Preplanning required images to avoid redundancy
   d. Utilizing magnification whenever possible

Answer Key

1. b   2. c   3. c   4. c   5. c

SUGGESTED READING

1. Cheon BK, Kim CL, Kim KR, Kang MH, Lim JA, Woo NS, et al. Radiation safety: A focus on lead aprons and thyroid shields in interventional pain management. Korean J Pain. 2018 Oct;31(4):244-252.
2. Frane N, Bitterman A. Radiation Safety and Protection. [Updated 2023 May 22]. In: StatPearls [Internet]. Treasure Island (FL): StatPearls Publishing; 2024 Jan-. Available from: https://www.ncbi.nlm.nih.gov/books/NBK557499.
3. Yoon I, Slesinger TL. Radiation Exposure in Pregnancy. [Updated 2023 May 1]. In: StatPearls [Internet]. Treasure Island (FL): StatPearls Publishing; 2024 Jan-. Available from: https://www.ncbi.nlm.nih.gov/books/NBK551690/

CHAPTER

5 Basic Imaging Techniques

"Mastering the basics of imaging is where a radiologist's true vision begins—because clarity in fundamentals leads to excellence in diagnosis."

INTRODUCTION

Radiology is a medical specialty that uses imaging techniques to diagnose and treat diseases within the body. A variety of imaging techniques are available, each suited for different applications and providing unique information. The continuous development and diversification of imaging techniques in Radiology are driven by several key factors, reflecting the evolving needs of medical diagnostics, treatment planning, and research. Here's classification of basic imaging techniques on the basis of technology and type of information they provided:

IONIZING RAYS BASED IMAGING

X-ray Radiography

- **Principle:** Uses X-rays to create images of the inside of the body. The X-rays pass through the body and are absorbed in varying amounts by different tissues, creating an image on a detector.
- **Applications:** Widely used for two-dimensional imaging of bones, detecting fractures, diagnosing lung and chest problems, and dental imaging (OPG).

X-ray machines can be mobile or fixed machine and can be conventional type or with CR system or full DR.

The key differences between mobile (portable) and static X-ray radiography described in **Table 5.1**.

Table 5.1: The key differences between mobile and static X-ray radiography.

Feature	*Mobile X-ray machine (Fig. 5.1)*	*Fixed X-ray machine*
Mobility	Highly mobile, can be moved to different locations (wards/rooms) easily	Stationary, installed in a specific location like a radiology room
Usage	Ideal for bedside examinations, emergency rooms, and in ICU for critically ill patients	Used for routine and specialized diagnostic imaging/procedures when patient mobility to the radiology department is possible
Size and portability	Compact and designed for portability. Often smaller than fixed units	Larger, more robust units with higher output capabilities

Contd...

Contd...

Feature	*Mobile X-ray machine (Fig. 5.1)*	*Fixed X-ray machine*
Image quality	Generally lower image quality	Higher image quality due to more sophisticated technology and stable imaging capabilities
Functionality	Primarily used for basic imaging tasks such as chest X-rays or limb trauma	Can handle a wider range of examinations, including specialized imaging like fluoroscopy, mammography, or angiography
Power and radiation exposure	May have lower power output, which can affect image quality and exposure times	Higher power output, enabling clearer images with potentially lower doses of radiation due to advanced technology
Cost	Generally less expensive due to smaller size and fewer features	More expensive, reflecting their advanced capabilities and the need for dedicated space and installation
Maintenance and setup	Easier to maintain and set up due to simplicity and mobility	Requires more complex maintenance and initial setup, often needing reinforced flooring and special electrical considerations (separate generator or transformer)

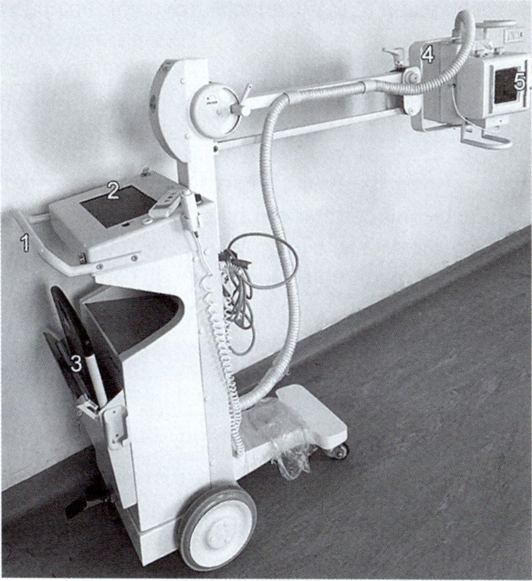

Fig. 5.1: Components of portable X-ray: (1) Transport handle, (2) Control panel, (3) Cassette compartment, (4) X-ray source assembly, (5) Collimator.

Computed Tomography (CT)

- **Principle:** A more advanced form of radiography that uses a series of X-ray images taken from different angles around the body and computer processing to create cross-sectional images (slices) of the bones, blood vessels, and soft tissues inside your body.
- **Applications:** Provides 3D images of all organs especially utilized for chest wall, Face, solid viscera, bones, and blood vessels.
- CT evolves in many ways like type of X-ray beam, type of table movement, number and arrangement of detectors and spiral technology, etc., creating various types of CT classifications.

Table 5.2 outlines the differences between single-slice CT scanners and multi-slice CT scanners whereas differences between non-HRCT and HRCT discussed in **Table 5.3**.

Table 5.2: The differences between single-slice CT scanners and multi-slice CT scanners.

Feature	*Single-Slice CT (axial scan)*	*Multi-Slice CT*
Number of detectors	One row of detectors	Multiple rows of detectors, capable of capturing multiple slices simultaneously
Image acquisition speed	Slower, as it captures one image slice per gantry rotation (step and shoot method)	Faster, as it captures multiple slices per gantry rotation, greatly reducing scan times
Volume coverage	Limited volume coverage per rotation, requiring more time to scan large areas	Increased volume coverage per rotation, ideal for scanning large areas quickly
Temporal resolution	Lower, not suitable for moving organs or fast-paced studies	Higher, excellent for imaging moving organs such as the heart
Spatial resolution	Generally lower as it captures less data per rotation	Higher, due to the ability to acquire more detailed cross-sectional images in a single pass
Reconstruction flexibility	Limited to images	High flexibility in reconstructing images at various planes and slice thicknesses due to extensive data collected
Radiation exposure	Can be higher as multiple passes may be needed for comprehensive imaging	Generally lower, as more efficient scanning reduces the need for multiple passes
Clinical applications	Suitable for basic diagnostic tasks and where high-speed scanning is not critical	Preferred for advanced diagnostic tasks, dynamic imaging of the heart and blood vessels, and comprehensive scans like whole-body trauma assessments
Cost and technological complexity	Less expensive and technologically simpler, making it accessible for basic medical facilities	More expensive and complex, requiring more advanced infrastructure and maintenance

Note: Spiral (Helical) CT is a scanning techniques that combines the rotation of tube with longitudinal movement of patient, so gives volumetric data with improved image resolution and lower radiation dose. Single and multi-slice CT, both utilizes this technology which was lacking in conventional CT machines.

Table 5.3: Differences between non-HRCT and HRCT.

Feature	*Non-HRCT*	*HRCT*
Resolution	Standard resolution	High resolution, focuses on fine detail
Slice thickness	Typically 5–10 mm	1–2 mm or less
Image reconstruction	Standard algorithms	Specialized algorithms that enhance edge definition
FOV	Broader	Focused FOV
Radiation	Might use higher dose per slice	Lower dose per slice
Primary indications	Routine assessments, broader pathologies such as tumors, infections, and large vascular abnormalities	Detailed assessment of the lung parenchyma, interstitial lung diseases, fibrosis, and early-stage emphysema, temporal bone, paranasal sinus, orbit,

Fluoroscopy

- **Principle:** Uses continuous X-rays (dynamic imaging) to create real-time video images of the internal structures of the body. It is often used a contrast agent that makes certain structures, such as the intestines, blood vessels, or joints, more visible. Difference between plain X-ray and fluoroscopic radiography tabulated in **Table 5.4**.
- **Applications:** Useful in guiding a variety of diagnostic and interventional procedures, including catheter insertion, gastrointestinal studies, MCU, HSG and orthopedic surgery and fluoroscopic radiography:

Table 5.4: Difference between plain X-ray and fluoroscopic radiography.

Feature	*Static X-ray radiography*	*Fluoroscopic radiography*
Image type	Produces static, single images	Provides real-time, continuous moving images
Usage and applications	Used for examining static structures (bones, chest)	Used for dynamic studies (GI tract, vascular imaging), and procedural guidance
Radiation exposure	Lower radiation dose due to brief exposure	Higher radiation dose due to prolonged exposure
Equipment complexity	Simpler equipment with stationary components	More complex utilizes image intensifier and movable components and capability for multiple viewing angles
Image quality and detail	Higher resolution images, better for detailed evaluation	Focuses on function, with slightly lower resolution due to continuous imaging
Operator skill and interaction	Less interaction needed once patient is positioned	Requires active management and manipulation during imaging

MAGNETIC RESONANCE BASED IMAGING (MRI)

- **Principle:** Uses a strong magnetic field and radio waves to generate detailed images of the organs and tissues in the body.
- **Applications:** Especially useful for imaging the brain, spine, muscle, tendon, meniscal and ligament. MRI is excellent for soft tissue contrast and is specially used in detecting tumors extension, brain disorders, and spinal cord pathologies.

SOUND BASED IMAGING

Ultrasound (Sonography)

- **Principle:** Uses high-frequency sound waves to create images of structures within the body. The sound waves echo off tissues with different reflections that are then converted into an image. Various ultrasound techniques discussed in **Table 5.5**.

Table 5.5: Differences between various ultrasound (USG) techniques.

Imaging technique	*Resolution*	*Imaging characteristics*	*Primary uses*
Conventional USG	Standard resolution	Uses sound waves of 3–5 MHz	General imaging for abdominal organs, obstetric scan, sometimes superficial organs in obese
HRUSG (High-Resolution Ultrasound)	High resolution	5–18 MHz	Detailed imaging of superficial body structures such as thyroid, breast, skin, and superficial blood vessels
Color Doppler	Standard resolution with flow mapping	Adds color imaging to show blood flow in real time, assessing velocity as PSV, and directions	Evaluation of blood flow and vascular structures; used in cardiology, vascular studies, and assessing blood flow in tumors
TVS (Transvaginal Sonography)	High resolution due to proximity	Transducer of 4–9 MHz inserted into the vagina for closer proximity to target organs	Gynecological assessments, early pregnancy scans, and evaluation of pelvic organs
3D USG (Three-Dimensional Ultrasound)	Variable resolution with 3D rendering	Provides three-dimensional images of the fetus or organs, allowing for volumetric assessments	Obstetric imaging to assess fetal an anamoly, complex gynecological issues, and in urology for assessing organ volume

- **Applications:** Commonly used in obstetrics for evaluating fetal development, but also for examining other organs like the liver, kidneys, and heart (Echocardiography).

NUCLEAR MEDICINE IMAGING

- **Principle:** Involves the administration of radiopharmaceuticals (radioactive substances) that accumulate in specific organs or lesions. Special cameras detect the radiation emitted by these substances to create images.
- **Applications:** Widely used in the diagnosis, staging and monitoring of cancer, heart disease, and certain neurological disorders by showing how tissues and organs are functioning.
- Includes positron emission tomography (PET) and single photon emission computed tomography (SPECT):
  - *Positron emission tomography (PET):* Uses short active radioactive tracers (e.g., fluorine 18) to visualize metabolic processes in the body, often combined with CT for detailed anatomical and functional information.
  - *Single photon emission computed tomography (SPECT):* Similar to PET but uses long active gamma emitting radioisotopes, e.g., Technitium 99m.

OPTICAL IMAGING

Not commonly used in radiology. It involves the use of light to visualize tissues, often on the surface of the body or via endoscopic procedures.

Endoscopy: Utilizes a lighted, flexible instrument to view the interior surfaces of organs directly. Endoscopic ultrasound is usually done for evaluation of pancreatobiliary disease and GI malignancies

HYBRID IMAGING TECHNIQUES

These combine two or more imaging modalities to provide comprehensive information about both the structure and function of body tissues.

1. **PET/CT:** Combines the functional imaging of PET with the anatomical detail provided by CT.
2. **SPECT/CT:** Offers combined functional and anatomical imaging similar to PET/CT but uses different tracers and technology.

CONTRAST MEDIAS AND COMMON CONTRAST PROCEDURES

All modalities can be done with or without contrast medias as per need of diagnosis. Contrast media (or contrast agents) are substances used in medical imaging to enhance the contrast of structures or fluids within the body, making them more visible on the images. These agents can significantly improve the accuracy of diagnostic imaging studies by highlighting features that might not be seen otherwise. The choice of contrast media often depends on the specific imaging requirements, patient history, and potential risk factors for adverse reactions. The development of newer contrast agents continues to focus on improving safety profiles and diagnostic efficacy.

Classification of Contrast Media

Based on the Imaging Modality

- **Radiopaque agents for X-ray and CT scans:** These agents absorb X-rays more effectively than the surrounding tissues. Commonly used agents include iodine-based and barium sulfate compounds.

Note: Barium studies are contraindicated in acute intestinal obstruction and bowel perforation. In these conditions either water soluble contrast like trazograph or urograffin, etc., can be used in place of barium or CT can be done if conditions are favorable.

- **MRI contrast agents:** These enhance the contrast in MRI scans and are primarily gadolinium-based. Rare complications is Nephrogenic systemic fibrosis.
- **Ultrasound contrast agents:** These are microbubbles of gas encapsulated in a shell, used to improve the echogenicity of blood or tissues, enhancing ultrasound images.

Based on Osmolality

- **High-osmolar contrast media (HOCM):** These are ionic agents that dissociate into two particles in solution, generally used less frequently today due to higher rates of adverse reactions.
- **Low-osmolar contrast media (LOCM):** Nonionic, do not dissociate into particles, associated with fewer adverse reactions and improved patient comfort.
- **Iso-osmolar contrast media (IOCM):** Have the same osmolality as blood plasma (i.e., 275–295 mOsm/kg) and are associated with the lowest risk of adverse reactions.

Based on Ionicity

- **Ionic:** Dissociate into anions and cations in solution, typically high-osmolar. Example: Sodium Diatrizoate (Trazograph) **(Fig. 5.2A)**.
- **Nonionic:** Do not dissociate, resulting in lower osmolality and reduced side effects. Example: Iohexol (Omnipaque), Iopromide (Ultravist) **(Fig. 5.2B)**.

Note: High osmolar ionic contrast media are no longer used intravascularly.

Based on Utilities

- **Iodinated contrast media (Figs. 5.2A and 5.2B):**
  - *Use:* Primarily used in CT scans and some types of X-ray imaging.
  - *Properties:* These are water-soluble substances that contain iodine, which is highly effective at absorbing X-rays. They can be administered orally, intravenously, or rectally.
  - *Varieties:* Include both ionic (high osmolality) and nonionic (low osmolality) agents. Nonionic agents are generally preferred due to their lower risk of adverse reactions.
  - *Common reactions:* Risk of allergic reactions, nephrotoxicity (kidney damage), particularly in patients with pre-existing kidney problems or dehydration are more with ionic contrasts.
- **Barium-based contrast media:**
  - *Use:* Specifically used for imaging the gastrointestinal (GI) tract in studies like barium swallows, enemas, and enterography **(Fig. 5.2C)**.
  - *Properties:* Barium sulfate is a radiopaque substance that is not absorbed by the body, providing clear images of the GI tract.
  - *Administration:* Taken orally or rectally, depending on the area of the GI tract being examined.
  - *Common reaction:* Risk of constipation or blockage; not to be used if there is suspicion of a GI tract perforation.
  - Commonly used in day-to-day practice due to easy steps, low cost and wider availability.

Single barium contrast is commonly done, but in few cases double contrast will be performed. Difference in both techniques are tabulated in **Table 5.6**.

- **Gadolinium-based contrast agents (GBCAs)**
  - *Use:* Employed to differentiate between normal and pathological tissues, especially in the brain, spine, liver, and to assess tumors and vascular diseases, e.g., optimark, Omniscan.

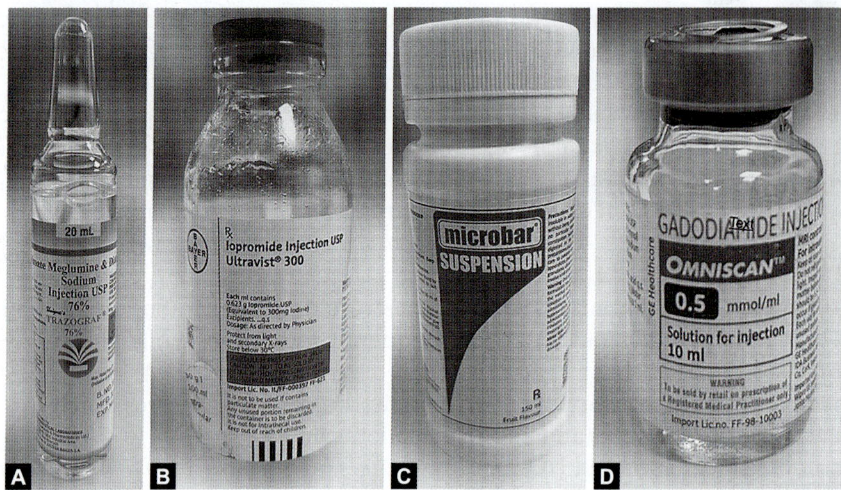

Figs. 5.2A to D: Various types of contrast agents: (A) Ionic type; (B) Nonionic type; (C) Barium suspension; (D) Gadolinium-based contrast agent.

Table 5.6: Differences between basic barium studies and double contrast barium studies.

Feature	*Basic barium studies*	*Double contrast barium studies*
Contrast material	Uses a single contrast agent, usually barium sulfate	Uses barium in conjunction with a gas-producing agent (like air or carbon dioxide)
Image detail	Provides a continuous coating of barium on the mucosal surface, highlighting large abnormalities	Provides detailed views of the mucosal lining by coating the walls with barium and distending the area with gas, enhancing the visibility of small lesions and fine mucosal details
Indications	Suitable for general examinations of the gastrointestinal tract, such as identifying large tumors or strictures	Ideal for detecting finer abnormalities like small polyps, early tumors, and minute changes in the mucosa
Procedure complexity	Less complex, generally easier to perform	More complex due to the need for precise timing and manipulation to achieve proper double contrast
Patient comfort	Generally more comfortable as it involves a simpler procedure with less manipulation	May be less comfortable due to the introduction of gas, which can cause distension and discomfort
Diagnostic accuracy	Good for large abnormalities but may miss finer details	Higher diagnostic accuracy for mucosal surface details and early-stage pathologies
Duration	Usually quicker as it involves a single type of contrast	May take longer due to the need for multiple phases and positions to ensure adequate double contrast
Cost	Generally less expensive due to the simplicity of the procedure and materials	More expensive due to the use of additional contrast materials and the complexity of the procedure

- *Properties:* Gadolinium is a heavy metal that affects the magnetic properties of water, enhancing the MRI signal.
- *Varieties:* Macrocyclic and **(Fig. 5.2D)** linear agents, with macrocyclic generally considered more stable and less likely to release gadolinium ions into the body.

- *Risk:* Rarely, can cause nephrogenic systemic fibrosis in patients with severe renal impairment. Newer agents have a lower risk.

- **Ultrasound contrast agents:**
  - *Use:* Enhance the echogenicity of blood, improving the visualization of blood flow and organs during ultrasound examinations. Commonly used in echocardiography to improve the visualization of cardiac structures, in liver imaging to detect lesions **Figures 5.3A and B**. Example: Definity, Optison, etc.
  - *Properties:* Consist of microbubbles containing gas that is encapsulated in a shell, enhancing the reflection of ultrasound waves.
  - *Administration:* Intravenous injection.
  - *Risk:* Generally well tolerated, with a low risk of adverse effects. Not suitable for patients with certain heart or lung conditions that could allow microbubbles to enter arterial circulation.

COMMON IMAGING PROCEDURES

Contrast X-ray procedures are commonly performed basic techniques of diagnostic radiology in day-to-day practice. They are related to various systems, discussed below.

- **GIT:** X-ray procedures done for study of GIT is known as Barium studies. It is of various types **(Table 5.7)**.
- **Urinary tract:** Commonly performed procedure is IVP which is base of CTU (also known as CT IVP). Here are common X-ray procedures related to urinary tract are as follows in **Table 5.8**.
- Some miscellaneous procedures are described in **Table 5.9**.
- Beside X-rays, few common radiological procedures are also performed with or without guidance of USG and CT which are described below in **Table 5.10**.

Table 5.7: Common X-ray procedures related to gastrointestinal tract.

Type of barium study	*Route and amount of barium*	*Common views*	*Indications*
Barium swallow (oropharynx to GE junction)	Mouthful/100–250 mL of 100 w/v	Plain AP followed by contrast, anterior-posterior, RAO, +/– lateral	Dysphagia, gastroesophageal reflux, structural anomalies of the esophagus
Barium meal (GE junction to DJ junction)	Per oral 250–400 mL	Plain AXR AP erect, followed by contrast supine AP (immediate, 15 minutes, 30 minutes), oblique, lateral, prone	Gastric and duodenal ulcers, motility disorders, malignancies, hiatus hernia, malrotation
Barium follow-through (DJ to IC junction)	Per oral 400–800 mL	Plain AXR AP erect, followed by contrast supine AP (30 minutes, 1 hour, 2.5 hours, 4.5 hours), oblique for IC junction	Small bowel disorders, Crohn's disease, tumors, malabsorption syndromes, intestinal TB
Barium enema (anal canal to ileocecal junction)	Per-rectal mechanical filling 500–1,500 mL	AXR erect, followed by contrast supine, left lateral, prone, oblique	Colonic tumors, polyps, inflammatory bowel disease, diverticulosis, Anorectal malformation, Hirschsprung disease

Table 5.8: Common X-ray procedures related to urinary tract.

Procedure	*Route and amount of contrast*	*Common views*	*Indications*
Intravenous pyelogram (IVP) or IVU, only performed after giving test dose if patient has no reactions **(Fig. 5.4)**	Water soluble ionic 76% or nonionic with IV dose of 1 mL/kg 50–100 mL	Plain AP abdomen supine, followed by contrast anterior-posterior (immediate, 10/15/30/60/120 minutes), 24 hours if suspected non-functioning, prone (differentiating functional or mechanical PUJ obstruction)oblique, lateral	Calculus, tumors, congenital abnormalities, hematuria, renal functioning
Retrograde pyelogram	Water soluble ionic 60% or nonionic, variable amount; directly instilled into ureters	Plain supine AP abdomen, followed by contrast anterior-posterior, oblique, lateral	Detailed outline of ureters and renal pelvis, especially when IVP is not feasible
Cystography	Water soluble ionic 60% or nonionic, per-catheter 250–500 mL	Plain supine AP pelvis, followed by contrast anterior-posterior, lateral, oblique	Bladder outline and integrity, vesicoureteral reflux, trauma to the bladder
Nephrostogram	Water soluble ionic 60% or nonionic, variable amount directly instilled into the renal pelvis via nephrostomy tube	Plain supine AP abdomen, followed by contrast anterior-posterior (immediate and delated up to 30 minutes or contrast reaches the bladder), lateral	Evaluation of renal pelvis and ureter, assessment of obstruction, post-surgical evaluation
Retrograde urethrogram (RGU) **(Fig. 5.5)**	Water soluble ionic 60% or nonionic, variable (10–30 mL with 10–15 mL in each view); either directly instilled into the urethra per 20 mL syringe or rarely by IV cannula if meatus is small (24 number)	Plain supine AP pelvis upto mid-thigh, followed by contrast anterior-posterior, oblique, lateral	Assessment of urethral structure, strictures, and trauma
Micturating cystourethrogram (MCU)	Water soluble ionic 60% or nonionic, variable (as per bladder capacity); directly instilled into the bladder by foleys catheter using 50 mL syringe	Plain supine AP abdomen and pelvis, followed by contrast anterior-posterior, oblique, lateral, in voiding phase and post-void AP view	Evaluation of the bladder and urethra during voiding, diagnosis of vesicoureteral reflux, assessment of urethral valves

Table 5.9: Miscellaneous group of contrast procedures.

Procedure	*Route and amount of contrast*	*Common views*	*Indications*
Sinogram	Water soluble ionic 60% or nonionic, variable (1–15 mL) directly instilled into sinus tracts by IV cannula (24 number)	Plain AP of that site, followed by contrast views specific to tract location, commonly AP and lateral	Investigation of sinus tracts, identification of connections to body cavities
Fistulogram	Water soluble ionic 60% or nonionic variable (10–50 mL) directly instilled into the cutaneous opening of suspected fistulous tract by IV cannula	Plain AP of that site, followed by contrast views specific to tract location, commonly AP and lateral	Diagnosis and mapping of fistula tracts, assessment of extent and depth commonly in anal region (replaced by MRI fistulography) and neck if suspected branchial fistula (replaced by CT sinogram)
T-tube Cholangiogram (contrast should fill biliary radicles and CBD draining into duodenum) **(Fig. 5.6)**	Water soluble ionic 60% or nonionic 5–20 mL per tube after clamping the tube close to skin	Plain supine AP followed by contrast abdomen, anterior-posterior, right oblique	Assessment of bile ducts post-surgery, check for leaks or obstructions. It is baseline technique for MRCP
Hysterosalpingography (HSG)	Water soluble ionic 60% or nonionic, 10 mL in each shot per cannula or catheter. First to see the uterine filling and second for fallopian tube patency	Anterior-posterior pelvis, sometimes lateral (commonly two X-rays are taken)	Investigation of choice for fallopian tube patency, also assess uterine cavity and post-surgical assessment to see recanalization

Table 5.10: Common procedures done on USG and CT.

Imaging technique	*Route and dose of contrast*	*Timing of images*	*Indications*
Sono-HSG	Uses ultrasound gel or normal saline instilling per catheter through vagina	Real-time ultrasound imaging done to see first filling of cavity followed by visualization of free fluid spillage adjacent to ovary or adnexa	Evaluation of the uterine cavity, i.e., endometrial pathology and fallopian tube patency in infertility assessment
CT triple phase	Nonionic (IV contrast)	Three phases: After NCCT, arterial phase (usually 15–30 seconds post-injection), portal venous phase (60–70 seconds post-injection), hepatic venous phase (2–3 minutes)	Liver lesions, characterization of masses, and vascular abnormalities
CT enterography	1.5–2 L neutral or low density oral and IV contrast	Delayed imaging (40–70 minutes after oral contrast intake)	Small bowel evaluation, particularly for Crohn's disease and other inflammatory bowel diseases

Contd...

Contd...

Imaging technique	*Route and dose of contrast*	*Timing of images*	*Indications*
CT angiography	Nonionic (IV contrast)	Timed post-contrast based on target vessels (e.g., arterial phase for arteries)	Assessment of vascular structures, aneurysms, dissections, and vascular malformations
CT enteroclysis (small bowel enema)	Infusion of contrast per tube/catheter	Delayed imaging (immediate to few minutes after infusion of contrast via a tube into the small bowel)	Detailed examination of the small intestine to identify mucosal and structural abnormalities
CT urography	Moderate (IV contrast)	Multi-phase imaging: Non-contrast, nephrogenic phase (100–180 seconds), and excretory phase (5–15 minutes)	Evaluation of the urinary tract, including kidneys, ureters, and bladder for tumors, stones, and structural anomalies
Note: Maximum dose of IV contrast in CECT is 1.5 mL/kg body weight. Contrast is injected by automatic pump injector after setting time and rate of contrast. All of the above procedures can also be performed by MRI.			

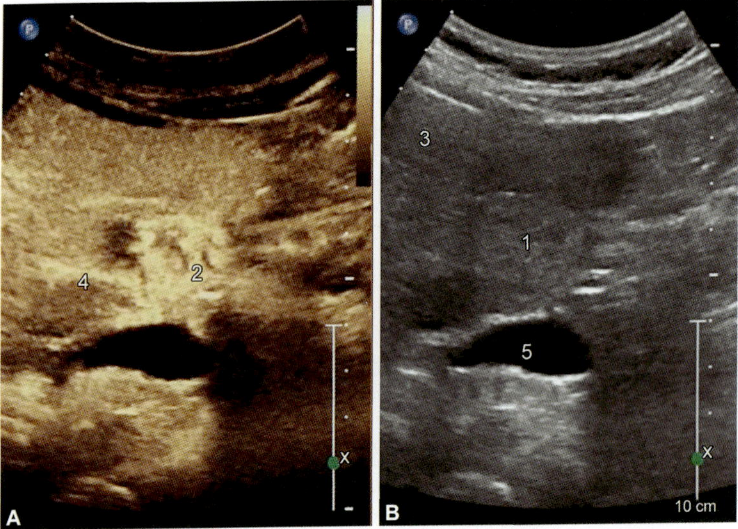

Figs. 5.3A and B: (A) shows contrast enhanced ultrasound image of hepatic solid lesion as a well-defined, more obvious and echogenic lesion (2) as well as contrast in portal vein radicle (4) as compared to image; (B) which is normal noncontrast 2D gray scale image showing liver (3), gallbladder (5) and iso-echoic solid lesion (1).

CONTRAST REACTIONS

It is an adverse events occurs after contrast medium is injected into the body.

Prevention and Management

It has to be managed at all steps of contrast procedure, i.e., pre-procedure, during procedure and sometimes post-procedure. Some common steps are:

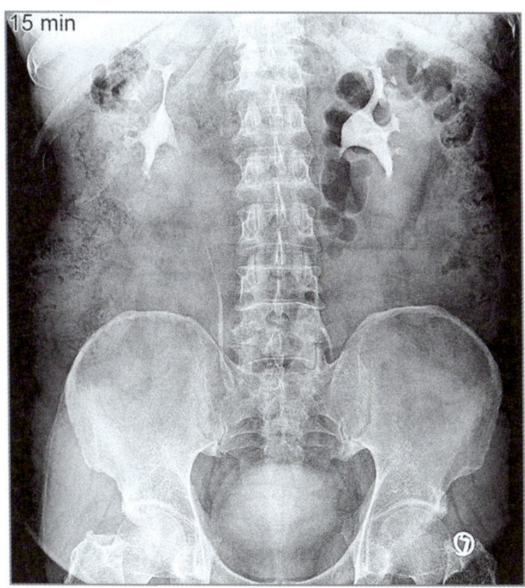

Fig. 5.4: Post-contrast view of IVP taken at 15 minutes showing contrast filling in PCS. Partial contrast is also visible in right ureter and bladder too.

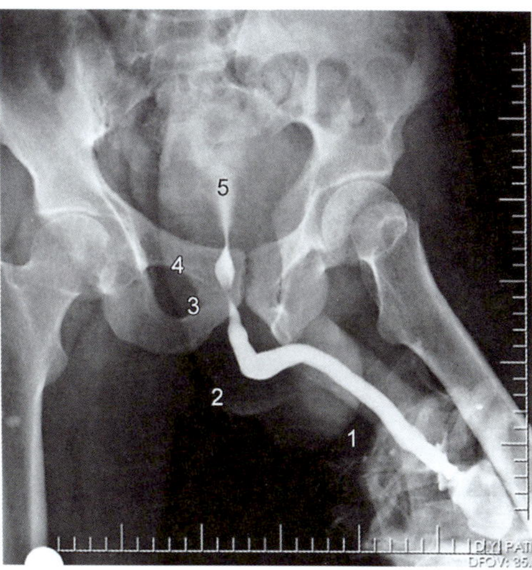

Fig. 5.5: Retrograde urethrogram (RGU): (1) Penile urethra; (2) Bulbous urethra; (3) Membranous urethra; (4) Prostatic urethra; (5) Contrast in urinary bladder.

Pre-screening

Identifying patients at risk for adverse reactions, such as those with a history of contrast media reactions, asthma, or significant allergies. It has to be managed as follows:

- **Premedication:** Administering steroids and antihistamines prior to contrast media administration in high-risk patients.
- **Using low or iso-osmolar nonionic contrast media:** These agents are associated with fewer adverse reactions and are preferred, especially in patients with a known risk of reaction.
- **Emergency preparedness:** Ensuring that facilities are equipped and staff are trained to handle severe reactions, including the availability of resuscitation equipment and medications.

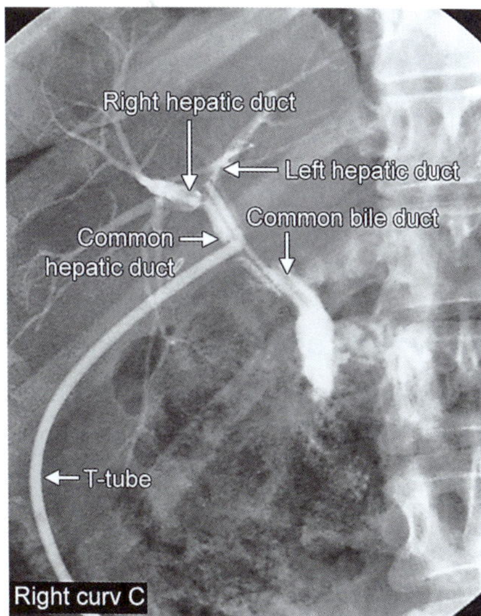

Fig. 5.6: T-tube cholangiogram.

Contrast reactions **(Table 5.11)** varied depending on type of contrast media used during imaging studies Reactions to contrast media can range from mild to severe and are generally less common with nonionic low-osmolar and iso-osmolar agent.

While working on the patient, Radiologist not only uses their knowledge skills but they have also to intervene for preprocedural patient preparation for best outcome and in the same time guide their technical staff for procedure too. Patient preparation before imaging procedures is crucial to ensure the safety of the patient, optimize the quality of imaging results, and reduce

Table 5.11: Description of common reactions to contrast media and their respective management strategies.

Contrast type	*Reaction type*	*Common reactions*	*Management strategies*
Iodinated contrast	Mild	Nausea, vomiting, warmth, metallic taste, urticaria	Often self-limiting. Symptomatic treatment may be required
	Moderate	Mild hypotension, tachycardia, bronchospasm,facial or laryngeal edema	Monitor closely, administer antihistamines, steroids, or bronchodilators as needed
	Severe	Anaphylaxis, severe hypotension, cardiac arrest, convulsions, respiratory distress	Immediate administration of epinephrine, oxygen, IV fluids, and steroids. Call for emergency support
Gadolinium-based	Mild	Nausea, headache, localized or mild allergic reactions	Symptomatic treatment with antihistamines or analgesics
	Moderate	Moderate allergic reactions, dyspnea	Administer antihistamines, steroids, and monitor patient closely
	Severe	Anaphylactoid reactions, severe hypotension	Immediate treatment with epinephrine, oxygen, IV fluids. Call for emergency support
Ultrasound contrast	Mild	Sensation of warmth, headache, nausea	Usually self-limiting. Monitor patient; symptomatic treatment may be required
	Moderate	Allergic-like reactions, flushing, dyspnea	Antihistamines and oxygen may be required. Monitor closely
	Severe	Anaphylaxis, cardiovascular collapse	Immediate epinephrine, oxygen, IV fluids, and call for emergency support

Note: Adrenaline dose is 0.3 to 0.5 mil of 1:1000 deep s/c or i/m repeated at 10–20 minutes

the likelihood of repeat scans. The specific preparations can vary significantly depending on the type of imaging procedure being performed. General overview of prerequisites and patient preparation steps for common imaging modalities are as follows:

X-ray and Computed Tomography (CT) Scans

- **Bowel preparation:** Ask the patient to take tablets of gasex and dulcolex after taking food like daliya and khichdi in last meal in case of IVP, barium studies and dedicated CT studies like enteroclysis, enterography, etc.
- **Fasting:** Patients may need to have a overnight fasting (usually 8–12 hours) before the scan especially if a contrast medium is to be used.
- **Allergies:** It is very important on a part of technical staff or even doctor to ask patient about any allergies, especially to iodine or shellfish, which might indicate a potential allergy to some contrast agents.
- **Medications:** Some medications may need to be temporarily discontinued, especially if they could interfere with the contrast agent or some medication hint the diseases. Diseases like Diabetes mellitus. Multiple myeloma, are relative contraindication of IVP.
- **Metallic objects:** Patients are usually asked to remove jewelery and wear clothing without metal fasteners to avoid harmful artifacts.
- **Pregnancy:** Always ask LMP in case of female patient to rule out possibility of pregnancy as X-rays related procedures are not recommended during pregnancy.

- **Blood test:** Serum creatinine should be normal as acute renal failure is contraindication for IVP and contrast CT studies. Procedure can only be performed after proper hydration followed by post procedural dialysis if imaging procedure is life saving for patient.
- Test dose of 1 mL should be given before all procedures where iv contrast has to be given.

Magnetic Resonance Imaging (MRI)

- **Metallic Implants:** Any metal implants, pacemakers, or other metallic objects are contraindication for MRI. Though MRI compatible implants made of Titanium or tantalum or nonmetallic are available but still patient should informed the healthcare provider about metallic objects.
- **Fasting:** Fasting may be required if a contrast agent is to be used.
- **Kidney function:** A blood test may be performed before the administration of gadolinium-based contrast agents to ensure that the kidneys can safely excrete the contrast.
- **Stillness:** Patients will be asked to remain very still during the scan to ensure image clarity. Claustrophobia is also contraindication for MRI

Ultrasound

- **Hydration and bladder preparation:** For KUBP and pelvic ultrasounds, patients has to drink 3–6 glass of water and not urinate before the exam to ensure a optimal full bladder, which provides better imaging of the uterus, ovaries, kidney, ureter, urinary bladder or prostate.
- **Fasting:** For abdominal ultrasounds, especially hepatopancreatobiliary scan, fasting for 8–12 hours or overnight is often required to reduce gas in the intestines and improve imaging quality.

Nuclear Medicine Imaging (PET, SPECT)

- **Fasting:** Patients are generally required to fast for a certain period before the scan, especially if it involves the use of a glucose-based tracer.
- **Medications:** Disclosure of all medications is important, as some may need to be adjusted or stopped temporarily.
- **Hydration:** Patients may be advised to drink plenty of water to help the flush of radioactive tracer from the body after the procedure.

General Preparations for all Imaging Procedures (Table 5.12)

- **Detailed health history:** Providing a detailed health history, including allergies, current medications, and prior surgeries, is essential.
- **Consent forms:** Patients may need to sign consent forms, especially when contrast agents are involved.
- **Clothing:** Wearing comfortable, loose-fitting cotton clothing is usually recommended. Patients may also be asked to wear hospital gown for the procedure/scanning.
- **Childcare:** If applicable, arranging for someone to care for young children during the imaging of their parents, as children are generally not allowed in imaging rooms. In case of scanning of child, parents especially mother is advisable to come with feed of child either in the form of breast feed or bottle of milk or some chips/toffee or rarely sedation is needed.

It is important for patients to closely follow the specific preparation instructions provided by their healthcare provider or imaging center, as these can vary based on the procedure and individual patient circumstances. Proper preparation helps ensure the safety and effectiveness of the imaging process.

Table 5.12: Description of various imaging techniques, their prerequisites, contrast used, reactions to contrast, and management of these reactions.

Name of procedure	*Prerequisites*	*Contrast used*	*Reaction*	*Management of reactions*
X-ray	Removal of jewelery and metal objects; informing about pregnancy	None usually; barium or iodinated contrast for specific studies (e.g., barium swallow)	Allergic reactions are rare; nausea or constipation with barium	Immediate cessation of procedure; administration of antihistamines, corticosteroids, or IV fluids as per severity
CT scan (Computed Tomography)	Fasting for a few hours if intravenous contrast is to be used; allergy history; renal function test for patients at risk of contrast-induced nephropathy, informing about pregnancy	Iodinated contrast	Mild: nausea, vomiting, warmth, or metallic taste; Severe: Anaphylaxis, contrast-induced nephropathy	Mild reactions often self-limiting; severe reactions require stopping contrast infusion, administering antihistamines, corticosteroids, or epinephrine, and supportive care for nephropathy
MRI (Magnetic Resonance Imaging)	Removal of metal objects; screening for implants (e.g., pacemakers, cochlear implants)	Gadolinium-based contrast agents	Mild: nausea, headache; Severe: Nephrogenic systemic fibrosis (NSF) in patients with renal failure	Mild reactions are managed symptomatically; NSF is rare but requires cessation of gadolinium use and potentially dialysis
Ultrasound	Fasting for abdominal scans to reduce gas; full bladder for pelvic scans to improve visibility	None usually; microbubble contrast agents for specific applications (e.g., echocardiography)	Allergic reactions to microbubble agents are rare	Monitoring and supportive care; use of alternative imaging modalities if severe reaction
PET scan (Positron Emission Tomography)	Fasting for a certain period before the test; avoidance of strenuous exercise a day before the scan	Radioactive tracers (e.g., FDG)	Allergic reactions are extremely rare; Risk of radiation exposure, though minimal	Supportive care for any allergic reactions; no specific management for radiation as exposure is low and controlled

LAST MINUTE REVISION

- IV test dose is always given prior to all contrast procedures using iodine-based contrast intravenously
- In case of ionic contrast 76% is used for IV route while 60% in case of non-IV use (though limited in use)
- Pregnancy and renal failure are contraindication for contrast procedures using X-rays
- Claustrophobia, non-titanium-based implants and pacemakers are contraindication for MRI
- Contrast dose in IVP is 1 mL/kg body weight while in CECT is 1–2 mL/kg or 1.5 mL/kg

REVIEW QUESTIONS

Multiple Choice Questions (MCQs)

1. **Which imaging technique is most commonly used to examine the structure of the heart and the flow of blood through its chambers?**
   a. X-ray
   b. Ultrasound
   c. CT scan
   d. MRI
2. **What type of contrast agent is typically used in a CT scan to enhance the visibility of blood vessels, gastrointestinal tract, and other specific areas?**
   a. Gadolinium-based agents
   b. Iodinated contrast materials
   c. Barium sulfate
   d. Microbubble contrast agents
3. **Which of the following imaging modalities does NOT use ionizing radiation?**
   a. CT scan
   b. MRI
   c. X-ray
   d. PET scan
4. **In ultrasound imaging, what property of tissues is primarily used to generate an image?**
   a. Electrical conductivity
   b. Thermal conductivity
   c. Density differences reflected in sound wave echoes
   d. Magnetic properties
5. **Which imaging technique uses radioactive tracers to visualize metabolic processes in the body?**
   a. MRI
   b. Ultrasound
   c. PET scan
   d. X-ray
6. **What is the main safety concern associated with MRI scans?**
   a. Exposure to ionizing radiation
   b. Allergic reactions to iodinated contrast material
   c. The presence of metallic implants in the body
   d. Exposure to ultraviolet light

Answer Key

1. b 2. b 3. b 4. c 5. c 6. c

SUGGESTED READING

1. Kim YH, Choi M, Kim JW. Are titanium implants actually safe for magnetic resonance imaging examinations? Arch Plast Surg. 2019 Jan;46(1):96-97. doi: 10.5999/aps.2018.01466. Epub 2019 Jan 15. PMID: 30685951; PMCID: PMC6369045.
2. Morcos SK, Thomsen HS, Webb JA; Contrast Media Safety Committee of the European Society of Urogenital Radiology. Prevention of generalized reactions to contrast media: a consensus report and guidelines. Eur Radiol. 2001;11(9):1720-8.

CHAPTER 6

Advanced Imaging Techniques

"Advanced imaging begins with mastering the basics—because in every slice, scan, and shadow lies the power of precise interpretation."

INTRODUCTION

The diagnosis and treatment of various diseases have been expedited with the help of medical imaging. Different medical imaging modalities are X-ray, ultrasound, computed tomography (CT), magnetic resonance imaging (MRI) and nuclear imaging. In the recent times with mounting innovations and advancements in technology, the medical diagnostic field has been revolutionized and has taken health care to new horizons. These techniques ensure accurate imaging with improved resolution, sensitivity, and specificity.

In this chapter, we enlist the advancements in each of the aforesaid modalities which are available to the clinicians for more refined and better patient management.

ADVANCED X-RAY TECHNIQUES

Since their discovery by Wilhelm Conrad Roentgen in 1895, X-rays have become the most widely available, typically fastest, and usually most cost-effective medical imaging modality. From the early radiographic approaches using X-ray films as detectors, the portfolio of medical X-ray imaging devices developed into a large range of dedicated instrumentation for various applications.

Some recent advances are:

- **3D x-ray imaging:** Traditional X-ray imaging provides only a 2D view, but advancements in technology now allow for high-resolution 3D imaging.
- **Low-dose X-ray imaging:** Concerns about radiation exposure have led to developments in low-dose X-ray imaging techniques. These advancements reduce the radiation dose while maintaining image quality, making it safer for patients, particularly in repeated imaging procedures.
- **Dual-energy X-ray imaging:** Dual-energy X-ray imaging involves the simultaneous acquisition of multiple X-ray images at different energy levels. This technique provides additional information about the composition of materials, allowing for improved tissue differentiation in medical imaging and enhanced material characterization in industrial applications. A computer then assembles the captured data to make cross-sectional images of the body that resemble "slices." A dual-energy CT scanner works similarly, but it also uses a second, lower-voltage X-ray tube in addition to the standard X-ray tube.

- **Phase-contrast X-ray imaging:** Phase-contrast X-ray imaging exploits variations in the phase of X-rays passing through an object, rather than just their absorption, resulting in higher contrast and resolution compared to traditional methods. This technique is particularly useful for imaging soft tissues in medical applications.
- **X-ray fluorescence imaging:** X-ray fluorescence (XRF) imaging combines X-ray excitation with the detection of characteristic fluorescence emitted by elements within a sample. This technique enables elemental mapping and quantitative analysis of materials, with applications in archaeology, art conservation, environmental science and forensics.
- **Synchrotron X-ray imaging:** Synchrotron radiation facilities produce intense and highly collimated X-ray beams, allowing for advanced imaging techniques such as microtomography, X-ray diffraction, and spectroscopy at the nanoscale level. These facilities enable research in diverse fields including materials science, biology and environmental science.
- **Dynamic X-ray imaging:** Dynamic X-ray imaging captures sequential X-ray images over time, allowing for the study of dynamic processes such as blood flow, joint movement, and cardiac function. This technique is valuable in both clinical diagnostics and research applications.
- **Portable X-ray devices:** Advances in miniaturization and portability have led to the development of handheld and portable X-ray devices. These compact devices are particularly useful in emergency medicine, fieldwork, and remote areas where access to static X-ray equipment may be limited **(Fig. 6.1)**.

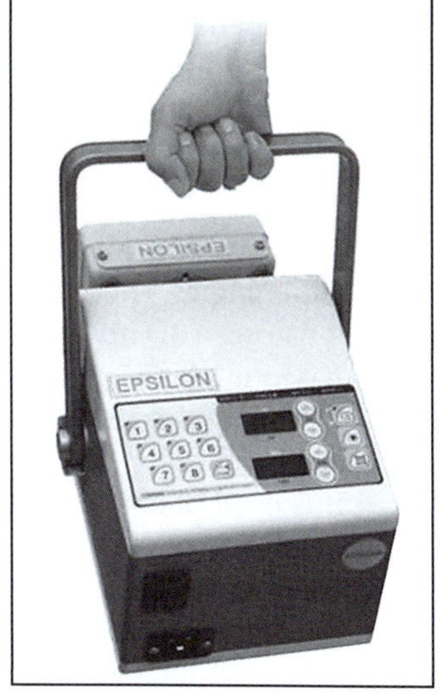

Fig. 6.1: Portable X-ray device.

- **Artificial intelligence in X-ray interpretation:** Machine learning and artificial intelligence algorithms are being increasingly integrated into X-ray interpretation software, aiding in the detection, classification, and analysis of abnormalities in medical images.
- **Tomosynthesis:** Tomosynthesis, an advanced type of digital mammography approved by the Food and Drug Administration (FDA) in 2011, goes by many names, including 3D mammography, breast tomosynthesis, and digital breast tomosynthesis (DBT). Sometimes, the flat images produced by conventional 2D mammography make it difficult for radiologists to detect cancer. This often leads to patients getting called back for additional tests. Tomosynthesis helps to avoid this using a different imaging approach. It creates multiple images of the breast using both 2D and 3D-like pictures, which are sent to a computer that uses algorithms to assemble the pictures, giving a more complete view of a patient's breasts. Tomosynthesis can increase accuracy overall, especially when combined with conventional mammography.

  Additional benefits include detection of breast cancer in the early stages, greater accuracy for breast cancer screening for people with dense breasts, reduction of callbacks and false-positive results **(Fig. 6.2)**.
- **Flexible X-ray imaging:** Until recently, most X-ray detector panels were flat and only capable of scanning X-rays in a 2D format. A large rotating gantry has allowed for 3D imaging to take place. However, due to the expense and equipment size, inventors have been looking for 3D imaging alternatives. One such alternative would be flexible imaging panels that curve around surfaces. In the last few years, several flexible panels have been invented that improve upon all currently available flat panels (direct and indirect types)

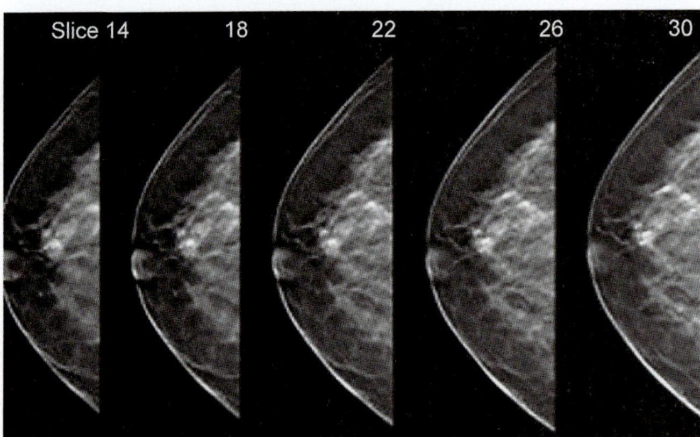

Fig. 6.2: Tomosynthesis providing slice by slice images of the breast.

used in medical imaging devices. Some of these new inventions are able to curve around surfaces and may even be worn by the patient for comfortable scanning of selective body regions for higher resolution.

ADVANCED ULTRASOUND TECHNIQUES

- **3D USG:** Works similar to traditional 2D USG except that ultrasound waves are directed from multiple angles. These waves are reflected back and captured to provide enough information to construct a 3D image.
  - It is multiplanar, gives high-spatial resolution, has less scan time and faster postprocessing (Tomographic ultrasound imaging [TUI], volume rendering (VR), and automatic slicing) can be done.
  - It is used in congenital uterine malformation. Characterization of adnexal masses and volume measurement.
  - It has added immense value in obstetrics to identify fetal face, cleft lip, and palate, nuchal thickness, cardiac, skeleton and neural tube defects.
- **Accelerated focused ultrasound imaging:** Permits high-speed 3D imaging of dynamic structures such as cardiac valves.
- **Volumetric ultrasound (4D = live 3D):** Volumetric ultrasound technology has been underdevelopment for the last several years. These innovative ultrasounds are used to create images with more depth and detail than traditional sonograms do. They can be used to identify tumors, analyze cardiac function, and more. This type of ultrasound gets its name from the ability to produce images with more visual volume, rather than a flat appearance, closely replicating the actual appearance of organs and systems **(Fig. 6.3)**.
- **Elastography:** Elastography looks specifically at the mechanical characteristics of tissues to better identify conditions, such as fibrosis of the liver, prostate cancer, and even breast lumps **(Fig. 6.4)**.
- **CEUS:** CEUS stands for "contrast-enhanced ultrasound." It's commonly used in scans of the digestive tract and heart. CEUS technology has been proved to be very effective at tumor detection, a task that usually requires more advanced tests, such as a CT or MRI.
- **AI and advanced pattern recognition algorithms:** Automation of time-consuming tasks, quantification and picking out the ideal image slice from a 3D dataset, visual mapping and annotation of screened anatomy, voice-recognition for hands-free operation is all being performed through artificial intelligence.

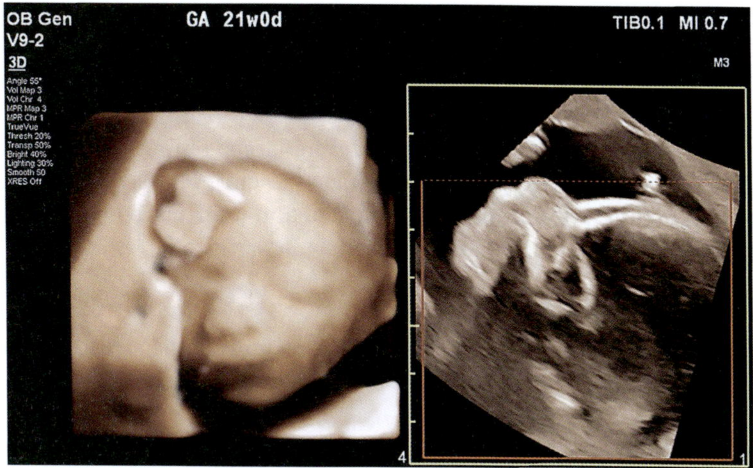

Fig. 6.3: Shows 3D view of fetal face performed by volumetric 4D probe.

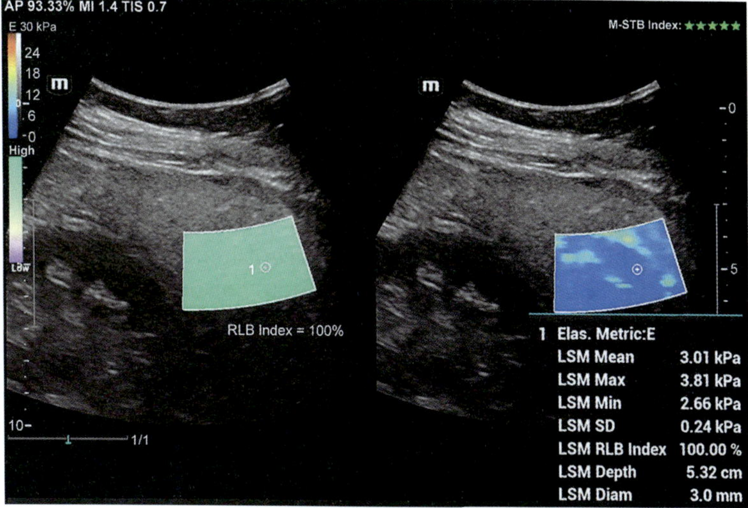

Fig. 6.4: Liver elastography.

- **Intravascular ultrasound (IVUS)**, laparoscopic ultrasound, contrast imaging and lately lung ultrasound are a few other advances in this field.
- **Ultrasound breast imaging:** This subspeciality has seen lot of modifications.

High Frequency Transducer

The transmission frequencies employed to scan breasts have increased through the years, moving from 7.5 MHz initially to 10–12 MHz and currently to 13–18 MHz. It provide increased axial and soft tissue resolution, permitting improved differentiation of subtle shades of gray, margin resolution, and lesion conspicuity in the background of normal breast parenchyma.

Extended Field-of-View Scanning

Extended FOV scans allow to display and measure large breast lesions. Additionally, it becomes possible to show the spatial relationship and the distance between a lesion and some anatomic landmarks, such as the nipple or between multiple lesions, as for multifocal/ multicentric cancer.

Automated Breast Ultrasound

ABUS allows a technologist to simultaneously acquire large volumes of tissue, from the skin to the chest wall, by using a large, specific transducer (15 cm). These volumes, consisting of a high number of thin scans, are stored to be visualized and reformatted by a doctor at another moment or another place.

Computer-assisted Diagnosis

This may allow for the simple and reproducible detection and characterization of breast lesions as well as the prediction of the response to treatment in patients with locally advanced breast cancer.

ADVANCED COMPUTED TOMOGRAPHY TECHNIQUES

The world's first computed tomography (CT) scan was performed in 1971.

CT technology has come a long way since its inception in the 1970s. This medical imaging technique uses X-rays and advanced computer algorithms to create detailed cross-sectional images of the body and has helped revolutionize diagnostics and treatment planning.

These advanced technologies continue to push the boundaries of what is possible in CT radiology, offering new opportunities for improved diagnostics, treatment planning, and patient outcomes.

The major advances in this field are:

- **Fast scanning protocols:** Techniques such as rapid acquisition and motion correction enable faster CT scans, reducing patient discomfort and improving output in busy clinical settings.
- **Reduced radiation dose:** Low-dose CT techniques and technologies, such as iterative reconstruction algorithms and automatic exposure control, have been developed to minimize radiation dose while maintaining image quality.
- **Artificial intelligence integration:** It is set to play a pivotal role in the evolution of CT technology. AI algorithms can assist radiologists in image interpretation, automating routine tasks such as organ segmentation, tumor detection and anomaly identification. This integration of AI not only improves diagnostic accuracy, but also increases efficiency, potentially reducing healthcare costs.
- **Spectral CT technology:** Spectral CT technology, also known as dual-source or dual-energy CT. It breaks down the X-Ray images at two different kV energies with a dual-source CT scanner. This technology is helpful in the automated bone removal in CT angiography, decrease metal device artifact, blood pool imaging, characterization of renal stones detection and quantification of urate crystals in Gout **(Fig. 6.5)**. It can also create contrast and non-contrast images with a single post-contrast scan.
- **Portable and point-of-care:** CT advancements in miniaturization and portable technology will likely lead to the development of compact, point-of-care CT scanners. These can be used in emergency rooms, ambulances and even remote locations, providing quick access to diagnostic imaging in critical situations.
- **Photon-counting CT:** This emerging technology uses photon-counting detectors to improve image quality, reduce noise, and potentially lower radiation dose further compared to conventional CT scanners.

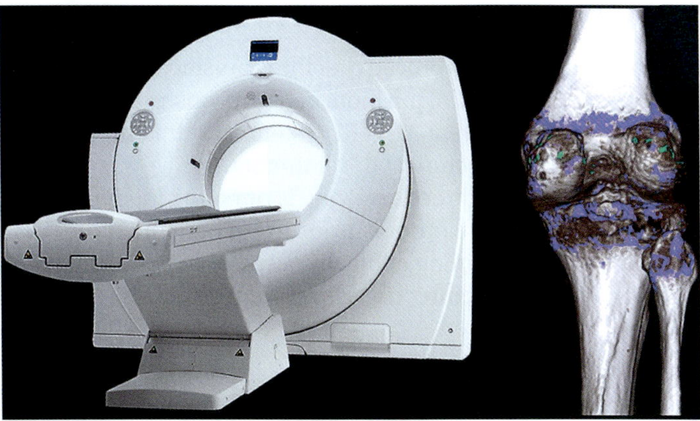

Fig. 6.5: Dual energy CT.

- **Dynamic CT imaging:** Dynamic CT imaging captures real-time changes in tissue perfusion and contrast enhancement, enabling better assessment of vascular diseases, tumors, and organ function.
- **Functional CT imaging:** Functional CT techniques, such as perfusion CT and CT angiography **(Fig. 6.6)**, provide information about tissue blood flow, oxygenation, and metabolic activity, aiding in the diagnosis and management of various diseases.
- **Cone-beam CT:** This technology is particularly useful in interventional radiology and image-guided procedures, offering real-time 3D imaging with a lower radiation dose compared to traditional CT scanners. Cone beam CT scan is also used commonly by dentists for planning dental procedures.
- **4D CT imaging:** 4D CT scans incorporate the element of time, allowing for the visualization of dynamic processes within the body, such as respiratory or cardiac motion, which is valuable for treatment planning in radiation therapy and other applications.

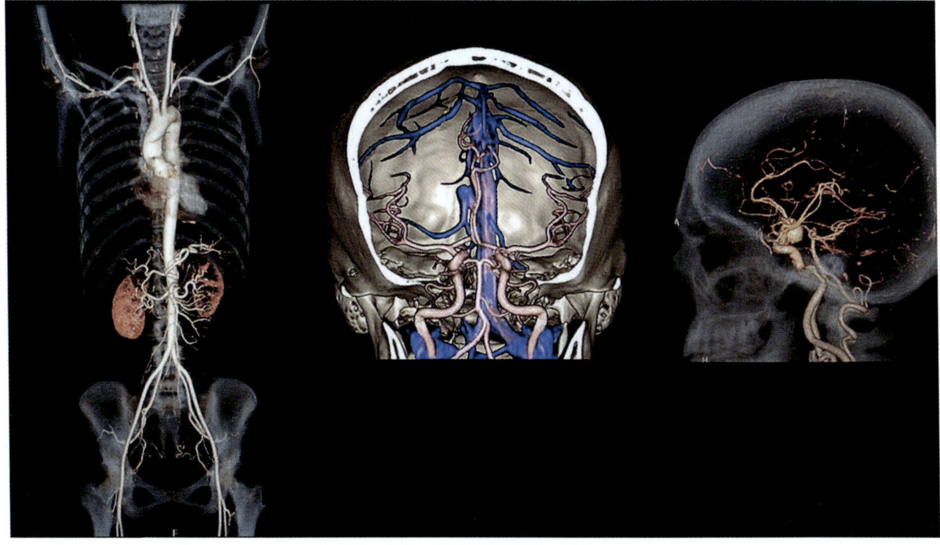

Fig. 6.6: CT angiography.

ADVANCED MAGNETIC RESONANCE IMAGING (MRI) TECHNIQUES

Clinical MRI systems have constantly improved over the years since their introduction in the 1980s. Immense development is seen in data acquisition, image reconstruction, and hardware systems.

Now, most academic centers have a 3T MRI system, and it is the main platform for both clinical practice and MR research/technical development.

3T MRI focuses on two different directions: One is pursuing higher system performance to achieve better image quality, and the other is prioritizing patient comfort, such as by using a wide bore MRI system while maintaining clinically acceptable performance.

The advancements are due to collective development in MR system, hardware, data acquisition and processing techniques.

Few of the newer applications are:

- **Dynamic contrast-enhanced MRI:** DCE-MRI helps in obtaining information about tissue perfusion and microvascular structure. It can assess tumor perfusion, microvascular vessel wall permeability and extravascular-extracellular volume fraction. It involves acquisition of serial images through the brain before, during, and after the injection of Gd-DTPA to evaluate the signal enhancement changes between intravascular and interstitial compartments. DCE-MRI primarily is used in oncology and to study response to chemotherapeutic agents **(Fig. 6.7)**.
- **Microstructural imaging by using DWI and diffusion tractography:**
  - Diffusion weighted imaging is based on the measurement of Brownian motion of water molecules.
  - *Diffusion tensor imaging (DTI):* It is an MRI technique that uses anisotropic diffusion to estimate the axonal (white matter) organization of the brain.
  - *Fiber tractography (FT):* It is a 3D reconstruction technique to assess neural tracts using data collected by diffusion tensor imaging.
  - Tractography is used in the assessment of the deformation of white matter by the tumors for presurgical planning, delineation of the anatomy of immature brains, neurogenerative disorders and in a few psychiatric conditions.

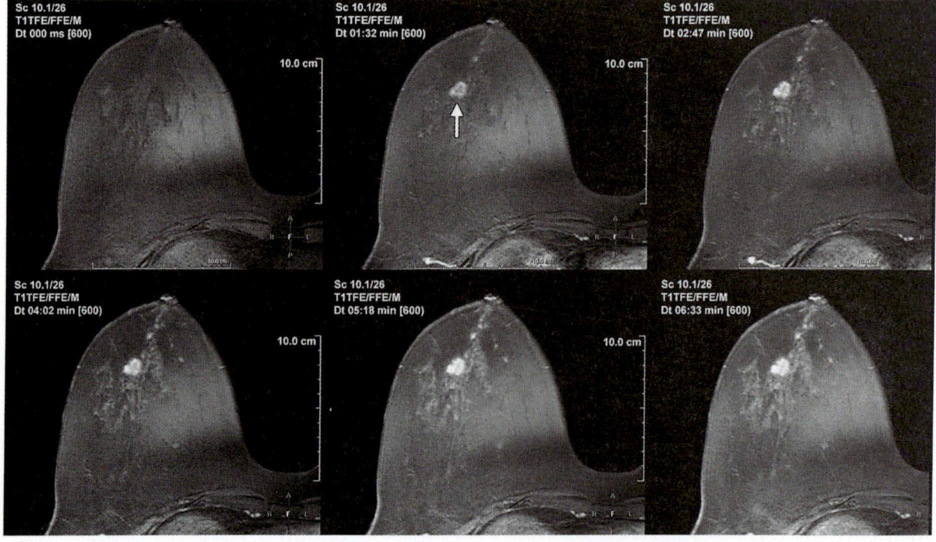

Fig. 6.7: Dynamic subtraction contrast enhanced MRI for small breast lesion.

- **Functional imaging using BOLD-MRI and perfusion weighted imaging:** Blood oxygenation-dependent imaging (BOLD) is a technique used to produce functional MRI (fMRI) images. fMRI is a technique used to obtain functional information by visualizing cortical activity. It detects subtle alteration in blood flow in response to stimuli or actions. It is used in presurgical patients aimed at localizing eloquent cortex.
- **Biochemical imaging using MR spectroscopy:** It provides metabolic information through electromagnetic signals in the radiofrequency range generated by atomic nuclei in molecules.
  - MRS can potentially differentiate primary brain tumors from other potential mimics, such as demyelinating disease, lymphoma, or infection. It helps to predict grades of glioma. As the grade increases, NAA and creatine decrease while choline, lipids and lactate increase.
  - MRS can also provide insight into whether treated tissue consists predominantly of radiation necrosis or tumor.
- **Multi-contrast MRI images from a single acquisition:** This technique gives users the flexibility to manipulate MR images retrospectively, leading to significant timesaving, fewer rescans and therefore cost savings.
- **Non-contrast vascular imaging and cardiac MRI**:
  - Non-contrast MRA is done without the contrast agent. It doesn't require infusion paraphernalia, renal function testing and venous cannulation.
  - Cardiac MRI plays an important role in the evaluation of cardiovascular diseases (CVDs), including ischemic heart disease, cardiomyopathy, valvular disease, congenital disease, pericardial disease, and masses.
  - Flow imaging enables accurate quantification of flow and velocities through valves, shunts, and surgical conduits.
  - Late gadolinium enhancement and parametric mapping techniques enable tissue characterization and yield prognostic information in ischemic heart disease.
- **Simplifying MRI-conditional implant scans:** MR-conditional implants include knee and hip replacements, spine implants, pacemakers and implantable cardioverter defibrillators (ICDs). More of these devices are becoming MR-conditional, which permits MRI scanning within certain parameter.
- **Evaluation of liver fibrosis using texture analysis on combined-contrast-enhanced magnetic resonance images at 3.0T.**
- **7T MRI system:** The added field strength allows for better visualization of smaller structures and subtle pathologies that may improve disease diagnosis.
- **The MR-guided focused ultrasound (MRgFUS) system:** Introduced for uterine fibroids treatment and then its application for essential tremor treatment was developed. MRI is used for the treatment planning and temperature monitoring in the MRgFUS intervention.

ADVANCED NUCLEAR MEDICINE AND MOLECULAR IMAGING

Nuclear medicine provides diagnostic, prognostic, predictive and intermediate endpoint biomarkers in oncology, cardiology, neurology and infectious and inflammatory disorders.

Current clinical applications of nuclear medicine include the ability to:

- Diagnose diseases such as cancer, neurological disorders (e.g., Alzheimer's and Parkinson's diseases), and cardiovascular disease in their initial stages, permitting earlier initiation of treatment as well as reduced morbidity and mortality.
- Non-invasively assess therapeutic response, reducing patient's exposure to the toxicity of ineffective treatments and allowing alternative treatments to be started earlier.

- Provide molecularly targeted treatment of cancer and certain endocrine disorders (e.g., thyroid disease and neuroendocrine tumors).

With the introduction of PET, and later hybrid imaging including SPECT/CT, PET/CT, and PET/MRI, nuclear medicine instrumentation has progressed over the last 2 decades. The more recent clinical translation of theranostics beyond thyroid treatment has triggered a dramatic transformation in nuclear medicine.

- **Positron emission tomography-computed tomography (PET-CT)**: It is an advanced medical imaging technique that combines the functional information from PET with the anatomical information from CT. PET-CT scans provide comprehensive images that can help diagnose, stage and monitor various diseases, including cancer, infections, neurological disorders and cardiovascular conditions.

  Advances in PET-CT scanners have led to improvements in image resolution, reducing image noise and enhancing overall image quality. This allows for better visualization of small lesions and improved accuracy in disease detection and staging.
- **Digital PET detectors:** Traditional PET detectors use analog photomultiplier tubes (PMTs) to detect gamma ray photons. Digital PET detectors, on the other hand, utilize semiconductor-based detectors, such as silicon photomultipliers (SiPMs) or avalanche photodiodes (APDs). Digital detectors offer higher sensitivity, improved energy resolution and faster timing characteristics compared to analog detectors, resulting in superior image quality and reduced scan times.
- **Total-body PET-CT**: Total-body PET-CT scanners are being developed to acquire PET and CT images of the entire body in a single scan session. These systems enable comprehensive assessment of disease burden, metastatic spread, and treatment response throughout the body, offering potential advantages in oncology, particularly for staging and monitoring advanced cancers **(Fig. 6.8)**.
- **Artificial intelligence (AI) applications:** AI algorithms are increasingly being integrated into PET-CT imaging workflows for tasks such as image reconstruction, noise reduction, lesion detection, and quantitative analysis. AI-driven approaches have the potential to improve diagnostic accuracy, streamline image interpretation and personalize treatment planning in various clinical settings.

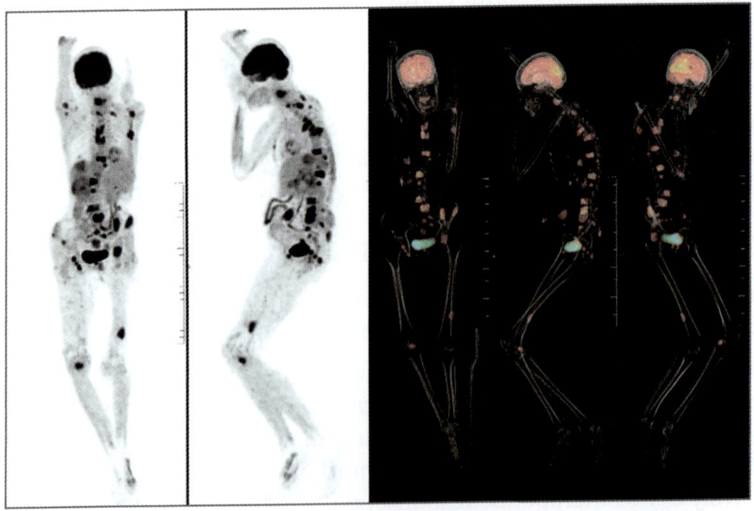

Fig. 6.8: Whole body PET-CT.

- **Theranostic imaging:** Theranostics involves the use of radioactive tracers for both diagnostic imaging and targeted therapy. PET-CT plays a crucial role in theranostic applications by enabling the visualization of disease-specific biomarkers and the assessment of treatment response. Advancements in theranostic agents and imaging protocols hold promise for personalized medicine approaches in oncology and other fields.
- **Hybrid imaging:** Similar to PET-CT, SPECT can also be combined with computed tomography (CT) to provide both functional and anatomical information in a single imaging session. This hybrid approach, known as SPECT-CT, enhances the diagnostic accuracy by correlating functional abnormalities detected on SPECT with the corresponding anatomical structures visualized on CT.

  SPECT is widely used in various medical specialties, including cardiology, neurology, oncology, and psychiatry. In cardiology, it is used for the evaluation of coronary artery disease, myocardial viability, and assessment of cardiac function. In neurology, it aids in the diagnosis of conditions such as stroke, epilepsy, and movement disorders. SPECT can help detect and stage tumors, assess treatment response, and monitor disease progression.
- **Several newer PET (Positron Emission Tomography) molecules:** newer molecules have emerged in recent years, expanding the capabilities of molecular imaging in various clinical and research applications. These molecules often target specific biological processes, enabling more precise diagnosis, treatment monitoring, and research into disease mechanisms.
- **PET-MRI:** It is a hybrid imaging technique utilizing the functional uptake information of positron emission tomography (PET) with the anatomical and soft tissue detail of magnetic resonance imaging (MRI).

  Early systems were tested in the late 2000s with commercial availability from 2010. The availability of PET-MRI remains limited, largely due to the costs and expertise required.

PET-MRI however, offers a lower ionizing radiation dose alternative with higher detection rates in a variety of studies when compared with the widely established PET-CT. It is of particular benefit to pediatric patients with chronic inflammatory conditions or malignancy, where serial follow up examinations following therapy are required **(Fig. 6.9)**. Beside post-surgery follow up it is used in dementia, epilepsy, myocardial viability and inflammatory conditions.

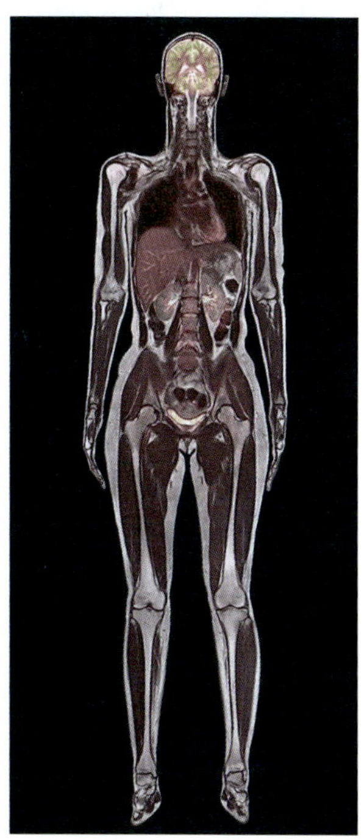

Fig. 6.9: Whole body PET MRI.

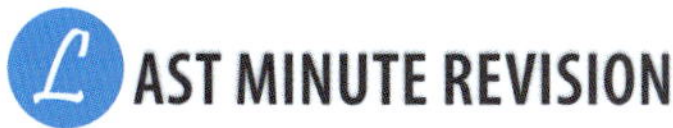

LAST MINUTE REVISION

- Advanced technology including AI are increasing day by day in all modalities.
- PET-CT and PET-MRI are hybrid type of imaging.
- DBT is three dimensional mammography.
- 4-D technology allows the scanning in live mode.
- Portable machines are available in DR as well as CT/MRI also.

REVIEW QUESTIONS

Multiple Choice Questions (MCQs)

1. **Tomosynthesis is used for:**
   a. Lung nodule
   b. Carcinoma cervix
   c. Breast mass
   d. Head injury
2. **Elastography can be used in:**
   a. Liver fibrosis
   b. Adrenal adenoma
   c. Intestinal TB
   d. Trauma
3. **Cone beam CT technology is used in:**
   a. Dental procedures
   b. Per-operative
   c. Bone fractures
   d. Mediastinal nodes
4. **Diffusion tractography is an advancement used in:**
   a. Identifying eloquent cortex
   b. White matter fiber tracts
   c. Assessment of metabolites
   d Vascular imaging
5. **DOTA is used in:**
   a. Contrast agent in CT scan
   b. Contrast agent in USG
   c. Molecular imaging in PET scan
   d. Contrast agent in MRI

Answer Key

1. c 2. a 3. a 4. b 5. c

SUGGESTED READING

1. Bolton TAW, Jochaut D, Giraud AL, Van De Ville D. Dynamic inter-subject functional connectivity reveals moment-to-moment brain network configurations driven by continuous or communication paradigms. J Vis Exp. 2019 Mar 21.
2. Krugh M, Langaker MD. Dual-energy X-Ray absorptiometry. [Updated 2023 Jun 5]. In: StatPearls [Internet]. Treasure Island (FL): StatPearls Publishing; 2024 Jan. Available from:
3. Smith H, Chieng R, Mellam Y, et al. Single photon emission computed tomography (SPECT). Reference article, Radiopaedia.org (Accessed on 27 Apr 2024).
4. So A, Nicolaou S. Spectral computed tomography: fundamental principles and recent developments. Korean J Radiol. 2021 Jan;22(1):86-96.

CHAPTER

7 Interventional Radiology

"Interventional radiology—where precision meets purpose, and every puncture paves the path to healing."

INTRODUCTION

Interventional radiology is subspecialty of radiology that uses imaging techniques like USG, CT, fluoroscopy/DSA to guide minimally invasive procedures, to either diagnose or treat various conditions without the need for or in addition to traditional surgery. Benefits of interventional radiological procedures include lesser procedural risk, faster recovery and better outcomes in many cases compared to surgical options. Spectrum of interventional radiology ranges from vascular and nonvascular interventions from head to toe, pain management, oncology, etc. In this chapter we provide a brief summary of some common interventional radiological procedures with emphasis on preparations/planning aspect of the same.

PREREQUISITES TO ANY INTERVENTIONAL RADIOLOGICAL PROCEDURE (TABLE 7.1)

Detailed evaluation of the patient including indications, excluding any contraindications is needed. It is generally advisable to prepare a preprocedure checklist that includes and is not

Table 7.1: Preprocedure checklist.

Preprocedure checklist
• Patient identification with correct site and side confirmation • Written informed consent • Relevant past medical history/comorbidity • History of allergy • Review of imaging • Review of medications • Laboratory parameters and coagulation profile • Need for intravenous fluids/blood products • Nil per oral (preoperative fasting) status • Prophylactic antibiotics • Sedation/anesthesia plan • Radiation safety • Pregnancy status (in females of reproductive age group) • Equipment for physiologic monitoring • Requirement of any special equipment • Specimen to be collected • Any anticipated adverse effect and safety equipment in place

limited to take a written informed consent, past medical history any drug and contrast allergies, laboratory parameters, current and past drug history especially history of antiplatelets and anticoagulants usage, nil per oral status, pregnancy status, and relevant hardware for the procedure.

Regarding coagulation parameter optimization, interventional radiological procedures are classified into low and high bleeding risk. For low-risk procedures like thoracocentesis, diagnostic biopsies of breast and thyroid lesions, if the patient has no known risk factors for bleeding; coagulation tests may be skipped and any antiplatelets may be continued. There is no INR cutoffs for low-risk procedures although a platelet count of at least 20 k is recommended. For procedures with higher risk of bleeding an INR cutoff of <1.5 and platelet cutoff of at least 50 k is recommended. For elective procedures with high-risk for bleeding, discontinuation of antiplatelets for 5 days is recommended.

Regarding vascular interventions in patients with renal disease decision making is based on eGFR (estimated glomerular filtration rate) values which can be determined by using patients' creatinine, age and sex. Patients with eGFR more than 45 are estimated to be at low-risk. Patients with eGFR between 30 and 45 are at intermediate risk and those with <30 are higher risk and may be started on fluid prophylaxis if no contraindications like cardiac failure. Renal replacement therapy should not be initiated or altered solely due to contrast use. When feasible in below diaphragmatic interventions alternate contrast media like CO_2 may be considered to reduce contrast dose.

MATERIALS

Materials required for interventional procedures vary widely based on both the type of procedure and operator preference/comfort and sometimes based on availability. A short summary of commonly used hardware for general use is provided. This list is neither exhaustive or complete and only provides an overall idea to orient the reader.

Contrast

Apart from iodinated contrast media commonly used in diagnostic radiology, other contrast like lipoidal, CO_2, tantalum powder, etc., are sometimes used. Lipoidal is used for lymphangiography, as a carrier for chemotherapy drugs and embolic agents like glue. CO_2 is used in patients with renal disease for below diaphragmatic vascular interventions, mainly lower limb arterial angioplasties.

Fine Needle Aspiration Cytology (FNAC)

It is usually done using a 22G or lower, spinal or Chiba needle. Core biopsies are usually done with Tru-cut needles of 20G or larger with either an automated or semiautomatic mechanism. Coaxial biopsy cannula can be used to take multiple samples and embolize biopsy tract to reduce risk of bleed.

Percutaneous Drainage

It is done using either using needles or catheters. Drainage catheters can be inserted using either trocar technique or Seldinger technique. Seldinger technique needs a needle, guidewire, tract dilator and drainage catheter.

Vascular Interventions

Needs the basic hardware consists of a vascular sheath, guidewire and diagnostic catheters. Vascular sheaths are used to secure vascular access and allow multiple exchanges or guidewires and catheters without causing blood extravasation or excess vascular injury at insertion site. They are generally sized according to the largest caliber catheter or device to be used.

Catheters: Most catheters for diagnostic angiograms are either 4 or 5F in diameter. Guide catheters are usually 6F or larger and allow check angiograms to be done and device passage within it. These diagnostic catheters come in various tip shapes for specific purposes like Simmons catheter, Cobra catheter, etc. Microcatheters are small size catheters, generally <3F that are intended to be passed coaxially within diagnostic or guide catheters for distal access into smaller vessels. Balloon catheters are used to provide luminal occlusion (compliant balloons) or angioplasty (semi and noncompliant balloons). Another type of commonly used catheters is side hole pigtail catheters for high volume angiograms like aortograms and side hole infusion catheters for catheter directed thrombolysis.

Embolic agents: Embolic materials are classified as either temporary agents like gel foam and autologous blood clot or permanent agents. Permanent agents can be either mechanical agents like coils or plugs, particulates like PVA or embospheres and liquid embolic agents like glue, onyx or sclerosants.

Stents: Are either bare metal, drug coated or covered? Bare metal stents are used to maintain vessel patency or in some cases to assist embolic material retention like intracranial stent assisted coil embolization. Drug coated stents reduce the thrombogenicity and intimal hyperplasia within the stent and are generally used for coronary vessels. Covered stents or stent grafts are intended to maintain vessel patency and treat bleeds.

With increasing use of MR imaging, most of the stents and coils are MRI safe. MR compatible biopsy guns are also available.

An interventional radiologist also needs to be familiar with commonly used drugs like local anesthetics, sedatives, antibiotics, vasodilators, anticoagulants, antiplatelets and thrombolytics. Heparin is the most commonly used anticoagulant for intravascular procedures and is generally administered as 2,500 U (40–50 U/Kg body wt) bolus followed by 1,000 U every hour and monitored using intraprocedural ACT (activated clotting time) measurement. Protamine sulfate is heparin antidote and is used to reverse the action of heparin. Most commonly used antiplatelets are aspirin, clopidogrel, ticagrelor and prasugrel. Intravenous antiplatelet like abciximab and tirofiban are also used.

All interventional radiologists are well aware of basic imaging, i.e., noninvasive imaging. Familiarity and understanding of noninvasive imaging modalities like CT, MR and USG forms a cornerstone of interventional radiological practice and provides an edge to a radiologist as compared to practitioners from other broad specialties. The ability to read source images of cross-sectional angiograms, using multiple imaging modalities in combination and techniques like in plane and out of plane USG guidance for procedures are needed to provide best outcomes. It is always prudent to evaluate the diagnostic imaging studies and perform any needed USG/ Doppler studies yourselves.

CLASSIFICATION OF INTERVENTIONAL PROCEDURES

Nonvascular Interventions

Amongst a large number of nonvascular interventions, here we will discuss a few common interventions in brief.

Percutaneous Aspiration and Drainage

It is the main line treatment for deep seated collections and abscesses. Either a single time drainage or more commonly a catheter placement for continuous drainage is done.

This catheter placement can be achieved either using Seldinger technique or trocar technique. In trocar technique a catheter with a sharp trocar within is directly guided into large and more easily accessible collections and trocar removed once tip is in collection to permit drainage. In Seldinger technique a needle (generally 18G) is placed in the collection under guidance, followed by passage of guidewire (generally a 0.035 inch), serial dilatation of tract over guidewire and finally placement of catheter. This is generally preferred in smaller and difficult to access collections and is generally more safer.

Postprocedure catheter care is needed to prevent secondary infections and displacement. Catheter needs to be flushed every 8–12 hours and is generally removed once collection subsides and output falls to below 10 mL/day.

Percutaneous Fine Needle Aspiration and Biopsy

This is done for sampling of solid lesions to aid in establishing diagnosis. FNA is generally done with a 22G or smaller needle, which is placed in a lesion of interest under imaging guidance, followed by aspiration of small amount of material, which is transferred onto a slide, fixed/air dried and sent to pathologist for analysis.

Percutaneous biopsy is generally done with a 20G or larger trocar system. It is preferable to use a coaxial system **(Fig. 7.1)** when multiple samples are needed in an intrapleural or intraperitoneal lesion. To prevent pneumothorax in lung lesion biopsy it is preferable to have single pleural puncture, avoid crossing fissures and emphysematous lung.

Percutaneous Biliary Drainage and Nephrostomy

In case of obstruction of biliary tree or urinary collecting system there can be proximal dilatation. Many of these obstructions can be crossed and recanalized through natural pathways like endoscopic ERCP and per urethral. In cases where these accesses fail, an interventional radiologist might be called upon for percutaneous access to decompress the system and if needed cross the stenosis and stent it.

Percutaneous access to both these systems is obtained under ultrasound guidance followed by further navigation under fluoroscopy. Safest access to these systems is obtained using commercially available micro puncture sets followed by serial dilatation of tract over guidewire and placement of drain. This access can be used for brush biopsy/sampling of stenotic site, balloon dilatation of stenosis, metallic or retrievable plastic stent across the lesion as appropriate.

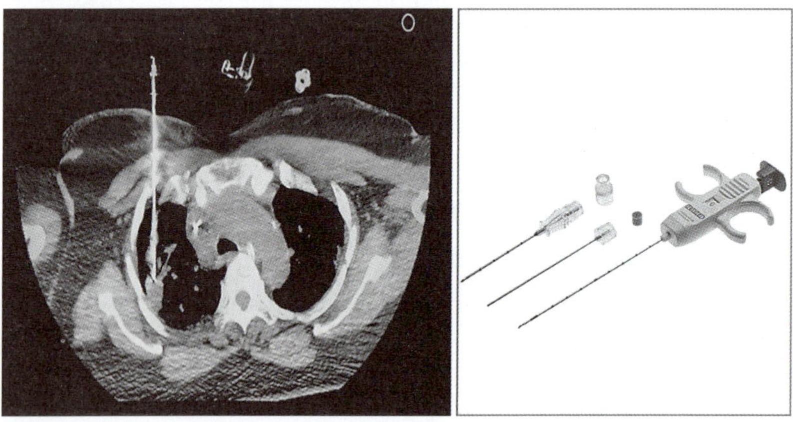

Fig. 7.1: CT guided biopsy of right lung nodule. The second image depicts the trucut biopsy gun with coaxial cannulas which permit multiple samplings.

Procedures for Pain Management

Multiple procedures for pain management can be done under image guidance including coeliac axis block for pancreatitis and upper GI malignancies, steroid/PRP/alcohol injections in many musculoskeletal pains, etc.

Other Procedures

Multiple other less common albeit important procedures like vertebroplasty for painful vertebral collapse **(Figs. 7.2A to E)**, RF/Microwave ablation for tumors and osteoid osteoma, feeding gastrostomy/jejunostomy, etc., are also available in an interventional radiologists arsenal.

Vascular Interventions (Figs. 7.3 and 7.4)

The spectrum of vascular interventions are large enough to fill up this entire book and still have something that might not be covered. Here we discuss a few common interventions in brief.

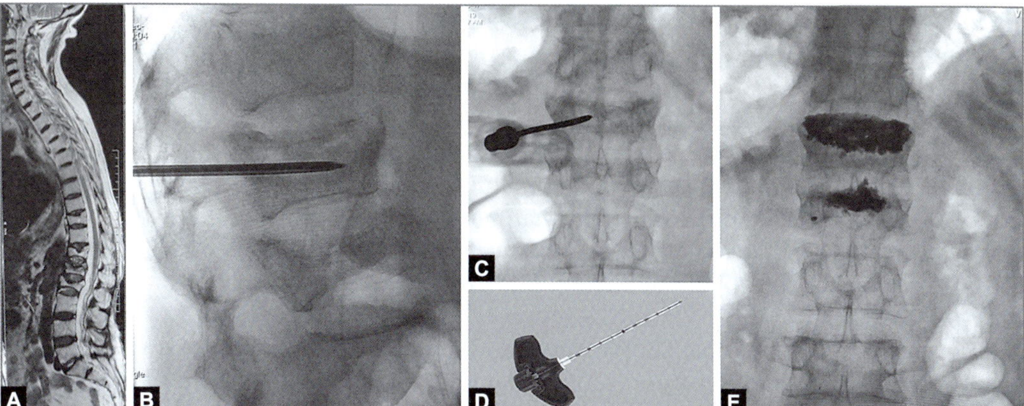

Figs. 7.2A to E: T2W Sagittal image showing partial collapse of L1 and L2. (A) Bone biopsy needle placed through transpedicular approach to anterior third of the vertebral body (B and C). needle shown in Fig. D and postvertebroplasty bone cement seen within the collapsed vertebral bodies (E).

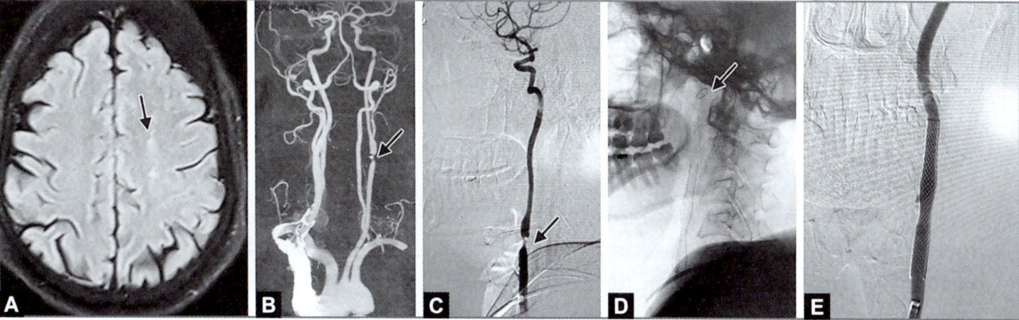

Figs. 7.3A to E: FLAIR MRI image showing watershed territory infarct (black arrow in Fig A) CT angiogram; (B) and left carotid DSA (C) showing focal more than 90% stenosis at left carotid bulb (black arrow in Fig. B and C). embolic protection device seen in Fig D (black arrow) with carotid stent and post stenting angiogram showing resolution of stenosis (E).

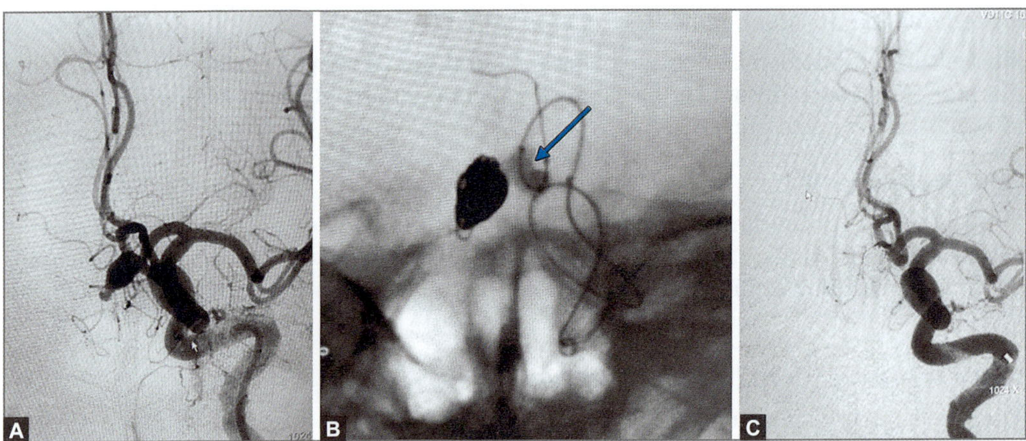

Figs. 7.4A to C: Acom Aneurysm (A) coiled with balloon assistance (blue arrow in B) and postcoiling angiogram (C) showing no filling of the aneurysm.

Diagnostic Angiography and Venography

Any vascular intervention begins with mapping of vessels by an angiogram/venogram. These images can be further supplemented by additional studies like cone beam 3D rotational angiograms, pressure studies, etc., when appropriate.

The first step in any such procedure begins with vascular access which is done using Seldinger technique. Initial vascular puncture (most commonly femoral artery/vein or radial artery) is done in retrograde or antegrade manner as appropriate using 18G needle followed by guidewire placement, tract dilatation and vascular sheath placement to secure the access. This can also be done with micropuncture sets that use a 21G needle in smaller vessels and high-risk scenarios.

Using multiple different shapes of catheters and guidewires the vessel of interest is accessed and contrast injected under fluoroscopy to obtain diagnostic images and guide further procedures.

Neurovascular Interventions

- **Stroke:** Mechanical thrombectomy is the standard of care in patients with ischemic stroke due to large vessel occlusions in window period of <6 hours. For patients presenting beyond 6 hours and <24 hours, a perfusion study can be used to delineate the penumbra that is potentially salvageable tissue to guide if there is potential benefit of intervention.
- **Carotid stenting:** In patients with either a TIA or stroke with >70% carotid stenosis or an asymptomatic patient with >90% stenosis benefit from carotid revascularization.
- **Aneurysms:** Endovascular treatment of intracranial aneurysms is generally achieved by packing the sac of aneurysm with detachable coils.
- **Arteriovenous malformations:** Intracranial arteriovenous malformations (AVM) are developmental lesions that are many times benign and incidentally detected. They have propensity to rupture and cause intracranial bleed. Unruptured AVM are generally managed symptomatically, however ruptured AVM needs treatment - generally achieved using endovascular embolization/open surgery/stereotactic radiotherapy, either individually or in combination. Liquid embolic agents like glue and EVOH copolymer (like onyx) are generally preferred embolic agents in these scenarios.

Gastrointestinal Vascular Interventions

- **Bleed embolization:** Most common sources of GI bleed requiring endovascular embolization are related to pancreatitis or due to vascular malformations. A preprocedure CT angiogram is generally needed to guide intervention as yield of diagnostic DSA is generally lower. Once source or probable site of bleed is established on CT angiogram, the relevant vessel is selectively and super selectively catheterized with microcatheters and embolized with various embolic agents as appropriate.
- **Portal hypertension and TIPSS:** The indications to intervene in portal hypertension is most commonly due to upper GI bleed that doesn't respond to endoscopic management. Multiple interventions are available in these scenarios, most commonly include BRTO (Balloon-occluded retrograde transvenous obliteration) and TIPSS (Transjugular intrahepatic portosystemic shunt).

BRTO is used to treat gastric varices by accessing the gastrorenal shunt via left renal vein, occluding outflow with a compliant balloon and sclerosing gastric varices with sclerosant-lipoidal emulsion.

TIPSS is used to reduce portal hypertension by creating a tract between hepatic vein and portal branch and securing the tract with a covered stent. Main indications for TIPSS are resistant variceal bleed and ascites requiring recurrent paracentesis.

Interventions in Liver tumor

- **Chemoembolization of liver tumor:** Main indications for chemoembolization are for early nonresectable HCC as bridge to transplant and for palliation in liver limited metastasis in GI malignancies like adenocarcinoma.
- **Portal embolization:** In cases where liver resection is planned but having insufficient functional liver residue, portal vein embolization can be done of resecting lobe to induce hypertrophy of residual lobe.

Aortic Aneurysms and Dissections

Stanford type B aortic dissections, thoracoabdominal aneurysms can be managed endovascularly using aortic stent grafts.

Renovascular Interventions

- **Renal artery stenting:** Renal angioplasty and stent placement is mainly indicated for resistant hypertension or recurrent flash pulmonary edema related to renal stenosis.
- **Renal embolization:** Renal embolization is generally done for management of post biopsy and post PCNL renal bleed. Other indications include large AML with or without bleed and preoperative embolization.

Visceral and Extremity Vascular and Lymphatic Malformations

Symptomatic high flow visceral and extremity malformations can be embolized endovascularly generally with liquid embolic agents.

Slow flow malformations and lymphatic malformations respond to either endovascular or percutaneous sclerotherapy with various agents like polidocanol, STS, bleomycin, etc.

- **Lymphangiography and thoracic duct embolization:** In patients with chylothorax or chylous ascites that don't respond to conservative management with fat free diet can be managed by lymphangiography and embolization. This is done with initial percutaneous access of inguinal lymph nodes and injecting lipoidal. Slow leaks generally stop by lymphangiography alone. High flow leaks generally need embolization.

- **Peripheral angioplasty:** Patients with peripheral arterial disease with critical limb ischemia or claudication not responding to conservative care generally benefit from percutaneous angioplasty and stenting when required. Long segment below knee vascular disease generally require longer balloons for angioplasty and stenting is avoided.
- **DVT and pulmonary embolism:** Patients with DVT that don't respond to heparin or those with contraindication to anticoagulation or with phlegmasia cerulea dolens can be managed by multiple endovascular means like catheter directed thrombolysis, pharmacomechanical thrombectomy devices and mechanical aspiration thrombectomy.

In patients with DVT with contraindication/resistance to anticoagulation an IVF filter can be placed to prevent pulmonary embolism.

In those that already have pulmonary embolism with cardiorespiratory failure pulmonary thrombectomy can be attempted to rapidly debulk the clot and revascularize the pulmonary circulation.

Dialysis Access Management

- **Tunneled dialysis catheters:** Tunneled dialysis catheters/Permcaths are used for long term dialysis in patients awaiting fistula maturation or in those with fistula failure. Compared to nontunneled catheters/central lines these catheters are more stable and less likely to get infected.
- **Dialysis fistula and central vein angioplasty:** Dialysis AV fistula are regarded as safest and best means for dialysis access. Due to hyperdynamic circulation/turbulence and repeated access they tend to dysfunction. These fistulas can be salvaged by angioplasty, embolization of collaterals, etc.

Varicocele Embolization and Pelvic Congestion Syndrome

In male patients with varicocele with hypofertility/pain and females with pelvic congestion syndrome, endovascular embolization of varices with coils and sclerosant offers a less invasive means of treatment compared to surgical ligation.

Uterine Artery Embolization

Patients with fibroids, postpartum bleed and uterine AVM that don't respond to conservative management, embolization of uterine arteries usually bilaterally can be done to help in hemostasis. For postpartum bleed temporary embolic agents like gel foam is preferred but for fibroid permanent agents like PVA particle of size around 500 μm is preferred to avoid embolizing ovaries via uterine ovarian anastomosis.

Varicose Vein

Symptomatic varicose veins can be ablated percutaneously with multiple techniques, most popular of which are using laser or RF ablation. For this a calf GSV is cannulated, and ablation catheter is placed within vein with tip around 2 cm from GSV, perivascular tumescence is administered to protect surrounding structures and compress the lumen, followed by retrograde ablation till access site.

RISK MANAGEMENT

The cornerstone of risk management in every interventional radiological procedure is obtaining an informed consent from the patient and/or the family. The task of obtaining consent should not be viewed as clerical or mechanical in nature but as an opportunity to educate the patient regarding the procedure, its expected benefits, and risks. It is preferable to obtain the procedural consent at least a few hours or a day prior to an elective procedure to allow the patient and family to process the information. It is always healthy to provide enough time and make the process of consent taking an interactive session where the queries of the patient are addressed rather than one sided lecture by the doctor. It is neither practical or necessary to explain every possible remote complication from the procedure but the common ones need to be explained. Informed consent needs to be taken in a language understood by the patient and preferably along with audio-visual recording.

Universal protocol for any interventional radiological procedure needs to be followed. It is a three-step process, includes multiple strategies to prevent wrong site, wrong procedure, and wrong patient errors:

1. Preprocedure verification.
2. Site marking.
3. Time-out.

Radiation safety principles need to be followed to protect both the operator and any assistants in the procedure room. This is mostly important for any fluoroscopy guided procedures. Basic principles of fluoroscopic radiation protection can be summarized by the acronym: TIDS—Time, Intensity, Distance, Shielding.

- **Time:** Limit the amount of fluoroscopy time. Use last image hold images or stored fluoroscopy loops instead of acquisitions when possible.
- **Intensity:** Use pulse fluro and minimum required MAs.
- **Distance:** Radiation dose reduces inversely with square of distance from source.
- **Shielding:** Use appropriate personal protective equipment. Regular maintenance of fluoroscopy equipment and protective gear also help. The biological effects of radiation need to be understood but detailed explanations are beyond the scope of this chapter and will be covered elsewhere in this book.

Need for infection control and asepsis in interventional radiological procedures cannot be over emphasized. Even though most of the procedures are minimally invasive and carry a lower risk of infection than most open surgical procedures, any breach in asepsis can lead to disastrous consequences in an otherwise technically successful procedure. Infection prevention starts from maintenance of IR suite to patient preparation to procedure technique and ends with optimal post procedure care. Both the primary operator and all staff need to be familiar with general surgical aseptic precautions.

Medical records for any admission need to be retained for at least 3 years as per NMC norms. As the field is rapidly expanding and new guidelines come out every few years it is imperative for a practitioner to stay abreast of current literature.

INTERVENTIONAL RADIOLOGY-INDIAN SCENARIO

Though interventional radiology training is a part of MD/DNB radiology curriculum, further training is generally necessary for dedicated interventional radiological practice. Many centers in India offer fellowship and PDCC (postdoctoral certification courses) training for 1 to 2 years, DM and DrNB courses in Interventional radiology and Neurointerventional radiology for 3 years. The number of centers and institutes offering these courses in India seems to increase in the past few years that will help bring increase the penetration of the field to many tier 2 and tier 3 cities and many of these places already have the required imaging modalities like USG, CT and even Cath labs and await a trained Interventional radiologist to set up his or her practice.

CONCLUSION

Interventional radiology remains a vibrant subspecialization which continues to evolve with ever expanding applications and innovative techniques limited only by imagination of the operator and current available technology. The field provides an opportunity to step away from the predominantly backstage role of a diagnostic radiologist into limelight as a clinician along with associated stress and risks. Common differences between interventional imaging and conventional imaging are as follows in **Table 7.2.**

Table 7.2: Difference between conventional imaging and interventional imaging.

Aspect	*Conventional imaging*	*Interventional imaging*
Safety	Lower/No risk of complications	Higher risk of complications
Patient comfort	More comfortable	Less comfortable
Detail and precision	Limited detail	High detail and precision
Therapeutic capability	Diagnostic only	Diagnostic and therapeutic
Preparation and recovery	Minimal preparation and recovery	Extensive preparation and longer recovery
Radiation exposure	Possible in X-ray and CT	Depends on the procedure
Cost	Generally lower	Higher cost
Complications	Minimal	Risk of bleeding, infection, adverse reactions
Uses	Broad range: bones, organs, soft tissues	Specific: blood vessels, internal organs, biopsies
Limitations	Depth penetration, motion artifacts, cost (MRI)	Invasiveness, resource-intensive, patient selection

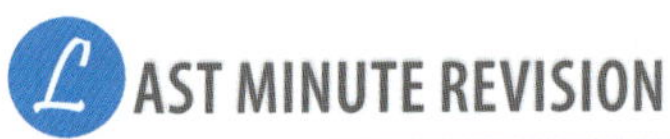

- Intenventional procedures can be done under guidance of all modalities as per demand of pathology and patient's condition.
- Major advantage of IR is it's therapeutic utility which can avoid the major open surgeries.

REVIEW QUESTIONS

Multiple Choice Questions (MCQs)

1. **For any vascular intervention which investigation is a prerequisite?**
    a. Serum creatinine
    b. Coagulation profile
    c. Serum bilirubin
    d. Both a and b
2. **Which is a correct statement for intracranial aneurysm interventions?**
    a. Web is an intraluminal device
    b. Coils are intrasaccular device
    c. Flow divertor are intrasaccular device
    d. Sceptre is a type of stent.
3. **In below knee peripheral vascular disease**
    a. Stenting can be easily done
    b. Has nothing to do with diabetes and Berger disease
    c. Long balloons are used for angioplasty
    d. Always use cutting balloons

4. **In stroke interventions which is true**
   a. Done within 3 hours of onset
   b. Stent retrievers are used in aneurysm coiling only.
   c. Aspiration of thrombus is the main goal
   d. Solumbra is combination used in aneurysm management.
5. **Indications for IVC filter include**
   a. DVT with contraindications to anticoagulation
   b. DVT progression on anticoagulation
   c. All cases of DVT
   d. Both a and b
6. **Which of these is a temporary embolic agent?**
   a. Glue
   b. PVA particles
   c. Coils
   d. Gelatin sponge/Gelfoam
7. **Which of the following is available in injectable form?**
   a. Aspirin
   b. Prasugrel
   c. Tirofiban
   d. Both a and c

Answer Key

1. d 2. b 3. c 4. c 5. d 6. d 7. d

SUGGESTED READING

1. Davenport MS. et al. (2020) `Use of intravenous iodinated contrast media in patients with kidney disease: Consensus statements from the American College of Radiology and the National Kidney Foundation', Radiology. 2020;294(3):660-68. doi:10.1148/radiol.2019192094.
2. Mukund A, Bhardwaj K, Mohan C. Basic interventional procedures: Practice essentials. Indian J. Radiol. Imaging. 2019;29(02):182-89. doi:10.4103/ijri.ijri_96_19.
3. Patel IJ. et al. Society of interventional radiology consensus guidelines for the periprocedural management of thrombotic and bleeding risk in patients undergoing percutaneous image-guided interventions --part II: Recommendations', J. Vasc. Interv. Radiol. 2019;30(8). doi:10.1016/j.jvir.2019.04.017.
4. Young S, Rostambeigi N, Golzarian J. The common but complicated tool: Review of embolic materials for the interventional radiologist, Seminars in Interventional Radiology. 2021;38(05):535-41. doi:10.1055/s-0041 -1736658.

CHAPTER

8

Career Opportunities in Radiodiagnosis

"In radiodiagnosis, every scan opens a door—not just to diagnosis, but to a world of endless possibilities."

INTRODUCTION

The allure of radiology as a postgraduate specialty has steadily grown among Indian medical graduates, becoming the zenith of preference for many who emerge victorious from the rigorous National Eligibility-cum-Entrance Test for Postgraduates (NEET-PG). This profound interest in radiodiagnosis is rooted in the promise of a multifaceted career, one that intertwines the precision of technology with the art of medicine. Radiodiagnosis stands as a testament to the dynamic nature of healthcare, offering a spectrum of opportunities that extend from the academic to the clinical realms, encapsulating the very essence of modern medicine.

The beauty of radiology is that it fits many career goals. Some radiologists open their clinics, turning their medical practice into a thriving business. Others prefer the steady work and fixed hours that come with a job in a large hospital or a big diagnostic company. This balance between independence and security makes radiology unique.

This chapter takes a closer look at these varied career opportunities. We'll explore how radiology is a field that lets doctors have a direct impact on patient care without the demanding hours of other specialties. Whether you're looking to be your boss or to work in a high-tech hospital setting, radiology offers a promising future.

In the coming sections, we'll dive into the different roles radiologists can take on, from academic research to clinical practice. We'll see how technology is changing the work they do and why radiology has become such a popular, attractive and fulfilling field for today's medical graduates.

ELIGIBILITY TO PURSUE A COURSE IN RADIODIAGNOSIS

Aspiring radiologists in India have a structured pathway to follow in their quest to enter this in-demand specialty. The nation presents a trio of postgraduate educational courses: a two-year Diploma in Medical Radio-Diagnosis (DMRD), alongside the more intensive three-year Doctor of Medicine (MD) and Diplomate of National Board (DNB) in Radiodiagnosis programs. Reflecting the trend observed in 2022, there are a substantial number of seats available across these streams—with 136 diploma and 4150 MD slots spread over private and public medical institutions.

To vie for these positions, medical graduates must navigate the competitive currents of the National Eligibility Cum Entrance Test for Post-Graduation (NEET-PG) or the Institute of National Importance Combined Entrance Test (INI-CET). Success in these examinations is a prerequisite to secure a coveted seat in one of the many esteemed institutes across India that offer these rigorous radiodiagnosis programs.

JOB OPPORTUNITIES IN RADIODIAGNOSIS

Radiodiagnosis professionals can explore a variety of career paths across different sectors. These opportunities can be broadly categorized into three main areas: private sector, industry, and academia.

Private Sector

Private diagnostic centers range from small clinics offering basic X-ray and ultrasound services to advanced centers equipped with sophisticated imaging technologies like CT and MRI scans, often requiring the collaboration of multiple radiologists. These settings offer radiologists the chance to work closely with patients and other healthcare professionals, providing diagnostic services that are integral to patient care. The work in private centers can be diverse, encompassing everything from routine imaging to complex interventional procedures.

Industry

The radiodiagnosis industry is vital to the healthcare sector, with companies that produce diagnostic equipment consistently seeking skilled radiologist. These professionals not only help in the development and refinement of imaging technologies but also play a key role in training, sales, and support for these products. Positions in the industry can be very rewarding, offering competitive salaries and the opportunity to be at the forefront of technological advancements in medical imaging.

Academia

Academic institutions are foundational to the training and development of new radiologists. As per the National Medical Commission (NMC) norms, each medical college is required to have a fully staffed department of radiodiagnosis to support their MBBS program. The staffing needs are based on the number of seats, with specific requirements for various academic posts as shown in **Table 8.1**.

WORK-LIFE INTEGRATION IN RADIODIAGNOSIS

Radiodiagnosis is increasingly recognized for offering a more favorable work-life balance compared to many other medical specialties. Its flexibility allows radiologists to tailor their

Table 8.1: Academic staff requirements and qualifications.

Designation	*Number required per 100 MBBS seats*	*Essential qualification*	*Minimum required experience*
Professor	1	MD/DNB in radiodiagnosis	3 Years as associate professor + 1 research publication in indexed journal
Associate professor	2	MD/DNB in radiodiagnosis	4 Years as assistant professor + 1 research publication in indexed journal
Assistant professor	3	MD/DNB in radiodiagnosis	1 year as senior resident from recognized medical college
Senior resident	3	MD/DNB in radiodiagnosis	Postgraduate in radiodiagnosis

careers according to personal needs and lifestyle choices. Many in the field take advantage of part-time work, nontraditional hours, or the growing field of teleradiology, which enables the reporting of CT and MRI scans from the comfort of one's home. This adaptability is one of the many reasons radiodiagnosis is an attractive career option for physicians seeking both professional fulfillment and personal well-being.

For those who thrive in high-pressure environments, there is the option to work in emergency radiology. This often involves working in an emergency department setting, where urgent imaging is required to make quick, sometimes critical medical decisions. The demand for these services typically means higher pay and the opportunity for those who choose it to make a significant impact in acute patient care.

Teleradiology

Teleradiology has revolutionized the practice of radiodiagnosis by allowing radiologists to interpret and report medical images from remote locations. This sub-specialty uses secure network technology to transmit image data and reports between different sites, offering a flexible work model that can significantly reduce the need for on-site radiologists, particularly after hours or in rural areas. Teleradiology not only improves service coverage but also enhances the work-life balance for radiologists, providing the freedom to work from virtually anywhere.

CHALLENGES AND CONSIDERATIONS IN RADIODIAGNOSIS

Like any branch of medicine, radiodiagnosis comes with its own set of challenges and considerations that prospective radiologists must be aware of. These challenges range from financial constraints to professional hazards, each impacting the field in unique ways.

Financially, establishing a private radiodiagnosis center requires significant investment. State-of-the-art radiological machines come with a high cost and necessitate dedicated space that adheres to the stringent guidelines set by the government. For instance, obtaining the Pre-natal Diagnostic Techniques (PNDT) certification is a time-consuming process essential for any center that conducts ultrasounds. Additionally, all radiological equipment must comply with the Atomic Energy Regulatory Board (AERB) standards to ensure safety and effectiveness. The need for compliance extends to the electrical department as well due to the high-power requirements of radiological machines.

On the professional front, radiologists face hazards related to radiation exposure despite rigorous safety protocols. The physical strain of the job is not to be underestimated either; long hours of neck flexion and continuous focus on high-resolution computer screens can lead to musculoskeletal and eye strain **(Table 8.2)**.

CONCLUSION

Radiodiagnosis stands as a cornerstone of modern medicine, offering a blend of technology and patient care that few other specialties can match. While it promises a rewarding career with ample opportunities for growth, innovation, and work-life balance through avenues like teleradiology and flexible working hours, it also presents unique challenges. These include the significant investment required to establish private practices, compliance with regulatory standards, and the physical and professional hazards associated with long hours of work and exposure to radiation. Navigating these challenges successfully requires a commitment to continuous learning, adaptability, and adherence to safety protocols, ensuring a fulfilling and sustainable career in radiodiagnosis.

Table 8.2: Detailed professional hazards and preventive measures for various radiological modalities.

Modality	*Hazards*	*Preventive measures*
CT/MRI	• Prolonged sitting leading to musculoskeletal problems • Eye strain from continuous screen viewing	• Ergonomic seating and workstations • Regular breaks and eye exercises • Use of anti-glare screens
Interventional radiology	• Radiation exposure • Repetitive stress injuries from equipment use • Long standing hours	• Lead aprons and thyroid shields • Proper hand positioning and ergonomic tools • Anti-fatigue mats and supportive footwear
Ultrasound	• Neck and shoulder strain from poor positioning • Wrist injuries from transducer manipulation • Eye strain	• Adjustable height tables and chairs • Proper technique for holding and moving the transducer • Frequent eye rest and focusing on distant objects
General radiography	• Radiation exposure • Back pain from bending and lifting patients	• Use of radiation badges and monitoring • Training in safe patient handling techniques • Ergonomic equipment
Mammography	• Repetitive motion injuries from positioning patients and equipment • Emotional stress from working with anxious patients	• Ergonomic positioning devices • Stress management techniques • Supportive patient communication training

LAST MINUTE REVISION

- Radiology is terminal and spinal branch which needs clinical sense with imaging findings for best outcome.
- Telereporting ease the task of reporting in remote areas.
- Developing the newer techniques to reduce professional hazards is main demand of this specialty (pathway for research and innovations)

REVIEW QUESTIONS

Multiple Choice Questions (MCQs)

1. Which certification is necessary for a center conducting obstetric ultrasounds in India?

a. AERB Certification
b. PNDT Certification
c. NOC from Electrical Department
d. ISO Certification

2. Which of the following is a professional hazard associated with performing ultrasound?

a. High radiation exposure
b. Neck and shoulder strain
c. Repetitive stress injuries from high-dose fluoroscopy
d. Minimal physical strain due to short procedure times

3. **Teleradiology allows radiologists to:**
   a. Operate radiological equipment remotely
   b. Interpret and report medical images from remote locations
   c. Perform remote surgeries
   d. Directly interact with patients online
4. **Which of the following is NOT a challenge associated with opening a private radiodiagnosis center?**
   a. High initial investment for radiological machines
   b. Obtaining a license to practice medicine
   c. Compliance with AERB guidelines for room sizes
   d. NOC from the electrical department due to high power requirements
5. **What advantage does a career in radiodiagnosis offer in terms of work-life balance?**
   a. Mandatory on-site presence at all times
   b. Flexible working hours and the possibility of teleradiology
   c. No need for continuous professional development
   d. High physical activity reducing the risk of sedentary lifestyle diseases

Answer Key

1. b 2. b 3. b 4. b 5. b

SUGGESTED READING

1. NMC Seats
2. AERB guidelines

UNIT 2

Core Radiological Anatomy and Specialized System Imaging

Unit Outline

CHAPTER

9

Radiological Anatomy

"Radiological anatomy is the foundation—because only when you know the map, can you read the journey of disease."

INTRODUCTION

Radiological anatomy, an integral facet of medical education and clinical practice, merges the precision of anatomical sciences with the technological advancements of radiology. This interdisciplinary approach provides healthcare professionals with an essential toolkit for accurate diagnosis and effective patient management. As we delve into this chapter, we aim to explore the fundamental principles of imaging techniques—X-rays, computed tomography (CT), magnetic resonance imaging (MRI), and ultrasound—and their pivotal role in visualizing human anatomy in health and disease.

The study of radiological anatomy is not merely about identifying structures; it's about understanding the living, dynamic human body as seen through the lenses of various imaging modalities. Each technique offers unique insights, from the dense calcified structures highlighted in X-rays to the detailed soft tissue contrasts provided by MRI. This chapter will guide you through these imaging modalities, emphasizing the correlation between anatomical details and their clinical implications.

Through a structured examination of different body systems, including the skeletal, thoracic, abdominopelvic, and neurological systems, this chapter will illustrate how radiological imaging is crucial in both routine clinical assessment and complex diagnosis.

To understand the various aspects of radiological anatomy we should have clear image of basic principle of all modalities (already discussed in Chapter 5) **(Table 9.1)**.

Table 9.1: Comparison of four primary imaging modalities.

Feature	*X-ray*	*Ultrasound (USG)*	*Computed tomography (CT)*	*Magnetic resonance imaging (MRI)*
Principle	Electromagnetic radiation passes through the body to create images based on tissue density	High-frequency sound waves reflect off tissues to create images in terms of echogenicity	X-rays rotate around the body to create detailed cross-sectional images in terms of density by Hounsfield unit	Strong magnetic fields and radio waves produce detailed images of organs and tissues in terms of intensity
Best for which structure	Bones, chest, and lungs, calcifications, air	Whole body except for bone and air	Detailed bone structures, chest, and abdomen	Soft tissues, brain, spinal cord, joints, and ligaments

Contd...

Contd...

Feature	*X-ray*	*Ultrasound (USG)*	*Computed tomography (CT)*	*Magnetic resonance imaging (MRI)*
Availability	Widely available and common in most medical facilities. Portable for bedside x-rays	Widely available, portable, and can be used at bedside	Available in most hospitals and imaging centers	Available in most hospitals and specialized imaging centers. Not as widely available as X-ray or CT
Cost	Low cost	Low to moderate cost, depending on the procedure	Higher cost than X-ray and USG, but less than MRI	Highest cost
Advantage	Quick and efficient for many diagnostic purposes	Safe, noninvasive, no radiation exposure, real-time imaging	Provides detailed images quickly, good for emergency diagnostics	Provides the most detailed images, no radiation exposure
Disadvantage	Radiation exposure, limited in evaluating soft tissues	Image quality affected by patient's body type, limited penetration depth, expertise dependent	High radiation dose compared to X-ray	Very expensive, contraindicated with certain implants, can be claustrophobic, noisy
Uses	Fractures, infections, e.g., osteomyelitis, consolidation	Pregnancy scans, abdominal organs, cardiac evaluations	Trauma assessment, cancer detection, vascular diseases	Neurological disorders, musculoskeletal conditions, detailed organ assessment

Radiological anatomy can be studied on all modalities, but for best diagnosis and management, minimum number of modality should be advised based on type of pathology and origin of pathology **(Table 9.2)**.

Table 9.2: Uses of basic modalities in different anatomical regions and systems.

Anatomical region/system	*X-ray*	*Ultrasound (USG)*	*Computed tomography (CT)*	*Magnetic resonance imaging (MRI)*
Head, face and neck	Dental, PNS, skull and skeletal imaging	Eye (B scan), Thyroid, salivary glands, neck vessels	PNS, neck mass, skeletal imaging	Soft tissue evaluation, nerve pathways, tumor staging
GIT	Erect abdomen for free air, (limited use)	Abdominal organs, free fluid assessment	Detailed intestinal imaging	Detailed soft tissue imaging (limited use)
Genitourinary	Kidney stones	Kidney, bladder, scrotum, prostate imaging	Detailed kidney and bladder imaging	Detailed imaging of pelvic organs
Hepatobiliary	Limited use	Liver, gallbladder, bile ducts	Liver and pancreas biliary tract evaluation	Detailed liver and biliary imaging
Bone	Fractures, alignment	Joint effusions, soft tissue evaluation	Detailed bone imaging, trauma	Bone marrow disorders, soft tissue detail
Brain	Limited use	Neonatal brain (through fontanelle, cranial USG)	Trauma, stroke, and anomaly detection	Detailed brain imaging, neurological disorders

Contd...

Contd...

Anatomical region/system	***X-ray***	***Ultrasound (USG)***	***Computed tomography (CT)***	***Magnetic resonance imaging (MRI)***
Spine	Alignment, fractures	Neonatal spine	Trauma, tumors	Disc disease, nerve impingement
Gynecological organs	Limited use	Uterus, ovaries, endometrial pathology	CT pelvimetry, tumors	Detailed imaging of pelvic organs, tumor staging
Breast	Mammography (special X-ray)	Breast cysts, solid masses	Limited use	Detailed breast tissue imaging
Obstetrics	Limited use	Fetal anatomy, amniotic fluid volume (best modality)	Limited use	Detailed assessment in specific indications, e.g, craniospinal anomaly
Lung and pleura	Infections, rib fractures	Pleural effusion, pediatric consolidation	Detailed lung imaging, pulmonary embolism	Cardiac and vascular imaging
Heart	Limited use	Cardiac function, valve abnormalities by echocardiography	Coronary calcium scoring, vascular imaging	Detailed cardiac structure and function

Deciding modality based on anatomical region is quite a hard decision. For early and best diagnosis, we should narrow down differentials on the basis of clinical scenario as well by knowledge of etiopathogenesis of various disease we can get best outcome by knowing the typical radiological appearance of various tissues and body structures **(Table 9.3)**.

Table 9.3: Appearance of various organs and body fluid on basic modalities.

Tissue/ anatomical structures	***X-ray***	***Ultrasound (USG)***	***CT scan***	***MRI***
Solid organs	Poorly visualized as soft density	Variable echogenicity pancreas > spleen > liver > renal cortex > renal medulla	Well visualized, varied density in terms of HU, seen in soft tissue window	Well visualized, variable signal intensity, commonly hypo on T1 and hyper on T2
Bone and calcifications	High density, well visualized	Poor visualization as hyperechoic giving acoustic shadowing	Excellent detail, high density, seen in bone window	Cortical bone hypointense on T1/ T2. Medullary bone T1 hyperintense and intermediate on T2. Calcification signal void or variable
Muscle	Soft tissue density, indistinct	Homogeneous, medium echogenicity	Isodense to slightly hyperdense	Intermediate T1, hyperintense T2
Fat	Low density, radiolucent	Variable, hyperechoic to anechoic	Negative Hounsfield units, clear contrast	High signal on T1, intermediate on T2
Fluid	Medium density (e.g., effusions)	Anechoic, no internal echoes	Water density	Low signal T1, high signal T2

Contd...

Contd...

Tissue/ anatomical structures	***X-ray***	***Ultrasound (USG)***	***CT scan***	***MRI***
Blood	Similar to fluid	Echogenic in acute, hypoechoic when chronic	High density in acute, isodense chronic	Variable in T1 and T2, depends on age. Best detection on GE sequence as signal void
Pus	Similar to fluid	Complex, variable echogenicity	Higher density than simple fluid	Variable T1, often bright on T2
Air/lung	Radiolucent, easily visualized	Poorly visualized, reverberation artifact	Radiolucent: well-visualized, seen in lung window	Signal void, no signal
Hyaline cartilage	Not visualized	Hypoechoic	Intermediate density	High T2 signal, intermediate T1
Ligament, tendon, menisci	Not visualized	Fibrous structures, echogenic	Not well visualized	Low signal on both T1 and T2
Nerves	Not visualized	Hypoechoic, surrounded by hyperechoic fat	Not well visualized	High T2 signal, intermediate T1
Vessels	Not visualized except calcified vessels	Hypoechoic; anechoic lumen shows flow (on Doppler)	Well visualized with contrast	Variable, often uses contrast enhancement

After understanding the uses of basic modality on the various anatomical regions or systems and suspected pathology, radiological anatomy becomes very easier to understand.

For example, comparison of radiological anatomy on four basic modalities in chest region is as follows **(Figs. 9.1A to F)**:

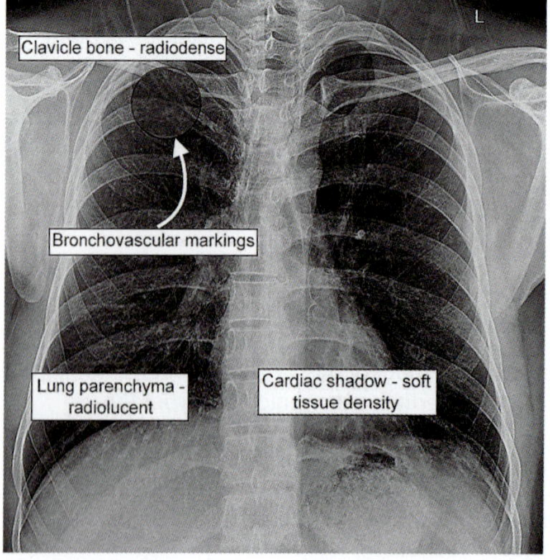

Fig. 9.1A: Chest PA view to show appearance of various anatomical structures in terms of density.

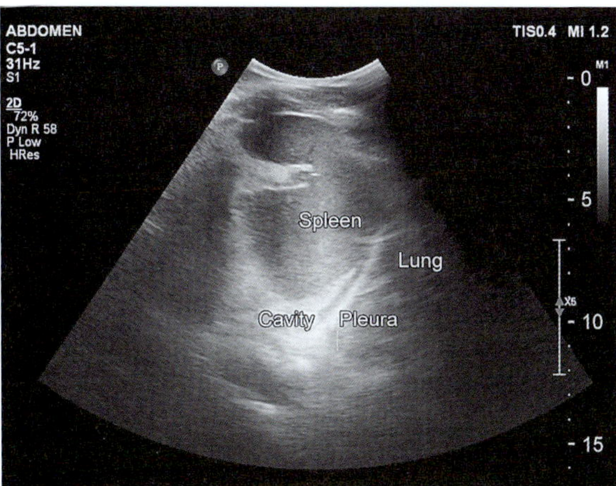

Fig. 9.1B: USG chest as viewed by convex probe.

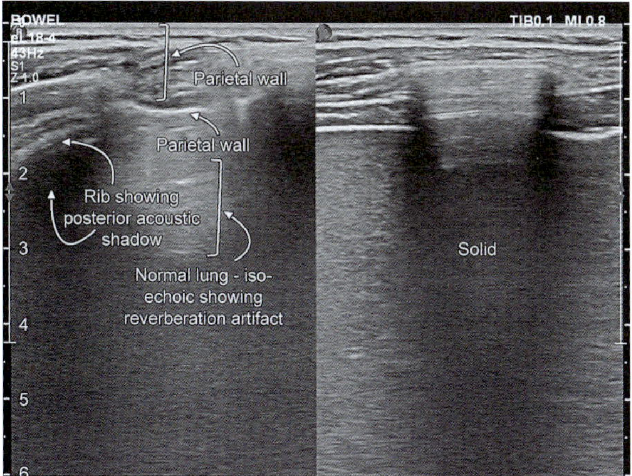

Fig. 9.1C: USG chest done by high resolution probe.

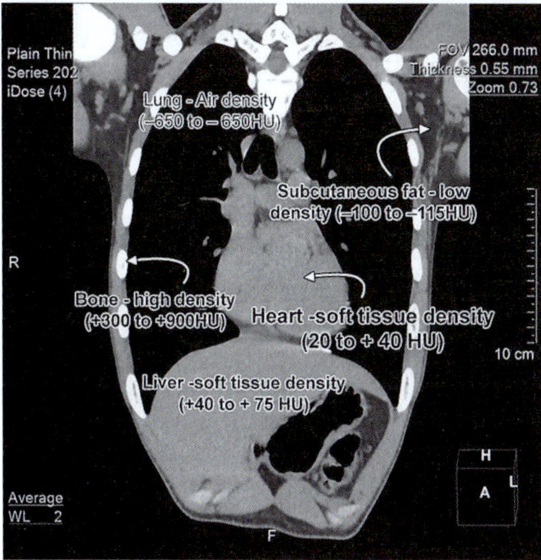

Fig. 9.1D: Coronal chest soft tissue window.

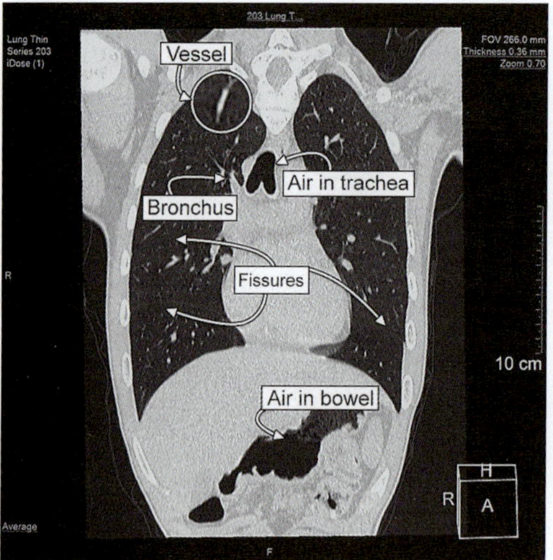

Fig. 9.1E: Lung window showing basic differences in appearance of same region on different CT window.

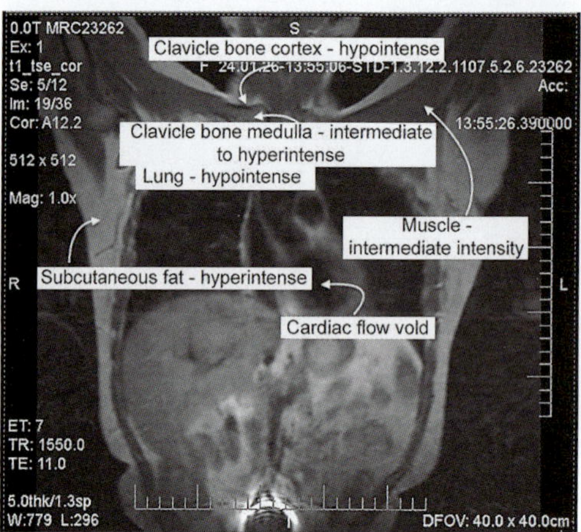

Fig. 9.1F: Coronal chest MRI.

LAST MINUTE REVISION

- **X-ray:** Best for bone and air. Other soft tissues are often indistinguishable unless contrast agents are used.
- **Ultrasound (USG):** Excellent for evaluating fluid collections, antenatal, pelvic, solid organs, and superficial structures like vessels and nerves with real-time dynamic assessment.
- **CT scan:** Provides excellent detail for solid organs, bone, calcification, air, vessels (with contrast), and acute hemorrhages; also great for evaluating complex anatomical regions.
- **MRI:** Superior for soft tissue contrast, such as in musculoskeletal imaging, neuroimaging, and assessing chronic blood or fluid collections.
- **Chronological arrangement as per HU:** Air (–1,000)>lung>fat>water>soft tissue>bone (+1,000)

REVIEW QUESTIONS

Multiple Choice Questions (MCQs)

1. **A 30-year male suffered from accident, after which he is unable to walk. X-ray of lower limb was apparently normal. Which imaging modality is best suited for the detailed evaluation of soft tissue structures such as the brain, spinal cord, joints, and ligaments?**
   A. X-ray
   B. Ultrasound (USG)
   C. Computed Tomography (CT)
   D. Magnetic Resonance Imaging (MRI)
2. **Which imaging modality is least suitable for evaluating structures surrounded by air, such as the lungs, due to reverberation artifacts?**
   A. X-ray
   B. Ultrasound (USG)
   C. Computed Tomography (CT)
   D. CECT
3. **In cases of suspected musculoskeletal conditions involving detailed bone structures and complex fractures, which imaging modality is preferred?**
   A. X-ray
   B. Ultrasound (USG)
   C. Computed Tomography (CT)
   D. Magnetic Resonance Imaging (MRI)
4. **For evaluating a pregnant woman's fetal anatomy and amniotic fluid volume, which primary modality is considered safe and effective?**
   A. X-ray
   B. Ultrasound (USG)
   C. Computed Tomography (CT)
   D. Magnetic Resonance Imaging (MRI)
5. **In the assessment of a patient with suspected coronary artery disease, which imaging modality is used for coronary calcium scoring?**
   A. X-ray
   B. Ultrasound (USG)
   C. Computed Tomography (CT)
   D. Magnetic Resonance Imaging (MRI)
6. **Which imaging modality is preferred for the assessment of the biliary tract and pancreatic pathology due to its detailed visualization capabilities?**
   A. X-ray
   B. PET-CT
   C. Computed Tomography (CT)
   D. Magnetic Resonance Imaging (MRI)

Answer Key

1. d 2. b 3. c 4. b 5. c 6. d

SUGGESTED READING

1. Chambers CH. Radiological anatomy. Med J Aust. 1973;1(16):816. doi: 10.5694/j.1326-5377.1973.tb110708.x. PMID: 4707806.
2. Woodard PK, Slone RM, Gierada DS, Reiker GG, Pilgram TK, Jost RG. Chest radiography: depiction of normal anatomy and pathologic structures with selenium-based digital radiography versus conventional screen-film radiography. Radiology. 1997;203(1):197-201. doi: 10.1148/radiology.203.1.9122392. PMID: 9122392.

CHAPTER

10 ENT and Face Imaging

"In every sinus, canal, and contour lies the radiologist's ability to restore voice, hearing, and breath."

INTRODUCTION

Ear, nose, and throat (ENT) and facial imaging are crucial components of radiology, particularly in diagnosing and managing conditions related to these regions. It covers disease of child to adult and from congenital to dreaded cancers of oropharyngeal region. As a student, understanding the basic principles, techniques, and applications of ENT and facial imaging is essential. This introduction aims to provide an overview of the common imaging modalities used, their indications, and the basic interpretation skills required for ENT and facial imaging. To understand complex anatomy and pathology of this region we should know gross radiological division of various parts and their embryological origin as well as appropriate used modalities as per need.

IMAGING MODALITIES

X-ray

- **Indications:** Basic evaluation of the bony structures of the face, sinuses, ear and mastoid air cells.
- **Techniques:** Waters view or occipitomental view [common paranasal sinuses (PNS) view] for maxillary sinuses, open mouth waters view for sphenoid sinus, Caldwell view for ethmoid and frontal sinuses, lateral view skull for fractures of facial bones/sella-turcica, X-ray nasal bone, modified Stenver's view for mastoids, soft tissue neck AP-lateral for adenoids/epiglottitis/foreign bodies, submentovertex/basal view for zygomatic arch, Townes view for occipital bone/mastoids.
- **Interpretation:** Identification of fractures, sinusitis, mastoiditis, and foreign bodies.

Ultrasound (US)

- **Indications:** Evaluation of superficial soft tissues, salivary glands, thyroid gland, and lymph nodes.
- **Techniques:** High-frequency linear probes, Doppler studies for vascularity.
- **Interpretation:** Cystic vs. solid lesions, abscesses, glandular pathologies (e.g., sialadenitis, thyroid nodules).

Computed Tomography (CT)

- **Indications:** Detailed assessment of bony structures, trauma, sinusitis, neoplasms, and preoperative planning.

- **Techniques:** Axial and coronal sections for middle ear, type of sinusitis, contrast-enhanced studies especially for neck tumors, 3D reconstruction for complex injuries.
- **Interpretation:** Fracture lines, sinus opacification, soft tissue masses, bony erosions.

Magnetic Resonance Imaging (MRI)

- **Indications:** Soft tissue evaluation, neoplasms, inflammatory conditions, and complex anatomical relationships.
- **Techniques:** T1, T2, FLAIR, STIR (sagittal in trauma and coronal in pott's spine) and contrast-enhanced sequences.
- **Interpretation:** Tumor characteristics (size, extent, invasion), inflammatory changes, vascular involvement, superior for soft tissue, inner ear, and nerve assessment.

Nuclear Medicine

Techniques such as positron emission tomography (PET) and Single photon emission computed tomography (SPECT) can be used to evaluate metabolic activity in tumors or infections.

RADIOLOGICAL EVALUATION

Ear Anatomy

As described in **Table 10.1**.

Table 10.1: Gross anatomy with relevant embryology and clinico-radiological aspects of normal ear (Figs. 10.1A and B).

Anatomical divisions	*Embryological origin*	*Best radiological modality*	*Radiological definition*	*Abnormal conditions*
External ear (auricle/pinna)	First and second pharyngeal arches	CT shows well-defined soft tissue structure with clear outline, symmetrical on both sides	The visible part of the ear that collects sound waves	Fractures (discontinuity), infection (swelling, increased density), tumors (masses), congenital anomalies (abnormal shapes)
External auditory canal	First pharyngeal cleft	CT shows well-defined tubular structure, patent canal, symmetrical on both sides	Tubular structure extending from the pinna to the tympanic membrane, through soft tissue and bone	Fractures (irregularity), infection (swelling, fluid), tumors (masses), foreign bodies (objects), congenital anomalies (atresia, stenosis)
Middle ear ossicles (malleus, incus, stapes) Chain of bones connect tympanic membrane to oval window of inner ear	Malleus and incus from the first arch, stapes from the second arch	HRCT shows clear, distinct high-density structures, properly aligned surrounded by temporal bone	Small, dense structures within the middle ear cavity that transmit sound vibrations	Fractures (discontinuity), dislocation (abnormal positioning), erosion (loss of bone density), congenital anomalies (abnormal shapes), otosclerosis (abnormal bone growth)

Contd...

Contd...

Anatomical divisions	*Embryological origin*	*Best radiological modality*	*Radiological definition*	*Abnormal conditions*
Tympanic membrane	First pharyngeal pouch	HRCT shows thin, intact, properly positioned at the junction of the external canal and middle ear	Thin, soft tissue structure separating the external auditory canal and middle ear cavity	Perforation (discontinuity), thickening (chronic inflammation), retraction (inward displacement), cholesteatoma (abnormal mass), infection (increased soft tissue density)
Eustachian tube	First pharyngeal pouch	CT shows well-defined tubular structure, patent lumen, intact surrounding bone	Narrow, tubular structure extending from the middle ear to the lateral wall of nasopharynx	Obstruction (narrowing or blockage), bony abnormalities (irregularities or erosions), soft tissue swelling, congenital anomalies
Inner ear (cochlea, semicircular canals, vestibule)	Otic placode	MRI shows clear, well-defined structures with normal morphology	Complex structures responsible for hearing and balance, within the temporal bone	Abnormal fluid collections (labyrinthitis), congenital anomalies (malformations), erosion or abnormal signal intensities (tumors or infections)

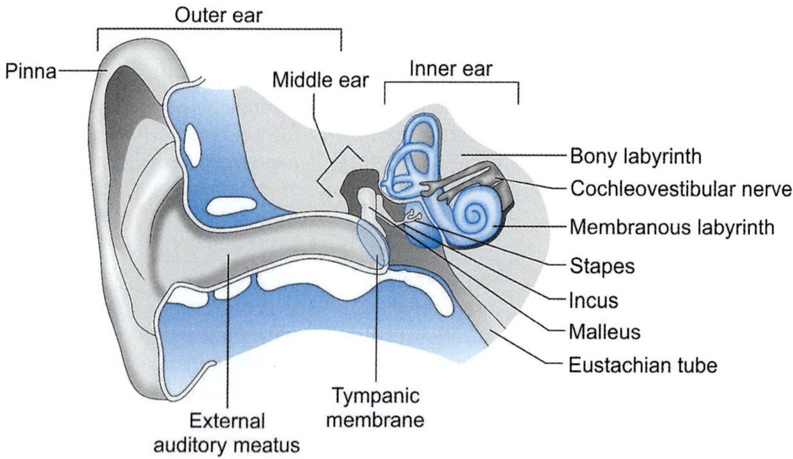

Fig. 10.1A: Shows parts of ear in pictorial manner.

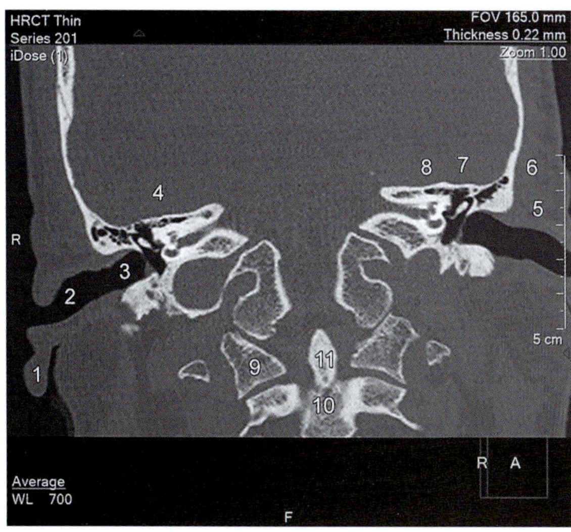

Fig. 10.1B: HRCT temporal bone (coronal section): (1) Pinna; (2) Cartilaginous external ear canal; (3) Bony external ear canal; (4) Petrous bone; (5) Tympanic membrane; (6) Middle ear ossicle; (7) Middle ear; (8) Epiglottis; (9) C1—Atlas vertebrae body; (10) C2—Axis vertebrae body; (11) Odontoid process of C2.

Nose and Paranasal Sinus Anatomy

As described in **Table 10.2**.

Table 10.2: Clinico-radiological aspects of nose and paranasal sinuses (Figs. 10.2A and B).

Anatomical part	*Embryological origin*	*Best radiological modality*	*Radiological definition*	*Abnormal conditions*
Nasal cavity	Nasal placodes, nasal pits	CT shows clear air-filled cavity, symmetric structures	Air-filled space above and behind the nose in the middle of the face	Obstruction (mass, polyp), deviated septum, thickened mucosa (inflammation), fluid collection (sinusitis)
Nasal septum	Frontonasal process	CT shows midline structure, straight and intact	Partition separating the two nostrils, composed of bone and cartilage	Deviated septum, fractures (discontinuity), perforation
Turbinates	Lateral nasal process	CT shows clear and well-defined, symmetric on both sides	Long, narrow shelves of bone that protrude into the nasal cavity, covered by mucosa	Hypertrophy (enlarged turbinates), mucosal thickening (inflammation)
Maxillary sinuses Present at birth and full developed at adolescent	Outpouchings of the nasal cavity	CT shows clear, air-filled sinuses with thin walls	Largest paranasal sinuses, located in the maxillary bones of the face (paired)	Opacification (sinusitis), fluid levels, mucosal thickening, polyps, tumors
Frontal sinuses Appear around 5–6-year and full developed at late teens	Outpouchings of the nasal cavity	CT shows clear, air-filled sinuses with thin walls	Paired sinuses located in the frontal bone above the eyes	Opacification (sinusitis), fluid levels, mucosal thickening, polyps, cysts Mucocele, osteoid osteoma

Contd...

Contd...

Anatomical part	*Embryological origin*	*Best radiological modality*	*Radiological definition*	*Abnormal conditions*
Ethmoid air cells Present at birth and fully developed by age of 12	Outpouchings of the nasal cavity	CT shows clear, air-filled cells with thin walls	Numerous small cavities in the ethmoid bone between the nose and the eyes	Opacification (sinusitis), mucosal thickening, polyps, cysts
Sphenoid sinus Appear around 3 year and full developed at adolescent	Outpouchings of the nasal cavity	CT and MRI shows clear, air-filled sinus with thin walls	Paired sinuses located in the sphenoid bone, behind the nasal cavity	Opacification (sinusitis), fluid levels, mucosal thickening, polyps, cysts
Nasal bones	Nasal placodes	CT and X-ray shows smooth, intact, and symmetric bones	Paired bones forming the bridge of the nose	Fractures (discontinuity), deformities (congenital or traumatic)
Nasal cartilage	Neural crest cells	MRI shows smooth and well-defined cartilage	Cartilaginous structures providing shape and support to the nose	Displacement, deformities, or signal changes indicating injury or disease
Nasal septum cartilage	Frontonasal process	MRI, straight and midline with smooth contours	Cartilaginous part of the nasal septum	Deviations, perforations, or signal changes indicating injury or disease
Olfactory bulb	Olfactory placodes	MRI, normal size and signal intensity, positioned above the cribriform plate	Neural structure responsible for the sense of smell, located above the nasal cavity	Atrophy, abnormal signal intensities indicating pathology (e.g., tumors, inflammation)

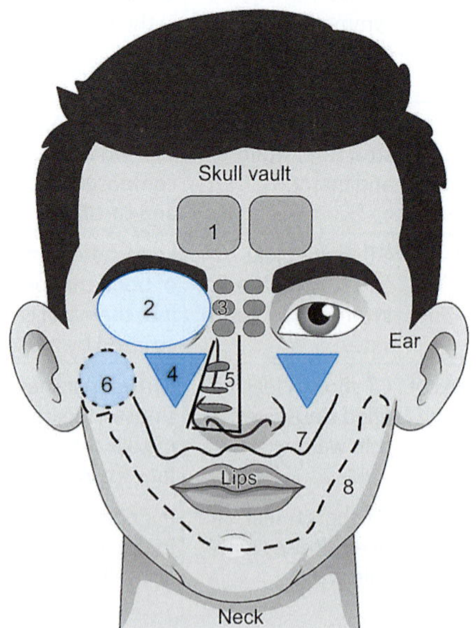

Fig. 10.2A: Radiological anatomy of face: (1) Frontal sinus; (2) Orbit; (3) Ethmoid sinus; (4) Maxillary sinus; (5) Nasal cavity with turbinates and midline septum; (6) Cheek (Zygoma); (7) Maxilla bone; (8) Mandible bone.

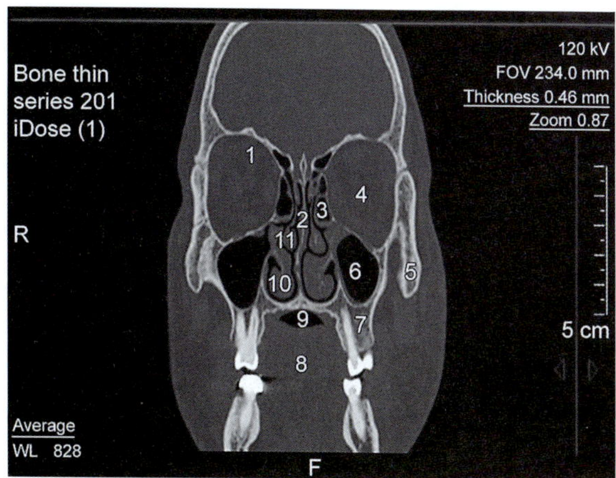

Fig. 10.2B: NCCT paranasal sinus (coronal section): (1) Superior rectus muscle; (2) Nasal septum; (3) Bulla ethmoidalis; (4) Orbit; (5) Zygomatic bone; (6) Maxillary sinus; (7) Body of maxilla; (8) Tongue; (9) Oropharynx; (10) Inferior turbinate; (11) Middle turbinate.

Throat Anatomy

As described in **Table 10.3**.

Table 10.3: Clinico-radiological features of neck anatomy (Figs. 10.3A and B).

Anatomical part	*Embryological origin*	*Best radiological modality*	*Radiological definition*	*Abnormal appearance*
Nasopharynx From base of skull up to C2 vertebrae	Endoderm of the foregut	CT, MRI shows clear air-filled space with normal soft tissue structures and no masses or swellings	Upper part of the pharynx, connecting with the nasal cavity above the soft palate	Masses (tumors, adenoids), asymmetry, fluid collections, or mucosal thickening
Oropharynx Opposite to C3 and C4 vertebrae, (hard palate to hyoid bone,)	Endoderm of the foregut	CT, MRI shows clear, air-filled space, normal tonsils, soft palate, and tongue base (root)	Middle part of the pharynx, located behind the mouth	Masses (tumors), asymmetry, mucosal thickening, or enlarged tonsils
Hypopharynx Posterolateral to larynx, opposite to C5 and C6 vertebrae	Endoderm of the foregut	CT, MRI shows clear air-filled space, smooth soft tissue contours, and normal bony structures	Lower part of the pharynx, extending from the hyoid bone to the esophagus and larynx	Masses (tumors), asymmetry, mucosal thickening, or foreign bodies
Larynx (voice box) Fibrocartilaginous tube for air extends from epiglottis to cricoid cartilage	Fourth and sixth pharyngeal arches	MRI, high-resolution CT, clear visualization of vocal cords, arytenoids, thyroid, and cricoid cartilage	Contains the vocal cords and responsible for sound production	Masses (tumors), vocal cord paralysis, asymmetry, thickening, or structural abnormalities

Contd...

Contd...

Anatomical part	*Embryological origin*	*Best radiological modality*	*Radiological definition*	*Abnormal appearance*
Vocal cords or vocal folds Anatomical division for laryngeal disease into supraglottic and infraglottic	Fourth and sixth pharyngeal arches	MRI, HRCT shows symmetric, thin, linear soft tissue structures within the larynx, extending from the thyroid cartilage to the arytenoid cartilages	Folds of tissue within the larynx that vibrate to produce sound	Paralysis, nodules, polyps, masses, or thickening
Laryngeal cartilages	Fourth (thyroid) and sixth (cricoid, arytenoids) pharyngeal arches	Clear, well-defined, and symmetric cartilages without erosion or masses	Cartilages forming the structure of the larynx, including the thyroid and cricoid cartilages	Fractures, erosions, masses (tumors), or asymmetry
Epiglottis cartilage located at the root of the tongue with clear attachment at hyoid bone and thyroid cartilage	Third and fourth pharyngeal arches	MRI, high-resolution CT shows smooth, well-defined, cartilage that are positioned over the larynx	Leaf-shaped flap that prevents food from entering the trachea during swallowing by covering glottis	Thickening, masses, or abnormal positioning (e.g., epiglottitis)
Piriform sinus	Endoderm of the foregut	CT, MRI shows clear recesses, symmetric on both sides, with smooth contours	Recess located on either side of the laryngeal orifice	Masses, asymmetry, mucosal thickening, or fluid collections
Cervical esophagus Muscular potential space for food	Endoderm of the foregut	CT, MRI, barium swallow shows smooth, well-defined lumen with normal peristaltic motion	The upper part of the esophagus, extending from the hypopharynx, C6 to the thoracic inlet, T1	Strictures, masses (tumors), diverticula (e.g., Zenker's), motility disorders, or foreign bodies

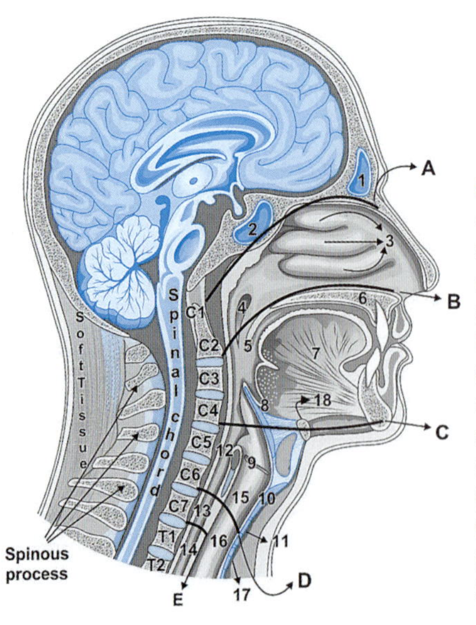

Fig. 10.3A: Pictorial representation of radiological anatomy of face and neck: (A) Plane along base of skull separating nasopharynx and brain; (B) Plane along hard palate dividing nasopharynx and oropharynx; (C) Plane along hyoid bone and tongue base dividing oropharynx and hypopharynx; (D) Plane along lower border of C6 vertebra dividing larynx and trachea; (E) Plane along lower border of C7 vertebra dividing cervical and thoracic esophagus; (1) Frontal sinus; (2) Sphenoid sinus; (3) Turbinates; (4) Eustachian tube opening; (5) Uvula (posterior tip of soft palate); (6) Hard palate; (7) Tongue; (8) Epiglottis; (9) Vocal cord; (10) Thyroid cartilage; (11) Cricoid cartilage (opposite to C6 vertebra); (12) Hypopharynx; (13) Cervical esophagus; (14) Thoracic esophagus; (15) Larynx; (16) Trachea; (17) Tracheal rings; (18) Hyoid bone.

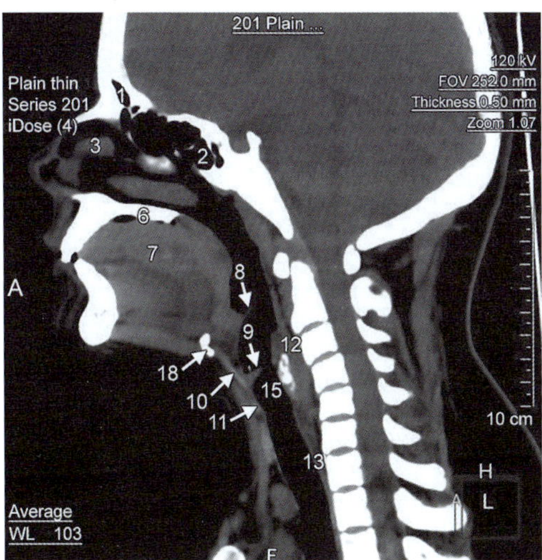

Fig. 10.3B: CT soft tissue window shows normal important landmark for understanding radiological neck anatomy.

Facial Anatomy

As described in **Table 10.4**.

Table 10.4: Clinico-radiological features of face related structures (Figs. 10.2A and B).

Facial structure	*Radiological division*	*Embryological origin*	*Best modality*	*Normal appearance*	*Abnormal appearance*
Frontal bone of skull	Bony structure enclosing the brain	Neural crest and mesoderm	CT, X-ray	Uniform bone density	Fractures, infective, tumor
Orbit	Bony cavity containing the eye and its structures	Neural crest	MRI, CT, USG (B scan)	Smooth, intact bony walls	Fractures, tumors
Maxilla	Upper jaw	Neural crest	CT	Uniform bone density	Fractures, cysts
Mandible	Lower jaw	Neural crest	Panoramic X-ray (OPG), CT	Uniform bone density	Fractures, cysts, osteomyelitis
Nasal cavity	Air-filled space surrounded nasal cavity	Neural crest	CT, MRI	Smooth turbinates on lateral wall with intact midline septum	Deviated septum, polyps
Paranasal sinuses	Air-filled spaces surrounding nasal cavity	Neural crest	CT	Clear sinuses	Sinusitis, masses, polyps
Temporal bone	Complex bone housing the ear	Mesoderm	CT, MRI	Detailed bone structure	Fractures, cholesteatoma

Contd...

Contd...

Facial structure	*Radiological division*	*Embryological origin*	*Best modality*	*Normal appearance*	*Abnormal appearance*
Oral cavity	Mouth including the teeth, gums, tongue, and salivary glands	Ectoderm (oral epithelium)	• X-ray for teeth (OPG) • CT/MRI for others	Uniform density, no caries	Caries, abscesses, tumors
Soft tissues	Skin, subcutaneous tissue, fat, muscles	Mesoderm	MRI, ultrasound	Homogeneous tissue	Masses, abscesses
Salivary glands	Glands producing saliva	Parotid from ectoderm, submandibular and sublingual from endoderm	MRI, ultrasound	Homogeneous tissue	Stones, tumors, inflammation
Muscles of mastication	Muscles for chewing	Mesoderm	MRI, CT, USG	Normal muscle morphology	Hypertrophy, atrophy, masses
Zygomatic bone	Cheek bone	Neural crest	CT	Uniform bone density	Fractures, lesions
Note: Few other bones contributing in facial skeleton: • **Lacrimal bones:** Small bones forming part of the medial wall of the orbit. • **Palatine bones:** Forming part of the nasal cavity and the hard palate. • **Inferior nasal conchae:** Curved bones within the nasal cavity. • **Vomer:** A thin, flat bone forming part of the nasal septum.					

COMMON PATHOLOGY

Infectious Pathologies

Ear and Face

- **Cellulitis (skin and subcutaneous tissue infection):** Ultrasound shows soft tissue thickening with increased vascularity, abscess formation. CT scan is needed to assess deep tissue involvement.
- **Dental infections:** Panoramic X-ray shows lucency in tooth, periapical thickening and abscess formation. CT scan may be needed for extensive infections.
- **Sinusitis:** X-ray PNS shows opacity in sinuses, nasal septum deviation and fluid level in acute infection. CT scan (noncontrast) shows mucosal thickening, **(Fig. 10.4)** turbinate hypertrophy, septum position as well as fantastic view of osteomeatal unit as well as anatomical variations of air cells in relation of sinuses which helps in planning of surgery (FESS). CT also aids in diagnoses of fungal sinusitis (hyphae are hyperdense) which can show expansion, erosion, rarely destruction of bones. MRI has limited role especially in severe cases for intraorbital and intracranial extension. Though MRI is IOC of post COVID mucormycotic sinusitis due to better soft tissue extension and assessment of necrosis and infarct as this fungus is angioinvasive.
- **Otitis media infection or inflammation of the middle ear:** Imaging is typically reserved for cases with complications or when the diagnosis is uncertain. High-resolution computed tomography (HRCT) of temporal bone shows fluid density within the middle ear cavity, **(Fig. 10.5)** thickening of the tympanic membrane, opacification or sclerosis of mastoid air

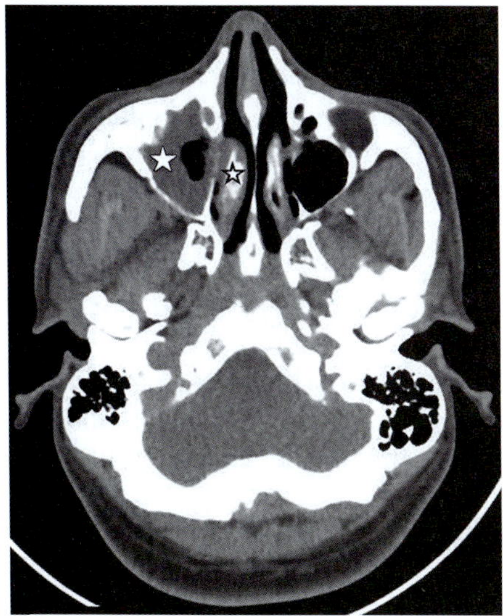

Fig. 10.4: Shows NCCT PNS with circumferential mucosal lining in the right maxillary sinus and right middle turbinate hypertrophy consistent with sinusitis.

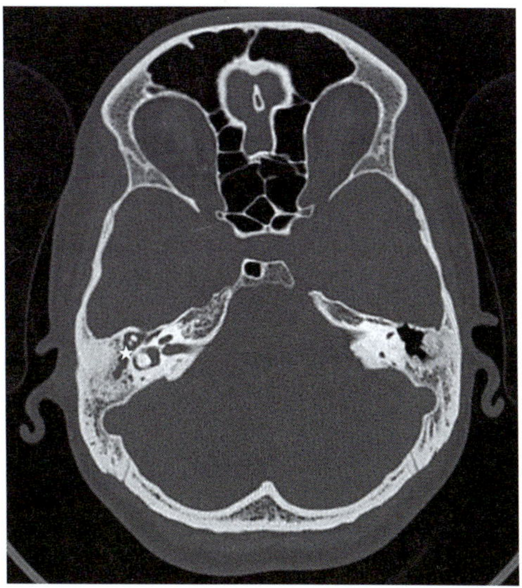

Fig. 10.5: HRCT temporal bone shows fluid density in right mastoid air cells and right middle ear cavity with sclerosis consistent with chronic oto-mastoiditis.

cells, presence of cholesteatoma. CT/MRI plays a very important role to rule out potential complications of otitis media, e.g., brain abscess, sinus thrombosis.

- **Cholesteatoma:** Abnormal growth of squamous epithelium in the middle ear commonly in epitympanum or mastoid that can cause destruction of local structures. Imaging is crucial for diagnosis, surgical planning, and follow-up. Nonenhancing isodense or slightly hypodense soft tissue mass with bony erosion, ossicular chain destruction, scutum blunting and tegmen tympani erosion.
- **Cholesterol granuloma:** A benign lesion that results from the accumulation of cholesterol crystals and granulomatous inflammation, often due to chronic inflammation or hemorrhage. CT shows typically hyperdense mass with possible fluid levels due to chronic bleeding.
- **Sialadenitis:** Inflammation of the salivary gland, often due to bacterial or viral infection or autoimmune conditions (e.g., Sjögren's syndrome). USG shows enlarged gland with heterogeneous enhancement; ductal dilation and sialoliths (stones) may be seen. Radiopaque stones visible on plain X-ray; cause ductal dilation and infection.

Infectious Pathologies of Neck

- **Lymphadenopathy:** Ultrasound (initial evaluation) to assess size (>10 mm in short axis diameter is significant), shape (round/oval) and internal characteristics like necrosis, calcification, hila intactness. CT is done for deep located nodes and staging of nodes. MRI **rarely use**, especially for differentiation of necrosis and caseation.
- **PET-CT** helps in assessing metabolic activity of enlarged lymph nodes with suspicious metastases, particularly useful in staging and monitoring malignancies.
- **Deep neck space infections:** CT scan with contrast.
- **Tonsillitis/pharyngitis:** Clinical diagnosis, ultrasound (if abscess suspected), CT scan (if complications are suspected like extension of parapharyngeal abscess).

Traumatic Pathologies

Face

- **Fractures:** CT scan (gold standard for bone fractures), X-ray (initial assessment).
- **Soft tissue injuries:** Ultrasound (for soft tissue evaluation), CT scan (if deeper injury suspected).

Neck

- **Blunt or penetrating trauma:** CT angiography (for vascular injury), CT scan (for structural damage).
- **Whiplash injury** (occurs due to rapid back-and-forth movement of the head and neck, often due to rear-end car accidents). MRI (if neurological symptoms are present) should include all basic scans in three planes and sagittal STIR, X-ray (initial assessment) should be done with immobilization technique.

Neoplastic Pathologies

Face

- **Benign tumors:** Hemangioma shows tubular spaces, phlebolith with vascularity on USG. Lipoma is well marginated homogenous commonly hyperechoic and in superficial plane. MRI for larger and deeper lesion (to delineate soft tissue involvement), CT scan (rarely for bone involvement), **Pleomorphic adenoma** is the most common benign tumor of the parotid gland: well-defined, lobulated mass, often with mixed echogenicity on ultrasound; T2 hyperintense and T1 hypointense on MRI with heterogeneous enhancement after contrast administration, **Warthin's tumor** common benign tumor, with male predilection typically seen in older adults and associated with smoking, well-defined having cystic and solid components, shows hyperintense cysts on T2-weighted MRI images.
- **Malignant tumors:** Clinical and histology is important for diagnosis of basal or squamous cell carcinoma though all imaging like MRI (soft tissue and extent evaluation), CT scan (for bone invasion), PET-CT (for metastasis) has role in comprehensive management.

  Choroidal melanoma is the most common primary intraocular malignancy in adults, arising from melanocytes in the choroid. Diagnosis is primarily made through clinical examination and imaging studies, particularly ultrasound and fundus photography. USG is primary modality of choice shows dome-shaped or mushroom-shaped mass with low to medium internal reflectivity and high vascularity.

  Mucoepidermoid carcinoma is the most common malignant tumor of the parotid gland. Poorly defined mass with heterogeneous enhancement; may show areas of necrosis and calcification.

Neck

- **Benign tumors:** Ultrasound (initial evaluation) for evaluation of thyroid nodule using TIRADS staging which stratify the risk of malignancy and guide management decisions, such as whether to perform fine needle aspiration (FNA) or follow-up imaging. In extrathyroidal pathology lesion is described in terms of location (e.g., paraganglioma/glomus tumors or carotid body tumor at carotid bifurcation with high vascularity,) plane of lesion (lipoma in subcutaneous plane), internal characters. CT/MRI done for its extent and internal component (e.g., light bulb sign for paragangliomas is due to intense enhancement

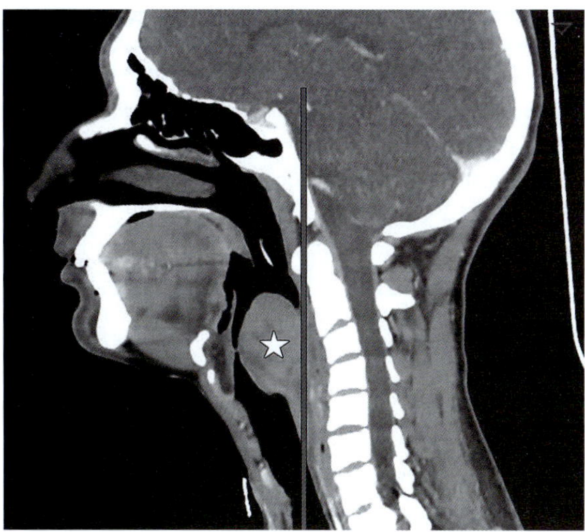

Fig. 10.6: CECT neck shows a large well defined round shaped heterogeneously enhancing soft tissue mass lesion in oro-hypopharynx region.

of vessels due to hypervascularity or T2 hyperintense due to cystic changes and myxoid degeneration).

- **Malignant tumor:** CECT is primary modality for evaluation of pharyngeal **(Fig. 10.6)**, laryngeal malignancy **and extension of suspected thyroid malignancy.** MRI and PET-CT (for metastasis).

Congenital and Developmental Pathologies

Face

- **Cleft lip and palate:** Cleft lip occurs due to the failure of fusion between the medial nasal prominence and the maxillary prominence, while cleft palate results from the failure of the palatal shelves (lateral palatine processes) to fuse. Prenatal diagnosis is on 4D USG, postnatal diagnosis is clinical, CT scan (for detailed anatomical planning).
- **Arteriovenous malformations (AVMs)** are rare, congenital vascular anomalies characterized by a complex tangle of arteries and veins connected by abnormal, high-flow shunts. Face is second most common site after brain.
  Ultrasound: Initial imaging to assess the flow characteristics and extent of the lesion.
  Doppler ultrasound shows high-velocity, turbulent blood flow within the AVM.
  CT angiography (CTA) provides detailed images of the blood vessels and can delineate the extent of the AVM and shows tangled mass of vessels with early filling of veins.
  MRI and MR angiography (MRA): Preferred for detailed soft tissue contrast and vascular mapping.
  Digital subtraction angiography (DSA): Gold standard for detailed vascular anatomy and planning interventional procedures.

Neck

- **Branchial cleft cysts** formed due to incomplete obliteration of the branchial clefts during embryonic development. Ultrasound (initial evaluation) shows well-defined, round or oval anechoic or hypoechoic structure with posterior acoustic enhancement and thin walls,

Table 10.5: Imaging characteristics for dermoid and epidermoid cysts.

Feature	*Dermoid cyst*	*Epidermoid cyst*
Content	Ectodermal and mesodermal elements (hair, fat and teeth)	Ectodermal elements (keratin, cholesterol)
Ultrasound	Heterogeneous with mixed echogenicity, posterior acoustic shadowing	Anechoic or hypoechoic, posterior acoustic enhancement
CT scan	Heterogeneous with fat density, often calcifications	Homogeneous low density, rarely calcifications
T1-weighted MRI	High signal due to fat, variable signal from other components	Low to intermediate signal, sometimes high due to dense keratin
T2-weighted MRI	Mixed signal, fat appears hyperintense	High signal due to fluid content, heterogeneous if proteinaceous material present
Fat suppression MRI	Fat suppression helps confirm fat content	No fat suppression needed
Diffusion-weighted imaging (DWI)	Typically not restricted, no specific high signal	Restricted diffusion with high signal on DWI, low ADC values
Contrast enhancement	Minimal to no enhancement of contents, capsule may enhance	Typically no enhancement of contents, slight enhancement of wall

located along the anterior border of the sternocleidomastoid muscle (usually in relation of one third). CT scan with contrast (for surgical planning) rarely needed.

- **Thyroglossal duct cyst:** Ultrasound (initial evaluation) shows midline/paramedian cyst round to oval anechoic to hypoechoic located in the usually between the hyoid bone and the thyroid gland. It shows posterior acoustic enhancement and may exhibit thin internal septations (if complicated). It often moves upward with swallowing or tongue protrusion, which is a characteristic feature. CT scan is needed (if infection or complications suspected).
- **Cystic hygroma:** A congenital lymphatic malformation, often multiloculated and found in the posterior triangle of the neck, USG is primary modality. CT is occasionally used, especially to assess bone involvement or in emergency situations to assess mass effect on airway.
- **Dermoid cyst and epidermoid cyst (Table 10.5).**

Inflammatory and Autoimmune Pathologies

Face

- **Sarcoidosis:** Chest X-ray (initial evaluation for pulmonary involvement), CT chest for pulmonary involvement, MRI (for CNS involvement).
- **Systemic lupus erythematosus (SLE):** Clinical diagnosis, MRI (for CNS involvement).

Neck

- **Thyroiditis:** Clinical diagnosis. Ultrasound (initial evaluation) shows enlarged gland (AP >18–20 mm) and isthmus thickness >6 mm (indicates diffuse involvement) and altered echogenicity. Vascularity may be increased in acute type and nodes can be enlarged in case of viral thyroiditis.
- **Sjögren's syndrome:** Ultrasound of salivary glands shows B/L enlarged parotid/submandibular glands, heterogeneous echo texture with multiple hypoechoic or anechoic

cystic areas, punctate or coarse calcifications, with or without enlarged nodes and altered vascularity.

Vascular Pathologies

Face

Hemangiomas: Already described in benign tumor

Neck

- **Carotid artery disease:** Doppler ultrasound shows wall thickening without or with luminal narrowing (stenosis) and altered velocity at different site, CT angiography/MR angiography for extent. Diffuse, symmetric wall thickening of carotid (giving macaroni appearance), aorta and its major branches in Takayasu arteritis.
- **Jugular venous thrombosis:** Doppler ultrasound, shows expansion of vein and iso to hypoechoic contents in it. CT venography/MR venography for extent.

Neurological Pathologies

Face

- **Bell's palsy:** Clinical diagnosis, MRI (if atypical presentation or prolonged symptoms).
- **Trigeminal neuralgia:** MRI (T1, T2, FLAIR, DW, T1 contrast) to rule out secondary causes with MRA for vascular assessment and CISS or FIESTA sequence for nerve visualization.

Neck

- **Cervical radiculopathy:** MRI to assess disc degeneration/bulge/protrusion, foramen narrowing and, nerve root compression.
- **Cervical myelopathy:** MRI (gold standard for spinal cord compression) shows T1 hypointense and T1 hyperintense signal.

Endocrine Pathologies

Face

- **Cushing's syndrome:** Clinical diagnosis, MRI (for pituitary adenoma).
- **Acromegaly:** MRI (for pituitary adenoma).

Neck

- **Goiter:** Ultrasound (initial evaluation), CT scan (if compressive symptoms or retrosternal extension).
- **Thyroid nodules:** Ultrasound (initial evaluation), fine needle aspiration (FNA) for cytology.

Miscellaneous Pathologies

Face

- **Temporomandibular joint disorders (TMJ):** MRI (gold standard for soft tissue and disc evaluation), X-ray OPG for initial assessment especially open-close mouth view for dislocation.
- **Eye globe:** B scan is primary modality of choice. In cataract USG shows thickened echoic capsule. It is also helpful in diagnosis of vitreous hemorrhage showing echoes in vitreous after history of injury and also in vitreous, retinal and choroidal detachment.

Neck

- **Cervical spondylosis:** X-ray (initial assessment) shows osteophytes and reduced IV disc in case of PIVD with adjacent end plate sclerosis, MRI (for detailed spinal cord and nerve root evaluation).
- **Torticollis:** Clinical diagnosis, ultrasound (for muscle evaluation in infants), MRI (if neurological symptoms are present). The sternocleidomastoid tumor, also known as a potato tumor, is a self-limiting benign mass found in the sternocleidomastoid (SCM) (mid to lower third) in infants with congenital muscular torticollis form due to birth injury leads to fibrosis and formation of a firm, palpable mass. USG is preferred imaging modality to confirm the diagnosis and rule out other neck masses. Muscle is enlarged, fibrotic with decreased muscle bulk and an isoechoic to hypoechoic intramuscular mass.

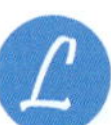

AST MINUTE REVISION

- MRI has limited but specific role in otitis media. It can assess intracranial complications (e.g., abscess, meningitis) and differentiates cholesteatoma from other soft tissues using non-EPI DWI, shows hyperintense signal on DWI, hypointense on T1, and variable on T2.
- Cholesterol crystals seen in thyroglossal cyst seen as echogenic foci with comet tail artifact.
- All cystic lesion shows posterior acoustic enhancement on USG.
- Thyroid nodule should be assessed in terms of composition, echogenicity, shape, margin, and echogenic foci to assess points for Thyroid Imaging Reporting and Data System (TI-RADS).

REVIEW QUESTIONS

Multiple Choice Questions (MCQs)

1. **A 25-year-old male presents with a history of facial trauma from a motor vehicle accident. He has severe facial swelling and pain, particularly around the nose and maxillary region. Which imaging modality is preferred for detailed assessment of the facial bones and detection of fractures?**
   a. X-ray b. Ultrasound
   c. Computed tomography (CT) d. Magnetic resonance imaging (MRI)
2. **A 45-year-old female complains of persistent swelling and pain in the region of the parotid gland. On physical examination, a firm, painless mass is palpated. Which imaging modality is initially preferred for evaluating the parotid gland and distinguishing between cystic and solid lesions?**
   a. X-ray b. Ultrasound
   c. Computed tomography (CT) d. Magnetic resonance imaging (MRI)
3. **A 50-year-old male presents with progressive hearing loss and tinnitus over the past few months. He is a known case of neurofibromatosis. Which imaging modality is preferred for evaluation of patient for detecting possible lesions?**
   a. X-ray b. Ultrasound
   c. Computed tomography (CT) d. Magnetic resonance imaging (MRI)
4. **A 35-year-old female presents with recurrent sinus infections and headaches. Physical examination reveals tenderness over the maxillary sinuses. Which imaging modality is preferred for a detailed assessment of the paranasal sinuses and planning for possible surgical intervention?**
   a. X-ray b. Ultrasound
   c. Computed tomography (CT) d. Magnetic resonance imaging (MRI)

5. A 50-year-old male presents with a painless, slowly enlarging mass in the midline of his neck that moves when he swallows. Which imaging modality is initially preferred for evaluating a suspected thyroglossal duct cyst?

a. X-ray
b. Ultrasound
c. Computed tomography (CT)
d. Magnetic resonance imaging (MRI)

Answer Key

1. c 2. b 3. d 4. c 5. b

SUGGESTED READING

1. Anbarasu A, Chandrasekaran K, Balakrishnan S. Soft tissue attenuation in middle ear on HRCT: Pictorial review. Indian J Radiol Imaging. 2012;22(4):298-304. doi: 10.4103/0971–3026.111483.
2. Kikkeri SN, Nagalli S. Trigeminal neuralgia. [Updated 2024 Mar 3]. In: StatPearls [Internet]. Treasure Island (FL): StatPearls Publishing; 2024.

CHAPTER

11

Neurological Imaging

"When the brain speaks in signals, it's the radiologist who interprets its silent cries."

INTRODUCTION

Neuroradiology is sub-specialty of radiodiagnosis that deals with diagnosis and intervention of diseases related to brain, spine, and peripheral nervous system. It encompasses a variety of techniques designed to image the structure and function of the brain and spinal cord. These imaging modalities are indispensable in modern medical practice, offering invaluable insights into neurological conditions and guiding treatment strategies. Neuroimaging techniques **(Tables 11.1 to 11.4)** range from those that provide detailed anatomical views to those that reveal functional and metabolic information about the nervous system.

INDICATIONS OF BRAIN IMAGING

- **Acute neurological events:** CT scans are often the first-line imaging for acute strokes or head injuries **(Figs. 11.1 and 11.2)**, detecting hemorrhages, fractures, and acute ischemic changes. MRI is used for more detailed evaluation in cases of diffuse axonal injury or to rule out stroke mimickers.
- **Chronic neurological conditions:** MRI is the modality of choice for chronic conditions like multiple sclerosis, where it can identify demyelinating plaques. It is also crucial in evaluating patients with chronic headaches or epilepsy.
- **Oncological applications:** Both CT and MRI are used to detect and monitor brain tumors. PET scans provide metabolic information that can help distinguish between tumor recurrence and treatment effects.
- **Neurodegenerative diseases:** Imaging plays a vital role in diagnosing conditions like Alzheimer's disease. MRI can show atrophy patterns, while PET scans can detect amyloid plaques and tau tangles characteristic of the disease.
- **Functional brain mapping:** fMRI is used in presurgical planning to map critical brain functions, minimizing the risk of postoperative deficits.

It is obvious that USG and X-ray has limited role in neuroimaging. Most of the brain pathology needs evaluation of brain on cross-sectional modality. Diagnosis can be made either of single modality or may need combination of both. Basic sections of brain includes axial with post-processing on CT and various planes in different sequences at predetermined anatomical levels at 3–5 mm thickness. While studying the images, following points should be considered: any loss of symmetry of various brain structure in both halves; location of lesion; single or

Table 11.1: Comparison of neuroimaging modalities.

Modality	*Uses*	*Advantages*	*Disadvantages*	*Normal imaging features*	*Abnormal imaging features*
X-ray (Fig. 11.1)	First choice for bony fractures, sinusitis, foreign body localization, postoperative metallic implant evaluation	Quick, inexpensive, widely available	• Limited to bone imaging, no soft tissue contrast, overlapping of structures present • Radiation risk • Cannot evaluate intracranial structures	Bone white dense structures, radiolucent air-filled sinuses (dark), other structures shades of grey	Fractures (seen as discontinuity/displacement of bone), bone lesions, deformities
Ultrasound (USG)	Neonatal brain imaging cranial USG, vascular assessment neck vessels Doppler, B-scan for eyeball	Fast, safe (no radiation), real-time dynamic imaging, portable, patient interaction possible	Limited by bone and air, operator dependent, limited soft tissue contrast	Low to moderate echogenicity of parenchyma, while septum/corpus/choroid/basal ganglia are echogenic and ventricles/cavum is anechoic **Note:** Vessels are echo-free, normal IMT <0.09 mm in carotid artery	Germinal matrix hemorrhage, periventricular cyst, hydrocephalus in neonates, plaques/Intima media thickness/stenosis in vessels **Note:** Vessels are echo free, normal IMT<0.09 mm in carotid artery
Computed tomography (CT) (Figs. 11.2 and 11.3)	Acute trauma and stroke, intracranial hemorrhage	Fast, best for air, bone, calcifications and acute bleeding, multiplanar with 3D reconstruction, no overlapping	Radiation exposure, limited soft tissue contrast, expensive	Clear differentiation of brain structures and ventricles; gray matter appears slightly denser (hyperdense) compared to white matter due to its higher cellular content and lower water content	Acute hemorrhage, fractures, mass effect, hydrocephalus, localize foreign body, CT angiography for aneurysm, space occupying lesions, AV malformations, AV fistula. CT perfusion commonly used for ischemic penumbra. CECT for tumors, infections etc.
Magnetic resonance imaging (MRI)	• Tumors, multiple sclerosis, chronic conditions, traumatic brain with normal CT appearance to detect diffuse axonal injury (DWI and SWI sequences) • Intraocular and globe pathology except foreign body • Carotid vessel disease (better extent and level)	• Superior soft tissue contrast, no radiation, multiplanar 3D, angiography without contrast, gradient commonly used to detect hemorrhage, calcification, and iron deposition • Functional MRI for brain activity • Diffusion perfusion weighted MRI (best) for ischemic penumbra	• Longer scan times, higher cost, bone and air-filled structures will show artifact • Absolute contraindications like ocular metallic foreign bodies, pacemakers, cochlear implants, aneurysm clips • Relative contraindications like first-trimester of pregnancy and claustrophobia	• Detailed brain anatomy, best white and grey matter differentiation, variable appearances on different sequences (described in **Table 11.2**)	• Tumors, plaques in MS, infarcts, demyelination • DW and ADC in infarct and tumor, MRS for differentiation of infection/tumor and differentiation of postoperative changes/residual tumor • MRA for AV malformations • Tractography to study tracts in vascular and demyelination disease

Table 11.2: Comparison of various sequences of brain MRI.

MRI parameters	*T1*	*FLAIR*	*T2*
TR	Short	Long	Long
TE	Short	Long	Long
FAT	Bright (hyperintense)	Variable, relatively bright	Intermediate
CSF	Dark (hypointense)	Dark (hypointense)	Bright (hyperintense)
Grey matter	Darker (hypointense)	Brighter (hyperintense)	Brighter (hyperintense)
White matter	Brighter (hyperintense)	Darker (hypointense)	Darker (hypointense)
Bone/air/calcification	Dark (hypointense)	Dark (hypointense)	Dark (hypointense)

Table 11.3: Comparison of various brain angiography.

Factors	*Digital subtraction angiography (DSA)*	*Contrast enhanced CT angiography (CECT ANGIO)*	*Contrast enhanced MR angiography (CE-MRA)*	*Time of flight MRI angiography (TOF MRA)*	*Phase contrast MRI angiography (PC MRA)*
Principle	More X-ray attenuation by iodinated contrast in blood vessels	Same as DSA but can also give detail in multiple planes and detail of adjacent structures	After IV contrast vessels are bright hyperintense on images than surrounding.	Moving blood has unsaturated proton than surrounding in-plane tissue and appear bright with dark background	Moving proton of blood has different phase shift compare to stationary proton while passing through the magnetic gradient Vessels are variable grayscale intensities based on flow velocity and direction
Contrast material	Iodinated water-soluble contrast material	Iodinated water-soluble contrast material	Gadolinium-based contrast	Not used	Not used
Advantage	Gold standard for any vascular pathology Therapeutic procedures can be performed	Gold standard and replacing DSA for diagnosis	No radiation risk	No radiation risk No contrast required	No radiation risk
Disadvantage	Radiation risk, contrast injection risk	Radiation risk, no provision of simultaneous intervention	Prolong scan time	Prone to artifact, prolong scan time	Prone to artifact, more technical and maximum scan time

Table 11.4: Comparison of brain imaging on CT and MRI.

Characteristic	*MRI*	*CT*
Strength	0.5, 1, 1.5 and 3, TESLA	16, 32, 64,128 slice
Modality	No radiation	Radiation
Examples of types	Diffusion, T2, T1, FLAIR, GRE, ADC	Soft tissue, window, bone, window, 3-D volume

Contd...

Contd...

Characteristic	*MRI*	*CT*
Parameter	TE, TR, slice thickness	KVP, mAs, slice thickness
Compact bone	Dark-hypointense	White Hyperdense
CSF	Hyperintense on T2/hypointense on T1 and FLAIR	Hypodense
Grey matter	Hyperintense on T2/hypointense on T1	Hyperdense
White matter	Hypointense on T2/hyperintense on T1	Hypodense
Subcutaneous fat	Hyperintense on T1, intermediate or relatively hyperintense on T2	Hypodense
Angiography	With or without contrast	Always with contrast

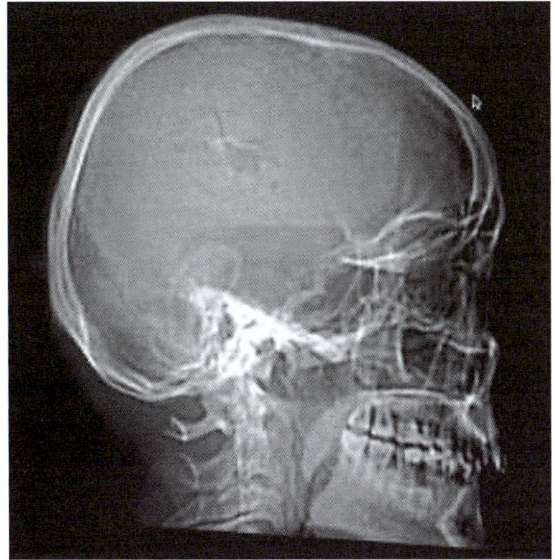

Fig. 11.1: X-ray skull lateral projection of a patient presented with head injury. The X-ray shows the fracture. However, the exact bone, site, size and underlying brain tissue cannot be evaluated accurately (Please see the CT section for further details).

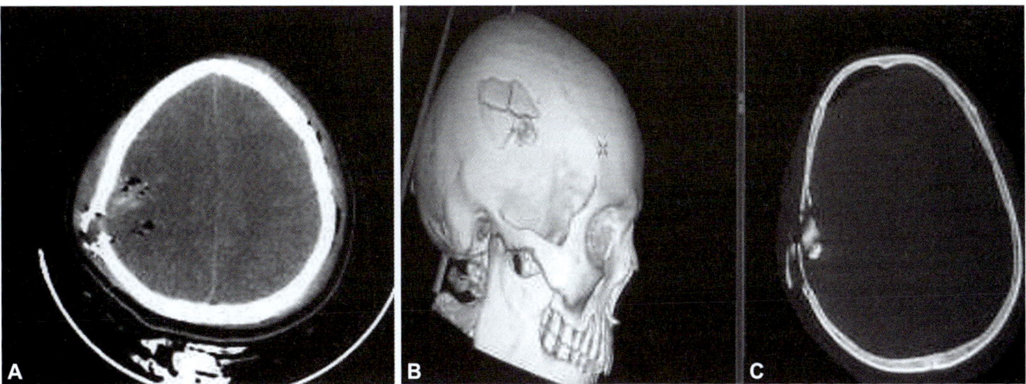

Figs. 11.2A to C: (A) Axial image; (B) 3D image; (C) Bone window settings. CT images from the same patient shown in **Figure 11.1**. See the superior bone and soft tissue details in CT as compared to X-ray.

multiple; midline shift; ventricles dilated or not; sulcal spaces prominent or effaced; symmetric or asymmetric distribution, with or without edema; type of edema, is there any hemorrhage, calcification or fat in lesion; contrast enhancement pattern; associated bony, vascular changes, CV junction, features of raised ICT and most important is significant relevant history.

Cytotoxic edema is seen in conditions like acute ischemic stroke, where there is cell swelling and reduced extracellular space, leading to restricted diffusion, i.e., hyperintense on DWI (low ADC). Also seen in encephalitis (inflammatory edema), epidermoid (due to thick content), high cellular tumors (lymphoma), abscess.

Interstitial edema seen in hydrocephalus is characterized by the accumulation of fluid in the brain's interstitial spaces. **Vasogenic edema** is a type of cerebral edema that occurs due to the breakdown of the blood-brain barrier (BBB), leading to the leakage of fluid into the extracellular space leading to no restricted diffusion, i.e., hypointense on DWI (high ADC). It is typically seen in conditions such as brain tumors, chronic infarct, and trauma. But vasogenic edema (reversible) in PRES appears hyperintense on DWI (also high ADC) primarily due to the dominant T2 shine-through effect due to excessive extracellular fluid, common in posterior parts of brain associated with hypertension, eclampsia and certain medications. Hence it is crucial to look at ADC maps alongside DWI to assess type of edema.

Common Pathologies

Hydrocephalus

- Dilatation of ventricular system, temporal horns of lateral ventricles >6 mm, anterior convexity of third ventricle and distention of third ventricular recesses, round frontal horn of lateral ventricles, periventricular seepage of CSF and effacement of CSF space.
- **Types of hydrocephalus:**
  - *Communicating hydrocephalus:* Obstruction is at the level of arachnoid granulation.
  - *Obstructive hydrocephalus:* External/internal lesion obstructing the CSF flow.
  - *Normal pressure hydrocephalus:* Due to altered CSF dynamics—Enlarged lateral and third ventricles disproportionate to cortical atrophy, *Evans' index* greater than 0.3, *Flow void sign i.e.,* Increased CSF flow void in the aqueduct on T2-weighted MRI.

Congenital Malformations of Brain

Joubert Syndrome

Absence of vermis with hypoplastic elongated cerebellar peduncle giving molar tooth appearance **(Fig. 11.3)**.

Corpus Callosal Agenesis

No midline coma-like white matter tract and periventricular fibers leads to parallel orientation of both lateral ventricles giving racing car sign, and high riding frontal horns giving Viking helmet sign.

Encephalocele

Herniation of cranial content through bony defect in skull. It can commonly congenital. Rarely can be acquired post-traumatic or post-surgery.

Craniosynostosis

Abnormalities in shape of calvarium due to premature fusion of cranial suture. Best evaluated using CT scan.

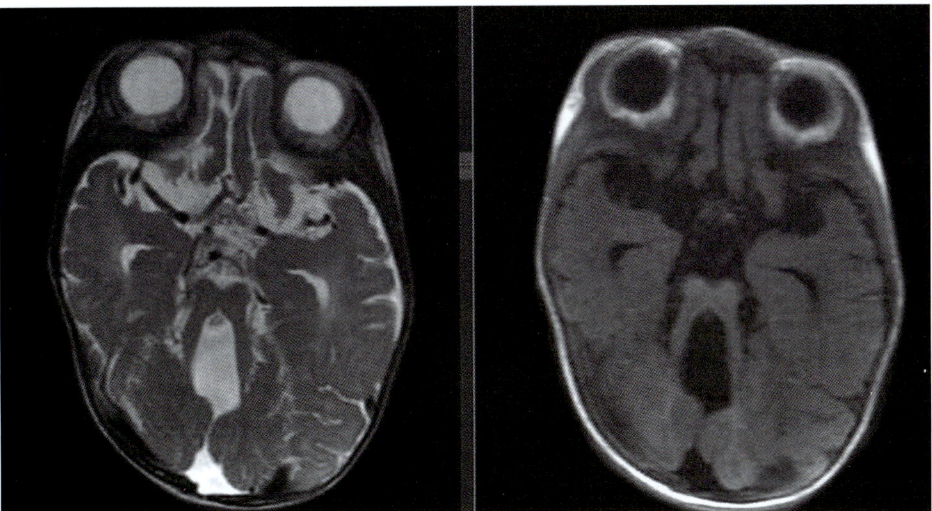

Fig. 11.3: MRI axial images shows absence of vermis (Molar tooth appearance).

- Scaphocephaly—premature fusion of the sagittal suture.
- Trigonocephaly—premature fusion of the metopic suture leading to a triangular forehead.

Chiari Malformation

Herniation of peg-like cerebellar tonsils, >5 mm through foramen magnum into cervical spinal canal with effacement of cervicomedullary junction. Commonly associated with syrinx formation, meningomyelocele and encephalocele.

Dandy-Walker Malformation

Vermian and cerebellar hypoplasia, posterior fossa cyst communicating with the 4th ventricle, enlarged posterior cranial fossa, upturning of torcula, associated with corpus callosal agenesis.

CNS Infections

- **Clinical presentations:** Fever, headache, altered level of consciousness, blurring of vision due to raised intracranial pressure; neck rigidity on clinical examination.
- **MRI brain with contrast is investigation of choice** for diagnosis, detection of raised ICT as it is contraindication for lumbar puncture and detection of complications like empyema, hydrocephalus and infarct.
- **Mode of spread:** Direct or hematogenous leading to breach in blood-brain/blood-CSF barrier and inflammation of brain covering meninges.

Leptomeningitis

Infection of arachnoid and pia mater—pyogenic (bacterial and tubercular)

On MRI

- FLAIR hyperintensity along sulci and gyri with effacement of CSF space and cistern.
- On post-contrast images there is branching linear enhancement of meninges with extension along the sulci and gyri complications:
  - Empyema—shows extra-axial diffusion restriction (bright on DW)
  - Ventriculitis—linear enhancement along ventricle wall with or without fluid level
  - Hydrocephalus

Pachymeningitis

Infection of dura—the enhancement pattern has linear thick line with no deep extension except along interhemispheric fissure and along tentorial leaves—infective/related to connective tissue disorders/IGG4 related.

Viral Encephalitis

Viral encephalitis can involve grey matter only (arbovirus, HSV) or white matter only (HIV, CMV) or both (measles, enterovirus)

- **Gray matter of medial temporal lobe and olfactory gyrus:** Herpes virus.
- **Deep gray matter nucleus with hemorrhage:** Flavivirus (dengue, Japanese encephalitis, etc.)
- Flavivirus encephalitis

Brain Abscess (Figs. 11.4A to D)

- T2 hyperintense lesion with perifocal edema, ring enhancement and central diffusion restriction.
- Stages of abscess formation—early cerebritis, late cerebritis, early abscess and capsular stage

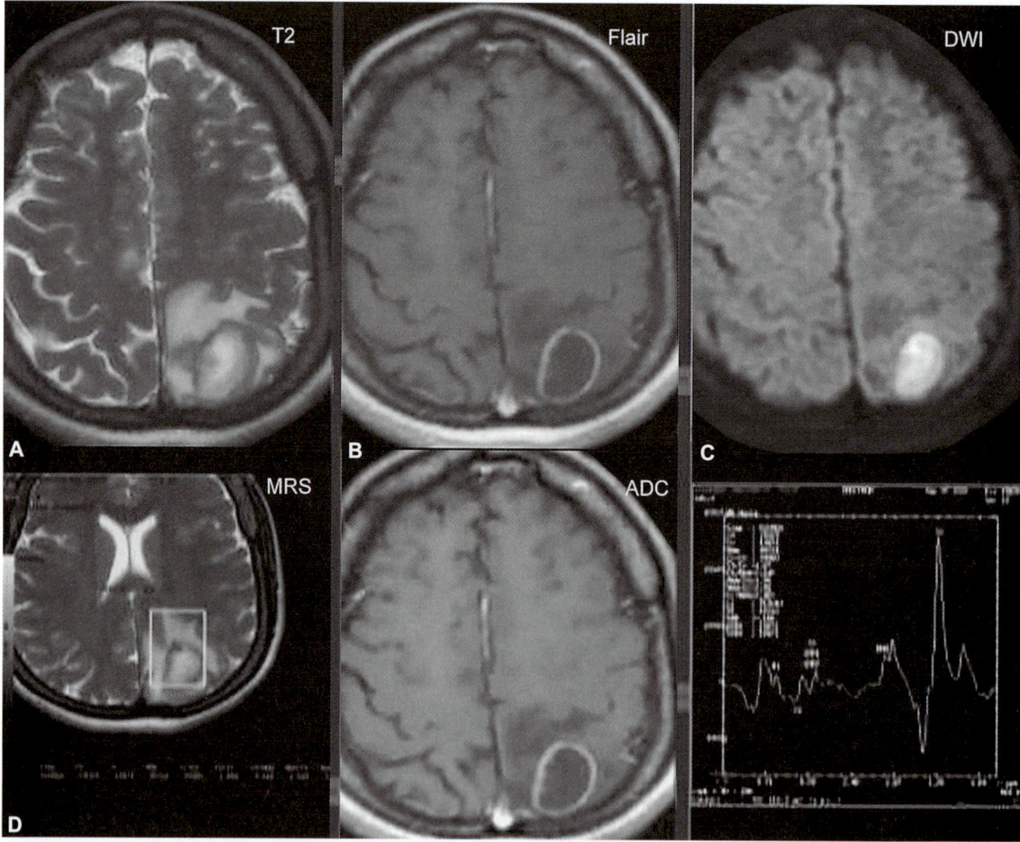

Figs. 11.4A to D: MRI brain axial sections shows brain abscess in left parietal lobe on various sequences: (A) T2 hyper-intense lesion with hypointense rim and significant perilesional edema; (B) FLAIR shows suppressed central content with hyperintense rim; (C) Central part shows diffusion restriction; (D) Amino-acid peak on MR-spectroscopy.

Tuberculoma (Figs. 11.5A to D)

- T2 hypointense lesion with rim enhancement and lipid-lactate peak on spectroscopy.
- Imaging findings depends on the degree of caseation **(Table 11.5)**.

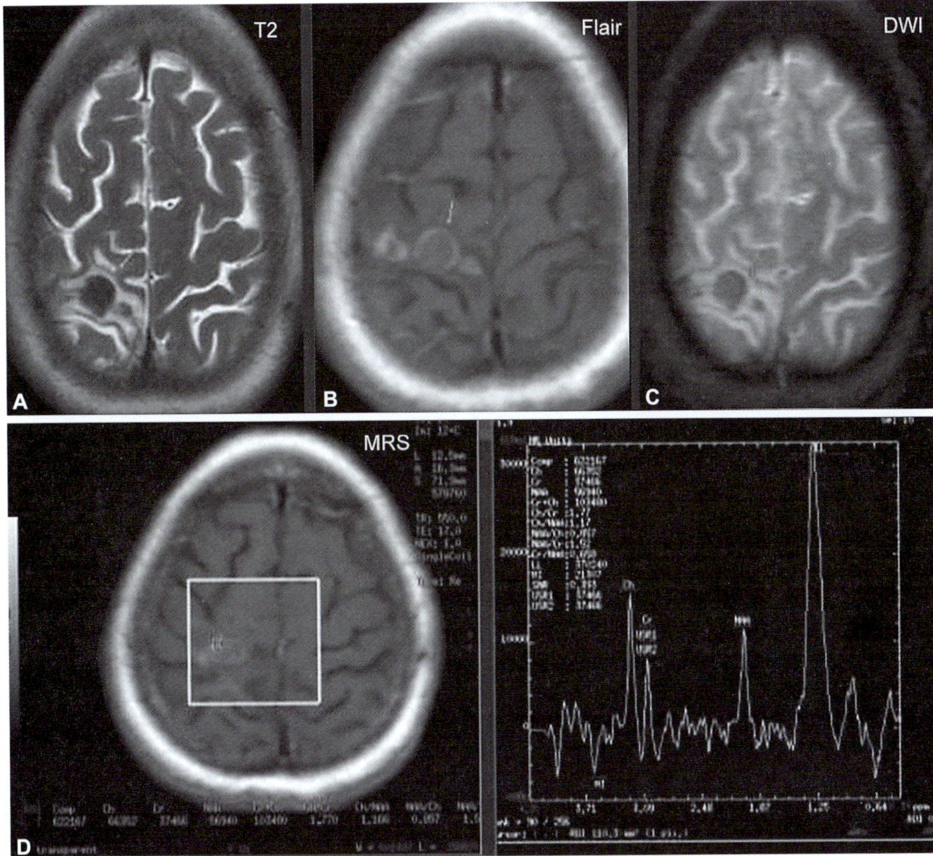

Figs. 11.5A to D: MRI brain axial sections shows appearance of tuberculoma in various sequences: (A) Small T2 hypointense lesion with mild perilesional edema; (B) On FLAIR appears hypointense with hyperintense rim; (C) Appears hypointense on DWI; (D) Shows lipid-lactate peak on MR-spectroscopy.

Table 11.5: Differential diagnosis for ring enhancing lesion.

Etiology	*T2*	*DWI*	*Post-contrast*	*Spectro*
Pyogenic	Hyperintense core/ hypointense rim	Central restriction, hyperintense	Thin or moderately thick ring enhancement/dual rim	Amino acid peak
Tuberculoma (Depends on caseation)	Hyperintense	No diffusion restriction	Solid	Lipid/lactate peak
	Hypointense	No diffusion restriction	—	Lipid/lactate peak
	Core hyperintense, rim hypointense	Restriction is variable	Irregular ring enhancement	Lipid/lactate peak

Contd...

Contd...

Etiology	*T2*	*DWI*	*Post-contrast*	*Spectro*
Tubercular abscess	Hyperintense core/ hypointense rim	Central restriction	Ring enhancement	Lipid/lactate peak
NCC	Hyperintense with dot	No	Ring enhancement	Amino-acid peak
Demyelination	Hyperintense	Restriction in acute (active disease)	Thin open ring	Variable
Glioblastoma	Hyperintense	Peripheral	Thick, irregular	Choline peak, reduced NAA, lipid/lactate peak
Metastasis	Hyperintense (+/– hemorrhage, calcification)	Variable	Solid/thick rim with necrosis	Choline peak, lipid in necrosis

Neurocysticercosis (NCC)

T2 hyperintense/FLAIR hypointense thin-wall-rim-enhancing lesion with cyst and dot appearance due to scolex.

Vascular Lesions

Infarction

Early signs on CT scan are: Hypodense parenchyma, loss of grey-white matter differentiation, hyperdense vessels, loss of normal definition of basal ganglia, insular ribbon sign, focal cerebral swelling (localized effacement of sulci).

Later on, obvious hypodense area is seen due to liquefactive necrosis of infarcted tissue on CT scan **(Table 11.6)**.

MRI appearance: Diffusion-weighted MR images can detect ischemic stroke as early as 30 minutes of onset of symptoms and before changes are perceptible by CT scan **(Figs. 11.6A to D)**.

Lacunar Infarct

- Less than 15 mm-sized infarct due to small perforator vessels occlusion
- Involve basal ganglia, thalamus, internal capsule, corona radiata and pons. Can be seen in ischemic stroke as well as infective (tuberculosis)

Table 11.6: Stages of ischemic stroke.

Stage	*CT scan*	*DWI*	*ADC*	*T2*	*FLAIR*
Hyperacute <6 hours	Normal	Restricted diffusion, hyperintense	Hypointense	Isointense	Isointense
Acute >6 hours	Hypodense	Restricted diffusion, hyperintense	Hypointense	Hyperintense	Hyperintense
Chronic >1 month	CSF density	Hypointense	Hyperintense	Hyperintense	Hypointense with surrounding hyperintense gliotic rim

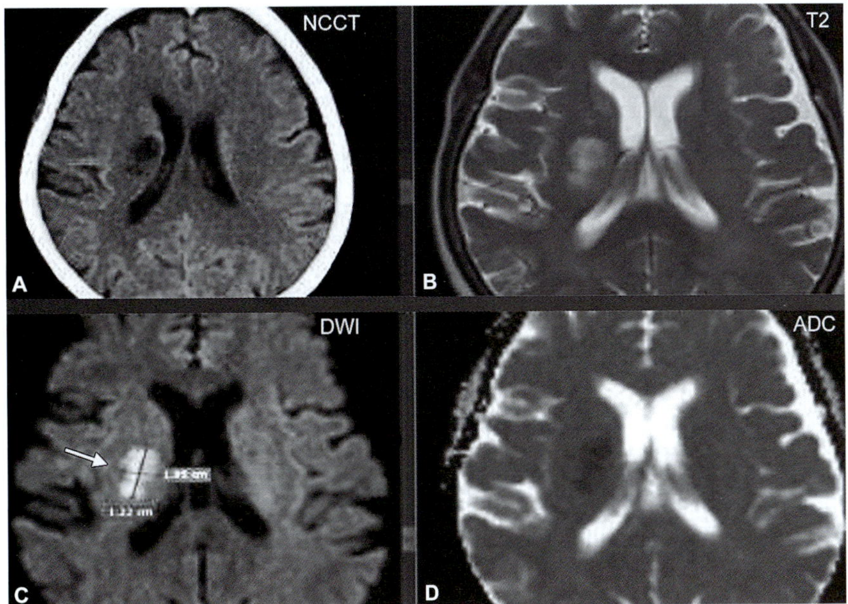

Figs. 11.6A to D: Shows appearance of acute infarct on axial section of NCCT and various sequences of MRI. (A) NCCT shows an ill-defined hypodense area in the right basal ganglia; (B) T2 hyperintense signal; (C) Lesion in right basal ganglia shows restriction on diffusion, i.e., bright on DWI; (D) Dark on ADC.

Hemorrhagic Infarct

- Venous infarcts are usually hemorrhagic and they do not correspond to arterial territorial distribution.
- Commonly associated with hypercoagulable conditions, pregnancy, etc.
- Secondary hemorrhage is also seen in arterial infarcts (hemorrhagic transformation).
- Imaging helps in detecting thrombosis of cerebral veins or dural venous sinuses.
- **CT scan:** Cord sign (hyperdense cerebral vein or dural venous sinus) on plain scans and empty delta sign on contrast scans.
- **MR venography** best depicts dural venous sinus or cerebral venous thrombosis.

Intracranial Hemorrhage

- Intracranial hemorrhage can be traumatic or nontraumatic (hypertensive bleed, aneurysm, vascular malformation, coagulopathy, tumor).
- According to location, it can be intraparenchymal, intraventricular, subarachnoid, extradural or subdural.
- If we see any hemorrhagic cerebral lesion, we should also consider other causes like hemorrhagic venous infarct, hemorrhage in arterial infarct, SOL with hemorrhage, etc.
- Acute hemorrhage is hyperdense (white) on CT scan and variable on MRI.
- Gradient Echo (GRE sequence) and susceptibility-weighted MR imaging are most helpful to detect hemorrhage **(Table 11.7)**.

Subarachnoid Hemorrhage (SAH)

- CT scan is primary investigation of choice for SAH.
- **Aneurysmal bleed:** Hyperdense area in sulci and CSF cistern with effacement.
- Sentinel clot adjacent to the target lesion.

Table 11.7: Stage of Blood in MRI and CT.

Stage	*CT*	*T1*	*GRE*
Hyperacute	Hyperdense	Isointense	Variable, rim blooming
Acute	Hyperdense	Isointense	Increased blooming, hypointense
Subacute	Isodense	Hyperintense	Increased blooming, hypointense
Chronic	Hypodense	Hypointense	Hypointense

- CT brain with angiography is the first choice for SAH detection, diagnoses, characterization of the lesion and post surgery follow-up.
- **MR angiography** can be done without the use of iodinated contrast media, but time-consuming.

Hypertensive Hemorrhage

- In uncontrolled hypertensive patients
- Presentation—with acute weakness.
- Typically involve basal ganglia, thalamus, pons and white matter
- May extend into ventricle.

Brain Tumor/Neoplasms

Investigation of choice is MRI brain with contrast. ***Basic approach includes*** *localize the lesion, extra-axial vs intra-axial, characterize the lesion with T2/T1/GRE signal/DW, describe the effect of lesion on surrounding, edema.*

Extra-axial lesion located outside the brain but within cranial cavity. Includes pathology related to meninges, blood vessels, nerves, interhemispheric fissure, cerebellopontine angle, ventricles and sellar region, etc. Features of extra-axial location include:

- CSF cleft between brain and lesion
- Vessels between brain and lesion
- Cortex between brain and lesion, clear distinct margin
- Dura (meninges) between brain and lesion

1. A common neoplastic lesion of skull in adult is multiple myeloma shows multiple punched-out lesion in inner and outer table of skull giving rain drop appearance **(Figs. 11.7A and B)**.

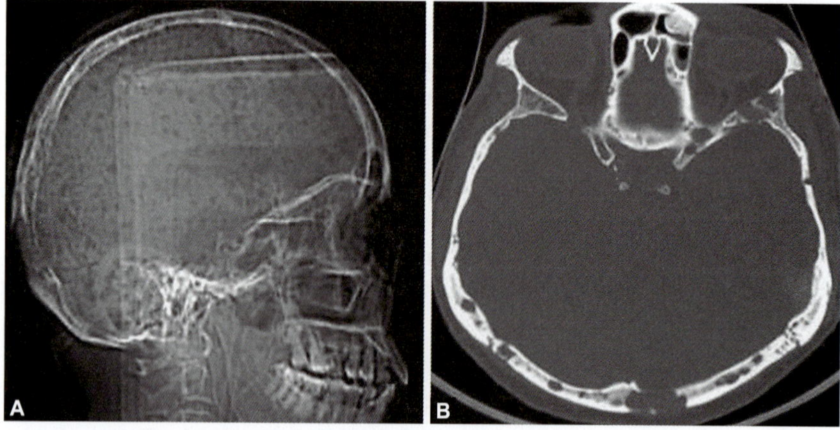

Figs. 11.7A and B: Multiple myeloma: (A) Showing multiple well circumscribed punched-out lytic lesions diffusely scattered in skull on X-ray skull lateral view; (B) Axial section, bone window on NCCT also confirmed it.

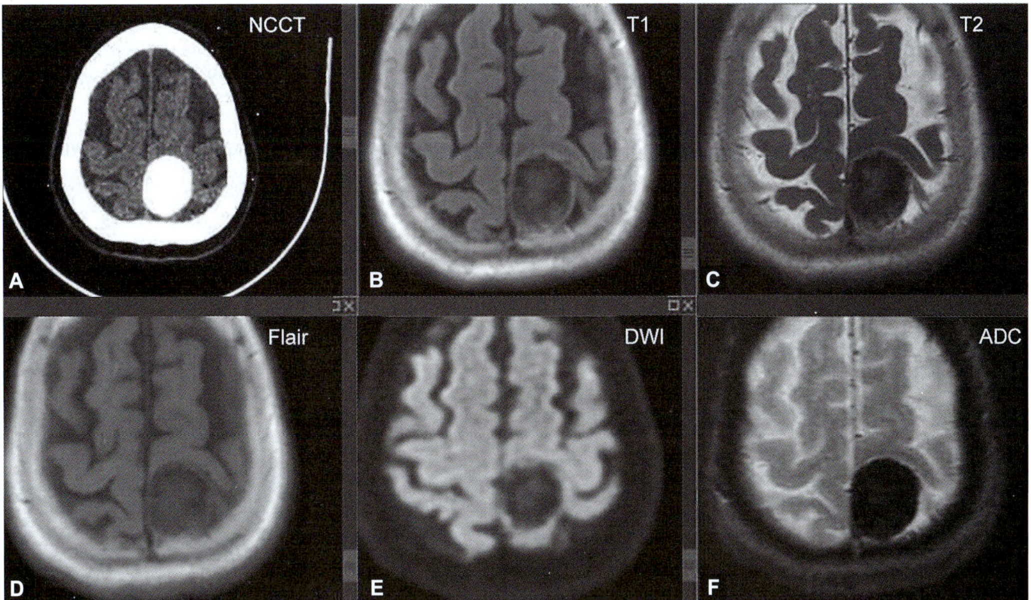

Figs. 11.8A to F: Shows appearance of calcified space occupying lesion, i.e., meningioma on axial section of NCCT and various sequences of MRI; A large, well-defined, extra-axial solid lesion which is hyperdense on NCCT (A); hypointense on T1 (B); T2 (C); FLAIR (D); DWI (E); ADC (F).

2. **Meningioma (Figs. 11.8A to F):**
   - An extra-axial lesion is broad-based, shows buckling of gray, white matter and CSF cleft sign.
   - Hyperdense on CT, T2 hypo/isointense with intense enhancement and thick dural tail sign and sclerosis (hyperostosis) of overlying bone.
   - Calcified meningioma is burned-out meningioma.
3. **CP angle cistern:**
   - Schwannoma in the right CP angle cistern, extra-axial, enhancing T2 hyperintense with extension in to internal auditory canal (ice-cream cone appearance)
   - Sclerosis of bone and dural tail sign—favors meningioma as a differential.
   - CP angle lesion following CSF signal and restricted diffusion—epidermoid cyst.

   If no diffusion restriction → arachnoid cyst.
4. Brain gliomas are a diverse group of primary brain tumors that arise from glial cells, which support and protect neurons. Gliomas are classified based on the type of glial cell they originate from (e.g., oligodendroglioma, astrocytoma, etc.) and their histological grade (Grade I low grade to high grade).

Seizure Disorders

- Children with NICU admission, failure to cry after birth and prematurity—hypoxic ischemic insult/encephalopathy is common cause
- Complex partial seizures refractory to antiepileptics: Common cause is mesial temporal sclerosis
  - MRI shows hippocampal atrophy with abnormal T2/FLAIR hyperintense signal.

- Seizures can also be presenting complaint in infection, tumor and congenital malformation
- **Schizencephaly**—the presence of CSF cleft lined with grey matter can extend from the pia mater to the lateral ventricles. Two types—open lip and closed lip schizencephaly, can be unilateral or bilateral.
- **Grey matter heterotopia**—ectopic normal grey matter along the normal path of neuronal migration.

Metabolic Encephalopathies

1. **Acute hypoxic:**
   - Involves parietal and occipital cortex, deep gray matter and perirolandic cortex
   - Appear hyperintense on T2, shows restricted diffusion and appear symmetrical
2. **Acute hypoglycemic:**
   - Patient with serum glucose <60 mg/dL
   - Involves posterior limb of internal capsule and thalamus with restricted diffusion.
3. **Hypertensive:**
   - Multiple foci of blooming in bilateral cerebral cortex, basal ganglia, thalamus and cerebellum: Hypertensive microangiopathy.
   - The differential is amyloid angiopathy which spares the basal ganglia.
4. **Liver disease:**
   - Asymmetrical involvement of insular cortex, anterior frontal lobe and medial temporal lobe. Raised serum ammonia level
   - Symmetrical T1 hyperintensity in basal ganglia and ventral aspect of midbrain due to manganese deposition in chronic liver disease.

Neurocutaneous Syndromes

Also known as phakomatoses. They are genetic disorders characterized by the involvement of both the nervous system and the skin. These syndromes often involve the development of benign and malignant tumors in various parts of the body, along with other abnormalities affecting the skin, eyes, and other organs.

Neurofibromatosis (optic gliomas, neurofibromas, vestibular schwannomas, meningiomas) Tuberous sclerosis (cortical tubers, subependymal nodules, SEGAs) Sturge-Weber syndrome (leptomeningeal angiomas, cortical atrophy, tram-track calcifications), Von Hippel-Lindau disease and Ataxia-Telangiectasia.

Neurodegenerative Disorders

A group of disorders characterized by the progressive degeneration of the structure and function of the nervous system. These diseases often lead to irreversible disability and can affect various parts of the nervous system, e.g.,

- **Alzheimer's disease:** Medial temporal lobe atrophy, enlarged ventricles, white matter changes
- **Parkinson's disease:** Subtle midbrain atrophy, iron deposition in substantia nigra, normal routine MRI
- **Huntington's disease:** Caudate nucleus atrophy, generalized cerebral atrophy

So after short discussion on common indications of neuroradiology, we can conclude utilities of various modalities as per clinical complaints as shown in **Table 11.8**.

Table 11.8: Shows the investigation of choice according to age and clinical presentation.

Complaints	*CT*	*Contrast CT*	*MRI plain*	*Contrast MRI*	*MRI brain with angiography*
Trauma	Yes	No	If CT is normal To detect diffuse axonal injury	No	
Epilepsy			Epilepsy protocol	Yes	
Infection				Yes	
Neoplasm				Yes	
Infarct	Yes		Yes		Yes
Pediatric trauma	Yes				
Child with developmental delay			Yes		
Dementia			Yes		

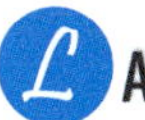

AST MINUTE REVISION

- CT is fast, can give excellent bone details and can detect hemorrhage, but has radiation risk
- MRI has no radiation risk, give excellent soft tissue detail, can also detect hemorrhage, but long acquisition time
- For infarct, MRI brain with diffusion and angiography is good choice.
- To rule out hemorrhage, CT is best and fast.
- Any given images of brain look for symmetry, midline shift, ventricles, CSF cistern, posterior fossa and cranio-vertebral junction.
- **Lesions showing restricted diffusion on MRI (hyperintense):** Acute infarct, epidermoid, abscess cavity, highly cellular tumor likely lymphoma, or medulloblastoma.

REVIEW QUESTIONS

Multiple Choice Questions (MCQs)

1. **Identify the given image plane, modality and name the labeled structure:**

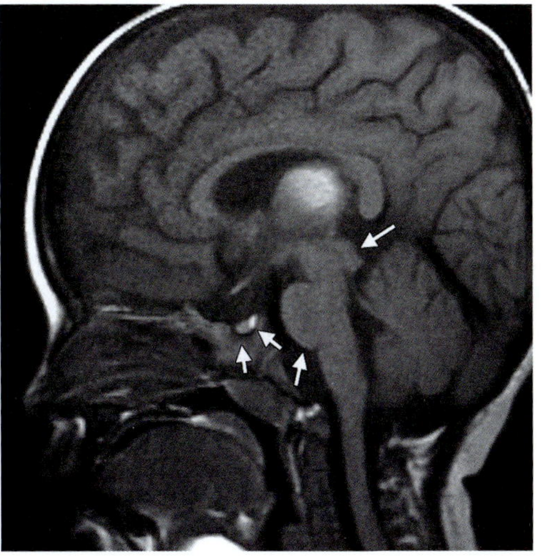

a. Axial T2 MRI showing pons and medulla
b. Axial CT showing cerebellum
c. DW MRI
d. Sagittal MRI of brain showing pituitary gland, pons and tectal plate.

2. **Identify the lesion in image, modality and diagnosis.**

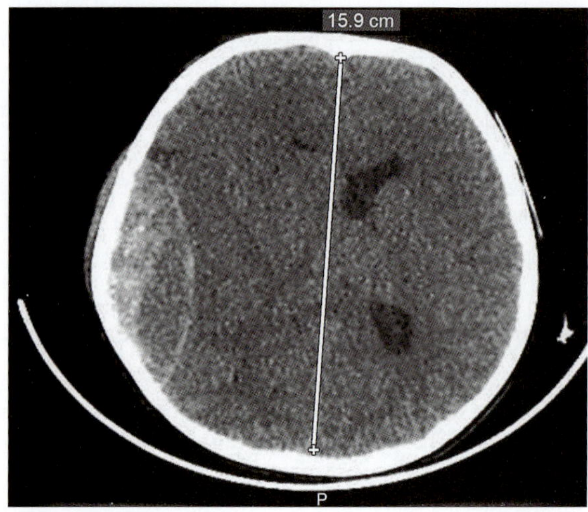

a. Axial CT brain showing acute infarct
b. MRI brain shows acute infarct
c. Axial CT of brain showing acute EDH with midline shift
d. Coronal MRI for pituitary adenoma

3. **Which of the following is not lesion of CP angle cistern?**
   a. Glioma
   b. Arachnoid cyst
   c. Schwannoma
   d. Meningioma

4. **Normal appearance of fluid on MRI:**
   a. T1 hyperintense
   b. T2 hypointense
   c. T2 hyperintense
   d. FLAIR hyperintense

5. **Modality of choice for hyperacute infarct:**
   a. CT
   b. MRI
   c. X-ray
   d. USG

Answer Key

1. d 2. c 3. a 4. c 5. b

SUGGESTED READING

1. Adam A, Dixon AK, Gillard JH, Schaefer-Prokop C, Grainger RG, Allison DJ. Grainger and Allison's Diagnostic Radiology. Elsevier Health Sciences; 2014.
2. Bailey and Love's Short Practice of Surgery, 27th edition. CRC Press. https://doi.org/10.1201/9781315111087
3. O'Connell PR, McCaskie AW, Williams NS. (Eds). 2018.
4. William E Brant, Clyde A Helms. Fundamentals of Diagnostic Radiology. Philadelphia, PA: Lippincott, Williams and Wilkins; 2007.

CHAPTER

12

Chest Imaging

"Chest imaging is the window to life—where every breath, vessel, and shadow tells a story waiting to be read."

INTRODUCTION

Chest imaging encompasses a range of diagnostic techniques used to visualize and assess the structures within the thoracic cavity, including the lungs, heart, and surrounding tissues. It is a fundamental component of medical diagnostics, providing critical information for the evaluation and management of various chest conditions. It is a very important region in all aspects as it deals with imaging of respiratory and circulatory organ, i.e., lung and heart. Besides this, not only radiologists but clinicians are also very keen to understand the basic modality of chest imaging, i.e., chest X-ray. In other systems of body though cross-sectional modality encompasses the 2D X-rays, it is one of the region where still X-ray play vital role in diagnosis as well as guider to select proper methodology to diagnose chest diseases. Other imaging modalities used in chest imaging are, computed tomography (CT), magnetic resonance imaging (MRI), ultrasound and PET scans.

MODALITIES USED IN CHEST IMAGING

Chest Radiography (X-ray)

Chest radiography is the most commonly performed imaging test for the evaluation of the thoracic cavity. It provides a quick and effective method for assessing the lungs, mediastinum and thoracic cage. X-rays are typically the first step in the diagnostic process for patients with symptoms such as cough, chest pain, trauma or shortness of breath. Reading of chest X-ray includes Airways, bones, Cardiac, Diaphragm, effusion, fields of lung, gastric bubble, hilum (ABCDEFGH). There are various views of chest X-ray as per requirements **(Table 12.1)**. These are as follows:

Commonly advised chest X-rays are AP and PA view **(Table 12.2)** which can be differentiating under these points.

Computed Tomography

Computed tomography (CT) scanning offers detailed cross-sectional images of the thorax and is particularly useful in evaluating complex thoracic pathology. It is the gold standard for diagnosing conditions such as pulmonary embolism, lung cancer, and interstitial lung disease. It also aids CT guided biopsies. High-resolution CT (HRCT) is specifically used for detailed assessment of lung parenchyma. Chest CT should be viewed in soft tissue as well as bone window. There are various protocols for doing chest CT which are as follows **(Table 12.3)**:

Table 12.1: Chest radiograph's view as per indications.

View	*Indications*
Posteroanterior (PA) view	Standard view for most diagnostic purposes, assessing heart and lungs
Anteroposterior (AP) view	Used when the patient is unable to stand (e.g., critically ill or immobilized patients), commonly done in wards/ICU, trauma patient
Lateral view	Provides additional information related to the extent and location of lesions, useful for assessing the retrosternal and retrocardiac spaces. Helps to divide the gross distribution of pathology in various mediastinal compartment and to assess vertebrae pathology
Lateral decubitus view	Evaluates pleural effusion by assessing fluid movement with gravity and detects small pneumothoraxes
Lordotic view	Evaluates the lung apices, useful for detecting apical tumors or tuberculosis

Table 12.2: Differentiating features of Chest X-ray PA and AP view.

Feature	*AP view*	*PA view*
Direction of X-ray beam	X-ray beam passes from front (anterior) to back (posterior)	X-ray beam passes from back (posterior) to front (anterior)
Patient position	Patient is usually lying down or seated	Patient is standing
Heart size appearance	Heart appears larger due to magnification	Heart size is more accurate due to less magnification
Scapulae position	Scapulae are often visible over the lungs	Scapulae are moved away from the lung fields
Usage	Used for bedridden patients or those unable to stand	Standard view for ambulatory patients
Clavicles	Clavicles often appear higher and more horizontal	Clavicles appear in a more natural position
Lung fields	Lung fields may appear less clear due to patient position and scapula overlap	Lung fields are clearer
Radiographic exposure	Typically, lower quality due to patient positioning and technical factors	Higher quality due to better patient positioning
Clinical situations	Intensive care units, emergency situations, immobile patients, trauma, especially for bony cage	Routine check-ups, outpatient settings
Diaphragm	Diaphragm appears higher and less sharply defined	Diaphragm appears lower and more clearly defined

Magnetic Resonance Imaging (Table 12.4)

Magnetic resonance imaging (MRI) is less commonly used in thoracic imaging compared to X-ray and CT due to its longer imaging times and higher cost. However, it provides superior soft tissue contrast and is valuable in evaluating thoracic outlet syndrome, cardiac conditions, and in some cases, lung and mediastinal tumors.

Table 12.3: Description of various types of chest CT.

Type of CT	*Indications*	*Advantages*	*Disadvantages*
Noncontrast chest CT	General chest evaluation, lung infections, interstitial lung disease, lung nodules/ masses, pulmonary embolism, trauma	Detailed images of chest anatomy, quick and widely available, good for a broad range of chest pathologies	• Radiation exposure • May require contrast for certain diagnoses • Limited detail for interstitial lung disease compared to HRCT
High-resolution CT (HRCT)	• Interstitial lung disease, pulmonary fibrosis • Small airways disease • Bronchiectasis	• High detail for lung parenchyma • Better evaluation of interstitial lung diseases	• Higher radiation dose due to multiple thin slices • Not ideal for general chest evaluation • Limited soft tissue and vascular detail
Contrast-enhanced CT (CECT) (Fig. 12.1)	• Pulmonary embolism • Lung cancer staging • Vascular abnormalities • Pleural disease • Lymphadenopathy • SPN and mediastinal mass	• Enhanced visualization of vessels and soft tissues • Improved detection of masses and lymph nodes	• Risk of contrast-induced nephropathy • Contrast allergy risk • Higher cost than non-contrast CT
3D CT (Fig. 12.2)	• Preoperative planning • Vascular imaging (e.g., aneurysms, embolisms) • Complex fractures • Congenital anomalies • Tumor assessment	• Enhanced anatomical visualization • Interactive viewing from multiple angles • Useful for surgical planning and complex anatomy	• Higher radiation dose • Requires advanced software and expertise • Higher cost
CT bronchoscopy (virtual bronchoscopy)	• Airway obstructions • Tracheobronchial pathologies • Preoperative planning for airway surgery • Foreign body detection • Evaluation of hemoptysis	• Noninvasive • Detailed airway visualization • No need for sedation/ anesthesia	• Cannot perform biopsies or therapeutic interventions • Limited by image resolution and quality • Radiation exposure

Table 12.4: Common indications of MRI chest.

Anatomical division	*Indications*	*MRI sequences*
Mediastinum	• Mediastinal masses (tumor characterization, cysts) • Lymphadenopathy • Thymic abnormalities	• T1-weighted imaging • T2-weighted imaging • Short tau inversion recovery (STIR) • Contrast-enhanced T1-weighted imaging
Chest Wall	• Tumor invasion (e.g., pancoast tumors) • Soft tissue masses • Inflammatory conditions	• T1-weighted imaging • T2-weighted imaging—STIR • Contrast-enhanced T1-weighted imaging
Lungs	• Parenchymal diseases • Tumor characterization and staging • Pulmonary hypertension	• T2-weighted imaging • Balanced steady-state free precession (BSSFP) • Contrast-enhanced MR angiography (MRA)

Contd...

Contd...

Anatomical division	*Indications*	*MRI sequences*
Heart	• Cardiomyopathy • Cardiac masses • Pericardial diseases • Congenital heart disease	• Cine MRI (balanced SSFP) • T1-weighted imaging • T2-weighted imaging • Late gadolinium enhancement (LGE)
Diaphragm	• Diaphragmatic paralysis • Diaphragmatic eventration	• Cine MRI • T1-weighted imaging
Vascular structures	• Aortic aneurysms • Aortic dissections • Congenital vascular anomalies	• Contrast-enhanced MR angiography (MRA) • Balanced SSFP

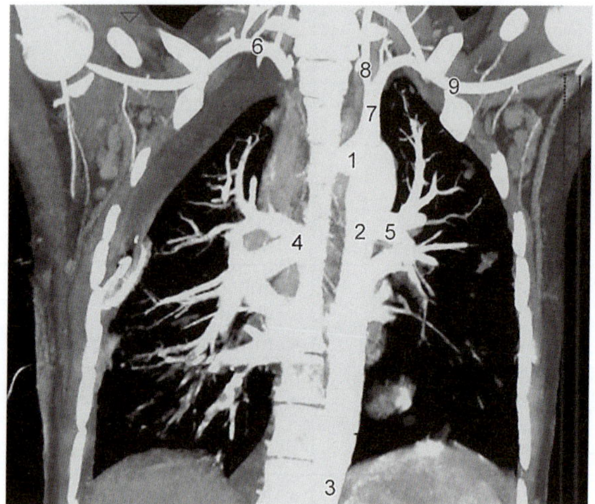

Fig. 12.1: CT Pulmonary angiography (coronal section) shows: (1) Arch of aorta; (2) Descending thoracic aorta; (3) Descending abdominal aorta; (4) Right main pulmonary artery; (5) Left main pulmonary artery; (6) Right subclavian artery; (7) Brachiocephalic artery; (8) Left common carotid artery; (9) Left subclavian artery.

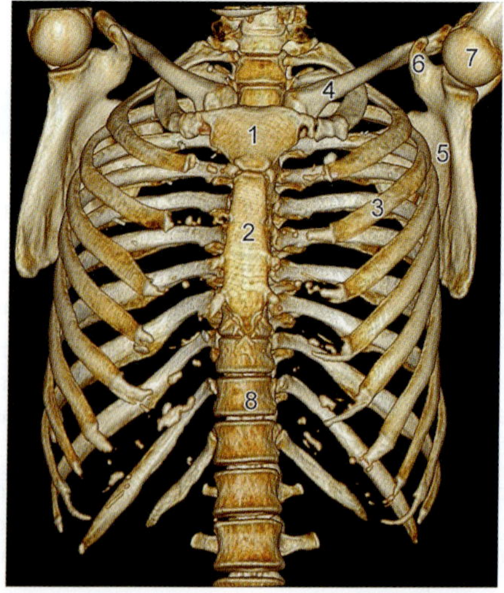

Fig. 12.2: 3D Volume CT chest (Coronal section) shows: (1) Manubrium sterni; (2) Sternum; (3) Rib; (4) Clavicle; (5) Scapula; (6) Coracoid process; (7) Head of humerus and (8) Vertebrae body.

Table 12.5: Features of thoracic ultrasound.

Category	*Details*
Equipment	• **Ultrasound machine:** High-resolution with thoracic imaging software • **Transducers:** Linear probe: 5–12 MHz, Curvilinear probe: 2–5 MHz, Phased array probe: For cardiac and deeper structures
Patient positioning	• **Sitting or semi-sitting:** For anterior and lateral chest wall evaluation • **Supine or semi-supine:** For posterior chest evaluation and bedridden patients • **Lateral decubitus:** For assessing pleural effusions and better visualization of lateral structures
Image acquisition	• **Scanning technique:** Systematic approach (anterior, lateral, posterior regions) • **Image orientation:** Correct probe marker orientation (towards head or right side) • **Depth settings:** Adjust for clear visualization • **Gain settings:** Adjust for optimal brightness and contrast
Common views	• **Longitudinal (sagittal) view:** Comprehensive overview • **Transverse (axial) view:** Detailed assessment of specific areas • **Oblique views:** For diaphragm and pleural spaces
Key structures	• **Chest wall:** Ribs, intercostal muscles, subcutaneous tissues • **Pleura:** Visceral and parietal pleura, pleural effusions • **Lungs:** Lung sliding, comet-tail artifacts, consolidation, air bronchograms • **Diaphragm:** Movement and integrity • **Mediastinum:** Large vessels and possible masses (limited view)
Artifacts	• **A-lines:** Horizontal reverberation artifacts (normal aerated lung) • **B-lines:** Vertical artifacts (interstitial syndrome or pulmonary edema) • **Lung point:** Transition point in pneumothorax • **Absence of lung sliding:** Suggestive of pneumothorax or pleural adhesions
Advantages	• **Noninvasive:** No ionizing radiation • **Bedside availability:** Useful in emergency and ICU • **Real-time imaging:** Dynamic assessment of lung and pleural movement
Limitations	• **Operator dependent:** Requires skill and experience • **Limited penetration:** Difficulty imaging deeper structures or through bone and air • **Subject to artifacts:** Interpretation challenges due to artifacts

Ultrasound

Thoracic ultrasound is frequently used for bedside evaluation in critically ill patients. It is particularly useful for diagnosing pleural effusions, pneumothorax, and guiding thoracentesis and biopsy procedures. Ultrasound is noninvasive, lacks ionizing radiation, and can be performed at the patient's bedside. It can also detect consolidation as well as used for POCUS in trauma patient. It needs very expertise and used in various positions by different probes as per requirements. These features are described in **Table 12.5**.

RADIOLOGICAL COMPARTMENTS OF CHEST

Chest imaging plays a crucial role in the diagnosis, management, and follow-up of a wide variety of thoracic diseases. Advances in imaging technology continue to enhance our ability to detect and characterize thoracic pathology, improving patient outcomes. For better and easy diagnosis, chest should be divided into basic three compartments **(Table 12.6)** which are as follows.

Table 12.6: Anatomical division of the thorax with imaging modalities, normal/abnormal appearance.

Compartment	*Structures included*	*Common pathologies*	*Preferred imaging modalities*	*Normal appearance*	*Abnormal appearance*
1. Lungs and pleura Origin: respiratory diverticulum and splanchnic mesoderm	**Lungs:** Lobes (right: 3, left: 2, divided by fissures), Bronchopulmonary segments (right: 10 and left: 8) contains segmental bronchi with associated vessels	Pneumonia, lung cancer, COPD, tuberculosis, bronchitis, lung nodules, interstitial lung disease	**Chest X-ray** Initial evaluation **CT scan:** Detailed assessment **HRCT:** Interstitial lung disease **Ultrasound:** Rarely advised for consolidation	Clear lucent lung fields, no opacities or masses, normal lung markings not extend in lateral one third and upper one third of lung field	Infiltrates, nodules, masses, consolidation, hyperinflation, interstitial opacities, fibrosis, atelectasis
	Pleura: Visceral pleura and parietal pleura with pleural space in between	Pleural effusion, pneumothorax, pleural thickening, pleural tumors	**Chest X-ray:** Initial detection **Ultrasound:** For effusions **CT scan:** In empyema, tumors	Pleural space barely visible, no fluid accumulation	Fluid accumulation, air in pleural space, thickened pleura, pleural masses
2. Mediastinum	**Anterior mediastinum:** Thymus, fat, lymph nodes	Thymoma, teratoma, lymphoma, thyroid masses	**CT scan:** Masses **MRI:** For extent and it's internal characteristics	Clear delineation of thymus and fat, normal size and shape of structures	Masses, enlarged lymph nodes, abnormal density or contrast enhancement
	Middle Mediastinum: Heart, pericardium, great vessels (aorta, pulmonary arteries/veins), trachea, main bronchi, lymph nodes, hila	Cardiac diseases, aortic aneurysm, pulmonary embolism (PE), lymphadenopathy	**CT scan:** Aortic aneurysm, pulmonary embolism (PE) **MRI:** Cardiac structures **Echocardiography:** Heart **PET-CT:** Lymphomas	Normal heart and vessel size and shape, clear trachea and bronchi, no lymphadenopathy	Enlarged heart or vessels, aortic dilation, filling defects in vessels (PE), masses, enlarged lymph nodes
	Posterior mediastinum: Esophagus, descending aorta, thoracic duct, sympathetic chain	Esophageal tumors, neurogenic tumors, aortic abnormalities	**CT scan:** Extent and nature of lesion **MRI:** Soft tissue characterization **Barium swallow:** Esophagus	Normal esophageal contour, normal aorta, no masses	Masses, abnormal esophageal contour or narrowing, aortic abnormalities
3. Chest wall and diaphragm	**Chest wall:** Ribs, sternum, intercostal spaces, muscles, skin	Rib fractures, chest wall tumors (sarcomas), infections (osteomyelitis)	**Chest X-ray (CXR):** Fractures **CT scan:** Bone and soft tissue lesion **MRI:** Soft tissue tumors **Ultrasound:** Solid vs cystic	Dense intact rib and sternum, no masses or abnormal shadows	Fractures, masses, osteolytic lesions, soft tissue masses or infections
	Diaphragm: Muscular structure separating thoracic and abdominal cavities	Diaphragmatic hernias, diaphragmatic paralysis, tumors	**Chest X-ray (CXR):** Initial evaluation **CT scan:** Hernias and masses **MRI:** Hernias and masses **Fluoroscopy:** Motion studies	Smooth, continuous diaphragmatic contour, normal motion during breathing	Disrupted or elevated diaphragmatic contour, hernias, abnormal motion, masses

Lung

On chest X-ray, lung is divided into three zones craniocaudal on the basis of anterior end of ribs (zone 1-anterior end of 2–4th rib, zone 2-anterior end of 4–6 rib and zone 3-anterior end

Table 12.7: Identification of normal and abnormal findings of lungs-radiographs.

Structures/lines	*Normal size/appearance*	*Abnormal appearance*
Trachea	Central or slightly to the right	Deviation can indicate a mediastinal shift or pathology
Aortic knob/knuckle	Visible as a smooth, rounded protrusion on the left	Enlargement can suggest aneurysm or hypertension
Heart size and borders	Cardiothoracic ratio in adult <50%, in child <60%	Cardiomegaly if ratio >50% in adult Cardiomegaly if ratio >60% in child
Hilar region	Symmetrical and slightly visible, left is slightly above	Enlargement can indicate lymphadenopathy or vascular congestion
Diaphragm	Right hemidiaphragm slightly higher due to liver than left, sharp costophrenic angles	Flattened diaphragm or blunted costophrenic angles, indicating hyperinflation or pleural effusion respectively
Ribs	Visible with no fractures or deformities	Fractures, lytic lesions, or deformities
Lung fields	Clear, with normal lung markings	Infiltrates, masses, pneumothorax, or increased interstitial markings
Mediastinum	Central with clear borders	Widening can suggest mass, fluid, or vascular enlargement
Costophrenic angles	Sharp and well-defined	Blunting indicates pleural effusion
Pulmonary vessels	Visible in the lower zones, tapering towards the periphery	Prominence or blurring indicates pulmonary hypertension or edema respectively
Clavicles	Symmetrical with even spacing	Fractures, displacement, or asymmetry can indicate injury or deformity
Spine	Visible through the heart shadow	Loss of clarity can suggest mediastinal or paraspinal mass
Paraspinal lines	Should be thin and uniform along the spine (less than 10 mm on left and less than 03 mm on right)	Widening can indicate aortic aneurysm, hematoma, or mass
Paratracheal lines	Normally 2–4 mm in thickness	Thickening (>5 mm) can indicate lymphadenopathy, fibrosis, or mass

of 6–8th rib). It should be read from periphery (chest wall) to central structures (trachea) or vice versa to see all normal anatomical structures, shadows and lines aiding in identification of normal and abnormal findings **(Table 12.7)**.

If there is any abnormality, then various radiological signs **(Table 12.8)** have to be studied that help to differentiate the origin of pathology in terms of parenchymal/extraparenchymal, pleural/extra pleural, lung/mediastinal location.

The mediastinum is the central compartment of the thoracic cavity, located between the two pleural sacs (the lungs). It extends from the sternum in the front to the vertebral column in the back and from the thoracic inlet above to the diaphragm below. Mediastinal pathologies are classified on the basis of location of abnormal findings in various mediastinum either in anterior or posterior or middle mediastinum for increasing diagnostic accuracy. Various types of classifications **(Table 12.9)** are developed to divide the pathology of mediastinum on Chest X-ray and CT scan. These are as follows.

Table 12.8: Various radiological signs related to chest imaging.

Sign	*Description*	*Indications for parenchymal pathology*	*Indications for extra parenchymal pathology (pleura and chest wall)*	*Indications for mediastinal pathology*
Hilar overlay sign	If the hilar structures are visible through a mass, it indicate that the mass is not located in the hilum (middle mediastinum)	Not applicable	Not applicable	Mass located anterior or posterior to hilum, differentiate hilar and nonhilar mass
Silhouette sign **(Fig. 12.3)**	Loss of normal borders between structures of the same radiographic density (e.g., heart, aorta) indicates the level of that pathology	Loss of heart border indicates adjacent lung pathology, i.e., middle lobe	Not applicable	Positive silhouette with adjacent mediastinal structures
Cervicothoracic sign	Upper mediastinal mass above the clavicles is likely in the neck (cervicothoracic junction)	Not applicable	Not applicable	Indicates a superior mediastinal or cervical mass
Extrapleural sign	Convex margin on the chest wall, tapering to the pleura	Acute angle	Smooth, well-defined borders, obtuse angles	Not applicable
Air bronchogram sign	Air-filled bronchi made visible by surrounding alveolar consolidation	Indicates lung consolidation	Not applicable	Not applicable
Continuous diaphragm sign	Continuous diaphragm without interruption suggests pneumomediastinum	Not applicable	Not applicable	Indicates presence of air in the mediastinum (pneumomediastinum)
Westermark sign	Decreased vascular markings distal to a pulmonary embolism	Not applicable	Not applicable	Suggestive of pulmonary embolism in the pulmonary vasculature
Juxtaphrenic peak sign	Elevated peak of diaphragm seen with lower lobe collapse	Indicates lower lobe atelectasis or effusion	Not applicable	Not applicable
Meniscus sign	Curved upper edge of pleural effusion seen on upright chest X-ray	Not applicable	Indicates pleural effusion	Not applicable
Fallen lung sign	Lung falls away from the hilum instead of collapsing towards it, indicating bronchial injury	Indicates severe lung trauma or bronchial disruption	Not applicable	Not applicable

Note:

- Hilar convergence differentiate nodal mass (negative) from vascular cause (positive)
- Right heart border forms by SVC, right atrium and IVC while left heart border forms by aortic knuckle, concavity of pulmonary trunk, left atrial appendage and left ventricle

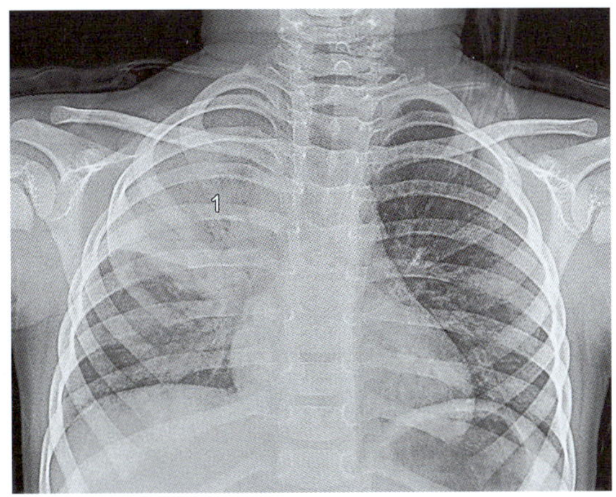

Fig. 12.3: Chest X-ray PA view showing consolidation in right upper lobe having air bronchogram (1) obscuring margin of adjacent structures (silhouette sign).

Table 12.9: Various types of classifications of mediastinal pathologies.

Type of classification	*Boundaries (will decide extent of disease)*	*Contents (will decide the origin of pathology)*
Sutton classification (anatomical classification)		
A. Superior mediastinum	Above upper level of pericardium and level of Ludwig (considered in anatomical classification)	Trachea, esophagus, arch of aorta and its vessels
B. Anterior mediastinum	In front of the anterior pericardium and trachea, behind the sternum	Thymus (particularly in children), lymph nodes, fat
C. Middle mediastinum	Within the pericardial cavity but includes trachea	Heart, pericardium, ascending aorta, pulmonary artery, lymph nodes
D. Posterior mediastinum	Behind the posterior pericardium, trachea and in front of the vertebral column	Descending aorta, esophagus, thoracic duct, lymph nodes
Felson classification (on chest X-ray lateral)		
A. Anterior mediastinum	Between sternum and posterior aspect of heart/great vessels	Thymus, lymph nodes, fat, connective tissue, heart
B. Middle mediastinum	Posterior to the heart and great vessels to a line drawn 1 cm posterior to the anterior edge of thoracic vertebrae	Trachea, bronchi, aortic arch
C. Posterior mediastinum	Space behind the posterior limit of middle mediastinum	Esophagus, descending aorta, azygos and hemiazygos veins, nerves, lymph nodes
ITMIG classification		
A. Prevascular compartment	• Superior—thoracic inlet • Inferior—diaphragm • Anterior—sternum • Lateral—parietal mediastinal pleura • Posterior—anterior aspect of pericardium	• Thymus, fat, lymph nodes • Left brachiocephalic vein
B. Visceral compartment	• Superior—thoracic inlet • Inferior—diaphragm • Anterior—posterior boundaries of prevascular compartment • Posterior—vertical line connecting a point on each thoracic vertebral body at 1 cm posterior to its anterior margin	• Vascular-heart, aorta, thoracic duct, SVC, intrapericardial pulmonary arteries • Nonvascular-trachea, main bronchi, esophagus, lymph nodes

Contd...

Contd...

Type of classification	*Boundaries (will decide extent of disease)*	*Contents (will decide the origin of pathology)*
C. Paravertebral compartment	• Superior—thoracic inlet • Inferior—diaphragm • Anterior—posterior boundaries of visceral compartment • Posterior—vertical line against the posterior margin of the chest wall at lateral margin of the transverse process of thoracic spine	Nerves (sympathetic chain), thoracic spine and paravertebral soft tissues

Common lines or structures **(Table 12.10)** to be noted to understand mediastinal diseases predominantly on CT.

Table 12.10: Common lines or structures.

Line/structure	*Description*	*Clinical utility*
Anterior junction line	Formed by the apposition of the visceral and parietal pleurae of the anterior mediastinum	Helps in identifying anterior mediastinal masses and abnormalities
Posterior junction line	Formed by the apposition of the visceral and parietal pleurae of the posterior mediastinum	Useful in differentiating posterior mediastinal pathologies
Aortopulmonary window	The space between the aortic arch and the pulmonary artery	Key area for identifying lymphadenopathy and masses
Cardiophrenic angle	The angle where the heart meets the diaphragm	Important for detecting pleural effusions and pericardial abnormalities
Costophrenic angle	The angle between the diaphragm and the chest wall	Useful in identifying pleural effusions and lung base pathologies
Oblique fissure	Divides the lobes of the lungs, visible on CT scans	Key in assessing lobar pneumonia, masses, and atelectasis
Horizontal fissure	Divides the upper and middle lobes of the right lung	Important for evaluating right upper and middle lobe pathologies
Thoracic inlet	The upper boundary of the thoracic cavity, includes structures entering the thorax	Useful in assessing masses or pathologies involving the thoracic inlet
Diaphragmatic crus	Muscular extensions of the diaphragm into the thoracic cavity	Important for identifying diaphragmatic and lower mediastinal pathologies
Sternum	The flat bone at the front of the chest	Key in assessing anterior mediastinal and chest wall pathologies
Spine	The vertebral column, visible in the posterior mediastinum	Useful for evaluating vertebral and paravertebral pathologies

COMMON CHEST PATHOLOGY

Lung Parenchyma

A. Infections

Common causes are bacterial pneumonia (consolidation either lobar or bronchopneumonia with air bronchogram), tuberculosis (tree-in-bud appearance) and viral (interstitial pneumonia

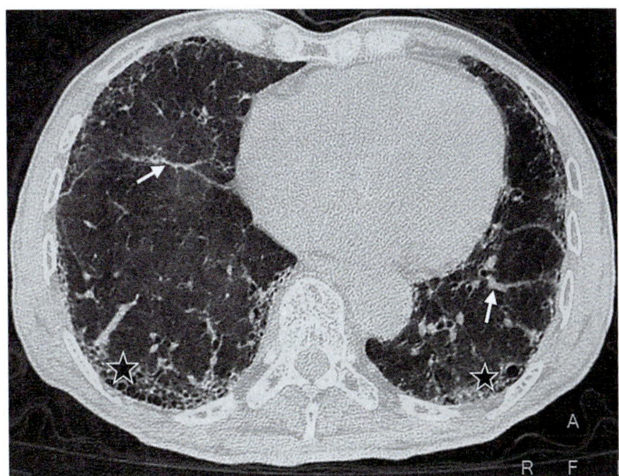

Fig. 12.4: HRCT Chest Lung window (axial section) shows: ★ More than 3 stacks of peripherally arranged small cysts in bilateral lung fields predominantly in lower lobes, →→. Multiple fibrotic bands causing tractional bronchiectasis in bilateral lung fields predominantly in lower lobes: Features are consistent with interstitial lung disease: UIP pattern.

as in SARS giving ground glass opacity). Primary modality is chest X-ray. CT is particularly useful to assess the type, extent of infection by seeing distribution and pattern of disease, complications of infections or when the X-ray results are inconclusive. May be associated with mediastinal lymphadenopathy and pleural effusion.

B. Interstitial Lung Disease (Fig. 12.4)

It encompasses a group of disorders that affect the lung parenchyma, primarily involving the interstitium—the space around the air sacs (alveoli) of the lungs. These diseases often lead to lung inflammation and fibrosis. Diagnosis of ILDs involves a comprehensive evaluation that includes clinical assessment, imaging, pulmonary function tests, and often histological examination (BAL and Transbronchial biopsy). HRCT is central to the evaluation process, providing critical information that helps to differentiate among various types of ILDs based on specific radiographic patterns. Typical findings include ground-glass opacities, reticular markings, traction bronchiectasis, and honeycombing.

C. Bronchiectasis

It is a chronic lung condition characterized by irreversible dilation and destruction of the bronchial walls. Can be congenital as in cystic fibrosis or acquired. Risk factors are infections like tuberculosis, fungal, COPD and smoking. Chest X-ray might show thickened bronchial walls, increased lung markings, and in severe cases visible dilated airways. It might also reveal other findings like hyperinflation or focal opacities due to infections. HRCT is the gold standard for diagnosing bronchiectasis, as it provides detailed images that allow for the accurate assessment of the airways (show signet ring sign, air trapping, mucus plugs) and surrounding lung parenchyma.

Pleural Disease

A. Pleural Effusion (Fig. 12.5) and Pneumothorax

Accumulation of fluid (effusion), air (pneumothorax), or blood (hemothorax) in between visceral and pleural layers of pleura. It can be caused by infections, systemic causes like CHF,

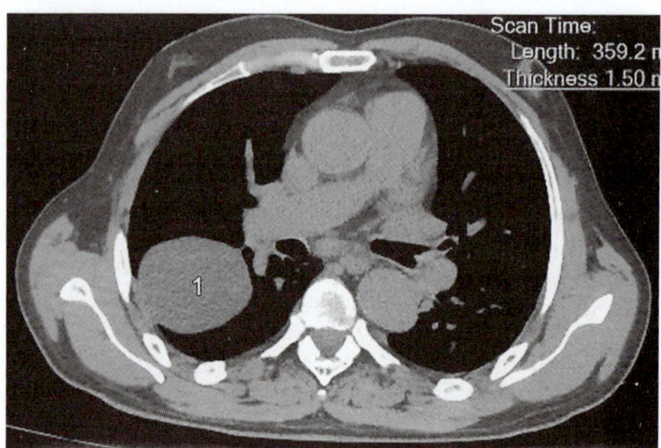

Fig. 12.5: HRCT soft tissue window (axial section) shows: (1) Well defined round fluid density (+10 HU) is noted along right oblique fissure, s/o encysted pleural effusion.

renal failure, trauma and rupture of cavity/bleb, etc. It can be unilateral or bilateral (especially in systemic diseases). Can be exudate (infections) or transudate (systemic causes). Chest is basic modality. USG is a highly sensitive tool, can detect 5–10 mL and also assess type of fluid. CT is indicated in Empyema necessitans, also known as "necrotizing empyema," a rare complication of empyema, (accumulation of pus in the pleural space). It occurs when the infection extends through the pleural layers and invades the surrounding tissues, including the chest wall and present with soft tissue mass in chest wall.

B. Mesothelioma

It is a rare and aggressive cancer associated primarily with asbestos exposure. It arises from the mesothelial cells that line the pleural cavity. CT is the primary imaging modality, shows irregular, nodular pleural thickening or mass lesion. MRI is particularly useful for assessing diaphragmatic invasion and differentiating between tumor and benign pleural thickening.

Mediastinal Disease

As mediastinum is divided into various compartments by various anatomical planes its pathologies are completely depend on contents of various compartments (as described in table of classification). Though few common entities are described below as:

A. Thymoma

Well-circumscribed, often lobulated mass in anterior mediastinum. Can be heterogeneous with areas of calcification or cystic change. May cause displacement of adjacent mediastinal structures. Show heterogenous enhancement. Chemical shift imaging can be useful in differentiating thymomas from thymic hyperplasia.

B. Lymphadenopathy (Fig. 12.6)

Considered pathological if SAD >10 mm. Can be primarily enlarged in lymphoma particularly Hodgkin lymphoma or secondarily enlarged in tuberculosis, sarcoidosis or due to metastases. Nodes are studied in terms of size, shape, necrosis, calcification, confluence of nodes and associated clinical features as well extent of other imaging findings. Can be seen in any mediastinum as mediastinal widening and enhancing soft tissue mass lesion.

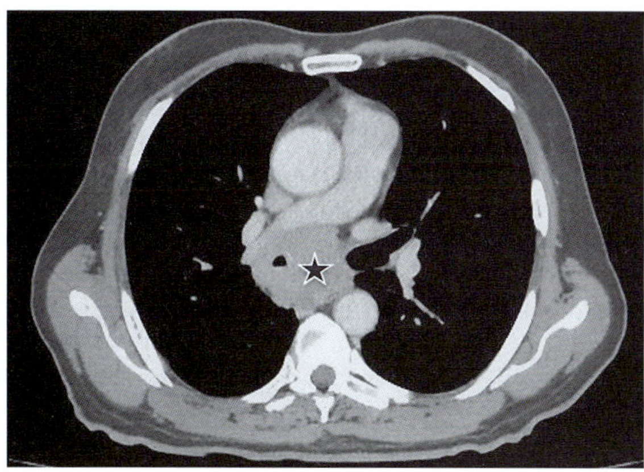

Fig. 12.6: CECT Chest soft tissue window (axial section) shows: ★Well-defined homogeneously enhancing soft tissue mass lesion centered in posterior mediastinum completely encasing carina and right main bronchus……features are consistent with lymphoma.

C. Neurogenic Tumor

Schwannomas and neurofibromas typically found in the posterior mediastinum, usually well-circumscribed and may have a "dumbbell" shape, extending through the intervertebral foramina.

D. Germ Cell Tumor

Most common type of germ cell tumor in the mediastinum is the teratoma. Present as well-defined mass in the anterior mediastinum on X-ray. **CT** provides more detailed imaging, revealing a complex, often cystic mass with possible calcifications, fat, and soft tissue components. It is excellent for evaluating the extent of the mass and its relationship to surrounding structures.

E. Mediastinal Cyst

Mediastinal cyst are shown **Table 12.11**.

Table 12.11: Mediastinal cyst.

Type of cyst	*Origin*	*Location*	*Imaging findings*
Bronchogenic cysts (most common)	Aberrations in the development of the tracheobronchial tree	Middle mediastinum, near trachea or main bronchi	Well-circumscribed, homogeneous, water-density lesions on CT. High signal on T2-weighted MRI images
Esophageal duplication cysts	Developmental malformation of the esophagus	Posterior mediastinum, adjacent to the esophagus	Smooth, rounded border, potential double-wall sign on CT
Pericardial cysts	Congenital malformations of the pericardium	Cardiophrenic angle, typically right side	Well-defined, water-density masses on CT. High T2 signal intensity on MRI
Thymic cysts	Congenital or acquired (often associated with inflammation)	Anterior mediastinum	Varies from simple, thin-walled cysts to complex cyst with septations or internal debris on CT/MRI
Neurenteric cysts	Congenital anomalies related to abnormal neural and gastrointestinal tract connections	Posterior mediastinum, often associated with the spine	Close association with the spine, features of both cystic and solid components on imaging

Common patterns of lung disease on chest X-rays are shown in **Table 12.12**.

Table 12.12: Common patterns of lung disease on chest X-rays.

Radiographic pattern	*Characteristics*	*Differential diagnoses*
Alveolar pattern	Patchy or confluent opacities, air bronchograms	Pneumonia, pulmonary edema, pulmonary hemorrhage, alveolar cell carcinoma
Interstitial pattern	Fine reticular, nodular, or reticulonodular opacities	Interstitial fibrosis, viral/atypical pneumonia, pulmonary edema, sarcoidosis
Nodular pattern	Well-defined, round opacities	Metastatic disease, granulomatous disease, primary lung cancer, benign tumors
Cavitary lesions	Nodules or masses with central lucency	Tuberculosis, lung abscess, necrotizing pneumonia, septic emboli
Hyperlucent areas	Areas appearing darker due to increased air content	Pneumothorax, emphysema, large bullae
Hilar enlargement	Enlarged hilum due to lymphadenopathy or mass	Lymphoma, sarcoidosis, bronchogenic carcinoma

Common patterns of lung disease on CT are shown in **Table 12.13**.

Table 12.13: Common patterns of lung disease on CT.

CT pattern	*Characteristics*	*Differential diagnoses*
Ground-glass opacity	Hazy increased attenuation of the lung with preserved bronchial and vascular markings	Viral pneumonias (e.g., COVID-19), interstitial lung disease, early pulmonary edema, alveolar proteinosis
Honeycombing	Clustered cystic air spaces typically subpleural and basal, with well-defined walls	Idiopathic pulmonary fibrosis (IPF), chronic fibrotic interstitial pneumonia, asbestosis
Tree-in-bud	Centrilobular small nodules with branching linear structures resembling budding trees	Endobronchial spread of infection (e.g., tuberculosis), bronchiolitis
Nodules	Well-circumscribed, round, or irregular opacities	Metastasis, granuloma (infectious or non-infectious), rheumatoid nodules, primary lung cancers
Consolidation	Homogeneous increase in pulmonary parenchymal attenuation that obscures vessel margins and airway walls	Bacterial pneumonia, organizing pneumonia, pulmonary contusion, lymphoma
Mosaic attenuation	Patchwork of varied lung densities due to air trapping or perfusion abnormalities	Hypersensitivity pneumonitis, airway disease (e.g., bronchiectasis), small airway obstructive diseases
Cystic air spaces	Rounded, circumscribed, air-filled spaces within the lung parenchyma	Lymphangioleiomyomatosis (LAM), honeycombing in fibrotic diseases, cystic bronchiectasis
Septal thickening	Thickening of the interlobular septa, often appearing as "septal lines"	Pulmonary edema, lymphangitic carcinomatosis, sarcoidosis, silicosis
Cavitary lesions	Air-filled spaces within pulmonary nodules or masses due to necrosis	Tuberculosis, necrotizing bacterial pneumonia, Wegener's granulomatosis, cavitary metastases

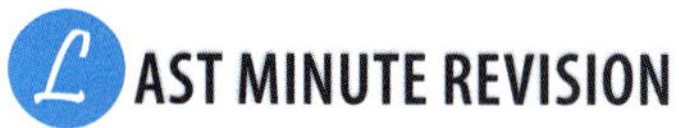

LAST MINUTE REVISION

- Commonly advised chest ray is chest X-ray PA view. It is the best view to study heart and lung diseases on X-ray.
- Air-filled regions are radiolucent on X-ray and CT while bones are radiopaque
- Air bronchogram is sign for consolidation which is indirect sign of patency of airway
- Silhouette sign will aid to diagnose/localize level of disease in chest
- Mediastinal pathology are studied with respect to compartment.
- Pathology related to aorta, enlarged lymph nodes and lipoma can be seen in all mediastinal compartments

REVIEW QUESTIONS

Multiple Choice Questions (MCQs)

1. **All are views of chest X-ray, *except*:**
   a. Chest PA
   b. Chest AP
   c. Chest lateral
   d. Chest prone
2. **Alveolar opacities are seen in:**
   a. Bacterial pneumonia
   b. Pulmonary edema
   c. Interstitial lung disease
   d. Pulmonary hemorrhage
3. **ITMIG classified mediastinum into various compartments, *except*:**
   a. Superior mediastinum
   b. Prevascular
   c. Visceral
   d. Paravertebral
4. **Lymphadenopathy can be seen in:**
   a. Anterior mediastinum
   b. Posterior mediastinum
   c. Superior mediastinum
   d. All of these

Answer Key

1. d 2. c 3. a 4. d

SUGGESTED READING

1. Keijsers RG, Veltkamp M, Grutters JC. Chest Imaging. Clin Chest Med. 2015 Dec;36(4):603-19. doi: 10.1016/j.ccm.2015.08.004. PMID: 26593136.
2. Ravin CE. Imaging of the chest. Acad Radiol. 1995 Sep;2 Suppl 2:S155-6. doi: 10.1016/s1076-6332(12)80064-x. PMID: 9419734.

CHAPTER

13 Spine Imaging

"Every vertebra holds a story of movement, strength, and sometimes pain—and radiologists are the storytellers."

INTRODUCTION

Spinal imaging is a critical tool in the diagnosis and management of various spinal disorders. It allows clinicians to visualize the anatomical structures of the spine and detect abnormalities that may be causing symptoms such as pain, neurological deficits, or deformity. Understanding the basic principles and applications of spinal imaging is essential for medical students, as it forms the basis for effective patient care and management in both acute and chronic settings.

COMMON INDICATIONS

Spinal imaging is utilized in a variety of clinical scenarios, including but not limited to:

- **Trauma:** Evaluating fractures, dislocations, and spinal cord injuries.
- **Degenerative diseases:** Assessing conditions like osteoarthritis, intervertebral disc herniation, and spinal stenosis.
- **Infections:** Identifying osteomyelitis, discitis, and epidural abscesses.
- **Neoplasms:** Detecting primary spinal tumors and metastatic disease.
- **Congenital anomalies:** Diagnosing conditions such as scoliosis, spina bifida, and other developmental abnormalities.
- **Pre- and postoperative assessments:** Planning surgical interventions and monitoring postsurgical outcomes.

IMAGING MODALITIES

X-ray

- **Description:** Basic imaging modality that provides a quick and inexpensive evaluation of the bony structures of the spine.
- **Indications:** Trauma, degenerative changes, alignment abnormalities, congenital anomalies.
- **Advantages:** Widely available, quick, and cost-effective.
- **Limitations:** Limited soft tissue visualization, exposure to ionizing radiation.
- **Common views:** Anteroposterior (AP), lateral, oblique, and special views like flexion-extension of specific spine as per clinical conditions.

Computed Tomography (CT)

- **Description:** Provides detailed cross-sectional images of the spine, offering excellent bone detail.
- **Indications:** Trauma (fractures), detailed bone assessment, surgical planning.
- **Advantages:** Superior bone detail, rapid acquisition.
- **Limitations:** Higher radiation dose compared to X-rays, limited soft tissue contrast.

Magnetic Resonance Imaging (MRI)

- **Description:** Provides high-contrast images of soft tissues, including the spinal cord, intervertebral discs, intervertebral foramen and ligaments.
- **Indications:** Disc herniation, classification of spinal cord pathology, infections, tumors, congenital anomalies.
- **Advantages:** Excellent soft tissue contrast, no ionizing radiation.
- **Limitations:** Longer acquisition time, higher cost, contraindications (e.g., pacemakers).
- **Common sequences:** T1, T2 in axial, sagittal planes with STIR as per indication, coronal for paravertebral structures.

Ultrasound

- **Description:** Utilizes high-frequency sound waves to visualize soft tissues and vascular structures.
- **Indications:** Limited use in spinal imaging, mostly for guided interventions (e.g., epidural injections), neonates spinal imaging like meningocele etc.
- **Advantages:** Real-time imaging, no ionizing radiation.
- **Limitations:** Limited field of view, operator dependent.

Nuclear Medicine (Bone Scintigraphy)

- **Description:** Involves the use of radioactive tracers to detect areas of increased metabolic activity.
- **Indications:** Detecting bone metastases, infections, and occult fractures.
- **Advantages:** High sensitivity for detecting pathology.
- **Limitations:** Low specificity, radiation exposure, and lower resolution.

APPLICATION OF IMAGING MODALITIES IN COMMON PATHOLOGY

- **Trauma**
  - *X-ray:* Initial assessment for fractures and alignment.
  - *CT:* Detailed evaluation of complex fractures and surgical planning.
  - *MRI:* Assessing spinal cord injury, ligamentous injury, and disc pathology.
- **Degenerative diseases**
  - *X-ray:* Detecting osteophytes, disc space narrowing, and spondylolisthesis.
  - *MRI:* Evaluating disc degeneration, herniation, spinal stenosis and compressive myelopathy.
- **Infections and inflammatory conditions**
  - *MRI:* Gold standard for detecting spinal infections (e.g., discitis, osteomyelitis) and inflammatory conditions.
  - *CT:* Assessing bony destruction and guiding biopsies.

- **Neoplasms**
  - *MRI:* Preferred for assessing spinal cord tumors, metastases, and primary bone tumors.
  - *CT:* Evaluating bony involvement and guiding biopsy.

RADIOLOGICAL ANATOMY

The spinal axis comprises both bony and soft tissue structures that work together to provide support, flexibility, and protection to the spinal cord and nerves.

Bony Structures Include

Vertebrae (C1-C7, T1-T12, L1-L5 and S1-S5 and Co1-Co4) having:

- **Vertebral body:** Main weight-bearing structure of the vertebra
- **Processes**
  - *Spinous processes:* Posterior projections from the vertebral arch.
  - *Transverse processes:* Lateral projections on each side of the vertebra.
  - *Articular processes:* Form the facet joints between vertebrae.
- **Facet joints:** Synovial joints between the articular processes of adjacent vertebrae.
- **Pedicles and laminae**
  - *Pedicles:* Bridge between the vertebral body and the transverse processes.
  - *Laminae:* Bridge between the transverse processes and the spinous process.
- **Vertebral arch:** Formed by the pedicles and laminae, encloses the vertebral foramen.

Soft Tissue Structures Includes

- **Spinal cord:** The central nervous structure running through the spinal bony canal, transmitting neural signals between the brain and the body. Terminate at L1-L2 in adult and up to upper border of L3 in neonate.
- **Nerve roots:** Extensions of the spinal cord that exit through the intervertebral foramina.
- **Ligaments**
  - *Anterior longitudinal ligament:* Runs along the anterior surface of the vertebral bodies.
  - *Posterior longitudinal ligament:* Runs along the posterior surface of the vertebral bodies inside the vertebral canal.
  - *Ligamentum flavum:* Connects the laminae of adjacent vertebrae.
  - *Interspinous ligaments:* Connect the spinous processes.
  - *Supraspinous ligament:* Runs along the tips of the spinous processes.
  - *Intertransverse ligaments:* Connect the transverse processes.
- **Muscles**
  - *Paraspinal muscles:* Support and move the spine.
  - *Erector spinae muscles:* Major muscle group that extends the spine.
  - *Multifidus:* Stabilizes the vertebrae during movement.
- **Intervertebral discs**
  - *Nucleus pulposus:* Soft, gel-like core providing cushioning.
  - *Annulus fibrosus:* Tough, fibrous outer ring.
- **Spinal meninges:** Protective layers around the spinal cord: dura mater, arachnoid mater, and pia mater forming subarachnoid space having CSF up to S2 and epidural space containing fat and blood vessels.

Embryology of the Spine

See **Table 13.1**.

Table 13.1: Description of spinal anomalies with reference to embryological development.

Developmental stage	*Process*	*Common pathologies*	*Radiological relevance and imaging*
Gastrulation (week 3)	Formation of three germ layers and the notochord	Neural tube defects (e.g., spina bifida)	Prenatal ultrasound and MRI can detect open neural tube defects and associated anomalies
Neurulation (weeks 3–4)	Formation and closure of the neural tube	Anencephaly, spina bifida	MRI and ultrasound reveal open or closed neural tube defects, malformations, and associated hydrocephalus
Somite formation (weeks 4–5)	Differentiation into sclerotome (vertebrae), myotome, and dermatome	Congenital scoliosis, vertebral segmentation defects	Ante-natal USG, X-rays, CT, and MRI show vertebral anomalies, curvature, and segmentation defects
Vertebral body formation (weeks 6–8)	Migration of sclerotome cells to form vertebral bodies and intervertebral discs	Hemivertebrae, vertebral malformations	Ante-natal USG, X-rays and MRI highlight hemivertebrae, segmentation issues, and incomplete vertebral formation
Chondrification (weeks 9–12)	Formation of cartilaginous vertebral models	Delayed ossification, vertebral fusion	MRI and CT can identify cartilaginous structures and any delay or anomalies in ossification
Ossification (weeks 13–24)	Endochondral ossification of vertebral bodies and arches	Congenital vertebral fusion, Klippel-Feil syndrome	X-rays and CT scans show ossified structures, vertebral fusion, and other ossification abnormalities
Postnatal development	Continuation of vertebral growth and secondary ossification centers appear	Scoliosis, spondylolisthesis	X-rays, MRI, and CT can detect growth abnormalities, vertebral slippage, and the degree of spinal curvature and deformity

COMMON PATHOLOGIES

Degenerative Disease

Most prevalent clinical conditions in the spine is degenerative disease, which affects the intervertebral discs, ligaments, and opposing vertebral endplates as well as the intervertebral posterior joints. The lower cervical and lumbar spine regions exhibit the most severe primary degenerative changes in the spine.

Two adjoining vertebrae, the intervertebral disc, spinal ligaments and facet joints among them represent a functional spinal unit. **Figures 13.1A to C** in diagrammatic representation as well as in MRI.

Based on the location and progression sequence, we propose a simple mnemonic and classification to make the description of spinal degenerative changes easier. These changes are divided into three categories: A, B, and C.

When imaging is performed, the degenerative process typically begins in the nucleolus pulposus (A-changes) and spreads to the adjacent vertebral bodies disc, annulus fibrosus (fissures and disc displacement), end plates, and bone marrow (B-changes). Progression of degeneration can eventually affect distant structures and result in osteoarthritis in the facet joints, hypertrophy of the ligamentum flavum, and spinal canal stasis (C-changes).

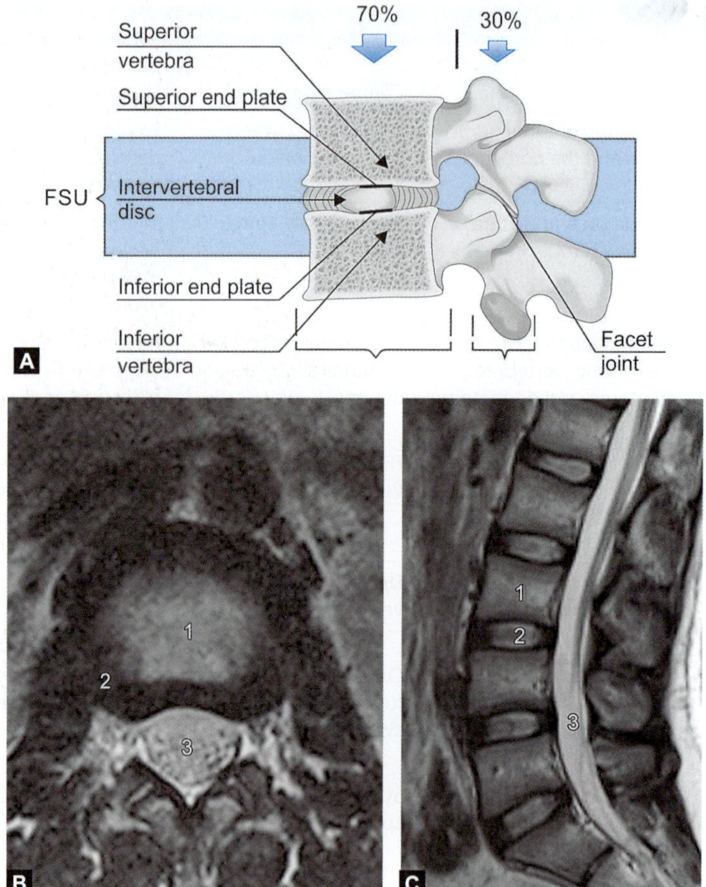

Figs. 13.1A to C: (A) Functional spinal unit (FSU). With biomechanical properties akin to those of the entire spine, the FSU is the smallest motion segment of the spine. The vertebral body and intervertebral discs transmit about 70% of applied axial compression, with the facet joints distributing the remaining 30% of the load; (B) MRI T2 weighted image of spine at IV disc level (axial section) shows: (1) T2 hyperintense—nucleus pulposus, (2) T2 hypointense—annulus fibrosus (concavity posteriorly), (3) T2 hyperintense CSF with multiple T2 hypointense dots s/o spinal nerves; (C) MRI T2 weighted image of spine (sagittal section) shows: (1) vertebrae body T2 isointense; (2) Intervertebral disc, T2 hyperintense—nucleus pulposus, T2 hypointense-annulus fibrosus; (3) Spinal canal, T2 hyperintense CSF with multiple T2 hypointense linear spinal nerves.

Disc herniation occurs when a segment of the nucleus pulposus separates and migrates out of its original intradiscal location. Herniation typically happens in patients who are still relatively young and have high intradiscal pressure. Disc herniation may cause protrusion, extrusion, or sequestration of the nucleus pulposus matrix, depending on the degree of focal migration of the nucleus pulposus. A disc herniation can happen in any direction **(Figs. 13.2A and B)**.

Note: Nucleus pulposus is slightly hyperintense on T1 and hyperintense on T2 as compared to annulus fibrosus with posterior concavity on axial scan.

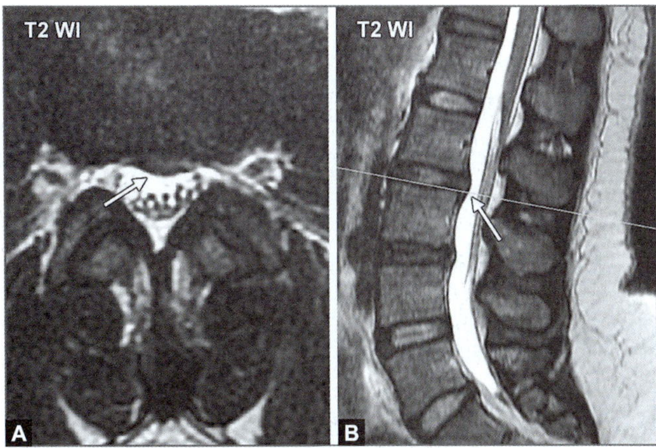

Figs. 13.2A and B: Focal disc displacement: protrusion.

Trauma

Spinal trauma is one of the common sites after head and extremities. It is one of the common indication of MRI spine after degenerative disease of spine. Common mode of injury is motor vehicle accident followed by fall, common in cervical region with male preponderance and bimodal age of presentation. Imaging play a vital role especially X-ray, CT for bony structures while MRI is modality of choice for spinal cord, IV disc, ligaments, nerve roots, etc. It is classified into stable and unstable injury depending on involvement of one column or unstable involving two or more column.

Infections

Spinal infections occur in 2–7% of cases of musculoskeletal infections. The distribution is bimodal, with one peak appearing before the age of 20 and the other between the ages of 50 and 70. The ratio of men to women varies from 2:1 to 5:1. The epidural space, meninges, spinal cord, vertebral bodies, intervertebral discs, and paraspinal soft tissues can all be affected by spinal infections. They are more frequently the consequence of hematogenous seeding from a distant site, though they can also be brought on by direct inoculation after spinal procedures. Viruses typically cause intramedullary infections while pyogenic bacteria are the most common cause of extradural and intradural extramedullary infections. Various infections can be differentiated based on characteristic imaging patterns, extent of disease and clinical scenario too. CEMRI is investigation of choice.

Pyogenic Spondylodiscitis

Pyogenic spondylodiscitis (vertebral osteomyelitis-discitis) is estimated to account for less than 2–4% of all osteoarthritis cases. It is believed to be caused by hematogenous spread from bacterial microemboli. The majority of these microemboli are found in the arterial system, where they lodge into one of the metaphyseal arteries, leading to infarction and infection. The most common cause of vertebral osteomyelitis is *Staphylococcus aureus*. Back pain is the most common presenting symptom, seen in nearly 90% of cases. Although plain radiography has a limited role in the evaluation of infectious etiologies, it is a common initial imaging step for patients with nonspecific back pain. The subtle radiographic indicator of a spine infection

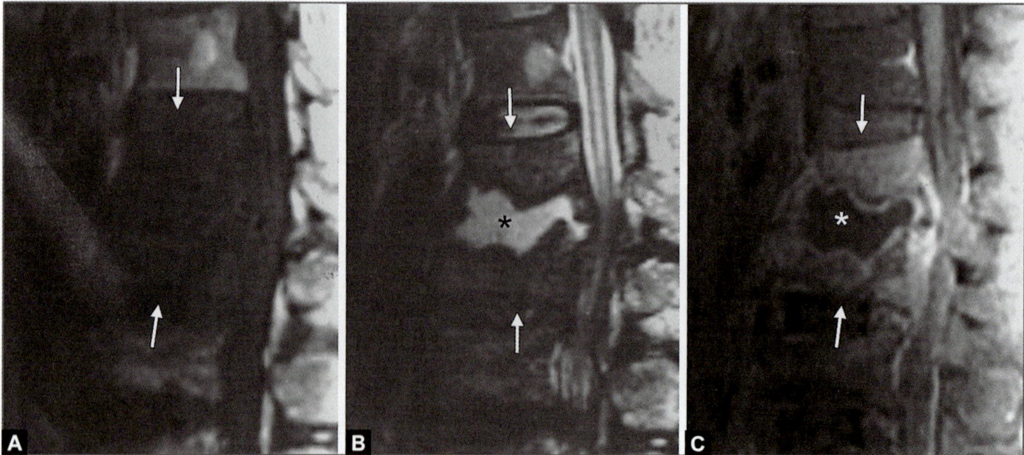

Figs. 13.3A to C: Pyogenic spondylitis in 66-year-old woman; (A) Sagittal T1-weighted image shows hypointense signal (*arrows*) in L2–L3 vertebral bodies; (B) On sagittal fast spin-echo T2-weighted image L2 and L3 vertebral bodies are isointense (*arrows*) to adjacent normal vertebrae with well-defined high signal (*asterisk*); (C) Sagittal fat-suppressed contrast-enhanced T1-weighted image shows heterogeneous enhancement (*arrows*) of L2 and L3 vertebral bodies with thin- and smooth-walled abscess (*asterisk*).

could be endplate irregularity. The endplate and nearby bone may erode more noticeably as the infection worsens. When assessing infectious discitis or osteomyelitis, magnetic resonance imaging (MRI) is considered the gold standard. Edema and the infiltration of inflammatory cells into the region are the primary causes of the early MRI findings of infection of the disc space and vertebral body. As a result, on T1-weighted images, the disc and surrounding vertebral bodies appear hypointense, and on T2-weighted images, they appear hyperintense **(Figs. 13.3A to C)**

Changes in infection on MRI might resemble those seen in degenerative spine conditions. The primary distinction between these two etiologies, however, is that the disc in the infected disc will have a higher signal and appear hyperintense on T2-weighted images, whereas the disc in the degenerative disease will appear hypointense on T2 due to loss of water content. Since spinal infections are almost always linked to the presence of paraspinal or epidural inflammation, as indicated by hyperintensity on T2-weighted images, this information is useful in making the diagnosis. The disc-endplate interface and/or the disc space itself are enhanced in T1-weighted scans carried out with Gd-DPTA contrast. Contrast studies can help differentiate between infectious and degenerative findings, such as Modic endplate changes, even though noncontrast studies might still be able to provide enough information for a diagnosis.

Epidural Abscess

An infection of the area between the dura and the vertebral periosteum is known as a spinal epidural abscess (SEA). It most frequently affects the thoracic spine. In most cases, *S. aureus* is the causative agent. Gadolinium (Gd) contrast-enhanced MRI is considered the gold standard for the imaging and diagnosis of SEA. On T1-weighted images, the abscess will appear hypointense or isointense in relation to the spinal cord, and on T2-weighted images it will appear hyperintense. The abscess will enhance peripherally with a central fluid signal after post-Gd T1-weighted imaging.

Tuberculous Spondylodiscitis (Figs. 13.4A to D)

The most frequent location of musculoskeletal involvement in tuberculosis is tuberculous spondylodiscitis, also referred to as Pott's disease. It is an infection brought on by *Mycobacterium tuberculosis* (*M. tuberculosis*), frequently as a consequence of hematogenous spread from the arteries. Patients with compromised immune systems and those living in endemic regions of the world are more susceptible to this infection, which primarily affects the thoracic spine. Notably, unlike many other organisms that may cause pyogenic spondylodiscitis, *M. tuberculosis* lacks proteolytic destructive enzymes. As a result, a significant imaging finding that could help distinguish tuberculous spondylodiscitis from pyogenic spondylodiscitis would be relatively minimal disc-space narrowing. Findings such as a thin and smooth abscess wall, the presence of a paraspinal or intraosseous abscess, involvement of multiple vertebral bodies, or subligamentous spread to three or more levels can help distinguish tuberculous spondylodiscitis from pyogenic spondylodiscitis. CT could be a good substitute, particularly in areas where MRI access is limited. In contrast to other pyogenic organisms, endplate destruction observed in tuberculous spondylodiscitis may be more fragmented. In cases of advanced disease, radiographs will show increased paravertebral soft tissue opacity without calcifications, vertebral body destruction, and kyphotic angulation.

Neoplastic

Spinal tumors are relatively uncommon, making up only 5–10% of all tumors of the central nervous system (CNS), with 70–80% of them thought to be intradural extramedullary (IDEM) in origin. Extradural and intradural are the two main categories, intradural lesions are further divided into: extramedullary and intramedullary.

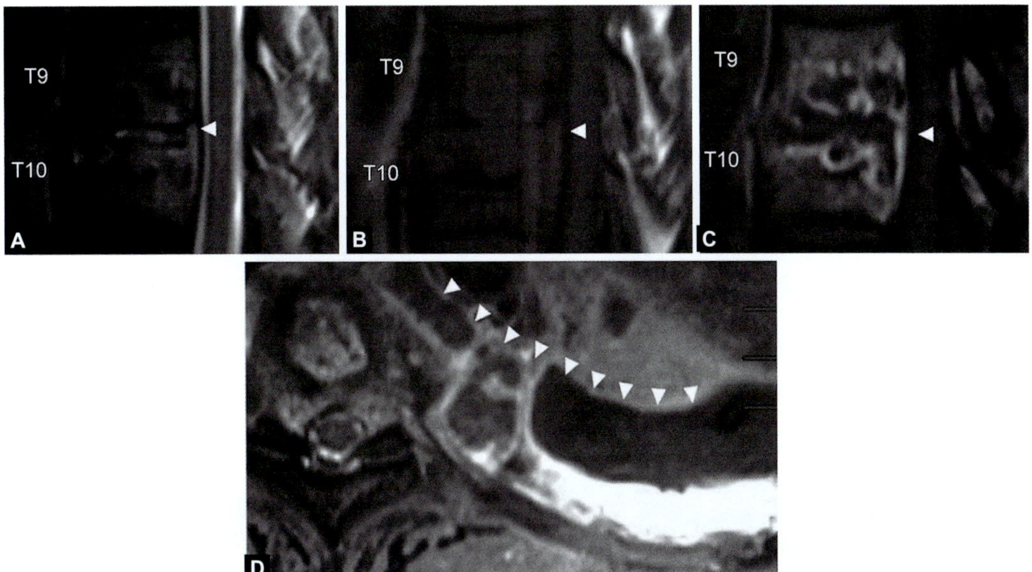

Figs. 13.4A to D: Imaging obtained in patient with thoracic tuberculous spondylodiscitis at T9–T10; (A) Sagittal T2-weighted MRI with hyperintense signal of the T9 and T10 vertebral bodies with vertebral body abscess with erosion into the disc space (arrowhead); (B) Sagittal T1-weighted MRI with hypointense signal of the T9 and T10 vertebral bodies (arrowhead); (C) Sagittal T1-weighted MRI postcontrast with enhancement of the T9 and T10 vertebral bodies with vertebral body abscess with erosion into the disc space; (D) Axial T1-weight MRI postcontrast with large multiloculated left paraspinal abscess with pleural extension and pleural effusion.

The standard approach in cases where there is a suspicion of spinal tumors is to use gadolinium-based contrast agents, which cause the spinal neoplasms to be enhanced. This aids in separating tumors from other differential diagnoses like reactive cysts and cord edema.

The two most prevalent intradural extramedullary tumors are meningioma and schwannoma, and both are linked to neurofibromatosis.

Schwannoma

Schwannoma is a tumor that originates from the nerve sheath's support cells. It is also referred to as neurinoma or neurilemmoma. About 25% of adult IDEM spinal tumors are of this type, making it the most prevalent tumor. A peak incidence occurs in the fourth to sixth decades of life, affecting both sexes equally. The most frequent presenting symptoms are radiculopathy and features of progressive myelopathy. The tumor may, however, range in size from a small intradural mass to a giant schwannoma, which is a large intraspinal or paravertebral mass extending beyond two vertebral segments. Roughly 15% of schwannomas appear as "dumbbell-shaped" transforaminal masses. In contrast to calcification and hemorrhage, which are uncommon and only observed in 10% of cases, cystic degeneration is extremely common, occurring in 40% of cases. Bone remodeling is linked to the transforaminal or intraspinal lesions. These lesions showed strong postcontrast enhancement and were predominantly isointense to the spinal cord on T1WIs and hyperintense to the cord on long TR images **(Figs. 13.5A to D)**.

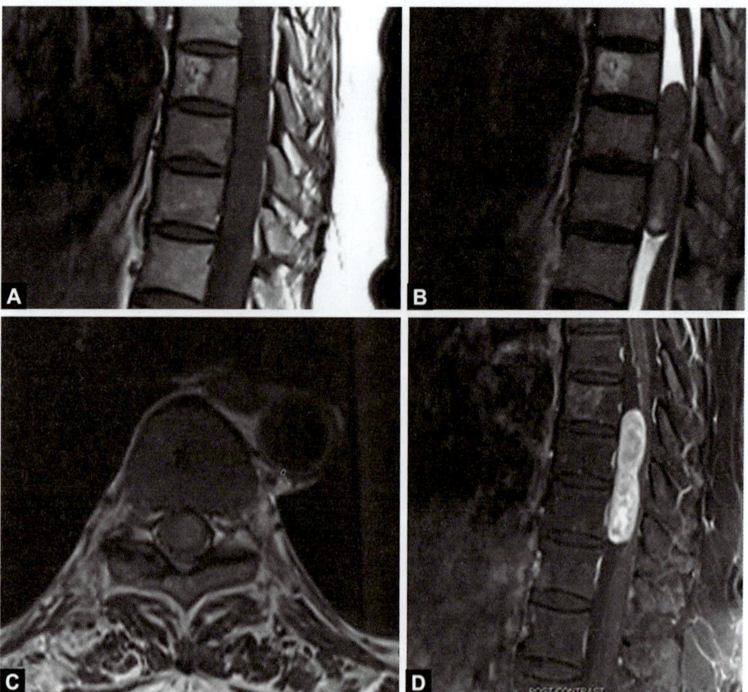

Figs. 13.5A to D: (A) T1 sagittal image demonstrating a dumbbell-shaped isointense intradural mass; (B) T2 sagittal lesion appearing iso to hyperintense; (C) T2 axial confirming intradural location; (D) Postcontrast T1 fat-saturated sagittal demonstrating avid homogeneous postcontrast enhancement. Histopathology reveals schwannoma.

Meningioma

Meningiomas, which make up about 25% of all spinal tumors, are the second most frequent tumors with IDEM locations. The following is the regional distribution of spinal meningiomas: 15% cervical, 3% lumbosacral, 2% foramen magnum, and 80% thoracic. Meningiomas are most common in the fifth and sixth decades of life, and they are strongly predisposed to affect women (80% of cases). The intradural compartment contains 90% of spinal meningiomas, the extradural compartment contains about 5%, and the remaining 5% encroaches on both the intradural and extradural compartments. There are similarities between the MRI results of spinal meningiomas and intracranial meningiomas. In most cases, spinal meningiomas on T1WIs and T2WIs are isointense to the cord. They frequently possessed a wide Dural attachment base. Following contrast administration, T1WIs shows moderate-to-intense enhancement **(Figs. 13.6A to D)**.

Note: T2 weighted central hypointensity = target sign, can be seen in schwannoma but common in neurofibroma.

Arachnoid Cyst

Spinal arachnoid cysts primarily affect children and adolescents, with a male predominance. These are identified as an incidental MRI finding. On the posterolateral aspect of the thoracic spinal cord, these cysts are frequently seen. Congenital lesions are believed to result from a dural defect caused by abnormality of the septum positum. Most cases are idiopathic. These cysts

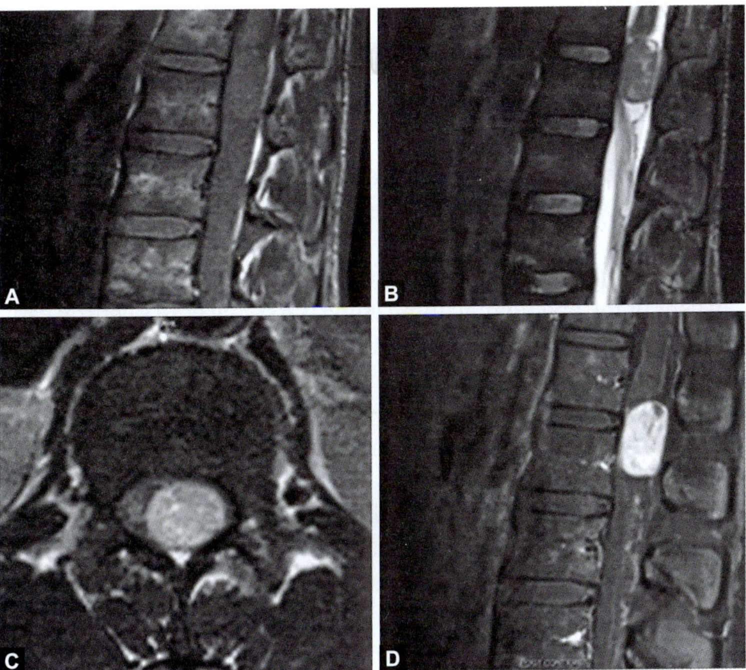

Figs. 13.6A to D: (A) T1 sagittal image demonstrating an oval-shaped isointense intradural mass; (B) T2 sagittal lesion appearing iso to hypointense; (C) T2 axial confirming intradural location; (D) Postcontrast T1 fat-saturated sagittal image demonstrating avid homogeneous postcontrast enhancement. Histopathology reveals meningioma.

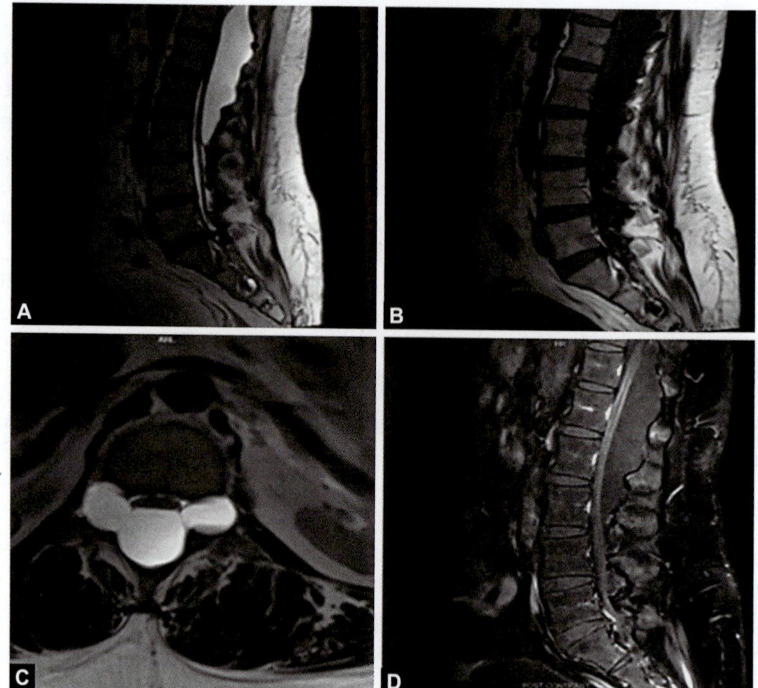

Figs. 13.7A to D: (A) T2 sagittal image demonstrating a hyperintense cystic-appearing lesion displacing and compressing the spinal cord; (B) T1 sagittal lesion appearing hypointense; (C) T2 axial intradural cerebrospinal fluid signal intensity lesion compressing the spinal cord; (D) Postcontrast T1 fat-saturated sagittal image demonstrating no obvious postcontrast enhancement. Histopathology reveals arachnoid cyst.

has long T1 and T2 relaxation times and appears isointense to the surrounding CSF because they contains CSF. There is no contrast enhancement visible in these lesions **(Figs. 13.7A to D)**.

Ependymal Tumors

Radial glial stem cells or the ependymal lining along the spinal cord's central canal are thought to be the source of intramedullary ependymal tumors.

Among adult infiltrative gliomas, ependymoma is the most frequent intramedullary spinal cord tumor. Consequently, an enhancing mass with well-defined margins that expands outward from the ependymal lining of the central canal and has a more centered than eccentric location is the classic appearance at imaging.

The features of signal intensity are comparable to those of ependymomas at other locations (such as the cerebral parenchyma and ventricular system): tumor heterogeneity with cystic or hemorrhagic components, such as polar cysts or the hemosiderin cap sign at the superior or inferior margins, as well as surrounding edema or syringohydromyelia. T1 hypointense to isointense; T2 isointense to hyperintense. Disruption of normal CSF flow is linked to syringx formation (syringohydromyelia) **(Figs. 13.8A to C)**.

Ependymoma is the most likely diagnosis if the tumor's epicenter localizes to the central canal.

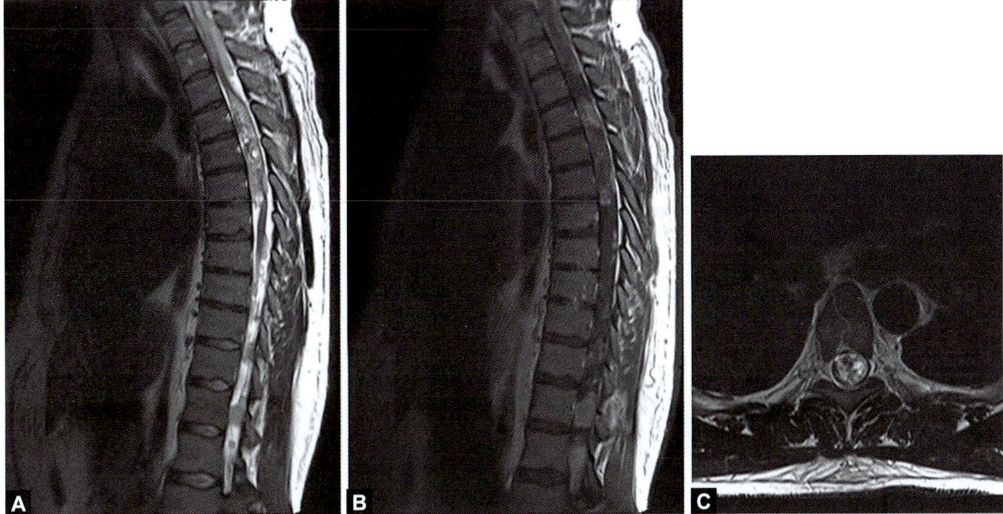

Figs. 13.8A to C: Anaplastic ependymoma in a 32-year-old man with progressive numbness and weakness in his lower extremities for 6 months and suspected neurofibromatosis type 2. (A, B) Sagittal T2-weighted; (A) and contrast-enhanced T1-weighted; (B) images reveal a large enhancing T2-hyperintense intramedullary mass in the upper thoracic spine and smaller enhancing extramedullary masses in the lower thoracic spine; (C) Axial T2-weighted image of the upper thoracic spine shows a heterogeneous partially exophytic mass centered in the spinal cord.

Note: The most frequent primary intra-axial tumor of childhood brain and spinal cord is pilocytic astrocytoma. Thus, majority of pediatric intramedullary tumors is astrocytoma (eccentric to spinal canal). After the basic discussion, it is clear that pathology of spine is commonly related to 3Ts. Their common differentiating features are:

Table 13.2: Differences between tuberculosis, tumor, and trauma in vertebral pathology.

Feature	*Tuberculosis (infections)*	*Tumor*	*Trauma*
Etiology	Mycobacterium tuberculosis infection	Primary (e.g., multiple myeloma) or secondary (metastatic) malignancies	Mechanical injury (e.g., falls, accidents)
Age group	Typically young adults to middle-aged	Varies: Primary: 50–70 years, Secondary: any age depending on primary cancer	Any age, depending on the nature and severity of the trauma
Clinical presentation	Gradual onset of back pain, fever, night sweats, weight loss	Progressive back pain, possible neurological deficits, weight loss, night pain, history of previous malignancy	Acute onset of pain, possible neurological deficits, history of trauma
Location	Thoracic and lumbar spine	Any part of the spine (thoracic, lumbar, cervical), commonly involved posterior arch in secondaries and body in primary lesion	Any part of the spine, depending on the mechanism of injury

Contd...

Contd...

Feature	*Tuberculosis (infections)*	*Tumor*	*Trauma*
Imaging findings: X-ray	Vertebral body destruction, loss of disc height, paraspinal abscess, "gibbus" deformity	Osteolytic lesions, vertebral collapse, "winking owl" sign (pedicle erosion), normal IV-disc height	Vertebral fractures, loss of vertebral height, misalignment, variable IV-disc height
Imaging findings: MRI	Hypointense on T1, hyperintense on T2, enhancement with contrast, paravertebral abscesses	Variable signal intensity, often hypointense on T1 and hyperintense on T2, enhancement with contrast, epidural mass	Fracture lines, bone marrow edema, retropulsion of bone fragments
Histopathological features	Granulomatous inflammation with caseous necrosis	Malignant cells, specific to the type of tumor (e.g., adenocarcinoma, myeloma cells)	N/A (histopathology not typically used for trauma diagnosis)
Treatment	Antitubercular therapy, surgical intervention for abscess drainage or stabilization	Depends on the type: surgery, radiotherapy, chemotherapy	Conservative management (e.g., bracing), surgical stabilization if necessary
Prognosis	Good with timely treatment, risk of deformity if untreated	Variable, depends on tumor type and stage	Generally good with appropriate management, but can vary depending on severity of injury

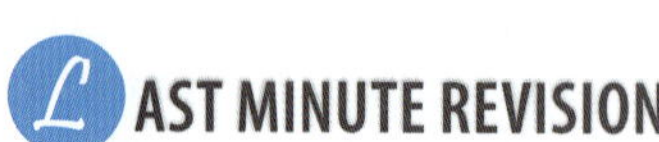

LAST MINUTE REVISION

- MRI provides excellent soft tissue contrast, making it ideal for evaluating intervertebral discs, spinal cord, ligaments, and detecting infections, neoplasms, and inflammatory conditions.
- Discogenic degeneration typically begins in the nucleus pulposus and progresses to the annulus fibrosus, vertebral bodies, and facet joints. While nondiscogenic degeneration initiates from posterior elements of vertebrae and it's ligaments.
- X-rays are used for initial assessment while CT provides detailed evaluation of fractures.
- MRI with gadolinium enhancement is investigation of choice for evaluating spinal tumors.

REVIEW QUESTIONS

Multiple Choice Questions (MCQs)

1. **Investigation of choice for imaging of spine:**
   a. X-ray　　b. CT scan
   c. Dexa scan　　d. MRI
2. **Most common spinal tumors are**
   a. Intramedullary　　b. Intradural extramedullary
   c. Extradural　　d. Meningeal
3. **Most frequent location of musculoskeletal involvement in tuberculosis:**
   a. Wrist　　b. Hip
   c. Spine　　d. Ankle

4. Signal intensity of spinal arachnoid cyst is equivalent to:

a. Muscles
b. CSF
c. Blood
d. Bone

5. Spinal ependymoma are:

a. Intramedullary tumors
b. Intradural extramedullary tumors
c. Extradural tumors
d. Bony tumors

Answer Key

1. d   2. b   3. c   4. b   5. a

SUGGESTED READING

1. Arbelaez A, Restrepo F, Castillo M. Spinal infections: clinical and imaging features. Top Magn Reson Imaging. 2014 Oct;23(5):303-14.
2. Kelly K. Koeller et al. Intradural Extramedullary Spinal Neoplasms: Radiologic–Pathologic Correlation Radiographics. 2019; 39:468-90.
3. Leonardi M, Simonetti L, Agati R. Neuroradiology of spine degenerative diseases. Best Pract Res Clin Rheumatol. 2002 Jan;16(1):59-87.
4. Sergiy V. Kushchayev et al. ABCs of the degenerative spine. Insights into Imaging. 2018;9:253-74.
5. Weishaupt D, Boxheimer L. Magnetic resonance imaging of the weight-bearing spine. Semin Musculoskeletal Radiol. 2003 Dec;7(4):277-86.

CHAPTER

14 Musculoskeletal Imaging

"Musculoskeletal imaging captures the essence of motion—bones, joints, and effort frozen in time for diagnosis."

INTRODUCTION

Musculoskeletal radiology is a subspecialty of diagnostic radiology that is involved in interpretation as well as performing image-guided procedures for all the pathologies pertaining to bones, joints, soft tissue and spine. It also includes sports injuries affecting pediatric as well as adult age groups. It is an important integral branch and has major implications in the management of patients.

Overview and History

Historically, there is a coincidence between the origin of musculoskeletal radiology and discovery of X-rays as the first human radiograph was of the hand which led to revolutionizing the modern healthcare and also revealed the potential of the radiographs in decrypting the restricted visual access to skeletal pathologies.

The musculoskeletal radiology encompasses a wide spectrum including imaging findings ranging from trauma, sports injuries, imaging of soft tissue and bone tumors. It is further involved in therapeutic decisions including guided injections, ablations, pain management and follow-up imaging.

Patients with musculoskeletal conditions are often managed with history and physical examination first. However, imaging plays an indispensable role for confirmation of the diagnosis, planning, management and also to ascertain predisposing factors in some situations.

Modern diagnostic imaging includes an armamentarium of modalities, including conventional radiography/X-rays, ultrasonography (USG), computed tomography (CT) scans, magnetic resonance imaging (MRI) and musculoskeletal interventional radiology. Sometimes combining two modalities may ascertain the diagnosis, as each modality has its own significance. The selection of the modality depends primarily upon the clinical question or query that needs to be addressed.

IMAGING MODALITIES

Radiographs/X-rays

Radiographs play a fundamental role in musculoskeletal radiology. They are the basic and first-line imaging modality, provide clear visualization of the bony anatomy and identify pathologies.

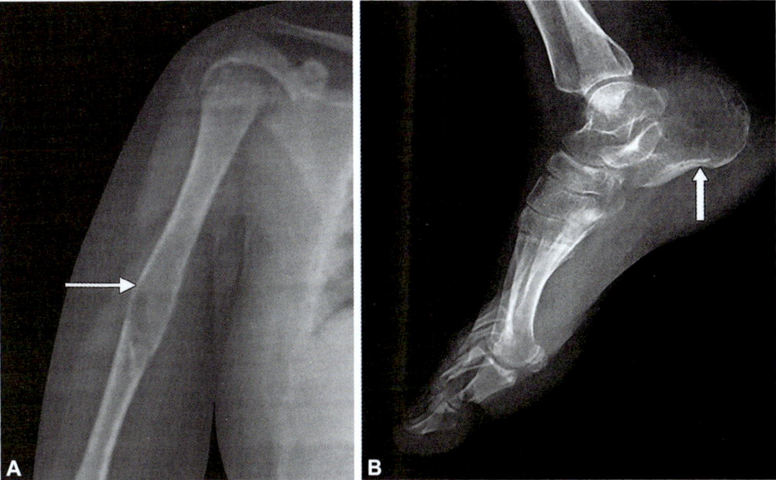

Figs. 14.1A and B: Radiographs showing osteolytic lesions with narrow zones of transition involving: (A) Mid-shaft of humerus (marked with arrow) suggesting simple cyst; (B) Involving calcaneum bone (marked with block arrow) suggesting benign bone tumor—Giant cell tumor.

Using radiographs one can identify and learn about the various anatomical landmarks of the bone, identify anatomical variations, and assess joint anatomy and articular surfaces. Radiographs play a vital role in assessment of fractures and their extensions, identifying patterns of dislocations, assessing benign and malignant bone tumors, osteoarthritis and are quite essential for almost all rheumatological pathologies especially osteoarthritis. **(Figs. 14.1 to 14.3)**. So, it plays an integral role in trauma, emergency and orthopedic settings and basic knowledge of the common fractures and their critical imaging points aids in urgent interventions and better patient care.

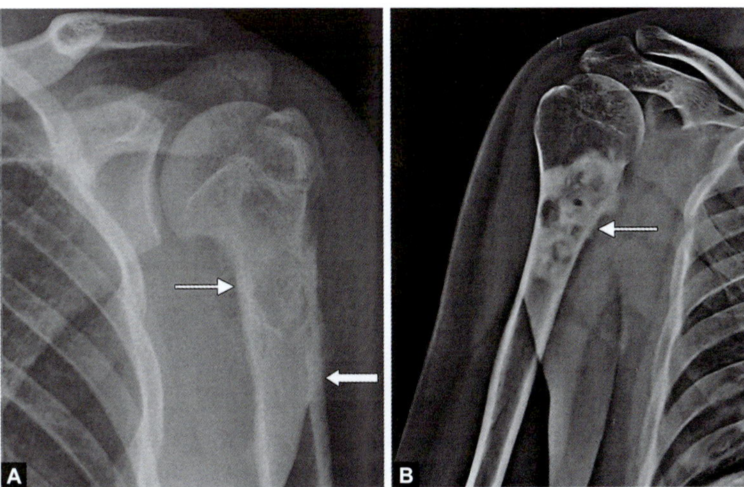

Figs. 14.2A and B: Anteroposterior radiographs of humerus showing lesions with wide zone of transition: (A) Osteolytic lesion involving proximal diaphysis of humerus (marked with arrow) with periosteal reaction (marked with block arrow) suggesting malignant bone tumor—Ewing's sarcoma; (B) Predominantly osteosclerotic lesion with extraosseous extension to adjacent soft tissue (marked with arrow) suggesting malignant bone tumor—osteosarcoma.

Radiographs are also used in multiple pediatric bony pathologies and skeletal dysplasia, but it is imperative to consider and remember the principle of radiation safety and protection, optimizing the dose and exposure to prevent inadvertent exposure to patients and doctors alike.

Radiographs are also useful in evaluation of bone density. Presence of osteopenia/osteoporosis or osteosclerosis can help in detection of multiple systemic abnormalities as well as metabolic disorders.

In summary, radiographs are vital to develop basic foundation and understanding of multiple musculoskeletal pathologies, normal anatomy and paves way to better understand the disorders clinically.

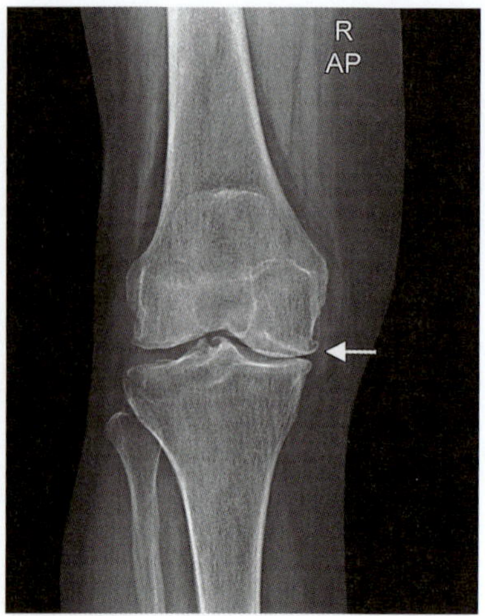

Fig. 14.3: Anteroposterior radiograph of right knee joint showing reduction in the joint space at medial compartment with marginal lipping (marked with arrow) suggest osteoarthritic changes.

Computed Tomography (CT)

It provides high-resolution images of the bones optimizing the detailed evaluation of deformities, fracture patterns, dislocations and aids in identifying subtle or occult bony abnormalities. Complex fracture patterns including intra-articular extensions can be made out easily with CT scans. CT scan also provide excellent visualization of the joint anatomy, aid in assessment of subchondral cysts in osteoarthritis and dual-energy CT scans may also quantify and ascertain the deposition of uric acid crystals in Gouty arthritis **(Fig. 14.4)**. Dynamic 4DCT helps in assessment of dynamic range of motions of multiple joints.

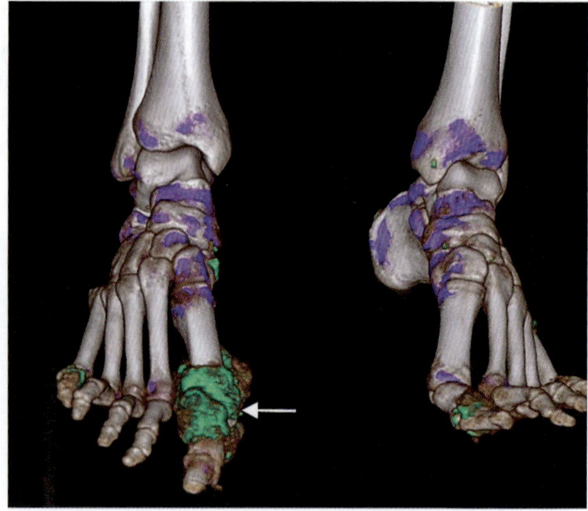

Fig. 14.4: Dual-energy CT scan showing areas of deposition of crystals in gouty arthritis (as marked by arrow).

Orthopedic surgeons frequently make use of CT scans as a roadmap for preoperative and presurgical planning, using which they can plan the optimum placement of the orthopedic hardware, determine best surgical approach and assess extent of bony involvement.

CT scans aid in characterization of bone tumors, provide information about size, location, extension and aid in diagnosis, guided interventions and treatment planning. CT also aids in guiding interventional procedures like aspirations, biopsies, injections and ablations (Radio frequency, microwave and cryoablations). Real-time visualization of the needle helps in precision needle placement, minimizes the risk of complication and leads to better patient outcomes **(Fig. 14.5)**.

CT scan is also useful in pain management in patients having spinal nerve root compression as it allows visualization of nerve root and provide excellent guidance for injection of steroid along with long-acting local anesthetic agent to provide immediate and long-term pain relief.

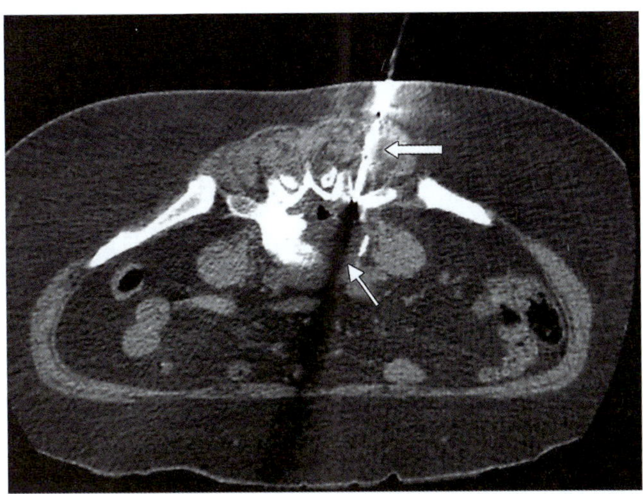

Fig. 14.5: CT guided biopsy from an osteolytic lesion involving vertebral body (marked with arrow). The biopsy needle is also seen (marked with solid arrow).

CT scan is extremely helpful in detection of condition like dystrophic ossification/myositis ossificans in patients who had history of prior trauma. MRI shows varied signals on various sequences in this condition and can misdiagnose it as aggressive soft tissue neoplastic lesion/malignancy.

CT also aids in assessment of traumatic and degenerative spinal pathologies, including fractures, ascertain bony cord compression, and also can be used to perform CT myelograms when suspecting traumatic or nontraumatic CSF leaks. Vascular relations and status can be assessed beautifully by using CT angiography.

Overall CT plays a crucial role by aiding in diagnosis and treatment planning of multiple musculoskeletal pathologies and guided interventional radiology procedures. It complements radiographs and MRI allowing comprehensive evaluation of various pathologies.

Ultrasound

It is a valuable tool for assessment of musculoskeletal pathologies as it provides real-time imaging, allowing dynamic assessment of structures including muscles, tendons, ligaments and joints which aids in assessment of soft tissue abnormalities, gliding of tendons and joint stability. It is an excellent tool to assess soft tissue pathologies including bursitis, tendonitis, soft tissue masses and grades of muscle tear **(Fig. 14.6)**. The soft tissue lesions can be assessed on the basis of size, shape, vascularity and can be classified into benign, malignant or indeterminate lesions.

It is a magnificent tool for guidance of injections and aspirations, again being real-time can increase accuracy for deployment of drugs and minimize risk of complications. Using USG, one can assess tendon movement, integrity and response of tendons to stress. Nerve ultrasound is a boon and aids in assessment of nerve entrapments, neuropathies, nerve tumors and evaluation of nerve injuries.

USG being ionizing radiation free acts as a frontline investigation for pediatric cases, with developmental dysplasia of hip (DDH), can aid in trauma settings such as contusions, strain and hematomas. USG also helps in guided biopsies.

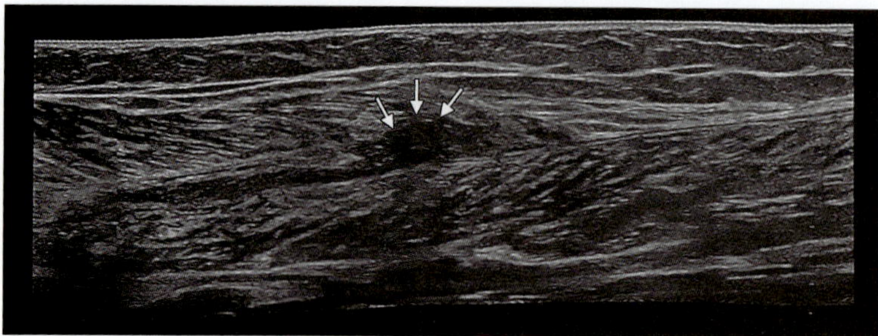

Fig. 14.6: USG panoramic image depicts disruption of normal pennate appearance of medial head of gastrocnemius muscle (<50% myoaponeurosis) and intervening hematoma (marked with arrows) along with plantaris injury.

MRI

MRI provides detailed visualization of soft tissue, assessment of muscles, tendons, ligaments, cartilage, and synovium. It provides superior soft tissue contrast than other modalities, specifically soft tissues and forms the workhorse of musculoskeletal imaging.

It is the best modality to assess articular structures like cartilage, meniscus, intra-articular ligaments and detect subtle abnormalities providing comprehensive information for diagnosis and treatment. Synovial abnormalities and bone marrow disorders can be assessed beautifully with MRI. It is highly sensitive for detection of marrow abnormalities including marrow edema, avascular necrosis, metastasis and tumors.

MRI uses various pulse sequences **(Table 14.1)** for evaluation of musculoskeletal abnormalities. Changes in MR signals of different bone and soft tissue pathologies in different MR sequences helps in diagnosing different abnormalities. The contrast enhanced MRI is done after intravenous injection of Gadolinium based contrast agents, which further help in characterization of soft tissue pathologies.

In patients of trauma, when Radiograph and CT scan do not show any fracture, MRI can still show bone marrow edema due to trabecular injuries, which usually corresponds to the site of pain.

It is the imaging modality of choice for evaluating spinal disorders including degenerative disc disease, disc herniations, spinal canal stenosis and spinal tumors (As described in chapter 13). It provides excellent details for facilitating accurate diagnosis and treatment planning.

MRI allows visualization of nerve roots in spine and provides information about exact level and degree of nerve root compression which is responsible for patient's symptoms that can be correlated as per the dermatome involvement.

It is gold standard for assessment of soft tissue tumors and masses, aids in sub-characterization of benign and malignant lesions and can also aid in guided biopsies.

Table 14.1: Various pulse sequences of MRI.

MRI sequence	*Utilities*
T1-weighted	Normal anatomy, anatomical variations, bone marrow abnormalities
T2-weighted	Pathologies, cystic lesions, muscle, ligament and tendon injuries
Proton density	Articular cartilage, ligament and tendon injuries
STIR	Bone marrow edema and subtle fractures

MRI can be used to monitor the response to treatment in musculoskeletal conditions such as inflammatory arthritis, tendonitis, and tumors. Serial MRI examinations can assess changes in disease activity, treatment efficacy, and tissue healing, guiding adjustments to the treatment plan as needed.

PET CT and PET-MRI

While CT scan and MRI have been used extensively for very long time in evaluation of different musculoskeletal disorders, hybrid imaging modalities like PET CT scan have been recently developed. These modalities combine the advantage of molecular information derived from PET and anatomical information derived from CT scan.

For evaluation of different diseases, various radio tracers are now available in PET CT. PET imaging provides functional information through the positron-emitting radiotracers which cannot be derived from CT scan. However, spatial resolution of PET CT is much lower compared to CT scan.

Fusion of the PET and CT scan data adds to the information given by single imaging modality and helps in better understanding of the musculoskeletal disorders for more effective treatment.

The most commonly used radiotracers for the evaluation of musculoskeletal disorders are 18F-fluorodeoxyglucose (18F-FDG) and 18F-sodium fluoride (18F-NaF). Out of these two, 18F-FDG is the most extensively used in clinical practice. Tumors, activated inflammatory cells and regions of infection have high glucose utility and show high avidity on PET images. 18F-NaF helps in evaluation of the blood flow as well as osteolytic and osteoblastic activity. The common utility of this radiotracer is in metabolic bone disease, fracture healing, osteonecrosis, tumors and bone graft viability.

The primary bone malignancies where PET CT scan is extremely helpful are osteosarcoma, Ewing's sarcoma, chondrosarcoma, primary bone lymphoma, multiple myeloma, etc. The PET CT scan helps in staging and grading of the tumors, monitoring of treatment response, follow-up and recurrence detection and in survival and prognostic stratification.

In patients of osteosarcoma, PET CT helps in local staging and evaluation of the metastasis. Reduction in the standardized uptake value (SUV) correspond to the response after chemotherapy. In patients having chondroid bone tumors, PET-CT helps to differentiate benign from malignant lesions. Higher SUVmax of more than 2.2–2.5 has 90% sensitivity for detection of chondrosarcoma. In patients with Ewing's sarcoma, higher SUV values correspond to the higher Tumor Grade. In patients with multiple myeloma, as bone scan is negative in many instances, PET-CT helps in determining the extent of the multiple lesions. PET CT scan also helps in detection of extraosseous deposits.

As many of these bone tumors are heterogeneous with areas of necrosis, PET CT has very important role in determining the areas of higher tumor activity to decide the biopsy site for more accurate results **(Fig. 14.7)**.

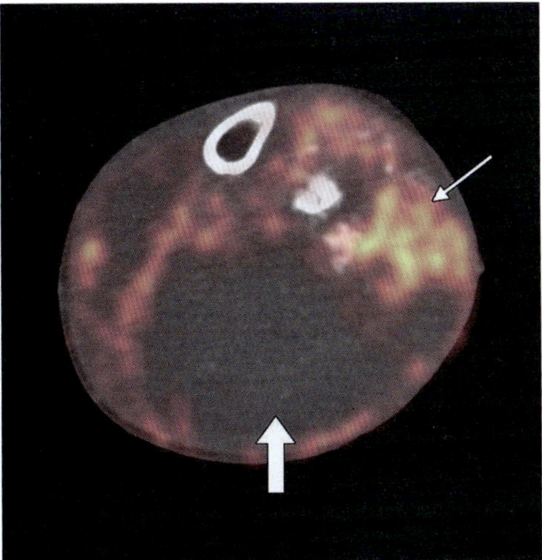

Fig. 14.7: PET-CT scan of a patient having osteosarcoma of fibula showing small peripheral areas of increased radiotracer activity (marked with arrow) and large central areas of necrosis (solid arrow).

In postoperative patients with metallic implants, MRI and CT scan can be of limited help due to artifacts. PET-CT scan can be of significant help in these patients to evaluate for infections and other postoperative complications.

In conditions like rheumatoid arthritis, osteoarthritis and metabolic bone disorders, PET CT scan helps in evaluation of severity of disease and response to treatment.

Recently, PET MRI systems have also been introduced to combine the advantages of PET and MRI as MRI has better soft tissue resolution compared to CT scan in evaluation of different musculoskeletal abnormalities. PET MRI also has advantage of lower radiation dose as compared to PET-CT scan.

COMMON INDICATIONS OF MUSCULOSKELETAL IMAGING

Evaluation of Sports Injuries

Imaging place a very important role in sports injuries by providing accurate assessment and prognosis of the injury. CT scan, MRI and X-rays are all commonly used in diagnosing and treating sports injuries.

X-rays are useful for the primary evaluation while MRI has a multifaceted role and it provides accurate diagnosis, prognostication for return to play and assessment of healing after injury.

MRI also has a very important role in differentiating acute injuries from chronic remodeling injuries which occurs in the presence of repetitive microtrauma in athletes.

Because of its ability to detect bone marrow edema very early, MRI can detect stress injuries in spine as well as various other bones, which if untreated can progress to fractures. Early detection of these injuries can help optimizing the patient care by providing rest that can result in early return to play and complete healing.

MRI is commonly used in sports injuries including muscle and ligament sprains, ligament tears, stress fractures and tendon injuries **(Figs. 14.8A and B)**. Detailed anatomical information and characterization of severity of injury aids in treatment planning and also estimating the return to play decisions for athletes. USG guided interventions including PRP (platelet rich plasma) injections can be done to facilitate healing and decrease off time for players.

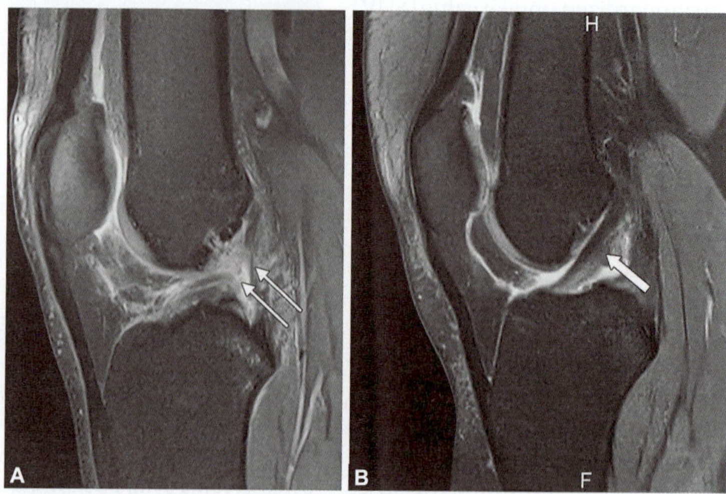

Figs. 14.8A and B: MRI in sports injuries: (A) Showing complete tear of anterior cruciate ligament (marked with arrows); (B) Compare it with the normal anterior cruciate ligament in a different patient (marked with block arrow).

Evaluation of Musculoskeletal Infections

Musculoskeletal infections include osteomyelitis, septic arthritis, soft tissue infections and tubercular infections. Because rich transphyseal vascular networks allow infections of the bone to cross the growth plate, (osteomyelitis and joint infections—septic arthritis) commonly coexist in newborn child. Osteomyelitis refers to infection of bone involving the medullary cavity that is typically bacterial. Usually, osteomyelitis results from hematogenous spread of infection. However, it can be due to direct extension from trauma or ulcers in some instances. Most common organism that causes osteomyelitis is *Staphylococcus aureus*. The common site of involvement can vary as per the age. In neonates, metaphysis and/or epiphysis are most commonly affected, while in children, the most common site of involvement is metaphysis. In adults, it commonly involves epiphyses and subchondral regions.

Radiographs are the first-line imaging modality for evaluation of osteomyelitis. In acute infections/acute osteomyelitis, common radiographic features are regional osteopenia, periosteal reaction—which can be aggressive including Codman's triangle, osteolysis/erosions and loss of trabecular architecture of bone. The aggressive looking appearance of acute osteomyelitis can mimic a bone tumor like round cell tumor.

In chronic infections/chronic osteomyelitis, the characteristic imaging features are sequestrum (a dense piece of devascularized bone that becomes separated from the remainder of the bone), involucrum is lucent (a thick sheath of periosteal new bone surrounding a sequestrum) and/or cloaca (a defect in the cortex of the affected bone).

USG helps in evaluation of associated soft tissue changes in form of edema and fluid collections. It also helps as guide for aspiration of the collection. Commonly used to detect joint effusion in viral arthritis of children.

CT scan is more sensitive than the radiograph for evaluation of periosteal reaction, sequestrum, cloaca and involucrum **(Figs. 14.9A and B)**. With addition of intravenous contrast, it can give further details of the collection/abscess in adjacent soft tissue.

MRI is most sensitive and specific imaging modality for diagnosis and evaluation of extent of bone involvement by osteomyelitis. It can detect the changes as early as 1 to 2 days of onset of infection. MRI also helps in evaluation of complications of osteomyelitis like involvement of

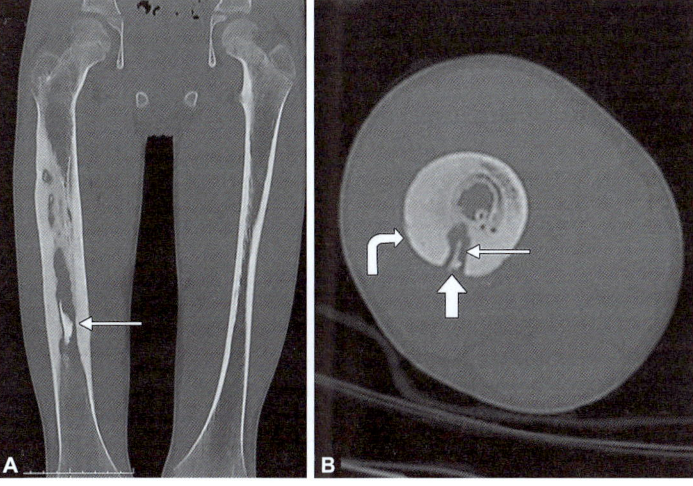

Figs. 14.9A and B: CT scan of femur (A and B) Coronal reformatted and axial images showing osteolytic lesion involving diaphysis of femur with periosteal reaction and sequestrum (marked with arrow), cloaca (marked with block arrow) and involucrum (marked with curved arrow).

joint or neurovascular bundle. MRI can also detect and characterize soft tissue infections like cellulitis and myositis.

Bone scintigraphy (Tc-99m), Indium-111 labeled WBC scintigraphy, Gallium-67 scintigraphy or PET CT can also be used for evaluation of osteomyelitis.

In tuberculous infections, patients can present with 'cold abscess' and localized swelling or discharging sinus. The infection can be multifocal involving multiple bones and joints at different parts of the body.

Evaluation of Bone Tumors

Imaging plays a crucial role in the management of patients with bone tumors. In spite of availability of highly advanced imaging modalities, even today radiographs remain the primary and most important tool for the diagnosis of a bone tumor. Radiographs are preferably obtained in two imaging planes—Anteroposterior and lateral or oblique for the site of clinical swelling or suspected bone lesion. The Mnemonic 'STAMPS' helps in remembering various features that need to be considered while analyzing a radiograph for bone tumor where 'S' stands for Solitary and Site, 'T' stands for Transitional zone, 'A' stands for Aggressiveness and Age, 'M' stands for Mineralization of the matrix, 'P' stands for Periosteal reaction and 'S' stands for soft tissue morphology **(Figs. 14.1 and 14.2)**. Limitations of radiographs include evaluation of lesions located at complex anatomic locations like spine, iliac bones and posterior elements of vertebrae where overlapping of structures limit the visualization of the lesions. Radiographs also have limitations in evaluation of soft tissue and extent of medullary involvement.

CT scan helps in evaluation of lesions at such complex regions and also allows visualization of minor bony changes, small calcifications, tumor mineralization, cortical changes and periosteal reactions. Still CT scan lacks in precise delineation of lesion extent due to inability to evaluate medullary involvement and soft tissue characterization.

MRI is considered as the best imaging modality for local staging of the bone tumors. The inherent capability of soft tissue characterization and extreme sensitivity for evaluation of bone marrow changes make it ideal for the complete evaluation of the extent of the lesion. MRI also helps in evaluation of the lesion extension up to articular margin and within the joint. The neurovascular structures and their encasement by the lesion can be accurately assessed with the help of MRI. Advanced MRI techniques like Diffusion Weighted Imaging (DWI) and Perfusion MRI are useful for differentiating benign from malignant bone lesions and in evaluation of treatment response.

FDG PET CT and PET MRI helps in distant staging of the lesion. They also help in predicting aggressiveness of the lesion as the malignant lesions are generally more FDG avid than benign lesions of same histological type. These molecular imaging methods also help in deciding biopsy site and evaluating response to treatment.

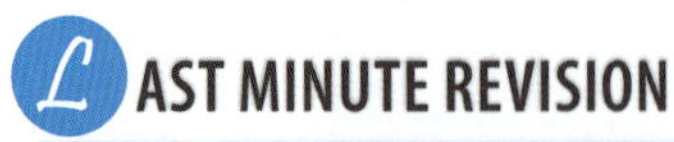

- Modern diagnostic imaging includes conventional radiography/X-rays, Ultrasonography (USG), computed tomography (CT) scans, Magnetic resonance imaging (MRI) and musculoskeletal interventional radiology.
- Radiographs play a vital role in assessment of fractures and their extensions, identifying patterns of dislocations, assessing benign and malignant bone tumors, skeletal dysplasia and almost all rheumatological pathologies.
- CT scan helps in detailed evaluation of deformities, fracture patterns, and aids in identifying subtle or occult bony abnormalities, complex fracture patterns providing preoperative roadmap, extension of bone tumors and to guide various interventional procedures like biopsies and injections.

- USG is useful as it provides real-time imaging, allowing dynamic assessment of structures including muscles, tendons, ligaments and joints. Excellent tool for guidance of injections and aspirations.
- MRI provides detailed visualization of soft tissue, muscles, tendons, ligaments, cartilage, and synovium. It is also useful for detection of bone marrow abnormalities.
- MRI uses different sequences for better visualization of different structures.
- Be careful while using radiographs and CT scan in pediatric patients, to keep the radiation dose as low as reasonably achievable while USG and MRI are safer options as they do not use radiation.
- PET CT is a hybrid imaging modality that uses different radiotracers and combines the advantage of molecular information derived from PET and anatomical information derived from CT scan.
- Main utility of PET CT in MSK imaging includes evaluation of bone and soft tissue tumors, infections, arthritis, guiding the biopsy and evaluation of response to treatment.

REVIEW QUESTIONS

Multiple Choice Questions (MCQs)

1. **Which of the following finding of radiograph is useful in identifying underlying metabolic disorders?**
   a. Fracture
   b. Osteopenia
   c. Bone tumor
   d. Bone infection
2. **Dynamic assessment of tendons and muscles is possible with which imaging modality?**
   a. CT scan
   b. Radiographs
   c. MRI
   d. Ultrasonography (USG)
3. **Which MRI sequence is most useful for evaluation of subtle fractures?**
   a. STIR
   b. T2 weighted
   c. Proton density
   d. None of the above
4. **A piece of devascularized bone that becomes separated from the parent bone is called:**
   a. Periosteal reaction
   b. Involucrum
   c. Sequestrum
   d. Sinus
5. **In which of the following 18F-FDG PET CT is not useful?**
   a. Bone tumors
   b. Infections
   c. Fractures
   d. Ligament injuries

Answer Key

1. b 2. d 3. a 4. c 5. d

SUGGESTED READING

1. Bohndorf K, Kilcoyne RF. Traumatic injuries: Imaging of peripheral musculoskeletal injuries. Eur Radiol. 2002 Jul;12(7):1605-16. doi: 10.1007/s00330-002-1461-8. Epub 2002 May 18. PMID: 12111052.
2. Dalinka MK, Boorstein JM, Zlatkin MB. Computed tomography of musculoskeletal trauma. Radiol Clin North Am. 1989 Sep;27(5):933-44. PMID: 2672082.
3. Renner JB. Introduction to musculoskeletal imaging. In: Esther, RJ. (Ed). Clinical Foundations of Musculoskeletal Medicine. Springer, Cham. 2021. https://doi.org/10.1007/978-3-030-42894-5_3
4. Shadpour D, Francis IB, Joshua GK, Elena G, Hamza AI, Kamyar M, et al. Musculoskeletal CT Imaging: State-of-the-Art Advancements and Future Directions. 2023;308:2.
5. WA Murphy, Jr. Introduction to the history of musculoskeletal radiology. RadioGraphics. 1990;10(5): 915-43.

UNIT 3

Obstetric and Gynecological Imaging

Unit Outline

CHAPTER

15

Basics of Obstetric Imaging

"In obstetric imaging, every heartbeat seen is a promise—radiologists bring the first glimpse of life into focus."

INTRODUCTION

Obstetrics imaging comprises primarily ultrasonography (USG). Ultrasonography is used widely for the prenatal evaluation as well as management of fetus. Various guidelines have been laid for fetal examination across each trimester. This chapter will discuss salient features of obstetrics ultrasound in each trimester along with Doppler assessment.

Techniques

Early first-trimester ultrasonography is commonly done through transvaginal route. 11–14 weeks scan (NT scan), anomaly scan, and growth scan are done via transabdominal route. The transvaginal route is also used to measure cervix length, scar assessment in previous LSCS and detailed evaluation of fetal anatomy. Sometimes high-frequency probe can also be used for dedicated study of fetal parts.

Obstetrics imaging comprises four basic scans:

1. Early first-trimester scan or viability scan or dating scan.
2. NT/NB scan or level 1 scan
3. Anomaly scan or level 2 scan or targeted imaging for fetal anomalies (TIFFA scan)
4. Third-trimester scan or growth scan

EARLY FIRST-TRIMESTER SCAN OR VIABILITY SCAN

It is performed between 7–10 weeks. The aim of early pregnancy scan is to locate early pregnancy such as intrauterine pregnancy (IUP) or ectopic pregnancy; viable versus nonviable IUP, IUP of uncertain viability and pregnancy of unknown location. It also confirm number of gestation, chronicity and correct dating. Beyond this, it can also assess any uterine anomalies, any associated uterine and ovarian pathologies.

It is essential to understand the chronological sequence of appearance of various embryonic structures **(Table 15.1)** in order to understand the diagnostic possibilities of early first-trimester scan, i.e., final outcome either normal healthy fetus or pregnancy failure.

Normal Pregnancy Changes in Early Intrauterine Pregnancy

- Fluid surrounding embryo and yolk sac is called amniotic cavity and chorionic cavity respectively.

Table 15.1: Chronological growth in early pregnancy.

Sonographic finding on TVS	*Time period of appearance in gestational age in weeks/technique to measure*	*Sonographic features*
Intradecidual sign	<04 weeks	Earliest sign of IUP seen on USG as an eccentrically located gestational sac within the echogenic decidua, with a relatively undisturbed collapsed uterine cavity visualized as a thin echogenic line **(Fig. 15.1A)**
Gestational sac (forming chorionic cavity)	4.5 weeks (measured in three orthogonal planes with calipers placed at the inner margins)	1–2 mm fluid collection surrounded by echogenic rim **(Fig. 15.1B)** Not extend beyond endomyometrial junction
Yolk sac	5–5.5 weeks (measured in three orthogonal planes with caliper placed at the inner margins)	Absolutely confirms IUP. Circular thick-walled anechoic structure having echogenic rim within the gestational sac **(Fig. 15.1C)**
Embryonic pole/CRL, i.e., crown-rump length. Embryo is up to 8 weeks of gestational age and afterwards called a fetus	6 weeks (midline sagittal section of embryo in neutral position, ideal orientation is horizontal, magnification, i.e., fill most of screen, endpoints clearly defined)	1–4 mm echogenic structure adjacent to yolk sac **(Fig. 15.1C)**
Cardiac activity	6 weeks or should be seen with CRL ≥6 mm	Flickering motion inside embryonic pole
Double sac sign (appearance helps to differentiate from pseudo sac or intrauterine fluid collection)	Definitive sign of IUP	Consists of two concentric echogenic rings surrounding the fluid collection and separated by a thin crescent of endometrial fluid
Amniotic cavity	Earliest seen at 6.5 weeks of gestational age	Thin membrane with fluid surrounding embryo

Note: Chorionic cavity: It is fluid containing cavity surrounding amniotic cavity. Amnion and chorion fuses with each other at 14–16 weeks with obliteration of chorionic cavity.

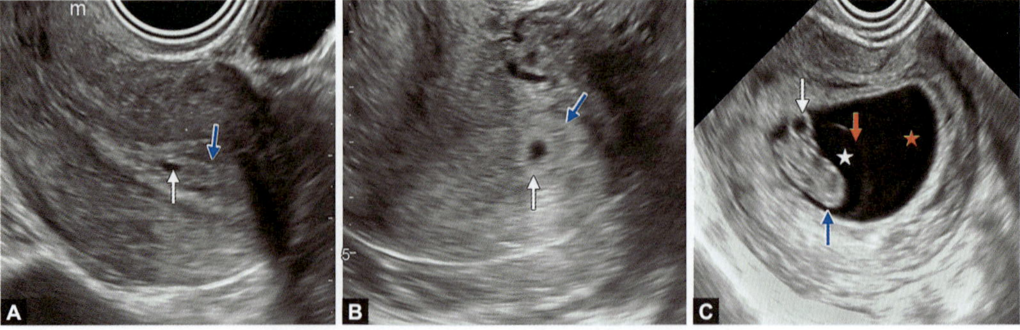

Figs. 15.1A to C: (A) Transvaginal USG showing 2 mm sized early gestational sac (white arrow) is embedded within decidua adjacent to endometrial cavity (blue arrow) also known as intradecidual sign; (B) Transvaginal USG showing double decidual sign comprising of inner echogenic rim (white arrow) representing decidua capsularis and outer echogenic rim (blue arrow) representing decidua parietalis; (C) Transvaginal USG showing yolk sac (white arrow), amnion (red arrow), chorionic cavity (red star), amniotic cavity (white star), and embryo (blue arrow) in 7 weeks of pregnancy.

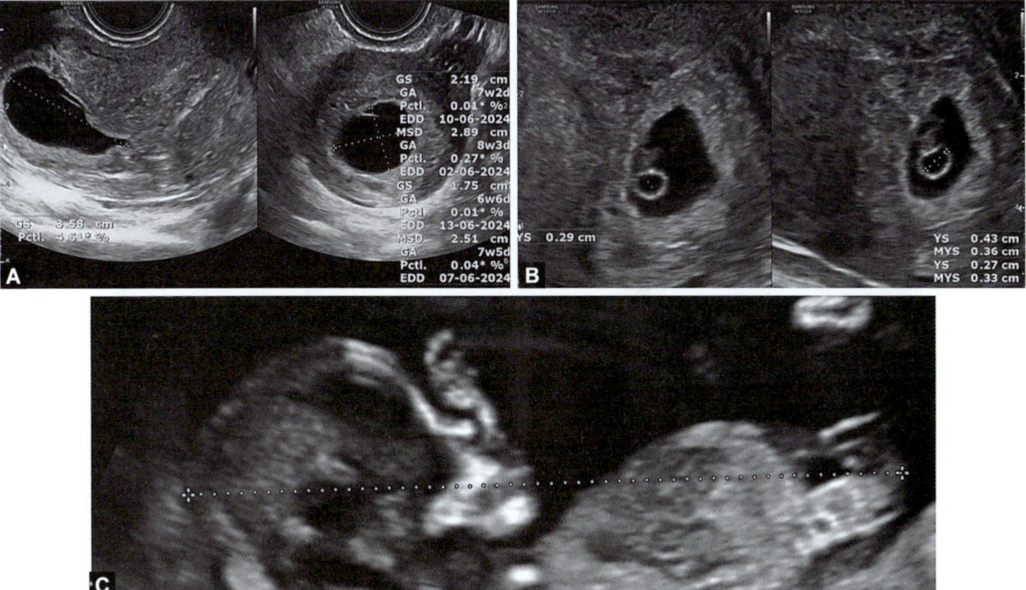

Figs. 15.2A to C: Showing measurement of mean sac diameter (A), yolk sac (B), and CRL (C).

- Accurate dating of the pregnancy by CRL measurement **(Figs. 15.2A to C)**.
- Detection of multiple pregnancies with reliable diagnosis of chorionicity: First-trimester is the best time to establish chorionicity and amnionicity. Gestational sac is precursor to the chorion or placenta; therefore number of gestational sac corresponds to the chorionicity. Number of yolk sac corresponds to amnion; therefore two yolk sac suggest diamniotic twin. Two gestational sac with two yolk sac suggests dichorionic diamniotic twin. Single gestational sac with two yolk sac suggests monochorionic diamniotic twin **(Figs. 15.3A and B)**.

Abnormal Early First-trimester Pregnancy

Abnormal early pregnancy findings includes.

Nonviable Pregnancy-diagnostic Criteria for Nonviable Pregnancy

If any one of ultrasonographic findings are present, it is a nonviable pregnancy or miscarriage:

- MSD ≥25 mm (with no obvious yolk sac or fetal pole)
- Embryo with CRL ≥7 mm without evidence of fetal heart activity
- MSD ≥18 mm without embryo, more than 70 days after LMP
- Embryo ≥3 mm without fetal heart activity, more than 70 days after LMP **(Fig. 15.4)**

Intrauterine Pregnancy of Uncertain Viability

Common findings that create suspicious, but not diagnostic of pregnancy failure or intrauterine pregnancy of uncertain viability.

- Enlarged yolk sac >7 mm
- Empty amnion sign
- <5 mm difference between MSD and CRL

If any of the above findings are present, follow-up ultrasonography after 7–10 days are advised to assess viability.

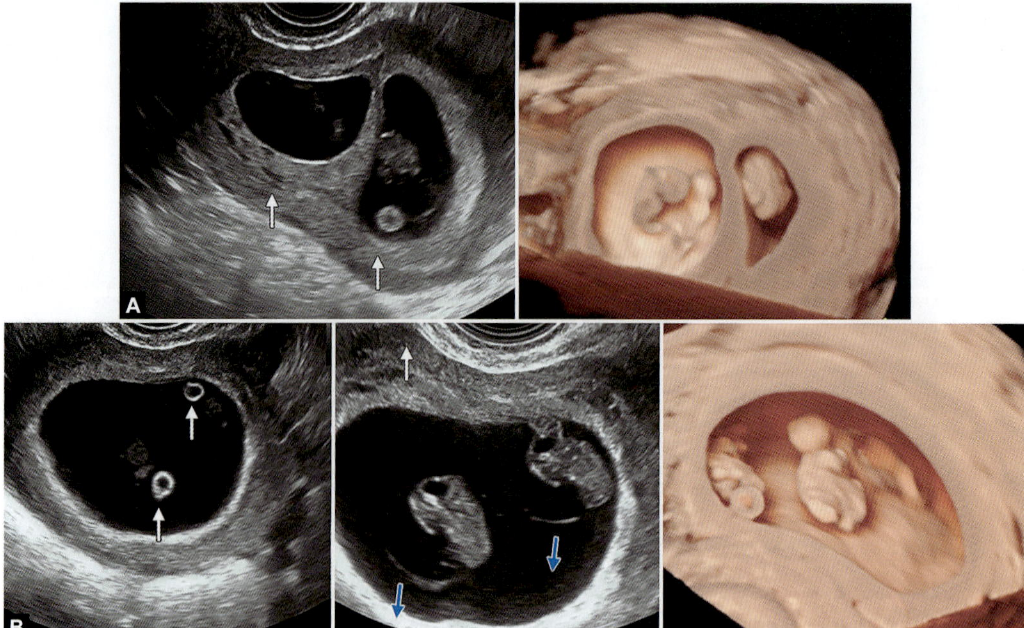

Figs. 15.3A and B: (A) Showing two separate gestational sac (arrow) with thick intertwin membrane suggesting dichorionic diamniotic twin gestation; (B) Single gestational sac with two yolk sac (white arrow) and two separate amniotic cavity (blue arrow) suggesting monochorionic diamniotic twin gestation.

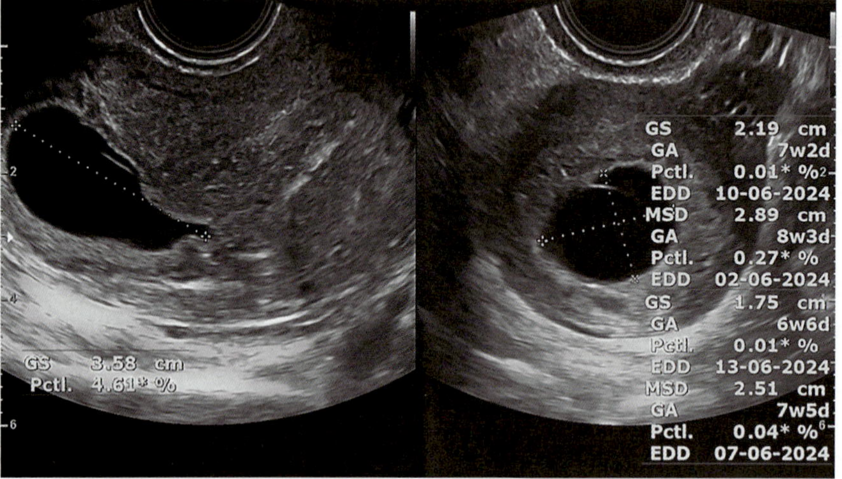

Fig. 15.4: Transvaginal USG showing irregular gestational sac, mean sac diameter measured more than 25 mm, embryo and yolk sac are not seen; findings suggesting nonviable pregnancy or miscarriage.

Pregnancy of Unknown Location

Pregnancy of unknown location (PUL) is the term given to the transient state of early pregnancy during which no definite IUP is visualized at US and the adnexa are normal or we can say normal pelvis USG findings.

At this stage, the three main possibilities include early IUP, occult ectopic pregnancy, and completed spontaneous abortion. Initial serum progesterone level, hCG ratio (hCG at 48 h/hCG at 0 h) and follow-up USG will help in determining outcome of PUL.

Ectopic Pregnancy

When pregnancy is located outside the uterine cavity, is called ectopic pregnancy. It can be uterine or extrauterine ectopic pregnancy. Extrauterine ectopic pregnancy includes tubal, ovarian, abdominal ectopic pregnancy. Uterine ectopic pregnancy includes intramural, caesarean, and cervical ectopic pregnancy.

NT/NB SCAN OR LEVEL 1 SCAN

It is performed between 11 and 13 + 6 weeks' gestation. It gives opportunities for:

- Assessing aneuploidy risk of common aneuploidies such as trisomy 13, 18, and 21.
- Early diagnosis of many major fetal abnormalities by detailed systematic examination of fetal anatomy such as head, neck, thorax, abdomen, spine and limbs.
- To identify women at increased risk for the development of preeclampsia in pregnancy by pulsatility index of uterine artery Doppler.

Aneuploidy Risk Assessment

There are many soft tissue sonographic markers for aneuploidy such as nuchal translucency, ossification of nasal bone, ductus venosus and tricuspid valve waveform assessment. Risk for common aneuploidies such as trisomy 13, 18, and 21 is calculated by combining USG marker and biochemical marker (beta HCG and PAPP-A = double marker done at 10–13 weeks) called as combined first-trimester screening test. We shall discuss in detail about sonographic aneuploidy markers.

Note: PAPP-A = Pregnancy associated plasma protein-A

Nuchal Translucency (NT)

It is the sonographic appearance of a collection of fluid under the skin behind the fetal neck in the first-trimester of pregnancy. It is one of the crucial component of first-trimester scan and has to be measured following strict guidelines given by Fetal Medicine Foundation. Even a slight error in measurements can lead to significant change in aneuploidy risk assessment. Normal value <3 mm should be measures from inner to inner border of lucency in neutral midsagittal view **(Fig. 15.5A)**.

Nasal Bone Criteria (Fig. 15.5A)

- In the assessment of the fetal nasal bone the gestation should be 11^{+0} to 13^{+6} weeks and the CRL 45–84 mm.
- The magnification of the image should be such that the head and upper thorax occupy the whole screen.
- A midsagittal view of the fetal profile should be obtained.
- When these criteria are satisfied, three distinct lines should be seen at the level of the fetal nose:
  - The top line represents the skin.
  - The bottom one, which is thicker and more echogenic than the overlying skin, represents the nasal bone.
  - A third line in front of the bone and at a higher level than the skin represents the tip of the nose.
- The nasal bone is considered to be present if it is more echogenic than the overlying skin and absent if it is either not visible or its echogenicity is the same or less than that of the skin.

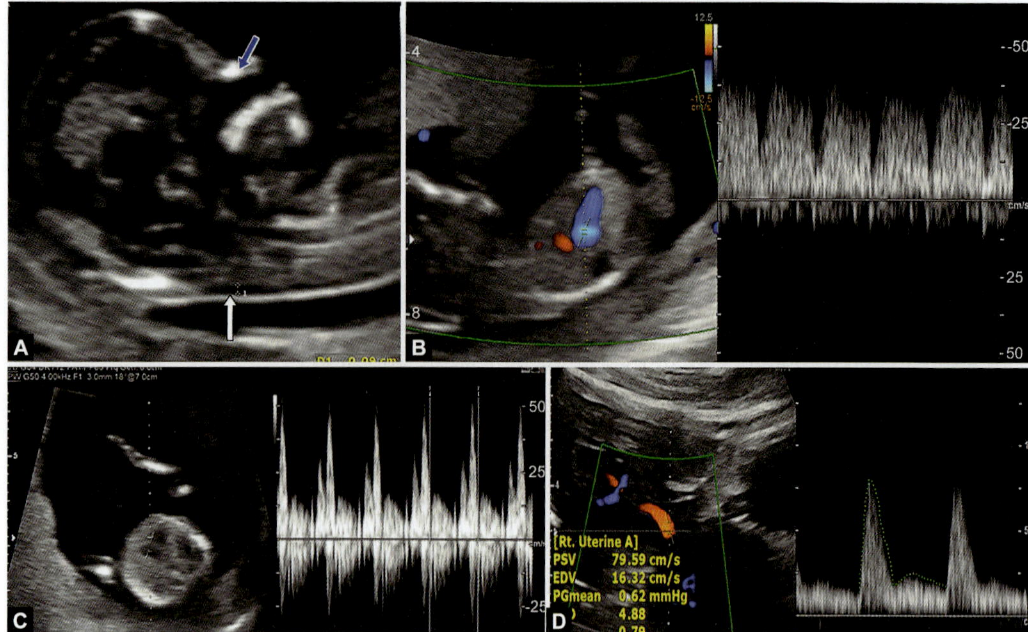

Figs. 15.5A to D: First-trimester aneuploidy marker assessment. (A) Showing measurement of nuchal translucency (white arrow) and assessment of nasal bone (blue arrow); (B) Showing ductus venosus waveform; (C) Showing tricuspid waveform; (D) Showing uterine artery Doppler in first-trimester.

Ductus Venosus (Fig. 15.5B)

- In the assessment of ductus venosus flow the gestation should be 11^{+0} to 13^{+6} weeks and the CRL 45–84 mm.
- The fetus should not be moving.
- The magnification of the image should be such that the fetal thorax and abdomen occupy the whole screen.
- A right ventral midsagittal view of the fetal trunk should be obtained.
- Color flow mapping should be used to demonstrate the umbilical vein, ductus venosus and fetal heart.

Tricuspid Flow (Fig. 15.5C)

In the assessment of tricuspid flow, it is important that the following criteria are observed:

- The gestation should be 11^{+0} to 13^{+6} weeks and the CRL 45–84 mm.
- The fetus should not be moving.
- The magnification of the image should be such that the fetal thorax occupies the whole screen.
- An apical four-chamber view of the fetal heart should be obtained.
- Color flow mapping should not be used because it is unreliable for the diagnosis of tricuspid regurgitation in the first-trimester.

Uterine Artery Doppler (Fig. 15.5D)

- Mean pulsatility index (PI) of both uterine arteries are measured for preeclampsia prediction.
- In the measurement of the uterine artery pulsatility index (PI) the gestation should be 11^{+0}–13^{+6} weeks and the crown-rump length 45–84 mm.

- A sagittal section of the uterus should be obtained and the cervical canal and internal cervical os identified.
- The transducer should be gently tilted from side to side and color flow mapping should be used to identify each uterine artery along the side of the cervix and uterus at the level of the internal os.

Fetal Biometry in First-trimester Scan

Crown Rump Length (CRL)

Already discuss in **Table 15.1 (Fig. 15.6A)**

Biparietal Diameter and Head Circumference (Fig. 15.6B)

It is measured at the level of thalami in axial plane. In measurement of BPD- Calipers should be placed at outer to inner margin of bone. Head circumference is measured by placing caliper at the outer margin of calvarium.

Abdominal Circumference (Fig. 15.6C)

It is measured in the axial section of abdomen at the level of stomach by placing caliper at the outer surface of skin by ellipse method or calculating from anteroposterior or transverse abdominal diameter.

Femur Length (Fig. 15.6D)

It is measured in the long axis plane of femur by placing calipers at the end.

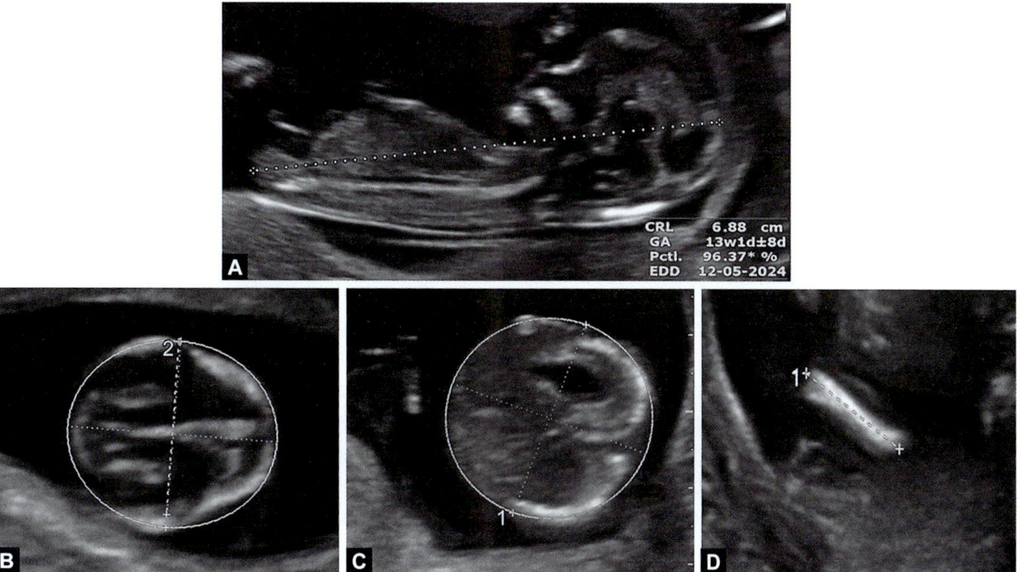

Figs. 15.6A to D: Fetal biometry in first-trimester. (A) Showing measurement of CRL; (B) Showing BPD and HC measurement; (C) Showing abdominal circumference measurement, and (D) showing femur length measurement.

ANOMALY SCAN OR LEVEL 2 SCAN OR TARGETED IMAGING FOR FETAL ANOMALIES (TIFFA SCAN)

It is mid-trimester scan performed between 18–22 weeks of period of gestation. Detailed anatomical evaluation of fetus is done in this scan. While assessing fetal structural anomaly environment surrounded the fetal are also studied. So, Components of anomaly scan includes:

- Fetal anatomy
- Assessment of amniotic fluid
- Placenta
- Fetal biometry
- Cervix
- Uterine artery Doppler
- Others—If any adnexal, myometrial or cervical pathologies to be reported.

Fetal evaluation at anomaly scan is performed according to ISUOG 20+2 plane approach. The key to the 20+2 planes approach is understanding the importance of knowing what the normal ultrasound appearances are in each plane of fetus from head to toe. This basic step helps in exclusion of a range of abnormal appearances/abnormalities, rather than 'making a diagnosis'.

Fetal Head

It is evaluated in three axial planes

Transventricular Plane (Fig. 15.7A)

It is at the level of lateral ventricle showing anterior and posterior part of lateral ventricle, Cavum septum pellucidum (CSP) in midline in anterior 1/3rd part interrupting midline falx. Width of lateral ventricle is measured in transventricular plane at the level of parieto-occipital sulcus. Its normal value is <10 mm. Ventriculomegaly is lateral ventricle width more than 10 mm.

Transthalamic Plane

(Biparietal diameter and head circumference are measured in this plane) **(Fig. 15.7B)**. It is acquired in axial plane inferior to transventricular plane by fulfilling following criteria:

- Transverse view of the fetal head at the level of the thalami
- Symmetrical appearance of both hemispheres
- Midline echo (falx cerebri) interrupted anteriorly by the cavum septi pellucidi
- Cerebellum not visible

Transcerebellar Plane (Fig. 15.7C)

It is obtained by slightly moving the probe caudal to transthalamic plane and tilting slightly posterior. Cerebellum, cistern magna is visualized in posterior fossa. Cerebellum appears butterfly shaped structure separated by echogenic vermis. Transcerebellar diameter and cisterna magna are measured in this plane. When cisterna magna measured >10 mm, it is called mega cisterna magna. Nuchal fold thickness is also measured (normal value <6 mm).

Head should also be assessed in sagittal and coronal plane corresponding to above mentioned axial plane.

Fetal Face (Figs. 15.8A to C)

It is evaluated in coronal to assess upper lip, orbit, nostrils and midsagittal facial profile.

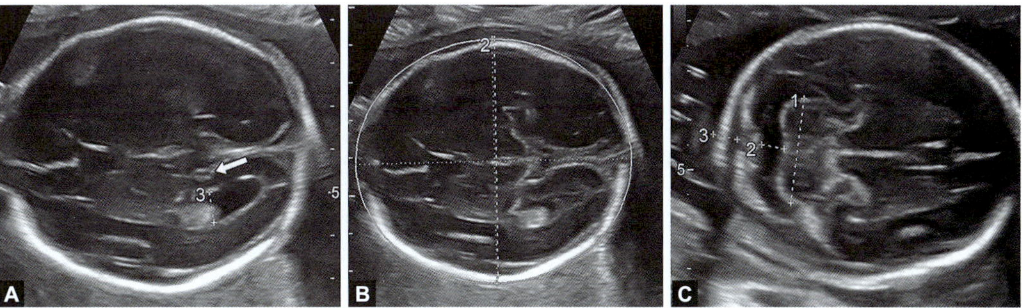

Figs. 15.7A to C: (A) Transventricular plane showing measurement of width of lateral ventricle at the level of parieto-occipital sulcus (arrow); (B) Transthalamic plane showing measurement of biparietal diameter and head circumference; (C) Transcerebellar plane showing measurement of transcerebellar diameter [1], cisterna magna [2], and nuchal fold [3].

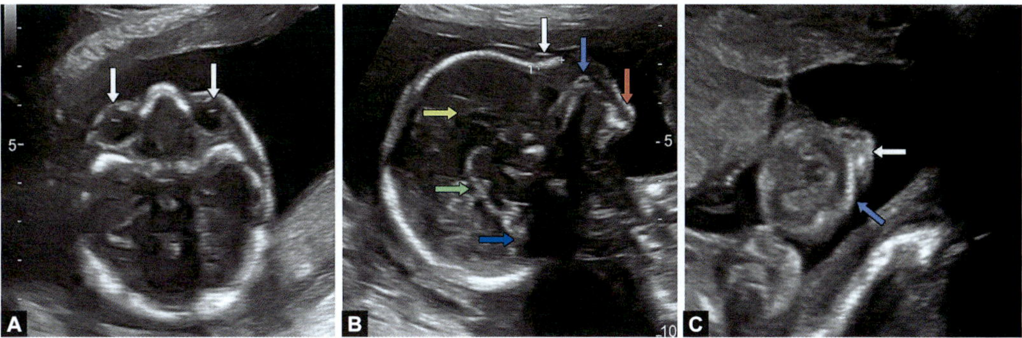

Figs. 15.8A to C: (A) Axial section of face showing bilateral orbits with lens (arrow); (B) Sagittal section or profile view of showing nasal bone (white arrow), palate (blue arrow), mandible (red arrow), corpus callosum (yellow arrow), midbrain (green arrow), and vermis (black arrow); (C) Coronal section of face showing nose (white arrow) and lip (blue arrow).

Fetal Neck

It is evaluated for any neck masses or fluid collection such as cystic hygromas, goiter or teratomas.

Fetal Thorax

It is evaluated for shape, ribs, any focal lesion involving lung such bronchopulmonary sequestration, congenital pulmonary airway malformation, masses and diaphragmatic hernia in 4 chamber view and coronal plane.

Fetal Heart (Figs. 15.9A to F)

Its evaluation includes situs, cardiac rate rhythm, axis, structural and functional abnormalities. Recommended planes are 4-chamber, outflow tracts, three-vessel view. Fetal heart rate ranged between 120–160 bpm normally. For normal situs, fetal heart in chest and stomach in abdomen should be positioned on the same side depending on lie and presentation of fetus. Normal fetal heart occupies 1/3rd area of chest and normal cardiac axis is 45 ± 20° towards the left side of the fetus.

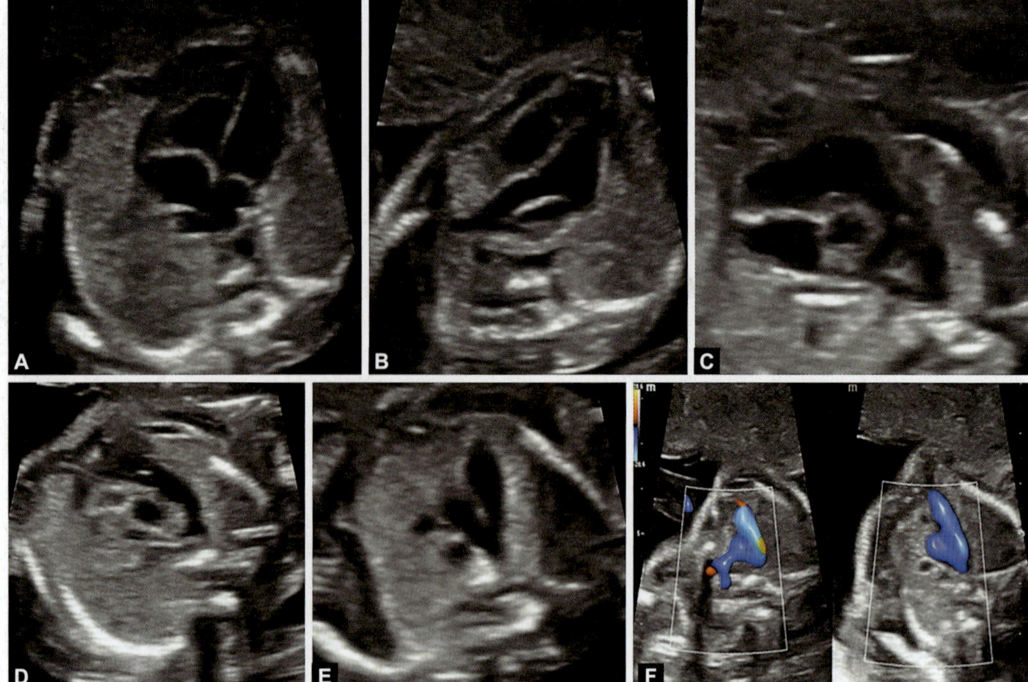

Figs. 15.9A to F: Various cardiac planes. (A) 4-chamber view; (B) Left ventricular outflow tract; (C) Right ventricular outflow tract; (D) 3-vessel view; (E) 3-vessel trachea view; (F) Colored arch view with normally oriented right subclavian artery.

Fetal Abdomen (Figs. 15.10A to C)

Abdominal situs, fetal stomach, gallbladder, umbilical vein, cord insertion, bowel echogenicity, any abnormal fluid collection, kidneys, and urinary bladder are mainly evaluated. Transverse section of abdomen is taken at the level of stomach, umbilical vein, at the level of umbilical cord insertion and transverse section of bilateral kidneys with renal pelvis.

Abdominal circumference is measured in axial section fulfilling following criteria:

- Transverse section of fetal abdomen
- As circular as possible
- Short length of umbilical vein at the level of portal sinus
- Stomach bubble visualized
- Kidneys should not be visible

Fetal Kidney (Fig. 10C)

Kidney are evaluated for its presence, kidney size, echogenicity, dilatation of renal pelvis, ureter, mass.

Fetal Pelvis

Urinary bladder is evaluated in transverse section of pelvis along with umbilical arteries adjacent to it. Fetal urinary bladder should not reach till the level of umbilicus and if its nonvisualized should prompt for abnormalities.

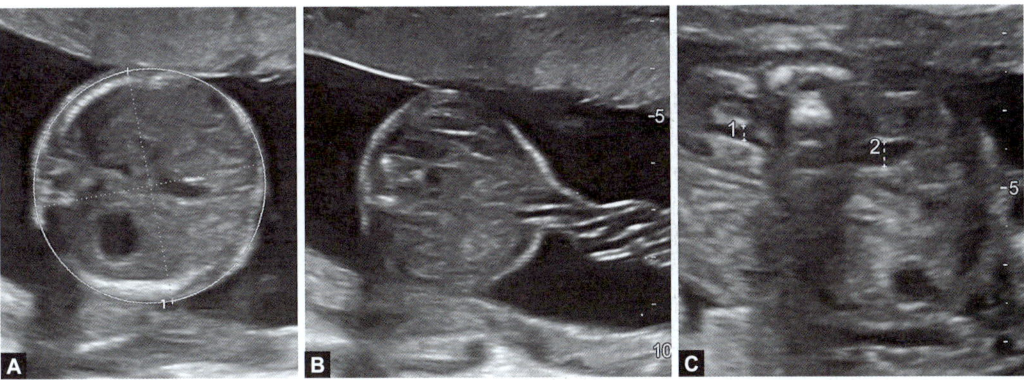

Figs. 15.10A to C: (A) Showing measurement of abdominal circumference; (B) Axial section of abdomen showing umbilical cord insertion; (C) Axial section of kidneys at the level of renal pelvis showing bilateral kidneys in paravertebral location.

Fetal Spine (Fig. 15.11)

Neural tube defect/spinal dysraphism (mainly spina bifida) commonly affect fetal spine. In sagittal plane, spine with intact skin should be demonstrated. In coronal view, vertebral body should be seen. If evaluated in all planes, spinal dysraphism, vertebral segmentation anomalies can be detected.

Limbs and Extremities (Figs. 15.12A to D)

Presence of all four extremities with feet should be documented. All long bones are assessed for their symmetry, length, shape, alignment, position and movement.

Femur length is measured in the following recommended plane:

- Imaged with both ends of the ossified diaphysis visible
- The longest axis of the ossified diaphysis is measured
- Excluding the distal femoral epiphysis if it is visible
- Excluding triangular spur artifacts that can extend the diaphysis length falsely.

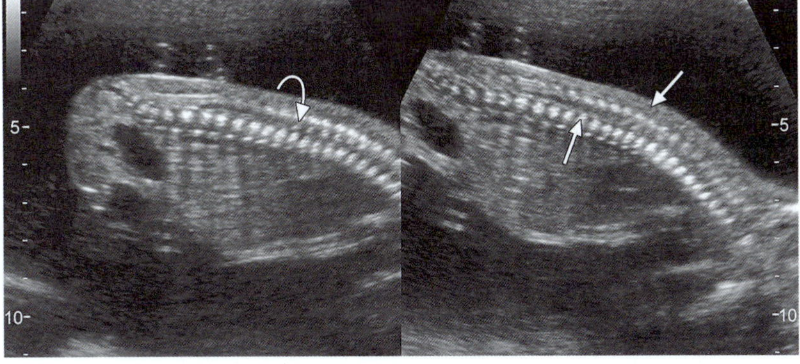

Fig. 15.11: Sagittal section of spine showing intact skin (white arrow), pedicle (curved arrow) and vertebral bodies (solid arrow).

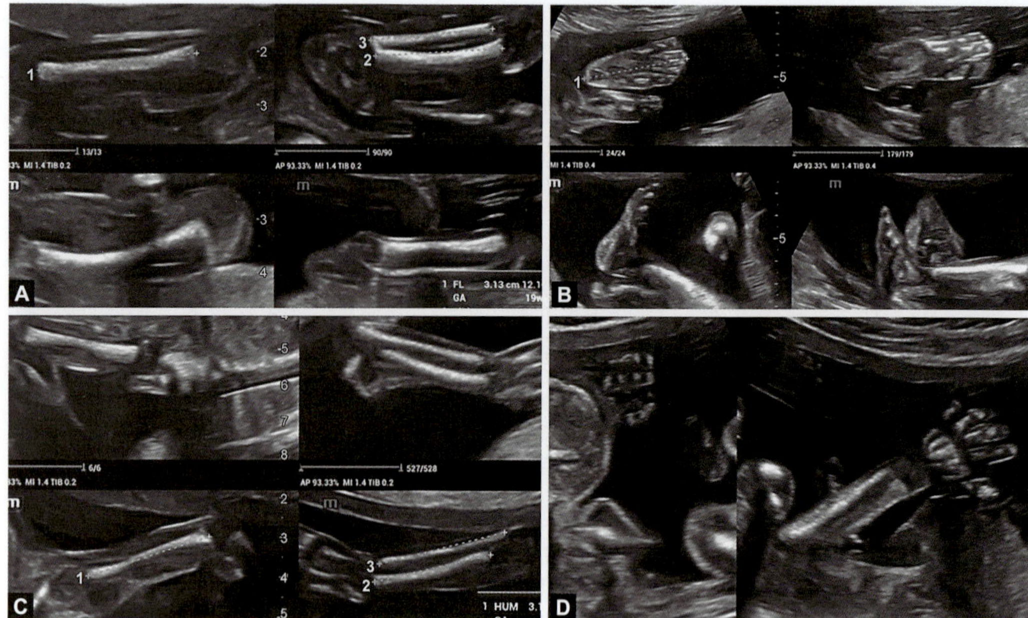

Figs. 15.12A to D: (A) Showing long bones of lower limb; (B) Feet; (C) Long bones of upper limb; (D) Hands.

Measurement of Amniotic Fluid Volume (Figs. 15.13A and B)

Many times it is subjective assessment, though measurement can be done either by deepest largest pocket or by amniotic fluid index.

Amniotic fluid index (AFI) may be preferable in assessing polyhydramnios, while deepest vertical pocket (DVP) may be preferable in assessing oligohydramnios.

For DVP, the largest vertical pocket free of umbilical cord or fetal parts is measured. DVP ≤ 2.0 cm is considered as decreased amniotic fluid volume, DVP > 2 cm and ≤ 8.0 cm as normal amniotic fluid volume, and DVP > 8 cm as increased amniotic fluid volume.

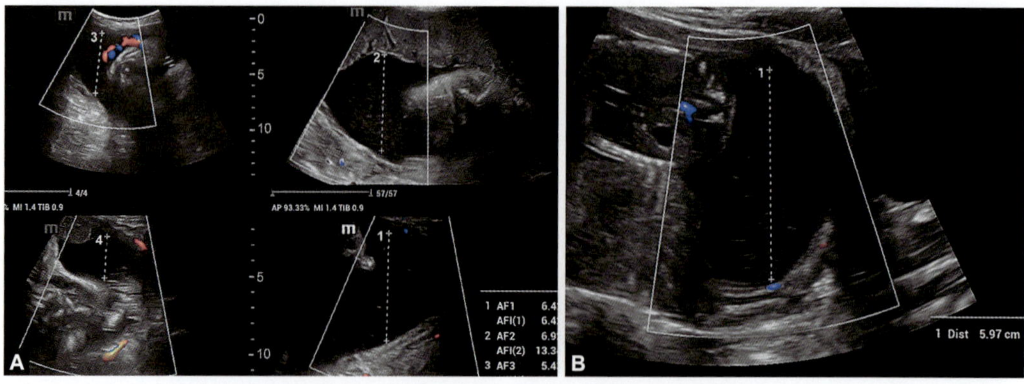

Figs. 15.13A and B: (A) Showing measurement of amniotic fluid index in four quadrants; (B) Showing measurement of single deepest pocket.

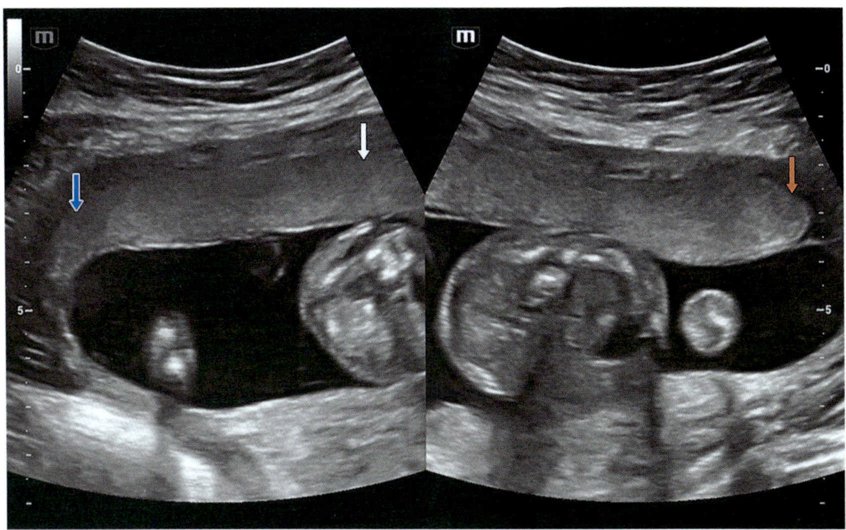

Fig. 15.14: Showing entire placenta (white arrow) with its upper (blue arrow) and lower edge (red arrow).

Placenta (Fig. 15.14)

Placenta location, appearance, size, focal lesion or mass, and its relation with internal os is assessed. When distance between lower edge of placenta and internal os is <2 cm, it is called as low lying placenta. When it covers internal os, it is called placenta previa.

Cervical Length Measurement (Fig. 15.15)

It is done by transvaginal route. When cervical length is <2.5 cm called as short cervix. Short cervix carries risk for preterm birth.

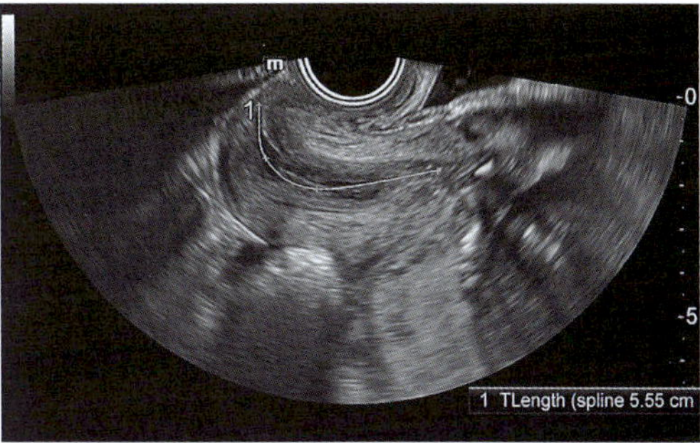

Fig. 15.15: Transvaginal USG showing measurement of cervical length along cervical mucosa.

THIRD-TRIMESTER USG OR GROWTH SCAN

It is performed mainly to assess fetal viability, presentation, anatomy and growth, amniotic fluid volume, placental location and fetoplacental Doppler. Other indications include antepartum bleeding, reduced fetal movements, preterm rupture of the membranes and suspected abnormalities of fetal growth based on physical examination, to estimate gestational age if earlier ultrasound is not done. Commonly performed between 32–36 weeks of gestation.

During this scan anomaly detected at level 2 are followed so, sometimes it is referred as level 3 scan too. Common points to be noted while doing this scan includes:

Fetal Biometry and Amniotic Fluid Volume

Technique of measurement is similar to second-trimester in according to standard guidelines.

Fetal Anatomy

There are certain anomalies which are detected in third-trimester as they develop or become visible after second-trimester. Genitourinary tract, central nervous system, and heart are commonly affected.

Placenta

It is evaluated for location and relationship with internal OS. Women diagnosed with a low-lying placenta or placenta previa at the routine second-trimester scan should have a follow-up assessment for placental location in the third-trimester. Transvaginal route is preferred especially for posterior placenta. If the leading placental edge is 20 mm or more from the internal cervical os, vaginal birth is considered a safe option. Features of placenta accreta spectrum should also be looked during third-trimester.

Color Doppler (Figs. 15.16A to D)

Uterine Artery

As it is used in all trimesters in preeclampsia screening, PI > 95th percentile alone is also predictor for preeclampsia and FGR too in third-trimester.

Umbilical Artery

Umbilical artery Doppler is measured in free loop as resistance is higher at placental and fetal abdominal end. However, in multiple gestation, fetal abdominal site is used for umbilical artery

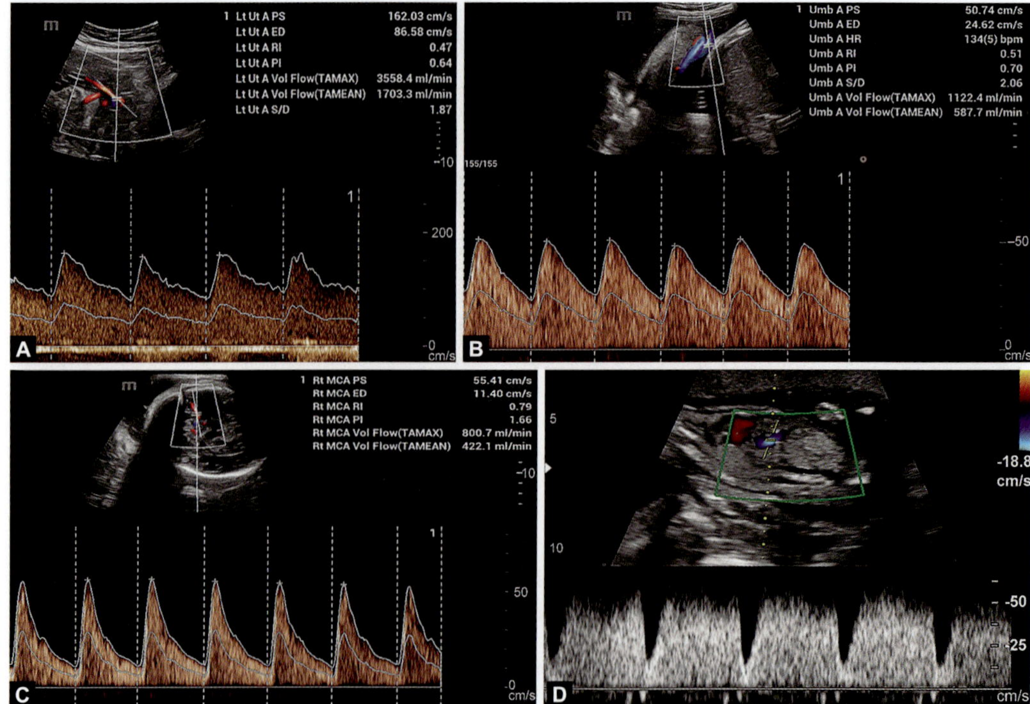

Figs. 15.16A to D: (A) Uterine artery at the level of crossing of iliac vessel with sample volume placed within 1 cm of crossing; (B) Umbilical artery Doppler in a free loop of umbilical cord; (C) Middle cerebral artery Doppler sample gate kept in the proximal part of middle cerebral artery; (D) Ductus venosus Doppler with sample volume kept at aliasing which represents ductus venosus.

Doppler as it eliminates ambiguity of assigning umbilical cord belonging to fetus. PI > 95th percentile is important factor to stage fetal growth restriction.

Middle Cerebral Artery

Middle cerebral artery is identified by color map in axial section in which sphenoid wing and thalami are visible, MCA is localized in circle of Willis. Sample volume is placed in the proximal 1/3rd of MCA close to origin. PI < 95th percentile is indicator fetal insufficiency in FGR or fetal hypoxia.

Ductus Venosus

Ductus venosus is a narrow-caliber vessel connecting umbilical vein with inferior vena cava. It is identified on color flow mapping demonstrating high-flow velocity in sagittal plane. Absent or reversal of A wave and high PI is supportive finding to assess risk for chromosomal, cardiac anomaly in first-trimester and as indicator of stage III FGR and termination of pregnancy in third-trimester.

LAST MINUTE REVISION

- **Intradecidual sign** is earliest sign of intrauterine pregnancy.
- **Transvaginal route:** Used for cervix length measurement, scar assessment (previous LSCS), placenta previa and detailed fetal anatomy.
- Ideal time for TIFFA scan is 18–22 weeks
- Commonly used indices for Doppler assessment in pregnancy is PI while PSV of MCA is used for detection and grading of fetal anemia.

REVIEW QUESTIONS

Multiple Choice Questions (MCQs)

1. **A 28-year-old woman presents at 8 weeks of gestation with lower abdominal pain and spotting. What is the most appropriate type of ultrasound to perform?**
   a. Early first-trimester scan
   b. NT/NB scan
   c. Anomaly scan
   d. Third-trimester scan
2. **A 32-year-old woman at 12 weeks of gestation comes for her routine checkup. Which ultrasound scan is typically performed at this stage to assess the risk of common aneuploidies?**
   a. Early first-trimester scan
   b. NT/NB scan
   c. Anomaly scan
   d. Third-trimester scan
3. **A 26-year-old pregnant woman at 20 weeks of gestation is scheduled for a detailed anatomical evaluation of the fetus. Which scan should be performed?**
   a. Early first-trimester scan
   b. NT/NB scan
   c. Anomaly scan
   d. Third-trimester scan
4. **A pregnant woman at 34 weeks of gestation with a history of low-lying placenta detected in the second-trimester comes for follow-up. Which scan is recommended to assess the placental location?**
   a. Early first-trimester scan
   b. NT/NB scan
   c. Anomaly scan
   d. Third-trimester scan

5. A 30-year-old woman at 6 weeks of gestation is found to have a yolk sac measuring 8 mm. What should be the next step in management?

a. Immediate termination of pregnancy
b. No further follow-up required
c. Follow-up ultrasonography after 7–10 days
d. Administration of progesterone supplements

Answer Key

1. a 2. b 3. c 4. d 5. c

SUGGESTED READING

1. Pedroso MA, Palmer KR, Hodges RJ, Costa FDS, Rolnik DL. Uterine Artery Doppler in Screening for Preeclampsia and Fetal Growth Restriction. Rev Bras Ginecol Obstet. 2018 May;40(5):287-93. doi: 10.1055/s-0038-1660777. Epub 2018 Jun 18. PMID: 29913544; PMCID: PMC10316938.
2. Souka AP, Pilalis A, Papastefanou I, Eleftheriadis M, Papadopoulos G. Quality assessment of the detailed anomaly ultrasound scan. J Matern Fetal Neonatal Med. 2019 Feb;32(4):666-70. doi: 10.1080/14767058.2017.1388366. Epub 2017 Oct 17. PMID: 29041834.
3. Stewart TL, Malone FD. First-trimester screening for aneuploidy: nuchal translucency sonography. Semin Perinatol. 1999 Oct;23(5):369-81. doi: 10.1016/s0146-0005(99)80003-2.

CHAPTER 16

Fetal Imaging: Developmental Anomalies

"Fetal anomaly scans aren't just about finding flaws—they're about empowering hope through early clarity and care."

INTRODUCTION

Fetal anomalies, also known as congenital anomalies or birth defects, are structural or functional abnormalities that occur during intrauterine development. Targeted imaging for fetal anomalies (TIFFA) is second-trimester anomaly scan done, to assess fetal anatomy and detect the presence of fetal anomalies. The second trimester extends from 13 to 27 weeks and 6 days of gestation, although the majority of these studies are performed between 18 and 22 weeks. Congenital defects can affect any system of fetus. Major defects include cardiac, neural tube defect, craniofacial along with subtle chromosomal anomalies and genetic syndromes. A systemic approach is very essential to rule out subtle markers of genetic abnormalities.

TECHNIQUES

- **Ultrasound**: Routine and specialized ultrasound scans (such as the TIFFA scan) are used to detect structural anomalies. Usually performed by convex probe with 3–5 MHz. 3D/4D should be done to confirm 2D findings and precisely diagnose the anomaly.
- **Maternal serum screening**: Blood tests that assess the risk of certain anomalies by measuring specific markers in the mother's blood, e.g. Triple marker (Alpha-fetoprotein, hCG, estriol). Quadruple (= Triple markers + InhibinA). Markers test done at 14 to 22 weeks of gestation.
- **Amniocentesis and chorionic villus sampling (CVS)**: Invasive tests that involve sampling amniotic fluid or placental tissue to detect genetic and chromosomal anomalies.
- **Noninvasive prenatal testing (NIPT)**: A blood test that analyzes fetal DNA circulating in the mother's blood to screen for chromosomal anomalies.

INDICATIONS OF TIFFA

- **Routine screening**: Typically performed between 18 and 22 weeks of gestation as part of routine prenatal care to check for congenital anomalies and ensure normal fetal development.
- **Abnormal findings in previous ultrasounds**: If earlier scans, such as the first-trimester ultrasound or nuchal translucency scan, show abnormal findings, a TIFFA scan is indicated for further evaluation.
- **Maternal age**: Advanced maternal age (35 years or older) increases the risk of chromosomal abnormalities, making a TIFFA scan advisable.
- **Abnormal maternal serum screening results:** If maternal serum screening tests (like the triple or quadruple test) indicate an increased risk for chromosomal abnormalities or neural tube defects, a TIFFA scan is recommended.

- **Family history of congenital anomalies**: A family history of congenital anomalies or genetic disorders warrants a detailed scan to rule out similar issues in the current pregnancy.
- **Maternal conditions**: Conditions such as diabetes, epilepsy, or exposure to teratogenic medications or substances during pregnancy can increase the risk of fetal anomalies, necessitating a TIFFA scan.

Steps in TIFFA

Biometry

Head circumference (HC), biparietal diameter (BPD), abdominal circumference (AC), femur length (FL) are routinely obtained to calculate estimated fetal weight (EFW) and expected date of delivery (EDD).

Morphological Assessment

Head to toe:

- **Fetal skull:** Integrity and shape
- **Fetal brain:** Cavum septum pellucidum
  - Ventricles and choroid plexus
  - Posterior fossa (diameters of transcerebellar diameter (TCD), cistern magna (CM)
  - Nuchal fold thickness (NFT)
- **Fetal face:** Profile and nasal views
  - Orbits and lenses (binocular distance BOD, interocular distance IOD)
  - Upper lip and palate, mandible
- **Fetal heart and chest:** Heart rate and rhythm
  - Cardiac situs, 4-chamber view, outflow tracts (LVOT, RVOT), aortic and ductal Arches
  - Shape of the thorax, diaphragm and lungs
- **Fetal abdomen:** Liver, stomach, kidneys and renal arteries, abdominal wall, umbilical cord insertion, urinary bladder and umbilical arteries, presacral space
- **Fetal musculoskeletal system, LIMBS:** Spine (sagittal and axial views)
  - Upper limb bones (humerus length–HL), radius, ulna, fingers and thumb, with open hands.
  - *Lower limb bones:* Femora (FL), tibia, fibula, orientation of ankles for talipes, feet
- **Other ancillary findings:** Fetal lie
  - Cervical length
  - Placenta (site and distance from the cervix), umbilical cord insertion site
  - Amniotic fluid index
  - Umbilical cord (number of vessels, knots)

ISUOG 20+2 PLANES APPROACH TO MIDTRIMESTER SCAN

It is a combination of 2 overview sweeps and 20 planes of fetus. Each plane related to a specific fetal section. Each plane has a number of structures to be evaluated. Criteria are specific. A combination of these planes enables the potential exclusion of 50 abnormal fetal appearances.

Overview 1: Sweep 1: Longitudinal head and body for initial orientation.
SPINE:

1. Sagittal complete spine with skin covering
2. Coronal complete spine
3. Coronal section of body

HEAD:

4. Transventricular plane
5. Transthalamic plane
6. Transcerebellar plane

THORAX:

7. Lungs, 4-chamber view of heart
8. LVOT
9. RVOT and crossover of LVOT
10. 3-vessel trachea (3VT) view of the heart

ABDOMEN:

11. Transverse section of the abdomen with stomach and umbilical vein
12. Transverse section of the abdomen at cord insertion
13. Transverse section of left kidney, pelvis, right kidney and pelvis.

PELVIS:

14. Transverse section of pelvis, bladder and both umbilical arteries

LIMBS:

15. Femur diaphysis length
16. 3 bones of both legs, both feet and normal relationship of both legs
17. 3 bones of both arms, both hands and normal relationship of both arms.

FACE:

18. Coronal view of upper lip, nose and nostrils
19. Both orbits and lenses
20. Median facial profile

Overview 2: Sweep 2: Transverse sweep of body from neck to sacrum, one vertebra at a time.

ULTRASOUND FEATURES OF COMMON ABNORMALITIES

Anencephaly (Figs. 16.1A to C)

No parenchymal tissue is seen above the orbits and the calvarium is absent. Parts of occipital bone and midbrain may be present. Exencephaly (presence of small amount of neural tissue) is considered a precursor. Small CRL and frog eye or Mickey Mouse appearance may be seen. Polyhydramnios is commonly present in anencephaly.

Gastroschisis (Fig. 16.2)

Herniated bowel appears free-floating rather than contained and is usually towards the right side of the umbilical cord. Small abdominal circumference. Accompanying oligohydramnios or polyhydramnios.

- **Complications:** In utero bowel obstruction, perforation, meconium peritonitis, necrotizing enterocolitis.
- **DDx:** Omphalocele (accompanied by surrounding membrane, with central cord insertion).

Edward's Syndrome (Trisomy 18)

CHD—ASD, VSD, PDA, dextrocardia

CNS/spinal abnormalities: Choroid plexus cysts (bilateral), agenesis of corpus callosum, Dandy Walker continuum, mega cistern magna, neural tube defects (myelomeningocele, spina bifida).

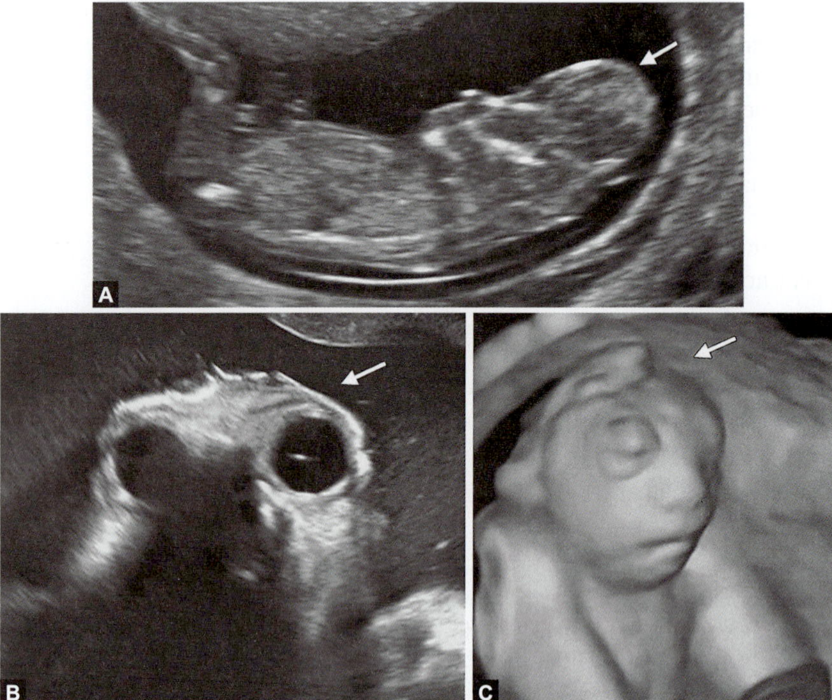

Figs. 16.1A to C: Shows small CRL in (A), frog eye appearance in (B), and anencephaly in 3D view in (C) image.

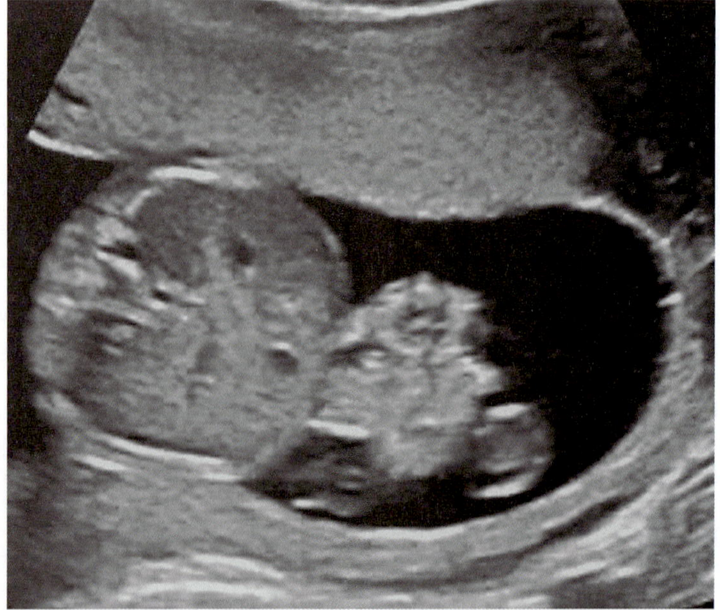

Fig. 16.2: Axial section of fetal abdomen showing free floating bowel in amniotic fluid with paracentral cord insertion (Gastroschisis).

Facial abnormalities, cystic hygroma, skeletal abnormalities (clenched hands, overlap of 2nd and 3rd digits, rocker bottom feet, clubfeet), single umbilical artery, umbilical cord cysts, CDH, omphalocele, renal abnormalities.

Patau's Syndrome

(Trisomy 13): Commonest autosomal trisomy. CHD, CNS abnormalities (holoprosencephaly, microcephaly), spinal abnormalities, early IUGR, facial and skeletal abnormalities (polydactyly), abdominal wall and GU abnormalities (cryptorchidism, cystic renal dysplasia) **(Fig. 16.3)**.

Bilateral Renal Agenesis—Potter's Syndrome

Fatal: Associated with trisomy 21, Turner's, 45 X mosaicism, 22q11 microdeletion. Lying down adrenal sign, oligohydramnios or anhydramnios, nonvisualization of the bladder.

Exomphalos (Fig. 16.4)

Midline sac containing bowel/liver with umbilical cord at the apex. High exomphalos may contain the heart (pentalogy of Cantrell), low exomphalos associated with cloacal abnormality and spina bifida. Associated with trisomy's 18, 13, cardiac defects.

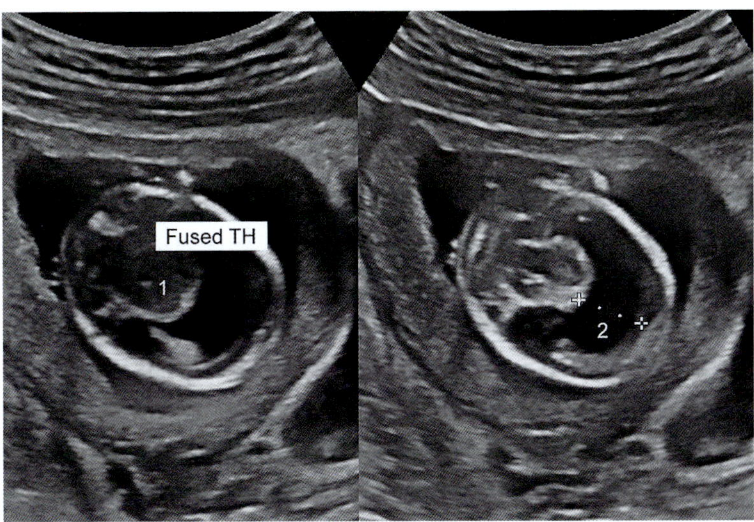

Fig. 16.3: Showing (1) fused thalamus and (2) monoventricle at gestational age of 16 weeks: Holoprosencephaly.

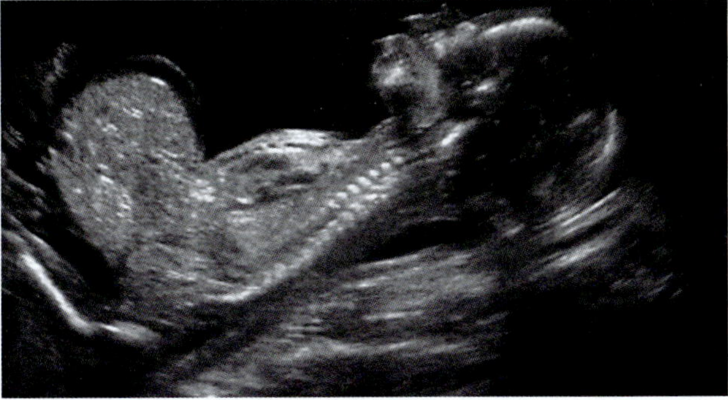

Fig. 16.4: Shows sac containing liver with cord insertion at apex (Exomphalos).

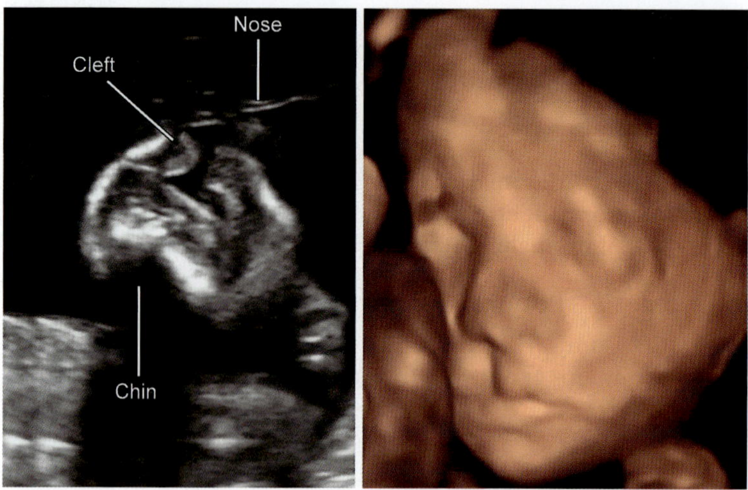

Fig. 16.5: Antenatal 2D coronal image of face shows defect in upper lip reaching up to nose which is beautifully depicted on 3D/4D coronal view of face (Cleft lip and palate).

Cleft Lip and Palate (Fig. 16.5)

Typical cleft lip appears as a linear defect extending from one side of the lip into the nostril. Both transverse and coronal planes are required for the diagnosis. Isolated cleft palate is difficult to diagnose. Associated with trisomy's 13, 18, and syndrome like Goldenhar, Treacher Collins, Pierre Robin anomaly.

Open Spina Bifida

Site lumbosacral (65%), sacral (24%), thoracolumbar (10%), cervical (1%). Associated with the Arnold Chiari malformation. Frontal bone scalloping (lemon sign), abnormal anterior curvature of cerebellar hemisphere (banana sign) can be seen. Contents can be meninges only (meningocele) or meningomyelocele.

Diaphragmatic Hernia (Fig. 16.6)

Polyhydramnios, cardiomediastinal shift, absent normal stomach bubble, reduced abdominal circumference, echogenic cystic lung mass are common antenatal USG findings.

Skeletal Dysplasias

Degree and distribution of shortening associated with fractures and bowing (osteogenesis imperfecta, thanatophoric dysplasia), degree and distribution of ossification (hypomineralization suggests achondrogenesis), polydactyly (short rib polydactyly syndrome, chondrodysplasia punctata) will support diagnosis of various types of skeletal dysplasias.

Down's Syndrome

Increased NT, echogenic intracardiac focus, ventriculomegaly, NFT > 6 mm, echogenic bowel, hypoplastic/absent nasal bone, short humerus, mild pyelectasia, short femur, aberrant right subclavian artery, cardiac defects, duodenal/esophageal atresia, omphalocele, sandal gap deformity, short maxilla, brachycephaly, abnormal ductus venosus waveforms are common features on antenatal ultrasound.

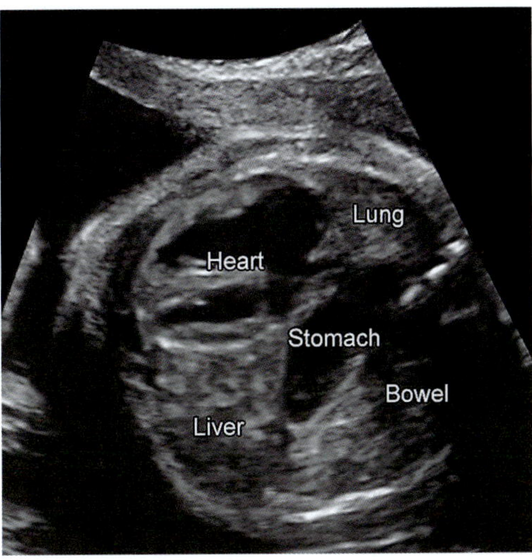

Fig. 16.6: Shows herniated fetal abdominal structures in thoracic cavity causing mass effect on heart consistent with diagnosis of congenital diaphragmatic hernia.

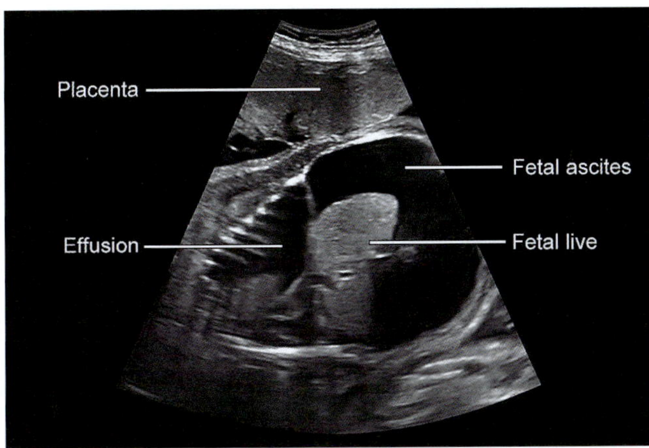

Fig. 16.7: Shows fluid collection in pleural and peritoneal cavity (Hydrops fetalis).

Hydrops Fetalis (Fig. 16.7)

Abnormal accumulation of serous fluid at the body cavities (pericardial, pleural or ascitic effusion) can be seen with RH incompatibility, maternal infections and many anomalies especially of cardiac origin etc. Commonly associated with placentomegaly and soft tissue edema.

LIMITATIONS OF THE ANOMALY SCAN

- White and grey matter forms in the brain only after the 7th month of gestation and it cannot be seen on the anomaly scan.
- IQ of the baby cannot be assessed.
- Degenerative disorders like Rett's syndrome, muscular dystrophies cannot be detected.
- Sensory conditions like hearing loss, blindness also cannot be detected.

Prenatal Genetic Screening Tests

QUAD test/quadruple blood test: Screens for Down's, Edward syndrome and neural tube defects. Done between 14–22 weeks of pregnancy.

Prenatal Diagnostics Tests

Amniocentesis: Done between 15–20 weeks of pregnancy.
Chorionic villus sampling: Done between 10–13 weeks of pregnancy

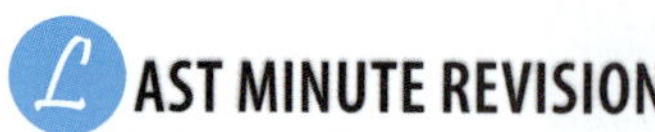

- Common anomalies are cardiac, neural tube defects and chromosomal anomalies.
- Ultrasound techniques used for diagnosis of congenital anomalies are 2D, 3D and 4D scan.
- ISUOG 20+2 planes approach is used for doing level 2 scan.

REVIEW QUESTIONS

Multiple Choice Questions (MCQs)

1. **Which scan plane is primarily used to measure the biparietal diameter (BPD) of the fetal head?**
   a. Transcerebellar plane
   b. Transthalamic plane
   c. Transventricular plane
   d. Sagittal plane
2. **The presence of a "banana sign" and "lemon sign" on ultrasound is indicative of which fetal anomaly?**
   a. Diaphragmatic hernia
   b. Gastroschisis
   c. Open spina bifida
   d. Anencephaly
3. **What is the typical sonographic finding of anencephaly?**
   a. Presence of a midline sac containing bowel/liver
   b. Absence of cranial vault above the orbits
   c. Cardiomediastinal shift with absent stomach bubble
   d. Polyhydramnios with a free-floating herniated bowel
4. **Which of the following sonographic markers is NOT typically assessed in the NT/NB scan?**
   a. Nuchal translucency
   b. Nasal bone
   c. Cisterna magna
   d. Tricuspid flow
5. **What is a key sonographic feature of gastroschisis?**
   a. Herniated bowel within a midline sac
   b. Free-floating herniated bowel to the right of the umbilical cord
   c. Absence of the umbilical vein
   d. Small AC with polyhydramnios
6. **A fetal ultrasound shows a linear defect extending from the lip into the nostril. This finding is suggestive of:**
   a. Down syndrome
   b. Cleft lip and palate
   c. Edwards syndrome
   d. Anencephaly

7. Which scan plane is used to measure the femur length (FL) of the fetus?

a. Transcerebellar plane
b. Sagittal plane of the femur
c. Transventricular plane
d. Coronal plane

Answer Key

1. b 2. c 3. b 4. c 5. b 6. b 7. b

SUGGESTED READING

1. Chaichanalap R, Hanprasertpong T. Success rate to complete optimal 20+2 ISUOG planes for foetal ultrasonographic structural screening during early second trimester pregnancy in Thailand. Ultrasound J. 2021 Aug 14;13(1):36. doi: 10.1186/s13089-021-00238-2. PMID: 34390410; PMCID: PMC8364586.
2. Tafuri SM, Lui F. Embryology, Anencephaly. 2023 May 1. In: StatPearls [Internet]. Treasure Island (FL): StatPearls Publishing; 2024 Jan–. PMID: 31424828.

CHAPTER 17

Fetal Imaging: Advanced Techniques

"With every 3D view and Doppler wave, radiologists redefine what's possible in seeing tomorrow's life today."

INTRODUCTION

Advanced imaging techniques have revolutionized the field of fetal pathology, providing detailed and accurate information crucial for diagnosis, treatment planning, and prognosis. The integration of these advanced imaging techniques enables comprehensive evaluation and improved outcomes for fetal pathologies. It can be classified as non-imaging and imaging techniques. Both techniques can be further divided into noninvasive and invasive type. Noninvasive techniques, includes ultrasound (US), magnetic resonance imaging (MRI), three-dimensional (3D) imaging, ECHO, NIPT and Marker assay. Invasive imaging techniques includes fetoscopy, amniocentesis and chorionic villi biopsy.

Comparison of advanced imaging modalities in fetal pathology shown in **Table 17.1**.

NONINVASIVE TECHNIQUES

Imaging Modalities

Ultrasound (US)

Ultrasound remains the first-line imaging modality in fetal pathology due to its real-time imaging capabilities, safety, and availability.

Techniques

- **2D ultrasound:** Standard initial assessment tool for fetal anatomy, growth, and development and also aids in fetal interventions.

Table 17.1: Comparison of advanced imaging modalities in fetal pathology.

Imaging modality	*Key use*	*Advantages*	*Limitations*
Ultrasound (2D, 3D, 4D)	Initial assessment, real-time imaging	Safe, widely available, cost-effective	Limited soft tissue contrast
MRI	Detailed anatomical evaluation	Superior soft tissue contrast, no ionizing radiation	Limited availability, cost, motion artifacts
3D imaging	Volumetric assessment	Detailed anatomical visualization	Requires specialized equipment
Fetal echocardiography	Detailed cardiac evaluation	High-resolution cardiac imaging	Requires expertise
Invasive techniques	Direct visualization and intervention	Allows for real-time diagnosis and treatment	Risk of complications

- **Doppler ultrasound:** Assesses blood flow in fetal and placental circulation, crucial for detecting abnormalities, such as intrauterine growth restriction (IUGR) and placental insufficiency.
- **3D and 4D ultrasound:** Provides detailed anatomical views and allows for real-time movement assessment, aiding in the diagnosis of structural abnormalities.

Magnetic Resonance Imaging (MRI)

Fetal MRI is used as a complementary tool to ultrasound, offering superior soft tissue contrast and detailed anatomical information without the use of ionizing radiation.

Techniques

- **T2-weighted imaging:** Provides high-resolution images of fetal anatomy, particularly useful for evaluating the brain, spine, and thoracic structures.
- **Diffusion-weighted imaging (DWI):** Assesses tissue cellularity and can help in detecting ischemic changes and certain types of tumors.
- **Functional MRI:** Investigates fetal brain activity and development.

Indications

- Detailed evaluation of central nervous system (CNS) anomalies (e.g., ventriculomegaly, brain malformations)
- Assessment of congenital diaphragmatic hernia and other thoracic abnormalities
- Diagnosis of abdominal and genitourinary malformations
- Evaluation of suspected placental abnormalities (e.g., placental invasion disorders)

Three-dimensional (3D) Imaging

3D imaging provides volumetric data that can be reconstructed to create detailed anatomical models, aiding in the visualization and understanding of complex fetal pathologies.

Techniques

- **3D ultrasound:** Enhances visualization of surface anatomy and spatial relationships between structures.
- **3D MRI:** Offers detailed volumetric assessment of internal structures, particularly useful for brain and organ anomalies.

Indications

- Comprehensive assessment of facial anomalies (e.g., cleft lip and palate)
- Detailed visualization of skeletal dysplasias
- Enhanced evaluation of complex congenital heart defects
- Presurgical planning for fetal interventions

Fetal Echocardiography

Fetal echocardiography is a specialized ultrasound technique focused on the detailed evaluation of the fetal heart.

Techniques

- **High-resolution imaging:** Allows for the assessment of cardiac anatomy, function, and hemodynamics.
- **Doppler studies:** Evaluate blood flow patterns and detect abnormalities, such as congenital heart defects and arrhythmias.

Indications

- Diagnosis of congenital heart defects (e.g., hypoplastic left heart syndrome, tetralogy of Fallot)
- Assessment of cardiac function and rhythm
- Monitoring of fetuses with a family history of congenital heart disease

Non-imaging Tests

Noninvasive Prenatal Testing (NIPT)

Noninvasive prenatal testing (NIPT) is a relatively recent advancement in prenatal screening that allows for the detection of certain genetic abnormalities in the fetus using a simple blood test from the mother. NIPT analyzes cell-free fetal DNA (cffDNA) circulating in the maternal blood, providing a highly accurate and safe method for early genetic screening.

It is a screening test, not diagnostic. Positive results should be confirmed with diagnostic procedures, such as amniocentesis or chorionic villus sampling (CVS).

Indications

NIPT is primarily used for screening common chromosomal abnormalities, including **trisomy 21 (Down syndrome), trisomy 18 (Edwards syndrome), trisomy 13 (Patau syndrome), Sex chromosome aneuploidies** (e.g., Turner syndrome, Klinefelter syndrome). It does not detect all genetic conditions or structural abnormalities.

Optimal timing: NIPT can be performed as early as 10 weeks of gestation. Though, it can be done any time later in pregnancy, but earlier testing allows for more options and timely decision-making.

Maternal Serum Marker Tests

Maternal serum marker tests are blood tests performed during pregnancy to screen for certain fetal conditions, including chromosomal abnormalities and neural tube defects. These tests measure specific substances in the mother's blood that can provide information about the health and development of the fetus.

Types of Maternal Serum Marker Tests

First Trimester Screening

Components: Pregnancy-associated plasma protein-A (PAPP-A)—a protein produced by the placenta in early pregnancy and **human chorionic gonadotropin (hCG)**—a hormone produced by the placenta.

- Performed between 11 and 14 weeks of gestation.
- Combined with maternal age and ultrasound findings, it assesses the risk for trisomy 21 (Down syndrome) and trisomy 18 (Edwards syndrome).

Second Trimester Screening (Quad Screen)

Components:

- **Alpha-fetoprotein (AFP):** A protein produced by the fetal liver.
- **hCG:** Also measured in the first trimester.
- **uE3 (Unconjugated estriol):** A hormone produced by both the fetus and the placenta.
- **Inhibin A:** A hormone produced by the placenta.

Ideal time: Performed between 15 and 20 weeks of gestation.

Indication:

Assesses the risk for:
- Trisomy 21 (Down syndrome)
- Trisomy 18 (Edwards syndrome)
- Neural tube defects (e.g., spina bifida, anencephaly)

Integrated and Sequential Screening

Integrated Screening

- Combines results from first trimester screening and second trimester quad screen.
- Provides a single risk assessment after all tests are completed.

Sequential Screening

- Involves performing the first trimester screening and then providing preliminary results.
- The second trimester screening is performed, and the final risk assessment is adjusted based on the combined results.

Timing

Combines tests conducted from 11 to 20 weeks of gestation.

Detection

Higher detection rates for chromosomal abnormalities compared to individual tests.

Interpretation of Results

- **Low risk:** Indicates a low probability of the fetus having the screened conditions, but does not rule them out entirely.
- **High risk:** Indicates an increased probability of the fetus having the screened conditions and may warrant further diagnostic testing, such as amniocentesis or chorionic villus sampling (CVS).

INVASIVE TECHNIQUES

Invasive imaging techniques, such as fetoscopy, are occasionally used in fetal pathology for both diagnostic and therapeutic purposes. Other include guided procedures, such as amniocentesis and chorionic villi biopsy.

Fetoscopy

Direct visualization of the fetus using a small endoscope, allowing for detailed assessment and intervention.

Indications

- Intrauterine surgery for conditions, such as twin-to-twin transfusion syndrome (TTTS).
- Fetal biopsy or direct sampling of tissues

Amniocentesis

Ultrasound-guided procedure done under local anesthesia. Needle is placed into amniotic fluid avoiding injury to the fetus and placenta.

Indications

- **Genetic testing:** To diagnose chromosomal abnormalities (e.g., Down syndrome), genetic disorders (e.g., cystic fibrosis), and neural tube defects.
- **Fetal lung maturity:** In cases where early delivery is being considered, to assess the development of fetal lungs.
- **Infection:** To diagnose intrauterine infections.
- **Treatment:** For therapeutic purposes, such as draining excess amniotic fluid in polyhydramnios.

Complications: Risk of miscarriage (0.1–0.3%), infection, and needle injury to the fetus.

Gestational Age

- Typically performed between 15 and 20 weeks of gestation.
- Early amniocentesis (before 15 weeks) is possible but associated with a higher risk of complications.
- Late amniocentesis can be performed after 20 weeks if indicated, such as for lung maturity testing or suspected infections.

Chorionic Villus Sampling (CVS): Done under Ultrasound Guidance Either Transabdominal (by Needle) and Transvaginal (Catheter) Route to Take Sample from Placenta

Indications

- **Genetic testing:** Similar to amniocentesis, CVS is used to diagnose chromosomal abnormalities and genetic disorders.
- **Earlier diagnosis:** Allows for earlier detection and decision-making compared to amniocentesis.

Gestational Age

- Typically performed between 10 and 13 weeks of gestation.
- Can be performed later if needed, but earlier procedures are preferred to allow for earlier diagnosis.

Comparison of NIPT, amniocentesis, and CVS shown in **Table 17.2**.

Table 17.2: Comparison of NIPT, amniocentesis, and CVS.

Feature	*NIPT (noninvasive)*	*Amniocentesis (invasive)*	*CVS (invasive)*
Indications	Common trisomies, sex aneuploidies, microdeletions	Genetic testing, fetal lung maturity, infection	Genetic testing
Gestational age	From 10 weeks onwards	15–20 weeks (can be earlier or later)	10–13 weeks (can be later)
Procedure	Maternal blood sample	Ultrasound-guided needle into amniotic sac	Ultrasound-guided catheter or needle into placenta
Risks	None	Miscarriage (0.1–0.3%), infection, Rh sensitization	Miscarriage (0.5–1%), infection, Rh sensitization
Accuracy	High sensitivity and specificity for common trisomies	High accuracy for detected conditions	High accuracy for detected conditions
Follow-up	Positive results confirmed by diagnostic tests	Rest, ultrasound monitoring, genetic results in 1–2 weeks	Rest, ultrasound monitoring, genetic results in 1–2 weeks

The Figures 17.1 and 17.2A to C depict the 2D, 3D USG and MRI.

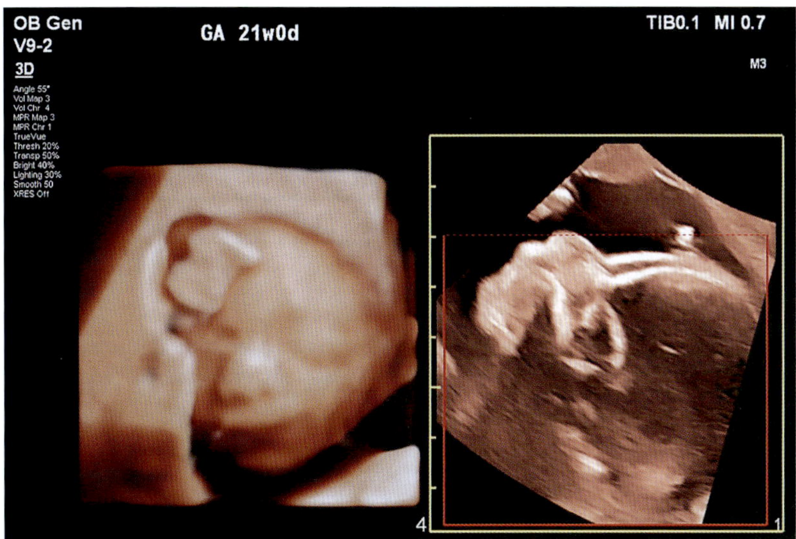

Fig. 17.1: 3D image shows normal fetal face showing upper-lower lips, nose and eyes as well as with hands lie on its cheek and forehead.

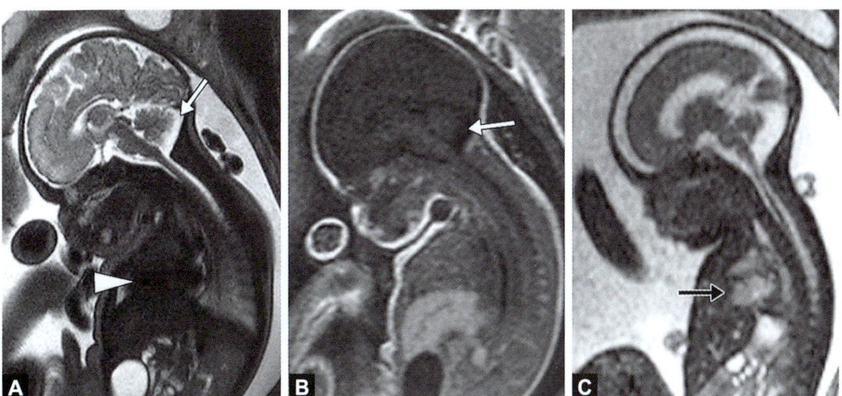

Figs. 17.2A to C: Sagittal T2-weighted single-shot fast spin-echo: (A) and T1-weighted gradient echo; (B) images of a fetus at 33 weeks of gestation. The fetal neuroanatomy is more prominently visualized on T2-weighted sequences compared to T1-weighted ones. The T1-weighted image exhibits lower spatial resolution and is more susceptible to motion artifacts relative to the T2 single-shot fast spin-echo. Cerebrospinal fluid appears hypointense on T1-weighted and hyperintense on T2-weighted images (indicated by arrows). Cardiovascular structures on the T2 single-shot fast spin-echo are hypointense (indicated by arrowhead); and (C) Sagittal balanced fast field echo of a fetus at 26 weeks of gestation offers image quality comparable to the T2 single-shot fast spin-echo.

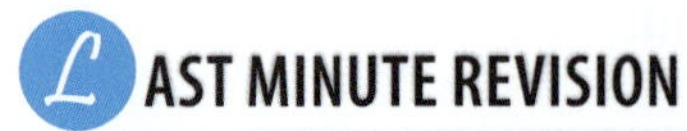

LAST MINUTE REVISION

- 3D and 4D ultrasound done for detailed anatomy and real-time movement.
- MRI is commonly done to confirm craniofacial anomaly and also in placenta accreta spectrum.
- NIPT is used to screen for genetic abnormalities using cell-free fetal DNA in maternal blood.

REVIEW QUESTIONS

Multiple Choice Questions (MCQs)

1. **A 28-year-old woman in her 16th week of pregnancy is advised to undergo a fetal anomaly scan. Which imaging modality would provide real-time assessment and is considered the first-line option?**
   a. MRI
   b. 2D ultrasound
   c. Fetal echocardiography
   d. 3D MRI
2. **A pregnant woman is referred for evaluation of suspected placental abnormalities. Which technique is best suited for detailed anatomical evaluation without ionizing radiation?**
   a. T2-weighted imaging
   b. Functional MRI
   c. Diffusion-weighted imaging
   d. CT
3. **Which test is ideal for early genetic screening and is performed from as early as 10 weeks of gestation using the mother's blood?**
   a. Amniocentesis
   b. Chorionic villus sampling
   c. Noninvasive prenatal testing
   d. Quad screen

Answer Key

1. b 2. a 3. c

SUGGESTED READING

1. Bulas D, Egloff A. Benefits and risks of MRI in pregnancy. Semin Perinatol. 2013 Oct;37(5):301-4. doi: 10.1053/j.semperi.2013.06.005. PMID: 24176150.
2. Harraway J. Noninvasive prenatal testing. Aust Fam Physician. 2017 Oct;46(10):735-9. PMID: 29036772.
3. Jindal A, Sharma M, Karena ZV, Chaudhary C. Amniocentesis. 2023 Aug 14. In: StatPearls [Internet]. Treasure Island (FL): StatPearls Publishing; 2024 Jan–. PMID: 32644673.

CHAPTER

18

Obstetric Emergencies

"In obstetric emergencies, time is life—radiologists lead the race with swift insight and accurate imaging."

INTRODUCTION

Obstetric emergencies are critical situations that arise during pregnancy, labor, or immediate postpartum, posing risk to both the mother and her baby. These emergencies require immediate medical/surgical interventions to prevent severe complications or death.

Pelvic pain and vaginal bleeding are the most common presenting complaints of women examined in emergency department. In addition to history, clinical examination and laboratory tests, sonography is the essential tool in evaluating pelvic pain and vaginal bleeding. Very rarely cross-sectional imaging is needed.

Furthermore, regardless of the indication, one should always perform a transabdominal ultrasound before considering transvaginal scanning (TVS) for establishing a correct diagnosis.

INDICATION OF ULTRASOUND IN OBSTETRIC EMERGENCIES

It can be divided as per various trimester, during labor and postpartum.

First Trimester

Emergency	*Clinical presentation (mother)*	*Clinical presentation (fetus)*	*Imaging modality*
Ectopic pregnancy	UPT positive patient with severe abdominal pain vaginal bleeding	Signs of intrauterine pregnancy are absent	(TVUS), transabdominal ultrasound
Abortions	Vaginal bleeding cramping	Fetal heartbeat assessment	Transvaginal ultrasound
Molar pregnancy	Excessive nausea, hyperemesis, disproportionate uterus size	Fetal parts are absent in complete mole	Ultrasound (snowstorm sign), avascular on USG
Subchorionic hematoma	Vaginal bleeding	Present in many emergencies, such as abortions, placenta previa, etc.	Transvaginal ultrasound, transabdominal ultrasound

Second Trimester

Emergency	*Clinical presentation (mother)*	*Clinical presentation (fetus)*	*Imaging modality*
Placenta previa (Also seen in third trimester)	Painless vaginal bleeding	Complete type is indication of cesarean delivery	Transabdominal ultrasound, transvaginal ultrasound

Contd.

Contd.

Emergency	*Clinical presentation (mother)*	*Clinical presentation (fetus)*	*Imaging modality*
Placental abruption (also seen in third trimester)	Severe abdominal pain, vaginal bleeding	Fetal distress	Ultrasound, MRI (if USG is inconclusive)
Preterm labor	Regular contractions, cervical dilation	Premature birth risk	Transvaginal ultrasound, transabdominal ultrasound
Cervical incompetence	Painless cervical dilation, pressure	Risk of preterm birth	Transvaginal ultrasound (short cervix)

Third Trimester

Emergency	*Clinical presentation (mother)*	*Clinical presentation (fetus)*	*Imaging modality*
Uterine rupture	Sudden severe abdominal pain, vaginal bleeding	Fetal distress	Ultrasound, MRI (if stable)
Amniotic fluid embolism	Sudden cardiovascular collapse, respiratory distress	—	Chest X-ray, CT pulmonary angiography
Preeclampsia/eclampsia	Severe hypertension, proteinuria, headache	Fetal growth restriction, distress	Ultrasound, MRI (for maternal cerebral involvement)
Chorioamnionitis	Fever, uterine tenderness	Fetal tachycardia	Ultrasound
Fetal distress	Decreased fetal movements, abnormal fetal heart rate	Signs of distress	Ultrasound

During Labor

Emergency	*Clinical presentation (mother)*	*Clinical presentation (fetus)*	*Imaging modality*
Obstructed labor	Failure to progress, severe pain	Fetal distress	Ultrasound
Shoulder dystocia	Difficulty delivering shoulders	Fetal distress	Ultrasound (for post-event assessment)
Cord prolapse	Visible/palpable cord, abnormal fetal heart rate	Acute fetal distress	Ultrasound
Uterine inversion	Severe pain, hemorrhage, visible uterus outside cervix	—	Ultrasound (if diagnosis is unclear), shows doughnut appearance

Immediate Postpartum Period

Emergency	*Clinical presentation (mother)*	*Imaging modality*
Postpartum hemorrhage	Heavy vaginal bleeding, signs of shock	Ultrasound (to assess retained products of conception)
Retained placenta	Incomplete placental delivery, bleeding	Ultrasound, shows echogenic placenta
Puerperal infection	Fever, uterine tenderness, discharge	Ultrasound, CT (if abscess suspected)
Pelvic hematoma	Severe pain, swelling, signs of shock	Ultrasound, CT (for detailed assessment)

COMMON OBSTETRIC EMERGENCIES

Ectopic Pregnancy

It refers to the implantation of a fertilized ovum outside of the uterine cavity. The most common site of ectopic pregnancy is the fallopian tube, accounting for nearly 95% cases. In the fallopian tube, the ampulla (70–80%) is the most common site, followed by isthmus (12%) and fimbria (5%).

Various types of ectopic pregnancy and their ultrasound appearances are discussed below **(Fig. 18.1)**.

Sonographic appearances include visualization of an extrauterine adnexal gestational sac containing a yolk sac or an embryo with/without a heartbeat is diagnostic of an EP.

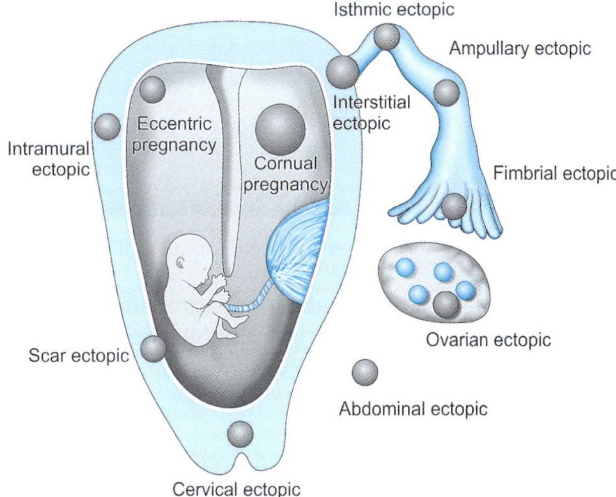

Fig. 18.1: Pictorial description of various sites of ectopic gestation.

- **Bagel sign**—adnexal tubal ring representing an empty gestational sac that appears as a round anechoic fluid collection with a thick echogenic rim.
- **Blob sign**—inhomogeneous adnexal mass.
- Hematosalpinx will appear tubular or ovoid in shape.
- In the setting of a positive pregnancy test and an empty uterus, any adnexal mass that is clearly not either an intraovarian corpus luteum, paraovarian cyst, or pedunculated myoma is diagnostic feature for ectopic pregnancy.
- There may be evidence of hemoperitoneum in case of rupture.
- 3D ultrasound is a useful because it may depict the precise location of the interstitial gestational sac and differentiate it from eccentrically located intrauterine gestational sac.

Color Doppler reveals hypervascular trophoblastic ring in the cervical region in case cervical ectopic. (Differential is miscarriage in progress, but it does not show vascularity)

In stable patients with unusual ectopic pregnancies, combined management can be tried. In this, we instill TVS guided Methotrexate (up to 50 mg) into gestational sac and intraembryonic KCL using 20–22 G long needle. Patient is also given systemic methotrexate. Local injection of MTX results in a higher MTX concentration and a more rapid termination of the pregnancy. **They are then followed by with weekly βhCG and ultrasounds. Depending on levels of βhCG, systemic methotrexate can be repeated. Resolution may take up to 2–4 months.**

Note: Heterotopic pregnancy is defined as the presence of multiple gestations, with one present in the uterine cavity and the other outside the uterus. There is an intrauterine gestation sac coexisting with an ectopic pregnancy. The most common ectopic site is the fallopian tube both in spontaneous and ART heterotopic pregnancies.

Subchorionic Hemorrhage (Fig. 18.2)

There is blood collection between the uterine wall and the chorionic membrane. It typically occurs within the first 20 weeks of gestation. Subchorionic hemorrhage places the gestation at

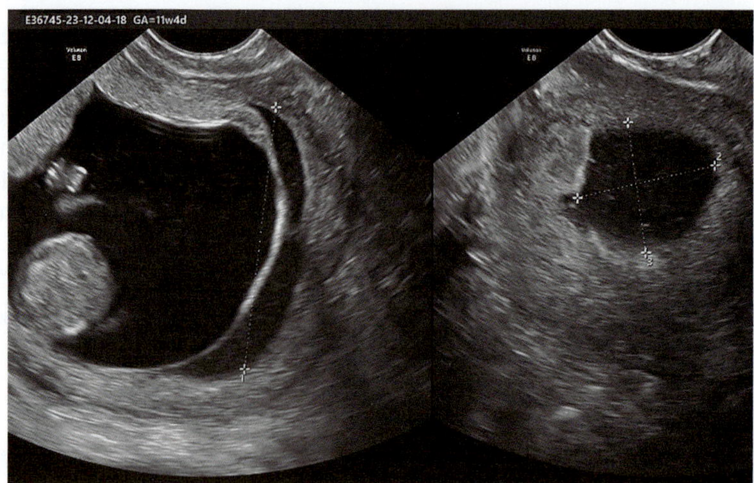

Fig. 18.2: Crescentic hypoechoic subchorionic collection—30% of size of sac s/o moderate collection.

increased risk of placental abruption, premature rupture of membranes (PROM) and preterm labor. Ultrasound reveals crescentic collection with elevation of the chorionic membrane

- In early pregnancy, a subchorionic hemorrhage is considered small if it is <20% of the size of the sac, medium-sized if it is 20–50%, and large if it is >50–66% of the size of the gestational sac.
- Large hematomas by size (>30–50%) and volume (>50 mL) worsen the patient's prognosis.

Antepartum Hemorrhage

Bleeding that occurs after the 20th week of gestation and before delivery. Common causes are placenta previa and placental abruption.

Placenta Previa (Fig. 18.3)

It should be used when the placenta lies directly over the internal os, low lying when the placental edge is less than 2 cm from the internal os, normal when the placental edge is more than 02 cm from the internal os.

Diagnosis of a PP is usually made during the second trimester scan. **Conclusive diagnosis of PP is possible only in the third trimester of pregnancies after 28 weeks**, because most low lying placentas will migrate to the uterine fundus with increasing gestational age.

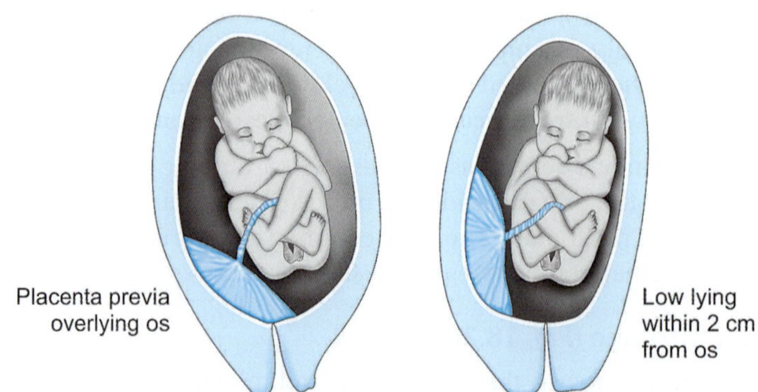

Fig. 18.3: Pictorial description of placenta previa and low-lying placenta.

Placental Abruption (Fig. 18.4)

Blood collection can be marginal, preplacental and retroplacental. Ultrasound detection rate is low, up to 50%. Normal ultrasound does not rule out an abruption. Given the low sensitivity of ultrasound in diagnosis, if there is a high clinical suspicion, then it is good practice to treat based on clinical suspicion. **Sonographic signs of placental abruption include:** Retroplacental hematoma (often poorly echogenic); intraplacental anechoic areas; separation and rounding of the placental edge (marginal); thickening of the placenta often more than 5.5 cm, thickening of the retroplacental myometrium.

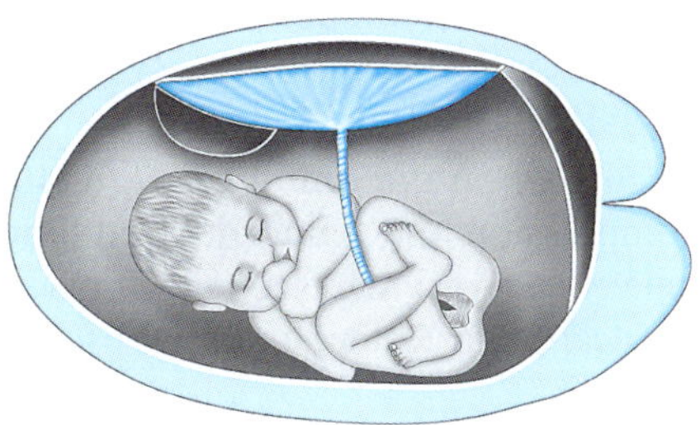

Fig. 18.4: Pictorial description of placental abruption—preplacental, retroplacental and marginal.

Larger the size of the abruption, greater the fetal and maternal morbidity. Small abruptions can be managed conservatively.

Vasa Previa

There are aberrant fetal vessels crossing over or in close proximity to the internal cervical os, ahead of the fetal presenting part. These vessels are within the amniotic membranes, without the support of the placenta. There is a high risk of tearing of these fetal vessels, if membrane ruptures. This can lead to serious fetal bleeding and unfortunately death.

Placenta Accreta Spectrum (Fig. 18.5)

Risk factors for placenta accreta includes: Prior cesarean delivery, placenta previa or low-lying placenta, history of prior uterine surgery, Asherman syndrome or pelvic radiation. Women with risk factors should undergo a targeted US assessment for possible placenta accreta in the mid trimester. Transabdominal and transvaginal US supplemented with Doppler should be carried out.

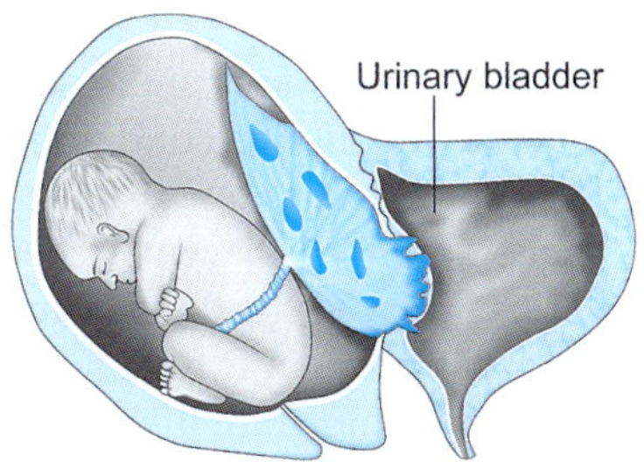

Fig. 18.5: Pictorial description of placenta accreta spectrum.

Ultrasound signs in suspected cases of placenta accreta spectrum are abnormal multiple (>4) placental lacunae; Loss of clear normal hypoechoic plane in the myometrium beneath the placental bed (focal placental adherence), Myometrial thinning <1 mm or undetectable; bulging of the placenta into surrounding organs adjacent to the uterus, causing a mass-like lesion protruding out from the uterine wall; bridging vessels often running perpendicular to myometrium.

When a placenta accreta occurs on the posterior or lateral walls of the uterus, it may be difficult to detect by ultrasound. MRI may be helpful in such cases.

Uterine Rupture

Most common cause (>90%) of uterine rupture is an old cesarean section scar. Uterine rupture may be limited to dehiscence of the ends of the cesarean scar with an intact overlying serosa layer. A full-thickness uterine rupture with direct communication of the uterine and peritoneal cavities results in massive hemoperitoneum, and carries high fetal and maternal morbidity and mortality. Classic scars are more likely to rupture before labor, whereas lower uterine segment scars tend to rupture after labor. Sonographic signs are protruding portion of the amniotic sac, hemoperitoneum or free fluid.

Prolapsed Umbilical Cord

Occurs when the umbilical cord slips ahead of the baby into the birth canal, leading to compression and reduced blood flow to the baby. This situation often requires immediate delivery via cesarean section. Ultrasound may show herniation of the umbilical cord into the cervical canal. Color Doppler is useful at confirmation.

Hypertensive Disorder of Pregnancy

Commonly presented as:

- **HELLP syndrome:** HELLP syndrome in a pregnant woman is characterized by hemolytic anemia, elevated liver enzymes, and a low platelet count. Ultrasound can exclude biliary tract disease and identify altered hepatic and renal echotextures. Possible US findings include—patchy areas of increased echogenicity in the liver, diffusely increased renal echotexture and size, perirenal fluid, and hepatic subcapsular hematoma.
- **Acute fatty liver of pregnancy:** It is a rare pregnancy-associated condition that manifests in the 3rd trimester of pregnancy or early postpartum period.
- Antepartum hemorrhage
- **Placental infarct:** On ultrasound, they appear hypoechoic with thick hyperechoic rim without Doppler signal or well-circumscribed mixed/hyperechoic mass, when hemorrhagic.
- Fetal growth restriction (FGR) with fetal distress

Trauma

The majority of injuries to the gravid uterus occurs in the third trimester. Patients can present with below-mentioned conditions to emergency department:

- Spontaneous abortion, Preterm labor, Premature rupture of membranes, Placental abruption (most common), Placental laceration and/or infarction, Uterine laceration and/or infarction.
- Direct injury to the fetus is uncommon as it is protected by the maternal abdominal wall, uterus and amniotic fluid. Injuries can occur in third trimester if there is oligohydramnios. Fetal head injury are the most common injuries are often due to maternal pelvic fracture.

Preterm Labor

According to the World Health Organization, a preterm birth (PTB) or delivery is defined as occurring between 20 + 0 and 36 + 6 gestational weeks. Cervical shortening **(Fig. 18.6)** is one of the common pathways for PTB. CL ≤25 mm can be used as a cut-off for the initiation of measures to prevent PTB in asymptomatic singleton pregnancies, irrespective of risk factors.

Amniotic Fluid Embolism (AFE)

A rare but serious condition where amniotic fluid, fetal cells, hair, or other debris enters the maternal bloodstream, causing an allergic-like reaction. Symptoms include sudden cardiovascular collapse, respiratory distress, and disseminated intravascular coagulation (DIC).

Acute Uterine Inversion

Ultrasound signs that suggests the diagnosis are:

- **On longitudinal scan:** Uterine fundus is upside down (fallen fundus sign).
- **On transverse scan:** A bull's eye or target-like appearance may be seen.

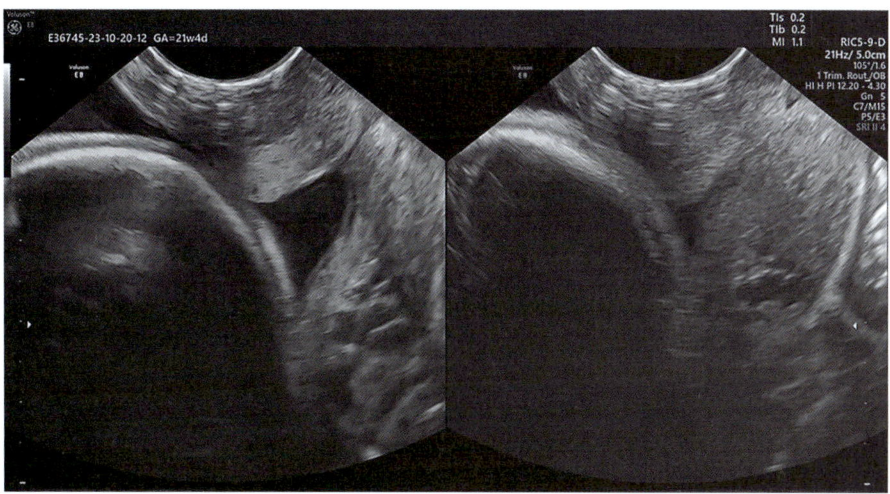

Fig. 18.6: Minimizing pressure reveals U-shaped funneling of internal os with cervical shortening.

Postpartum Hemorrhage (PPH)

Refers to uterine bleeding after delivery primary postpartum hemorrhage is defined as the loss of ≥500 mL of blood from the birth canal within 24 hours of birth. Secondary postpartum hemorrhage defined as abnormal or excessive per vaginal bleeding between 24 hours and 12 weeks postnatally.

- Ultrasound is done to find the possible correctable cause for the PPH.
- Uterine atony is the most common cause.

Retained Products of Conception (Figs. 18.7A and B)

Ultrasound is first-line investigation in suspected retained products of conception: Various imaging appearances are echogenic or heterogeneous contents within the endometrial cavity. Color Doppler shows presence of vascularity within the endometrial contents but the absence of color Doppler flow has a low negative predictive value as retained products of conception may be avascular.

Note: Succenturiate lobe of placenta **(Fig. 18.8)** (smaller separate lobe connected by vascular membrane to the main placenta). It can get retained and result in PPH.

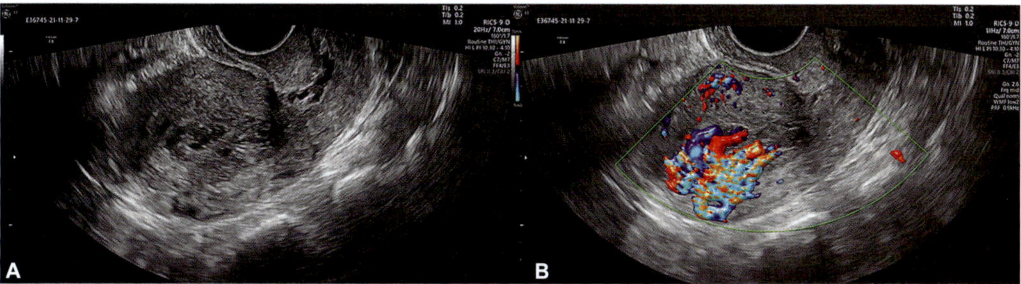

Figs. 18.7A and B: Vascular retained products of conception in endometrial cavity with enhanced myometrial vascularity of posterofundal myometrium.

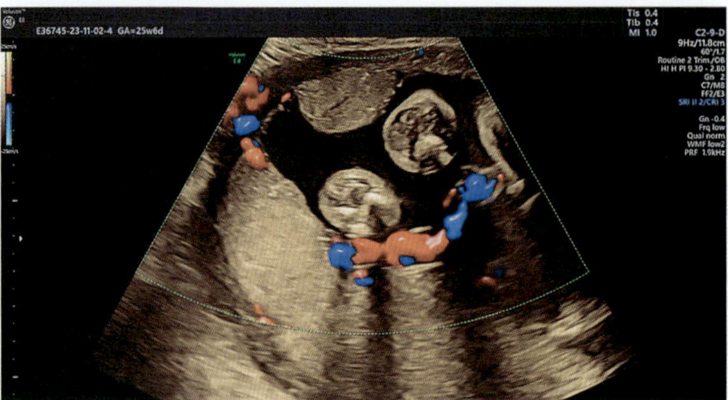

Fig. 18.8: Posterior placenta with succenturiate lobe along anterofundal wall.

Most obstetric emergencies present with signs and symptoms suggesting acute medical/surgical emergencies, where successful outcome depends on prompt diagnosis. The use of ultrasound in obstetric emergencies is well established. This tool should be used by skilled trained ultrasound specialist for establishing correct diagnosis so that timely management can be provided by healthgiver. One missed or wrong diagnosis costs us two lives and hence everyone should be well versed with the imaging appearances of various emergency conditions in pregnant and postpartum patient.

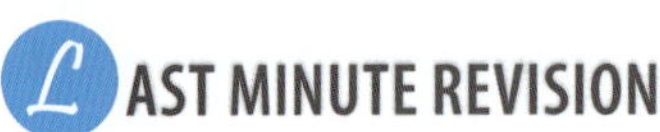

LAST MINUTE REVISION

- **Ectopic pregnancy** is diagnosed by transvaginal ultrasound (TVUS) by identifying extrauterine gestational sacs, often with visible yolk sac or embryo.
- **Molar pregnancy:** Diagnosis via ultrasound where fetal parts are absent in a complete mole; uterus appears disproportionately large for gestational age.
- **Subchorionic hematoma:** Identified on ultrasound as a crescentic collection elevating the chorionic membrane.
- **Uterine rupture:** Ultrasound used for detecting signs, such as protrusion of the amniotic sac and free fluid suggesting hemoperitoneum.
- **Amniotic fluid embolism (AFE):** Diagnosed primarily via clinical presentation; imaging used for pulmonary assessment (e.g., chest X-ray, CT pulmonary angiography).
- **Preeclampsia/eclampsia:** Ultrasound for fetal assessment; MRI may be utilized for evaluating maternal cerebral involvement.
- **Vasa previa** can be detected on transvaginal ultrasound with color Doppler to visualize aberrant fetal vessels crossing the internal cervical os.

REVIEW QUESTIONS

Multiple Choice Questions (MCQs)

1. **A 25-year-old woman presents to the emergency department with sudden, severe pelvic pain and vaginal spotting. She is known to be six weeks pregnant. Which imaging modality should be initially used to evaluate for a possible ectopic pregnancy?**

   a. Transabdominal ultrasound
   b. Transvaginal ultrasound
   c. MRI of the pelvis
   d. CT scan of the abdomen and pelvis

2. **A 32-year-old pregnant woman presents with painless vaginal bleeding in the second trimester. Which condition must be excluded first, and what is the preferred initial imaging technique?**
   a. Placental abruption; MRI
   b. Placenta previa; transvaginal ultrasound
   c. Uterine rupture; transabdominal ultrasound
   d. Placenta previa; transabdominal ultrasound
3. **During routine prenatal care, a 19-week gestation ultrasound reveals a crescentic collection under the chorionic membrane. What is the most likely diagnosis, and what is the implication of this finding?**
   a. Molar pregnancy; indicates invasive growth
   b. Subchorionic hematoma; risk of placental abruption and preterm labor
   c. Placental abruption; immediate delivery may be necessary
   d. Ectopic pregnancy; surgical intervention required

Answer Key

1. b 2. d 3. b

SUGGESTED READING

1. Cali G, Forlani F, Lees C, Timor-Tritsch I, Palacios-Jaraquemada J, Dall'Asta A, et al. Prenatal ultrasound staging system for placenta accreta spectrum disorders. Ultrasound Obstet Gynecol. 2019;53:752-60.
2. Kamaya A, Petrovitch I, Chen B, Frederick C, Jeffrey R. Retained Products of Conception: Spectrum of Color Doppler Findings. J Ultrasound Med. 2009;28(8):1031-41. doi:10.7863/jum.2009.28.8.1031 - PubMed.
3. Lee W, Lee VL, Kirk JS, Sloan CT, Smith RS, Comstock CH. Vasa previa; prenatal diagnosis, natural evolution and clinical outcome. Obstet Gynecol 2000;95:572-6.
4. Nadim B, Infante F, Lu C, N Sathasivam G. Condous Morphological ultrasound types known as 'blob' and 'bagel' signs should be reclassified from suggesting probable to indicating definite tubal ectopic pregnancy Ultrasound Obstet Gynecol, 51 (2018), pp. 543-549.

CHAPTER

19

Gynecological Imaging

"Gynecological imaging is more than diagnosis—it's about dignity, care, and seeing women's health with empathy and precision."

INTRODUCTION

Gynecological imaging is a cornerstone in the diagnosis and management of various conditions affecting the female reproductive system. The goal of this chapter is to provide a comprehensive overview of the primary imaging modalities used in gynecology, including ultrasound (US), computed tomography (CT), and magnetic resonance imaging (MRI), and to detail their application in diagnosing congenital, inflammatory diseases, infertility, and malignancies. Understanding the strengths and limitations of each modality is crucial for effective patient care and optimal clinical outcomes. Normal appearance of female genital organs on various modalities are shown in **Table 19.1**.

Table 19.1: Normal appearance of female genital organs on various modalities.

Organ	*Modality*	*Normal appearance*
Uterus	X-ray	Not visualized unless calcifications are present, e.g., in fibroid
	USG	Homogeneous myometrium, central echogenic line representing the endometrium varies with menstrual cycle. Uterine size and shape are well assesed on USG
	CT	• Isodense to muscle, homogeneous myometrium, with low attenuation endometrial canal • On Enhancement cervical fibrous stroma enhances < myometrium > endometrium
	MRI	• Clear delineation between the myometrium and endometrium especially on T2. Myometrium is intermediate signal on T1 and T2; endometrium is low signal on T1 and high on T2 • Junctional zone (innermost myometrium) is hypointense on T2 due to less water content
Ovaries	X-ray	Not visualized unless calcifications or large ovarian masses are present
	USG	Ovoid structures with follicles, which are anechoic (fluid-filled). Size may vary with age and menstrual cycle
	CT	Soft tissue structures, follicles as small low-density areas. Enhancement varies. Typically located superolateral to uterus, posterior to external iliac vessel and anterior to internal iliac vessels
	MRI	Intermediate signal intensity on T1-weighted images; high signal on T2-weighted images with follicles appearing as hyperintense on T2

Contd...

Contd...

Organ	*Modality*	*Normal appearance*
Vagina	X-ray	Not visualized
	USG	Seen as a collapsed, hypoechoic tubular structure with central echogenic mucosa
	CT	Soft tissue structure, typically collapsed, seen as a low-density tubular structure
	MRI	T2-weighted images, show bright mucosa with intermediate signal intensity vaginal wall
Fallopian tubes	X-ray	Not typically visualized unless calcified or filled with contrast material (e.g., hysterosalpingography)
	USG	Not typically visualized unless pathologically dilated
	CT	Not typically visualized unless pathologically dilated or filled with fluid or blood
	MRI	Not typically visualized unless pathologically dilated, appearing as fluid-filled structures with low signal on T1 and high signal on T2
Adnexa (ligaments and other surrounding structures)	X-ray	Not visualized
	USG	Adnexa are normally evaluated for the presence of ovaries and any paraovarian masses; the normal adnexa is difficult to isolate if not pathologically enlarged
	CT	Typically appears as normal soft tissue, evaluation is focused on identifying masses or abnormalities
	MRI	Normal adnexa may not be distinctly visualized if not pathologically involved

MODALITIES

Ultrasonography (US)

Ultrasonography is the primary imaging method for patients exhibiting clinical symptoms, such as abnormal uterine bleeding, endocrine dysfunction, pelvic pain, gynecologic infections, and pelvic lump. For a comprehensive evaluation of pelvic and abdominal organs, a combination of transabdominal (TAUS) and transvaginal US (TVUS) is required. Its main role is to broadly classify pathology as uterine or extrauterine in origin. It plays a significant role in diagnosing gynecologic diseases, such as infections. For instance, pelvic inflammatory disease (PID) can be identified using US by detecting findings, such as thickened, fluid-filled fallopian tubes, the presence of tubo-ovarian abscesses, and increased vascularity of pelvic tissues. TVUS is particularly useful for evaluating endometritis, which may present as an irregular or thickened endometrial lining with fluid or gas within the endometrial cavity.

In the context of infertility also, ultrasonography is a critical diagnostic tool. TVUS is used to evaluate ovarian follicles and its reserve (antral follicle count), endometrial thickness, and uterine abnormalities, such as fibroids or polyps. It also assists in monitoring ovulation and follicular development during fertility treatments. Sono-Hysterosalpingography, (Sono-HSG) where saline is infused into the uterine cavity during ultrasound, can provide detailed images of the uterine cavity, helping diagnose conditions, such as intrauterine adhesions or polyp extent. Not only this TVS 3D/4D provides very good detail especially in congenital uterine anomalies and fibroid extension.

Computed Tomography (CT)

CT is extensively used for cancer staging and evaluating complex pelvic pathologies, mostly in collaboration with USG. It offers detailed cross-sectional images of the body, making it effective in identifying the extent of disease spread. CT is particularly useful in assessing the presence of lymph node involvement and distant metastases. However, CT involves exposure to ionizing radiation and is less effective than MRI in soft tissue characterization.

Magnetic Resonance Imaging (MRI)

MRI provides superior soft tissue contrast compared to CT, making it invaluable in the assessment of complex gynecological conditions. It is particularly useful for evaluating the extent of tumors, detecting deep infiltrative endometriosis, and assessing congenital anomalies. MRI techniques, such as Dynamic Contrast Enhancement (DCE) and Diffusion Weighted Imaging (DWI) enhance the detection and characterization of various pathologies, offering detailed information on tissue composition and vascularity. Malignant tumors, for example, are more likely to show a high-intensity signal on DWI at a high b (1000) value and appear dark on ADC (Apparent Diffusion Coefficient) maps. MRI combined with DWI allows for better characterization and assessment of tumor stage and extent, including the detection of subtle peritoneal disease, as well as the assessment of tumor response and recurrence.

Despite its advantages (no ionic radiation and better soft tissue visualization), MRI has some disadvantages, such as low availability, higher cost, long image acquisition time leading to motion artifacts, reduced patient cooperation, and MRI safety issues.

COMMON PATHOLOGIC CONDITIONS

Imaging in Congenital Anomalies

Mullerian duct anomalies occurs due to non-development and varying degree of non-fusion or non-resorption of Mullerian ducts. These anomalies are associated with menstrual disorders, such as primary amenorrhea (e.g., in agenesis, gonadal dysgenesis), infertility (e.g., in unicornuate), pain (vaginal septum with hematocolpos), obstetrics complication, such as recurrent abortion in septate uterus and renal anomalies. USG and MRI are main modalities for its diagnosis. Various types of congenital anomalies are related to the arrest in the various steps of embryonic development, which are tabulated as follows **(Table 19.2)**:

Table 19.2: Normal embryologic origin of the female pelvic organs with corresponding anomalies that may arise due to arrest.

Structure	*Embryologic origin*	*Arrest in developmental step*	*Manifested anomalies*
Uterus	Paramesonephric (Müllerian) ducts	Arrest in fusion and absorption of Müllerian ducts	Uterus didelphys, bicornuate uterus, unicornuate uterus, septate uterus
Ovaries	Primordial germ cells migrating from the yolk sac to the gonadal ridge	Arrest in germ cell migration or gonadal ridge formation	Gonadal dysgenesis, streak ovaries, Turner syndrome
Vagina	Upper portion: Paramesonephric ducts Lower portion: Urogenital sinus	Arrest in fusion of Müllerian ducts or urogenital sinus development	Vaginal agenesis, vaginal septum, transverse vaginal septum, Mayer-Rokitansky-Küster-Hauser (MRKH) syndrome

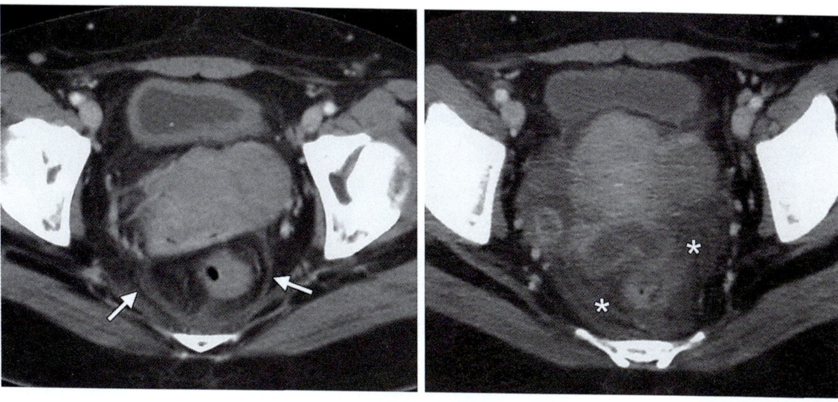

Fig. 19.1: Thickening of the uterosacral ligament and increased haziness of the presacral and perirectal fat planes on contrast-enhanced CT indicating PID.

Imaging in Inflammatory Diseases

Inflammatory diseases of the female genital organs, such as pelvic inflammatory disease (PID) **(Fig. 19.1)**, are common and can lead to serious complications if not promptly diagnosed and treated. These conditions often result from ascending infections and can affect the uterus, fallopian tubes, and ovaries.

Pelvic Inflammatory Disease (PID)

PID is primarily caused by sexually transmitted infections (STIs), such as *Chlamydia trachomatis* and *Neisseria gonorrhoeae*. It can lead to severe complications, including tubo-ovarian abscess (TOA), peritonitis, and infertility.

Imaging in PID

- **Ultrasound (US):** US is typically the first imaging modality used in diagnosing PID. It can reveal thickened, fluid-filled fallopian tubes (hydrosalpinx) and detect tubo-ovarian abscesses.
- **Computed tomography (CT):** CT is useful for evaluating the extent of infection and identifying complications, such as abscess formation. Common findings include thickening of the fallopian tubes, uterosacral ligament thickening, and pelvic fat stranding.
- **Magnetic resonance imaging (MRI):** MRI is often used as an adjunct to US and CT for detailed evaluation. It provides excellent soft tissue contrast and can detect subtle signs of inflammation and abscesses with high accuracy.

Other Inflammatory Conditions

- **Cervicitis:** Inflammation of the cervix, often diagnosed clinically. Imaging findings include an enlarged, hyperemic endocervical canal on CT or MRI.
- **Endometritis and uterine empyema (Fig. 19.2):** Endometritis involves inflammation of the endometrium, whereas uterine empyema is the accumulation of pus within the uterine cavity. CT and MRI can show fluid collections and abnormal enhancement of the endometrium.
- **Salpingitis and tubal empyema:** Salpingitis is the inflammation of the fallopian tubes, which can progress to tubal empyema if untreated. Imaging shows thickened, fluid-filled tubes with pus.

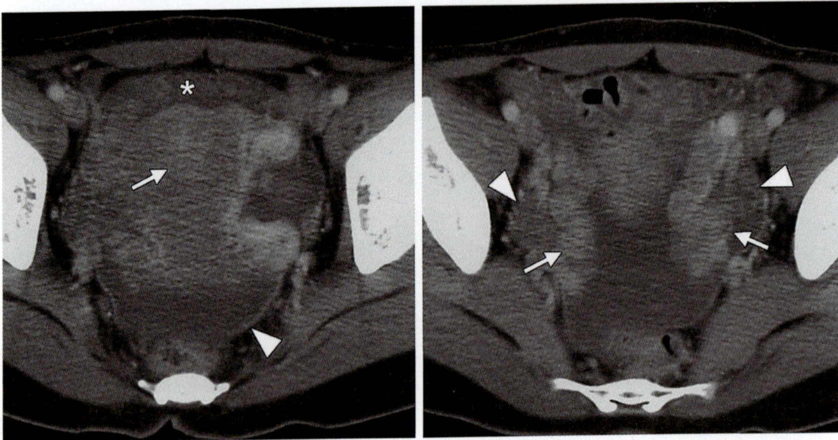

Fig. 19.2: Contrast-enhanced CT showing endometrial enhancement indicating potential endometritis and bilateral tubal thickening consistent with salpingitis.

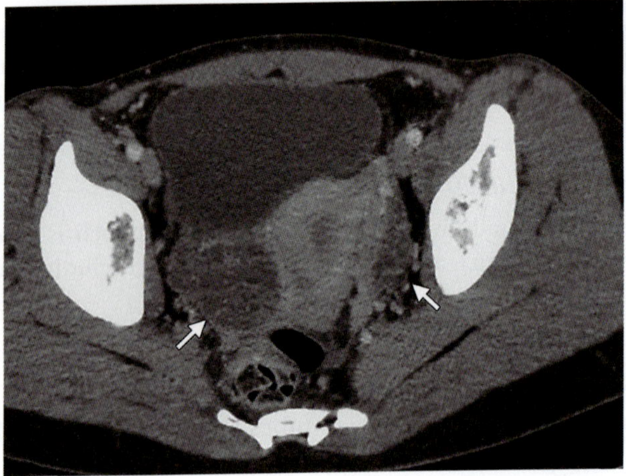

Fig. 19.3: Contrast-enhanced CT image showing enlargement of the bilateral ovaries indicating oophoritis.

- **Oophoritis (Fig. 19.3):** Inflammation of the ovaries often associated with salpingitis. MRI and US can reveal normal or enlarged polycystic ovarian appearance with surrounding edema and hyperemia.

Imaging in Infertility

Infertility is a significant concern in gynecology, affecting many couples worldwide. Imaging plays a crucial role in diagnosing the underlying causes of infertility, including structural abnormalities, tubal factors, and ovarian dysfunction. TVUS is the primary imaging modality for evaluating infertility. It assesses ovarian follicles (by follicular or ovulation study and antral follicle count), endometrial thickness, and uterine anomalies. Hysterosonography (S-HSG) can further enhance the evaluation of the uterine cavity while X-ray HSG provide detail about the patency of tubes.

Common Infertility Issues (Tables 19.3 and 19.4)

- **Tubal factor infertility:** Often caused by PID, resulting in blocked or damaged fallopian tubes. Hysterosalpingography (HSG) is a specialized X-ray technique used to evaluate tubal patency.

Table 19.3: Imaging findings in infertility.

Condition	*Imaging findings*
Tubal factor infertility	Blocked fallopian tubes, hydrosalpinx
Ovarian factor infertility	Multiple small follicles (PCOS), ovarian cysts
Uterine factor infertility	Uterine anomalies, fibroids, polyps

Table 19.4: Common causes of infertility and their imaging modalities.

Condition	*Primary imaging modality*	*Additional imaging*
Tubal factor infertility	HSG (X-ray)	MRI
Ovarian factor infertility	TVUS	MRI
Uterine factor infertility	TVUS, S-HSG	MRI

- **Ovarian factor infertility:** Conditions, such as polycystic ovary syndrome (PCOS), cysts, etc., can be diagnosed with TVUS, which shows multiple small ovarian follicles **(Figs. 19.4A to D)**.
- **Uterine factor infertility:** Congenital anomalies, fibroids, and polyps can be evaluated with US and MRI. MRI is particularly useful for detailed assessment of uterine structure.

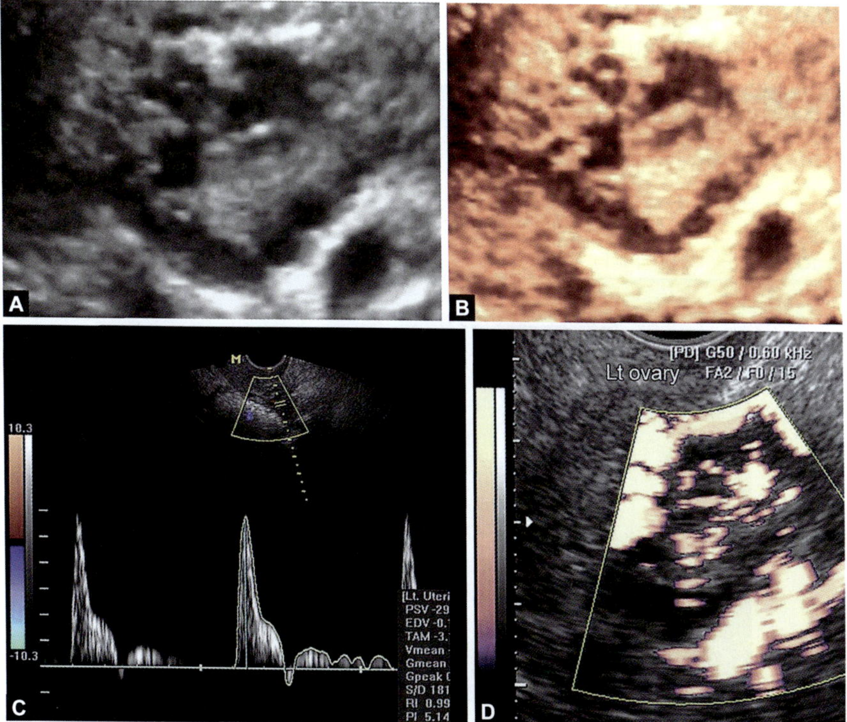

Figs. 19.4A to D: Polycystic ovary. Three-dimensional grayscale (A) and color; (B) image shows a polycystic ovary. Spectral Doppler; (C) and power Doppler; (D) image show reduction in diastolic flow, reverse diastolic component, and increased stromal vascularity in polycystic ovary.

Malignancies (Table 19.5)

Gynecological malignancies, including ovarian, endometrial, and cervical cancers, are significant health concerns requiring accurate diagnosis and staging for effective management. Imaging plays a vital role in the detection, characterization, and staging of these malignancies.

Ovarian Cancer

Ovarian cancer is often diagnosed at an advanced stage due to non-specific symptoms. Early detection and accurate staging are crucial for effective treatment.

Imaging in Ovarian Cancer

- **Ultrasound (US):** US is the first-line imaging modality for suspected ovarian cancer. It can identify complex adnexal masses, septations, and solid components suggestive of malignancy.
- **Computed tomography (CT) (Fig. 19.5):** CT is essential for staging ovarian cancer, evaluating the extent of disease spread within the abdomen and pelvis. It helps in detecting peritoneal implants, lymph node involvement, and distant metastases.
- **Magnetic resonance imaging (MRI):** MRI provides superior soft tissue contrast and is used to further characterize adnexal masses. It is particularly useful in differentiating benign from malignant lesions and assessing local invasion.

Endometrial Cancer

Endometrial cancer is typically diagnosed early due to abnormal uterine bleeding. Imaging is crucial for staging and treatment planning.

Table 19.5: Imaging modalities and their use in gynecological malignancies.

Cancer type	*Primary imaging modality*	*Additional imaging*
Ovarian cancer	US, CT	MRI
Endometrial cancer	TVUS, MRI	CT
Cervical cancer	MRI, CT	US

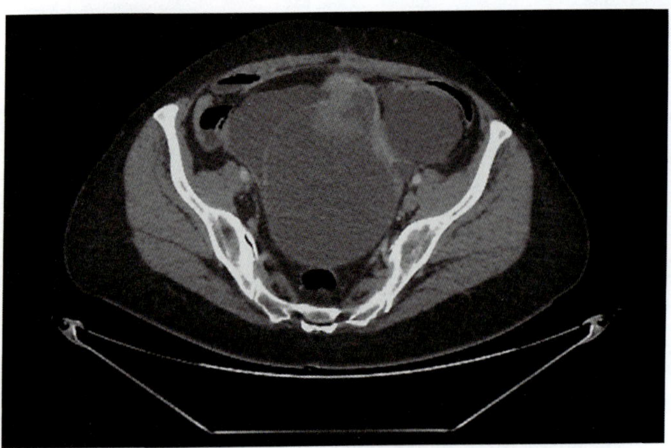

Fig. 19.5: CT scan showing complex adnexal masses with septations indicative of ovarian cancer.

Imaging in Endometrial Cancer

- **Ultrasound (US):** TVUS is used for initial evaluation, measuring endometrial thickness and detecting abnormal growths.
- **Computed tomography (CT):** CT is used for staging and detecting metastases. It provides a comprehensive overview of the disease spread.
- **Magnetic resonance imaging (MRI):** MRI is the modality of choice for local staging, assessing myometrial invasion, and detecting cervical involvement. It offers detailed images of the uterus and surrounding structures.

Cervical Cancer

Cervical cancer screening and early detection have significantly improved outcomes. Imaging is essential for staging and evaluating the extent of disease spread.

Imaging in Cervical Cancer

- **Ultrasound (US):** US is limited in evaluating cervical cancer but can be used to assess large pelvic masses.
- **Computed tomography (CT):** CT is valuable for staging, identifying lymph node involvement, and detecting distant metastases.
- **Magnetic resonance imaging (MRI):** MRI is the preferred modality for local staging, assessing tumor size, parametrial involvement, and detecting pelvic lymph node metastases. It provides detailed images of the cervix and adjacent structures.

Gestational Trophoblastic Diseases (Table 19.6)

It represents a spectrum of tumors originating from abnormal proliferation of trophoblastic tissue, encompassing both benign and malignant conditions.

Table 19.6: Gestational trophoblastic diseases.

Type of GTD	*Diagnostic features*	*Characteristic blood test findings*
Hydatidiform mole (HM)	**Complete mole:** Enlarged uterus, no fetal parts, "snowstorm" appearance on ultrasound	Extremely high hCG levels, typically >100,000 mIU/mL
	Partial mole: Presence of fetal parts, abnormal placenta, "Swiss cheese" appearance	Moderately elevated hCG levels, lower than complete moles
Invasive mole	Invasion into the uterine wall, abnormal bleeding, mass in the uterus	Persistently elevated hCG levels after molar pregnancy
Choriocarcinoma	Aggressive tumor, can metastasize to lungs, brain, liver, vaginal bleeding, hemoptysis	Very high hCG levels, often >100,000 mIU/mL
Placental-site trophoblastic tumor (PSTT)	Slow-growing tumor, irregular vaginal bleeding, months to years after pregnancy	Low to moderately elevated hCG, high hPL levels
Epithelioid trophoblastic tumor (ETT)	Discrete nodules or masses in uterus, abnormal vaginal bleeding	Low hCG levels, high hPL levels, unlike other GTNs

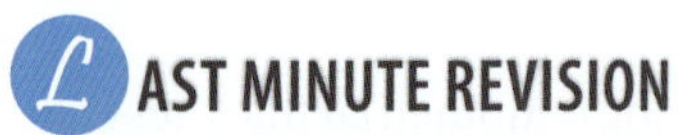
AST MINUTE REVISION

- USG is crucial in classifying gynecologic diseases into uterine or extrauterine. It is first line investigation in all gynecologic conditions.
- MRI is invaluable tool in assessing especially deep infiltrative endometriosis, congenital anomalies, and malignancies.
- Diseases of female pelvis should be approached predominantly at two different levels, such as age (unmarried, reproductive and menopausal female) and presenting complaint, such as pain, menstrual irregularities, infertility, lump, etc.
- CT should be done only in restricted conditions of pelvic diseases due to radiation and suboptimal soft tissue contrast.

REVIEW QUESTIONS

Multiple Choice Questions (MCQs)

Clinical history: A 28-year-old woman presents with primary amenorrhea and cyclical pelvic pain. A physical examination suggests the presence of a transverse vaginal septum.

1. **What is the most likely diagnosis, and which imaging modality is preferred for further evaluation?**
   a. Diagnosis: Polycystic ovary syndrome (PCOS); Modality: CT
   b. Diagnosis: Vaginal agenesis; Modality: US
   c. Diagnosis: Transverse vaginal septum; Modality: MRI
   d. Diagnosis: Endometriosis; Modality: Hysterosalpingography (HSG)

Clinical history: A 35-year-old woman presents with lower abdominal pain, fever, and a history of recent pelvic surgery. The clinician suspects pelvic inflammatory disease (PID) with a tubo-ovarian abscess.

2. **What is the most appropriate initial imaging modality to confirm the diagnosis?**
   a. Ultrasound (US)
   b. Computed tomography (CT)
   c. Magnetic resonance imaging (MRI)
   d. X-ray

Clinical history: A 42-year-old woman with a history of irregular menstruation and infertility undergoes an ultrasound that shows multiple small ovarian follicles.

3. **What is the most likely diagnosis, and which imaging modality was used?**
   a. Diagnosis: Endometrial cancer; Modality: MRI
   b. Diagnosis: Ovarian cancer; Modality: CT
   c. Diagnosis: Polycystic ovary syndrome (PCOS); Modality: US
   d. Diagnosis: Cervical cancer; Modality: X-ray

Clinical history: A 60-year-old woman presents with postmenopausal bleeding. Ultrasound reveals a thickened endometrium.

4. **What is the most likely diagnosis, and which imaging modality should be used next for staging?**
   a. Diagnosis: Ovarian cancer; Modality: CT
   b. Diagnosis: Endometrial cancer; Modality: MRI
   c. Diagnosis: Cervical cancer; Modality: US
   d. Diagnosis: Fibroid; Modality: X-ray

Clinical history: A 30-year-old woman presents with severe dysmenorrhea and deep pelvic pain, particularly during menstruation. The clinician suspects endometriosis.

5. Which imaging modality is preferred for the detailed assessment of this condition?

a. Ultrasound (US)
b. Computed tomography (CT)
c. Magnetic resonance imaging (MRI)
d. X-ray

Clinical history: A 25-year-old woman with a history of pelvic inflammatory disease (PID) presents with infertility. Hysterosalpingography (HSG) shows blocked and dilated fallopian tubes.

6. What is the most likely cause of her infertility, and which imaging modality confirmed other findings?

a. Cause: Ovarian cysts; Modality: MRI
b. Cause: Tubal factor infertility; Modality: USG
c. Cause: Uterine fibroids; Modality: US
d. Cause: Endometrial polyps; Modality: CT

Answer Key

1. c 2. a 3. c 4. b 5. c 6. b

SUGGESTED READING

1. Shibuki S, Saida T, Hoshiai S, Ishiguro T, et al. Received: 17 September 2023/Accepted: 20 November 2023/Published online: 2 January 2024
2. Steinkeler JA, Woodfield CA, Lazarus E, Hillstrom MM. Female Infertility: A systematic approach to radiologic imaging and diagnosis. Radiographics. 2009;29:1353-70.
3. Suneja G, Viswanathan A. Gynecologic Malignancies. Hematol Oncol Clin North Am. 2020 Feb;34(1):71-89. doi: 10.1016/j.hoc.2019.08.018. PMID: 31739953

UNIT 4

Pediatric Radiology

Unit Outline

CHAPTER

20 Basics of Pediatric and Neonatal Imaging

"Neonatal imaging is more than technique—it's a tender lens into the earliest days of life."

INTRODUCTION

Radiological investigations are indispensable in the healthcare system, providing vital diagnostic information. In pediatrics, however, imaging presents unique challenges due to the specific needs and characteristics of children. This chapter explores the distinct aspects of pediatric imaging, including environment setup, equipment and protocols, training, quality assurance, and radiation protection. It also covers the clinical applications of various imaging modalities in pediatric care.

CHALLENGES IN PEDIATRIC IMAGING

Environment

Acquiring quality images in pediatric patients hinges on gaining the child's trust and cooperation. Children are often irritable and wary of strangers and unfamiliar environments. To create a child-friendly radiology department, walls can be painted with colorful characters, and the waiting room can feature children's books or a small aquarium **(Fig. 20.1)**. Parental involvement is crucial, though sedation or immobilizers might be necessary for longer studies such as MRI **(Fig. 20.2)**. Common sedatives for pediatric imaging include diazepam, midazolam, and ketamine. Minimizing the need for sedation is essential due to its potential harmful effects **(Table 20.1)**.

Equipment and Protocols

A dedicated pediatric imaging department with specialized pediatric CT technologists can enhance compliance with pediatric protocols and significantly reduce patient doses. Facilities should cater to children of all sizes, from premature infants to adult-sized teenagers, with child-focused imaging tailored to their age. Standardization of techniques and protocols for all modalities is crucial. Adhering to low radiation dose protocols can be challenging in high-volume radiology departments that scan both pediatric and adult patients.

Training

Only appropriately trained staff should perform pediatric imaging, with regular performance reviews. Unfortunately, there is little incentive for radiographers to specialize in this area, resulting in a shortage of dedicated pediatric radiographers. Radiologists interpreting pediatric

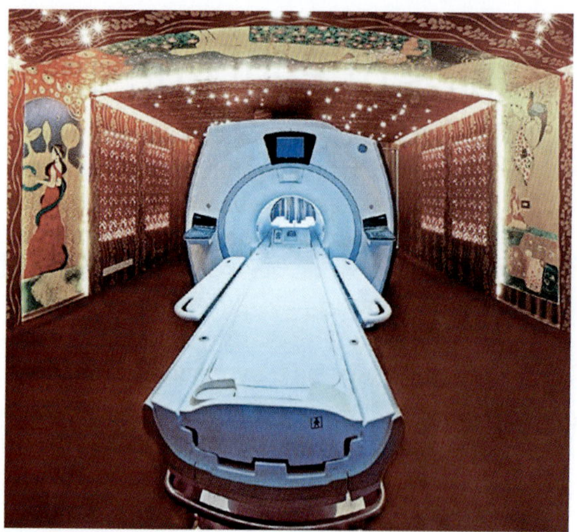

Fig. 20.1: Gantry room for pediatric imaging.

Note: Gantry and surrounding are colorful, this makes the environment friendly for the children and helps in receiving their cooperation.

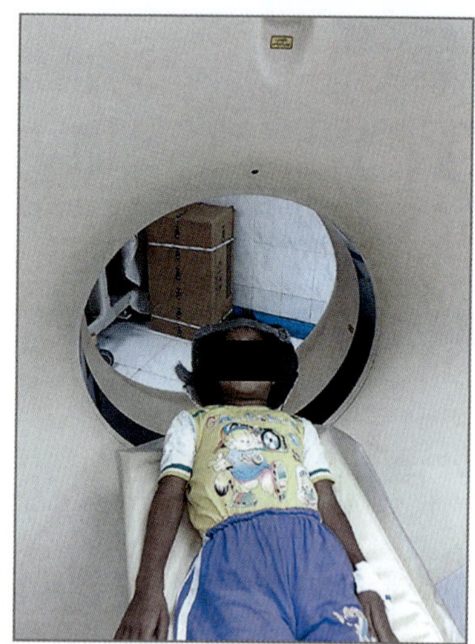

Fig. 20.2: Pediatric scanning with head immobilizers to avoid motion artifacts and repeat scan.

Table 20.1: Sedation agents commonly used in pediatric imaging.

Sedation agent	*Indication*	*Common dosage*
Diazepam	Longer imaging procedures	0.2–0.5 mg/kg orally
Midazolam	Short imaging procedures	0.05–0.1 mg/kg IV
Ketamine	Procedural sedation	1–2 mg/kg IV

cases must possess in-depth knowledge and expertise, as pediatric pathologies differ significantly from adult conditions. Familiarity with normal anatomical variants in children is crucial to avoid misdiagnosis. Pediatric radiologists should recommend the appropriate modality for specific cases.

Radiation Protection (Table 20.2)

Radiation protection is a primary concern for pediatric imaging due to the higher risk of cancer induction in children, estimated to be about ten times higher than in adults. Children's longer life expectancy also increases the potential for radiation-related harm. The literature suggests that CT usage should be controlled, and the ALARA (As Low As Reasonably Achievable) principle should be strictly followed. The appropriate imaging modality should be selected based on clinical indications, such as using ultrasound instead of CT for suspected

Table 20.2: Radiation protection measures in pediatric imaging.

Measure	*Description*
ALARA principle	Keeping radiation "As low as reasonably achievable"
Beam filtration	Reducing low-energy photons with aluminum and copper
Anti-scatter grid	Removing for younger children to reduce patient dose
Protective shields	Using gonadal, thyroid, and breast shields appropriately

appendicitis. MRI is preferred over CT for most cross-sectional imaging in children, except in trauma cases.

TECHNICAL CONSIDERATION

Conventional Radiography

Guidelines ensure acceptable quality diagnostic radiography in children, aiming to produce adequate images, provide accurate interpretation, and use low radiation doses. Recommendations include:

- Use computed or digital radiography to optimize exposure factors and avoid repeats.
- Use high-contrast, high-resolution films.
- Use low-absorption cassette or image plates and table-tops.
- Stringent exposure parameters.
- Proper positioning, centering of the beam, collimation, and restraining methods.
- Fine focus techniques to reduce radiation dose without losing detail.
- Minimize projections to visualize the area of interest.

Ultrasound

Pediatric ultrasound is safe, inexpensive, and readily available, with no radiation risks. It is suitable for repeated follow-up studies. Special pediatric probes should be used, and warming the gel and towels can make the process more comfortable for the child **(Fig. 20.3)**. Aseptic procedures must be maintained to prevent infections in infants.

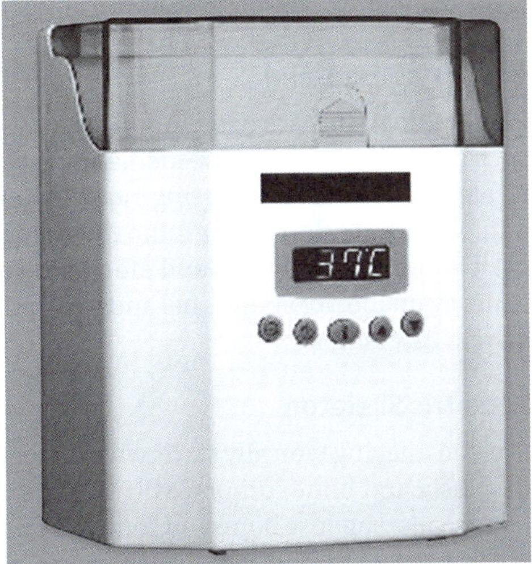

Fig. 20.3: Gel warmer must be used in cold environment to prohibit the uncomfortable cold sensations to child while using ultrasound gel.

Computed Tomography

CT's primary concern is radiation exposure. Optimization of scan parameters includes reducing rotation time, detector coverage, field of view, and kilovolts, and using smart milliamperes/auto milliampere options. CT angiography in children requires reduced contrast volume, appropriate injection rates, and timing of scans, dose minimization, and consideration of breath-holding abilities. Neonates should be adequately insulated from room temperature (18–22°C) using blankets or warmers to prevent hypothermia.

Magnetic Resonance Imaging

Magnetic resonance imaging (MRI) often requires sedation or general anesthesia in younger children. Smaller anatomical structures necessitate a higher signal-to-noise ratio, achieved with pediatric-specific coils, high-field strengths, and optimized field of view and slice thickness. Physiological factors, such as heart rate, breathing, and blood-flow rates, etc., influence image acquisition and contrast injection rates. Respiratory gating can help mitigate motion artifacts. Antenatal MRI is valuable for evaluating congenital anomalies detected on ultrasound, but contrast agents are not administered to pregnant mothers and should be avoided in the first trimester.

Safety issues in children include a higher risk of radiofrequency heating effects and the need to avoid MR contrast agents in children under 2 years.

CLINICAL APPLICATIONS

Pediatric Brain

Ultrasound is preferred for infants due to its safety and availability. Cross-sectional imaging, such as MRI, is required for older children once the fontanelles are closed. MRI is invaluable for investigating brain anatomy and development, while CT is reserved for trauma evaluation. For patients with ventriculoperitoneal shunts, a low-dose "shunt protocol" CT head is used to monitor ventricle size and shunt catheter location. Other neurological indications are served by MRI as described below **(Table 20.3)**.

Pediatric Chest

Radiographs are the primary technique for chest evaluation, but challenges include achieving inspiration, minimizing motional blur, and reducing radiation dose. Helical CT provides detailed images of the thoracic bony cage, vascular, and pulmonary architecture. MRI distinguishes between mediastinal fat, blood vessels, and soft tissues, useful for cardiac anomalies, mediastinal masses, and chest wall lesions. Functional lung imaging with MRI is now possible, and PET/CT is increasingly useful for lymphoma imaging in children.

Pediatric Abdomen

Plain radiographs are used for initial assessment of abdominal disease. Fluoroscopic studies, such as upper GI or contrast enema, are essential for neonatal GI obstruction workup. Ultrasound is safe and reliable for assessing intra-abdominal organs, diagnosing conditions like appendicitis and ovarian torsion, and guiding procedures like intussusception reduction. CT is used for evaluating trauma injuries and preoperative tumor assessments. MRI has significantly advanced in the evaluation of abdominal and pelvic diseases, including biliary tract, pancreas, and urinary system assessment.

Pediatric Skeleton

Skeletal imaging typically starts with radiography, crucial for detecting and categorizing skeletal dysplasia and bone tumors. MRI stages diseases and monitors follow-up, while radionuclide bone scans diagnose bone and soft-tissue infections and assess occult trauma. Bone scintigraphy is also used for evaluating suspected non-accidental injury and unexplained bone pain. Proper technique is essential for obtaining high-quality diagnostic images.

Table 20.3: Comparison of imaging modalities for pediatric brain.

Modality	*Advantages*	*Disadvantages*
Ultrasound	Safe, no radiation, bedside availability	Limited use once fontanelles are closed
MRI	Detailed anatomy and functional imaging	Requires sedation, longer duration
CT	Fast, good for trauma evaluation	High radiation exposure

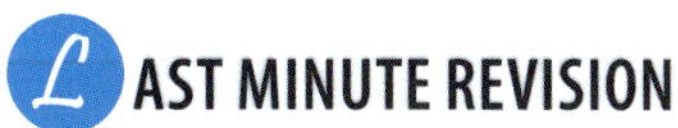

LAST MINUTE REVISION

- Create a child-friendly radiology department to gain children's trust and cooperation.
- Use specialized pediatric equipment and standardized protocols to enhance image quality and reduce radiation.
- Ensure only trained staff with expertise in pediatric imaging, perform and interpret scans.
- Follow the ALARA principle to minimize radiation exposure in pediatric imaging.
- Tailor the use of imaging modalities to the clinical situation, prioritizing safety and diagnostic efficacy.

REVIEW QUESTIONS

Multiple Choice Questions (MCQs)

1. **A 5-year-old child presents to the emergency room with a head injury after falling off a bicycle. He is conscious but complains of a headache and vomiting. What is the most appropriate imaging modality for initial evaluation?**
   a. MRI　　b. CT Scan
   c. Ultrasound　　d. X-ray
2. **A 2-year-old girl presents with a painful, swollen abdomen and a high fever. The clinician suspects appendicitis. What is the best initial imaging modality?**
   a. MRI　　b. CT Scan
   c. Ultrasound　　d. X-ray
3. **A newborn presents with signs of respiratory distress. The clinician suspects a congenital diaphragmatic hernia. What is the best initial imaging modality?**
   a. MRI　　b. CT Scan
   c. Ultrasound　　d. X-ray
4. **A 7-year-old child presents with severe right lower quadrant pain and tenderness. The clinician suspects intussusception. What is the best initial imaging modality?**
   a. MRI　　b. CT Scan
   c. Ultrasound　　d. X-ray
5. **A 3-year-old child presents with a limp and pain in the hip. The clinician suspects a hip joint effusion. What is the most appropriate imaging modality for initial evaluation?**
   a. MRI　　b. CT Scan
   c. Ultrasound　　d. X-ray

Answer Key

1. b　2. c　3. d　4. c　5. c

SUGGESTED READING

1. Tajaldeen A, Kheiralla OAM, Alghamdi SS, Alsleem H, Al-Othman A, Abuelhia E, et al. Evaluation of Pediatric Imaging Modalities Practices of Radiologists and Technologists: A Survey-Based Study. J Multidiscip Healthc. 2022 Mar 5;15:443-53.
2. Thukral BB. Problems and preferences in pediatric imaging. Indian J Radiol Imaging. 2015 Oct-Dec;25(4):359-64.

CHAPTER

21

Pediatric Neuroimaging

"Pediatric neuroimaging explores the growing mind—each scan a chance to guide a child's path before words are even spoken."

INTRODUCTION

During the neonatal period, encompassing the first month of life, a substantial proportion of infant mortalities and persistent neurological issues originate from adverse incidents. Premature infants are particularly susceptible to brain damage during this critical time. Imaging is pivotal for diagnosing and comprehending such injuries and for predicting neurodevelopmental outcomes. Cranial ultrasound is typically the initial imaging modality employed due to its portability. It is effective in monitoring conditions, such as germinal matrix hemorrhage, hydrocephalus, and significant brain malformations. However, ultrasound may not be as effective as computed tomography (CT) or magnetic resonance imaging (MRI) in detecting small calcifications or subtle brain malformations. CT is generally reserved for cases requiring confirmation of specific conditions, such as intracranial calcifications. MRI, on the other hand, is the most advanced technique for evaluating the neonatal brain. Advanced MRI techniques, such as diffusion-weighted imaging (DWI) and functional magnetic resonance imaging (fMRI) offer valuable insights into brain physiology and function. Furthermore, arterial spin labelling allows for noninvasive assessment of neonatal brain perfusion.

IMAGING TECHNIQUES

When assessing the pediatric brain, different imaging modalities provide unique insights into the developing neural structures. This overview outlines the key characteristics and considerations of ultrasound, CT, and MRI for pediatric brain imaging.

Ultrasound

- **Advantages:** Ultrasound is a noninvasive imaging modality that offers high-resolution images for evaluating superficial brain structures, particularly in neonates.
- **Limitations:** Ultrasound may struggle to visualize deeper brain structures, such as the cerebellum and posterior fossa, due to limited penetration depth and reduced visibility of more intricate details.
- **Applications:** Primarily used for neonatal brain screening, such as evaluating for intraventricular hemorrhage and periventricular leukomalacia. Accessible and quick, it is suitable for bedside use.

Computed Tomography (CT)

- **Advantages:** CT provides increased tissue contrast and can visualize deep brain structures, making it useful for assessing hemorrhage, fractures, and acute injuries.
- **Limitations:** Concerns about radiation exposure limit its use in pediatric patients. It is generally reserved for specific cases where rapid imaging is needed or when MRI is contraindicated.
- **Applications:** Commonly used for evaluating acute brain injuries, cranial trauma, and potential abnormalities requiring immediate assessment.

Magnetic Resonance Imaging (MRI) (Figs. 21.1 and 21.2)

- **Advantages:** MRI is the most sensitive modality for detecting abnormalities in the pediatric brain. It offers superior soft tissue contrast and can utilize various imaging sequences to optimize visualization.
- **Limitations:** MRI can be time-consuming and may require sedation in younger children to minimize movement. It is also more expensive and less readily available in emergency situations.
- **Sequences:**
  - *T1-weighted:* Provides detailed anatomical images, particularly useful for assessing myelination and brain maturation.

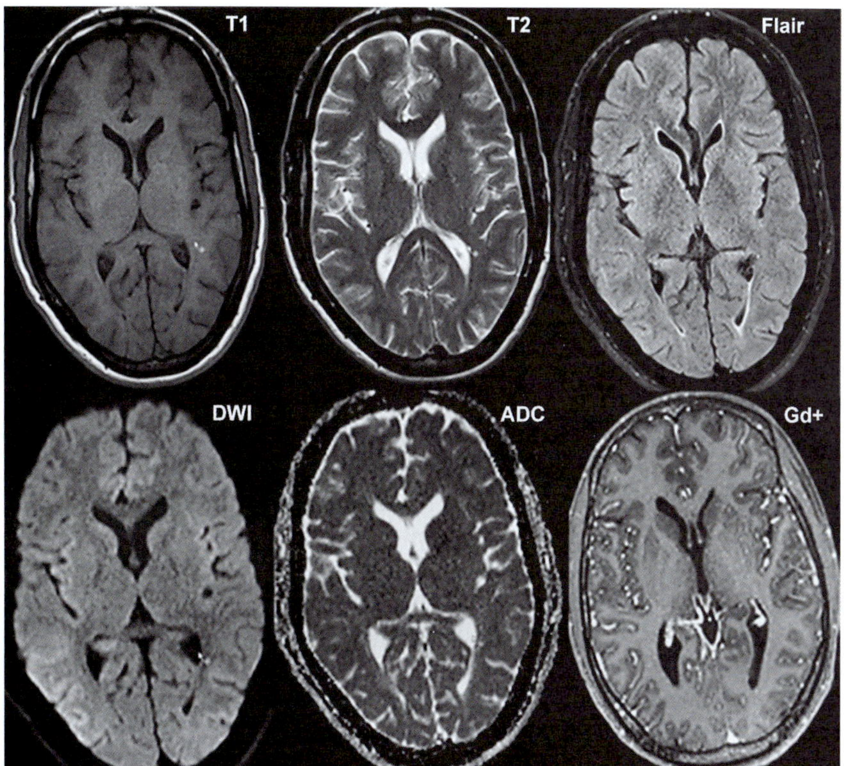

Fig. 21.1: MRI images of a patient showing T1-weighted, T2-weighted, fluid-attenuated inversion recovery (FLAIR), diffusion-weighted image (DWI), apparent diffusion coefficient (ADC) map and Gd+ (post-gadolinium) contrast-enhanced images.

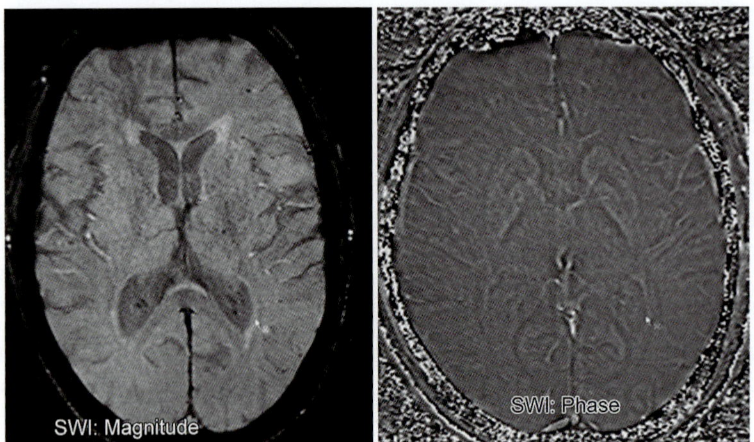

Fig. 21.2: Susceptibility-weighted images of a patient (magnitude and phase images).

- *T2-weighted:* Excellent for detecting water content and fluid changes, such as edema and inflammation.
- *Diffusion-weighted imaging (DWI):* Useful for evaluating brain ischemia, infarction, and white matter tract integrity.
- **Gradient-Echo:** Helpful for detecting microbleeds and vascular malformations.

- **Optimization:** Adjustments in scan parameters, such as longer echo times and inversion times for T1-weighted scans, enhance the quality of neonatal imaging. Dedicated neonatal MR head coils improve image quality, contrast, and resolution for smaller field of view imaging, aiding in better visualization of critical structures like the brainstem and posterior fossa.

Overall, each imaging modality has its strengths and weaknesses in pediatric brain assessment. A careful choice based on the clinical scenario and correct selection of modality as per patient needs can provide the most accurate and safe diagnosis.

COMMON PATHOLOGY

Hypoxic Ischemic Encephalopathy

Brain injury in term neonates can vary significantly and is affected by the severity and duration of the insult. Imaging results may vary based on when they are conducted, with studies before 72 hours potentially underestimating injury severity due to delayed cell death, such as apoptosis, peaking around the 72-hour post-insult. Therapeutic hypothermia, typically initiated within 6 hours of birth and maintained for 72 hours, can prolong this process.

Hypoxic-ischemic encephalopathy (HIE) typically arises from severe asphyxia, causing sudden blood supply disruption and resulting in oxygen and glucose deprivation in the neonatal brain. Structures with high metabolic demands, including the thalami, basal ganglia, and brainstem, are particularly susceptible to hypoxia and ischemia. The ventral lateral thalami, posterolateral lentiform nuclei, posterior midbrain, hippocampi, lateral geniculate nuclei, and perirolandic cerebral cortex are notably vulnerable regions. Profound asphyxia is associated with conditions, such as quadriparesis, choreoathetosis, seizures, mental retardation, and cerebral palsy.

- Ultrasound and CT often show transient or persistent hyperechogenicity in deep brain structures, potentially progressing to cavitation, especially in basal ganglia and thalami.
- MRI is the preferred imaging for neonatal encephalopathy; MRS at 24 hours post-insult is sensitive to hypoxic-ischemic injury, indicating elevated lactate and reduced N-acetyl-aspartate (NAA), with lactate peaking 3–5 days post-event.
- DWI is highly sensitive for acute brain injury, detecting lesions in deep gray and perirolandic gray matter earlier than conventional MRI.
- Conventional MRI progresses from unremarkable to increased T1-weighted signal and decreased T2-weighted signal in the subacute phase, followed by increased T2-weighted signal in the chronic phase.

Prematurity

Premature birth, especially very preterm birth (before 32 weeks of gestation), can lead to various neurological features and imaging findings due to the immature development of the central nervous system. Some common neurological features of prematurity along with associated imaging findings are as follows:

Intraventricular Hemorrhage (IVH)

- IVH can lead to intracranial hemorrhage, presenting with symptoms, such as lethargy, apnea, seizures, or a sudden change in mental status.
- **Imaging findings:** Cranial ultrasound (CUS) typically reveals echoic or echo lucent areas within the ventricles, depending on the stage of hemorrhage. Severe IVH may progress to hydrocephalus or periventricular hemorrhagic infarction.

Periventricular Leukomalacia (PVL)

- PVL is characterized by white matter injury and can lead to developmental delays, spasticity, motor deficits, and cognitive impairment later in life.
- **Imaging findings:** CUS initially shows echoic periventricular areas, later progressing to cystic lesions or gliosis. MRI is more sensitive and can demonstrate diffuse or focal areas of signal abnormality in the periventricular white matter.

Cerebral White Matter Injury

- White matter injury is associated with motor and cognitive deficits, including cerebral palsy and learning disabilities.
- **Imaging findings:** MRI reveals abnormal signal intensity in the cerebral white matter, typically involving periventricular regions. Diffusion-weighted imaging (DWI) may show restricted diffusion in acute injury, while T2-weighted or FLAIR sequences demonstrate hyperintense signal changes in chronic injury.

Intracranial Hemorrhage

- Intracranial hemorrhage can lead to symptoms, such as seizures, irritability, poor feeding, or altered consciousness.
- **Imaging findings:** CUS or MRI can reveal hemorrhage within the parenchyma, subarachnoid space, or ventricles. Hemorrhages may resolve or evolve into complications, such as hydrocephalus or porencephaly.

Congenital Brain Malformations

Chiari Malformations

Chiari malformations are a group of defects associated with congenital caudal 'displacement' of the cerebellum and brainstem.

- **Chiari I malformation** is the most common form, characterized by the displacement of peg-like cerebellar tonsils (>5 mm) into the upper cervical canal through the foramen magnum.
- **Chiari 1.5 malformation** is described both as a separate condition and a variant of Chiari I malformation, involving caudal descent of cerebellar tonsils and brainstem.
- **Chiari II malformation** involves the displacement of the medulla, fourth ventricle, and cerebellar vermis through the foramen magnum, often associated with a lumbosacral spinal myelomeningocele.
- **Chiari III malformation** shares similarities with Chiari II, but includes an occipital and/or high cervical encephalocele.
- **Chiari IV malformation** presents with severe cerebellar hypoplasia without displacement of the cerebellum through the foramen magnum, possibly a variation of cerebellar hypoplasia.
- **Chiari V malformation** is characterized by the absence of the cerebellum and herniation of the occipital lobe through the foramen magnum.
- **Chiari 0 malformation** refers to the presence of a syrinx without cerebellar tonsillar or brainstem descent, is infrequently used and considered confusing, and it is advised to avoid it, particularly in light of reports indicating syrinx improvement after posterior fossa decompression.

Dandy-Walker Continuum

The Dandy-Walker continuum encompasses two main conditions: the Dandy-Walker malformation and the Dandy-Walker variant.

Dandy-Walker Malformation

- This condition involves either complete or partial absence (agenesis) of the vermis, along with cystic enlargement of the fourth ventricle.
- It leads to an enlarged posterior fossa with displacement of the torcula (a structure at the back of the head where dural sinuses converge).
- Often, supratentorial hydrocephalus (build-up of cerebrospinal fluid within the brain's ventricles) accompanies this malformation.
- Roughly 70% of patients also exhibit associated anomalies, such as abnormal or absent corpus callosum (a structure connecting the brain's hemispheres), callosal lipoma (fatty tissue in the corpus callosum), and neuronal migration anomalies.

Dandy-Walker Variant

In this variant, there is underdevelopment (hypoplasia) of the inferior portion of the vermis, coupled with non-obstructive cystic enlargement of the fourth ventricle.

- Unlike the malformation, the posterior fossa appears normal or slightly enlarged.
- In contrast to the Dandy-Walker continuum, two other conditions should be kept in mind:

Posterior Fossa Arachnoid Cyst

- This condition involves a cystic space filled with cerebrospinal fluid (CSF) in the posterior fossa.
- It does not affect the formation of the cerebellum and typically causes anterior displacement of the fourth ventricle and cerebellum.

Mega Cisterna Magna

- In this condition, there is enlargement of the CSF spaces (>10 mm) behind the cerebellum.
- It does not exert pressure on surrounding structures and does not affect the development of the cerebellum.

Inborn Errors of Metabolism

Metachromatic Leukodystrophy

- Metachromatic leukodystrophy (MLD) is characterized by a deficiency in arylsulfatase A enzyme, leading to cerebroside sulfate accumulation in lysosomes.
- **MLD has four subtypes:** Congenital, late infantile, juvenile, and adult. The late infantile subtype is most common, typically appearing between 14 months to 4 years of age.
- Symptoms include initial unsteady gait progressing to severe ataxia, flaccid paralysis, dysarthria, mental retardation, and decerebrate posturing.
- Imaging shows marked T2 hyperintensity of white matter fiber tracts with diffuse involvement, sparing subcortical white matter initially.

Infections

Neonatal brain infections pose a significant risk for long-term neurological issues, being caused by viruses, bacteria, and parasites transmitted during different stages of development—in utero, during labor and delivery, or after birth.

Bacterial and fungal infections commonly transmit during labor or postnatally, while infections, such as toxoplasmosis, syphilis, rubella, and cytomegalovirus (CMV) are often transmitted in utero. Herpes simplex virus (HSV) and human immunodeficiency virus (HIV) can be transmitted during any stage.

Bacterial Infections

- Common bacteria causing neonatal brain infections include group B streptococcus, *Escherichia coli, Streptococcus pneumoniae, Haemophilus influenzae* type B, and *Listeria monocytogenes.*
- Ventricular enlargement, due to impaired CSF absorption from inflammatory exudate, is common in meningitis but does not necessarily indicate ventriculitis.
- **Ventriculitis** is characterized by ependymal enhancement and sometimes pus-fluid levels, often accompanied by hydrocephalus and intraventricular abscesses.
- **Sterile subdural effusions** are common in neonatal meningitis, but about 2% of cases progress to **empyemas**, identified by distinct signal intensity from CSF and peripheral enhancement.
- **Cerebritis,** evidenced by vasogenic edema with/without patchy enhancement, may appear on autopsy despite normal in vivo imaging findings.
- As the disease progresses, enhancing areas may merge, forming a **cerebral abscess** with restricted water diffusivity and an enhancing capsule.

CNS Tuberculosis

It may present as focal lesions, such as tuberculomas or tuberculous abscesses, or more widespread conditions, such as meningitis and arachnoiditis.

Tuberculomas and Tuberculous Abscesses

- Tuberculomas constitute the majority of focal TB lesions and are usually devoid of tuberculous meningitis (TBM).

- On CT, tuberculomas appear iso- or hyperdense to cortex before contrast administration, often exhibiting ring or nodular enhancement with surrounding edema.
- They typically show low signal on T2-weighted images and isointense signal on T1-weighted images, with rim enhancement post-contrast administration.
- TB abscesses are larger lesions, also rim-enhancing, but with low density centrally, similar to pyogenic abscesses.

Tuberculous Meningitis (TBM)

- TBM is the most severe form of TB in children, presenting with diffuse involvement of the CNS, which can be asymmetrical, unilateral, or focal.
- MRI is excellent for detecting basal enhancement and infarctions but may have limited impact due to availability constraints, especially in resource-limited areas.

Complications of TBM

Includes vasculitis (can lead to infarcts), hydrocephalus, spinal arachnoiditis.

Viral Encephalitis

Herpes Simplex Virus Type 2 (HSV-2) Infection

- Outbreaks during pregnancy increase the risk of miscarriage or delivering a low birth weight baby.
- Neonatal transmission commonly occurs during birth but in utero transmission is possible.
- HSV-2 encephalitis poses a serious risk to the newborn.
- Diagnosis is typically made through viral culture or PCR of CSF.
- Imaging may reveal cortical hemorrhagic foci, leptomeningeal enhancement, and cystic white matter changes.
- Findings are typically normal in neonates.
- Late findings include atrophy, delayed myelination, and CNS lymphoma.

Japanese Encephalitis (JE)

- It is a viral infection transmitted by arthropods, belonging to the flavivirus family, and is associated with significant mortality and morbidity.
- Recurrent outbreak of JE are reported annually, between the month of July and October from the districts of upper Assam of Northeast India.
- Abnormal T2 and FLAIR hyperintensities indicative of Japanese encephalitis (JE) are commonly observed in the thalami, substantia nigra, basal ganglia, hippocampus, pons, and occasionally in cortical and subcortical regions, as well as cerebellar hemispheres.
- DWI's sensitivity to cytotoxic edema, an early indicator of encephalitis, makes it superior in detecting early-stage JE cases but less effective in later stages.
- During the acute stage of JE, DWI typically shows diffusion restriction with low apparent diffusion coefficient (ADC) values, which gradually increase during the late acute and chronic stages.

Neurocysticercosis (NCC)

- It is a parasitic infection affecting the nervous system, resulting from the presence of cystic larvae of *Taenia solium*.
- It represents the most prevalent helminthic infection of the nervous system in humans and is a primary contributor to epilepsy incidence in tropical regions, particularly noted as the leading cause of focal seizures in children from North India.

Table 21.1: Difference between neurocysticercosis and CNS tuberculosis.

Neurocysticercosis	*CNS tuberculosis*
Lesions are generally smaller than 2 cm and often multiple	Lesions are often multiple, >2 cm because of conglomeration
Meningitis is not a prominent feature	Meningitis with basal exudates and hydrocephalus is usually associated
Generally present at gray white matter junction and can also involve eyes, muscles and subcutaneous tissue	Generally posterior fossa is involved
T2W image shows hyperintensity with hypointense scolex	T2W image shows can show hypo- or hyperintense lesion without any mural nodules
Lesions show less edema and less midline shift	Lesions show more edema and more midline shift
MRS shows multiple amino acid peak	MRS shows lipid peak
Raised ICP is transient	Raised ICP is present
Constitutional symptoms usually absent	Constitutional symptoms usually present

- **Location of cysts:**
  - Cysts can be found anywhere within the neuroaxis and may be intra-axial or extra-axial
  - Most commonly, cysts are located in the parenchyma.
  - In the subarachnoid space over the cerebral hemispheres, cysts can attain significant size.
  - Ventricular involvement is also observed.
- Difference between neurocysticercosis and CNS tuberculosis shown in **Table 21.1**.
- **Stages of infection:** Each stage exhibits distinctive imaging features, although there is no clear demarcation between them.
  a. *Vesicular stage:*
    - Characterized by cysts with dot sign, CSF density/intensity, and occasionally an eccentric hyperintense scolex on T1.
    - Typically, no enhancement is observed, although faint enhancement of the wall and scolex may occur.
    - Absence of surrounding vasogenic edema.
  b. *Colloidal vesicular stage:*
    - Marked by turbid cyst fluid, appearing hyperattenuating to CSF on CT and hyperintense on T1 MRI.
    - Surrounding edema is evident, and the cyst and wall become thickened and enhance brightly.
    - The scolex may initially be visible but gradually diminishes.
  c. *Granular nodular stage:*
    - Edema diminishes, and the cyst retracts, eventually becoming a small enhancing nodule.
    - Persistent but less marked enhancement is observed.
  d. *Nodular calcified stage:*
    - Represents the end-stage with quiescent calcified nodules.
    - No edema is present, and there is no enhancement on CT.
    - Signal drop-out on T2 and T2* sequences, with some intrinsic high T1 signal.
    - Long-term enhancement on MRI may predict ongoing seizures.

Epilepsy

It is very common presenting complaints in childrens. Causes are innumerable (e.g., infections, congenital causes, prematurity, tumors, etc.). Few common causes are described below:

Focal Cortical Dysplasia

The exact mechanism of epilepsy in FCD is not fully understood, but possible factors include abnormal firing from dysplastic neurons, dysfunctional synaptic circuits, and disorganized inhibitory interneurons.

- FCD can occur in any cerebral cortex and vary in size, ranging from one gyrus to multiple lobes.
- MRI features of FCD include increased cortical thickness, blurring of cortical-white matter junction, and abnormal signal intensities in T2 or FLAIR sequences in cortex and subcortical white matter, along with abnormal sulcation and gyration pattern.

Lissencephaly

In lissencephaly, MRI typically shows a smooth brain surface with a lack of normal convolutions or gyri. The cortex appears thickened and lacks the usual sulci and gyri, resulting in a characteristic "smooth brain" appearance.

Pachygyria

Pachygyria is characterized by broad and abnormally thick gyri. On MRI, the cortex appears thicker than normal, with fewer and larger gyri than expected. This can result in a "pebbled" or "cobblestone" appearance of the brain surface.

Polymicrogyria

Polymicrogyria is characterized by an excessive number of small, irregular gyri. On MRI, the cortex appears densely folded with numerous small gyri, giving a "bumpy" or "spongy" appearance to the brain surface.

Heterotopia

Heterotopia refers to clusters of neurons that have migrated abnormally and are located in the wrong brain regions. On MRI, heterotopias appear as focal areas of abnormal signal intensity within the white matter or along the ventricular walls (Iso-intense to grey matter on all sequences).

Schizencephaly

Schizencephaly is characterized by clefts or cleft-like openings in the cerebral cortex that extend from the surface of the brain to the ventricular system, always lined by grey matter. On MRI, these clefts are visualized as linear clefts of CSF signal intensity extending from the brain surface to the lateral ventricles, often associated with abnormal cortical development around the clefts.

Phakomatosis

Tuberous Sclerosis

- Tuberous sclerosis complex (TSC) is an autosomal-dominant neurocutaneous syndrome affecting multiple systems including the brain, eyes, heart, kidney, skin, and lung.
- Seizures are prevalent in 80–90% of TSC patients, with 25–30% experiencing intractable seizures.

- Medically refractory epilepsy in children with TSC often involves multiple cortical/subcortical tubers characterized by broad gyri, thick cortex, and abnormal signal in cortex and subcortical white matter.
- Cortical/subcortical tubers in TSC may occasionally exhibit calcification and cystic degeneration.
- Subependymal nodules, common in TSC, often calcify.
- Subependymal giant cell astrocytomas, another manifestation of TSC, frequently occur near the foramen of Monro.

Neurofibromatosis Type 1

Neurofibromatosis Type 1 (NF1) patients face an elevated risk of developing primarily benign tumors affecting the nervous system:

- Optic pathway gliomas (OPGs) represent the most common central nervous system tumors in NF1 children under seven years old, with an incidence of 15–20%.

Epilepsy-associated Tumors

Epilepsy-associated tumors constitute a significant portion, potentially up to two-thirds, of the pathological substrate for epilepsy surgery. These tumors arise within the cortex and are clinically characterized by seizures, typically displaying benign behavior with low proliferation rates, although malignant transformation can occur in rare instances.

Ganglioglioma (Fig. 21.3)

- Gangliogliomas commonly present with seizures, particularly complex partial seizures that are often medically refractory.
- They tend to be larger in children than in adults and are predominantly located in the temporomesial or temporolateral regions.
- Comprised of both glial and neuronal elements, gangliogliomas can manifest as solid masses, cysts, or mixed lesions, often causing remodeling of adjacent bone due to their cortical location.

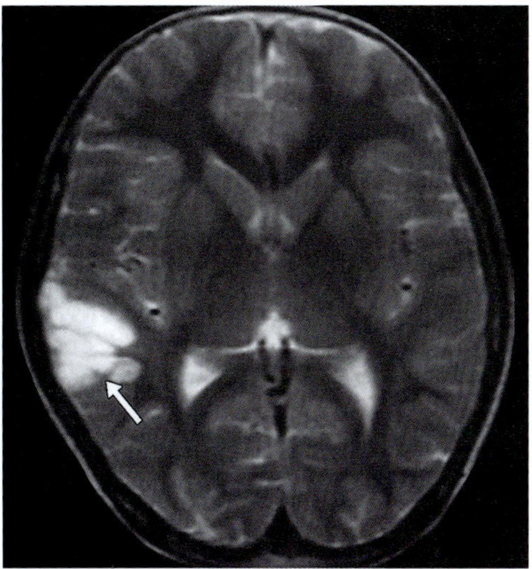

Fig. 21.3: T2 hyperintense mass involving cortex of right temporal lobe suggestive of ganglioneuronal tumor.

- Imaging characteristics include hypodensity on CT in a majority of cases, with varying degrees of density and frequent calcification. On MRI, the solid portion typically appears hypointense or isointense on T1-weighted images and hyperintense on T2-weighted images, often with enhancement.

Dysembryoplastic Neuroepithelial Tumor (DNET)

- DNET is a benign cortical tumor typically found in the supratentorial region, showing a predilection for the temporal lobes
- It may present with a well-demarcated margin or slightly blurred margins, along with associated gyral broadening, sulcal effacement, ventricular distortion, and skull remodeling.
- On imaging, DNET tends to appear hypodense with a cystic appearance on CT, with reported calcifications in a portion of cases. MRI typically shows a low T1 and high T2 signal, often with multicystic features and possible enhancement, extending into the ventricle in some instances (soap bubble/bubbly appearance).

Brain Neoplasm

Medulloblastoma

- It is the most prevalent childhood posterior fossa tumors, account for approximately 38% of all such tumors and 15–20% of pediatric brain tumors.
- Medulloblastomas typically originate midline within the vermis, causing obstructive hydrocephalus as they grow into the fourth ventricle, though they may localize to the cerebellar hemispheres in older patients or those with the desmoplastic subtype.
- Imaging features include hyperdensity on CT while T1 and T2 hypointensity relative to gray matter with homogeneous enhancement on MRI. Elevated taurine content on MRS may also be observed.

Craniopharyngiomas

- Craniopharyngiomas are slow-growing, benign tumors located in the sellar and parasellar regions, comprising 3–10% of all pediatric brain tumors.
- They are WHO grade I tumors, originating from ectodermal remnants of the Rathke's pouch, with a bimodal incidence in the first and fifth decades of life. The adamantinous type is more common in children, while the squamous-papillary variant is predominant in adults
- Imaging typically reveals mixed cystic and solid components, with high signal intensity on both T1- and T2-weighted MRI images in areas with high protein content or subacute hemorrhage. Hypointensity on T1-weighted images may indicate the presence of keratin within cysts. Calcifications are commonly demonstrated on CT scans, aiding diagnosis and surgical planning.

Astrocytomas

The modified WHO classification categorizes astrocytomas into low grade (grades I and II) and high grade (grades III and IV), with grading predictive of patient survival.

- Pilocytic astrocytomas, classified as grade I WHO tumors, represent 20–30% of childhood brain tumors and typically manifest within the first two decades of life.
- These tumors commonly arise in various locations, such as the optic pathways, hypothalamus, thalamus, basal ganglia, cerebral hemispheres, cerebellum, and brainstem, with patients with NF1 having an elevated risk, especially for optic pathway tumors.
- On imaging, grade I astrocytomas usually exhibit well-defined lesions with contrast enhancement of the solid component, possibly accompanied by cystic components. Increased ADC values within these lesions aid in differentiation from higher grade astrocytomas.

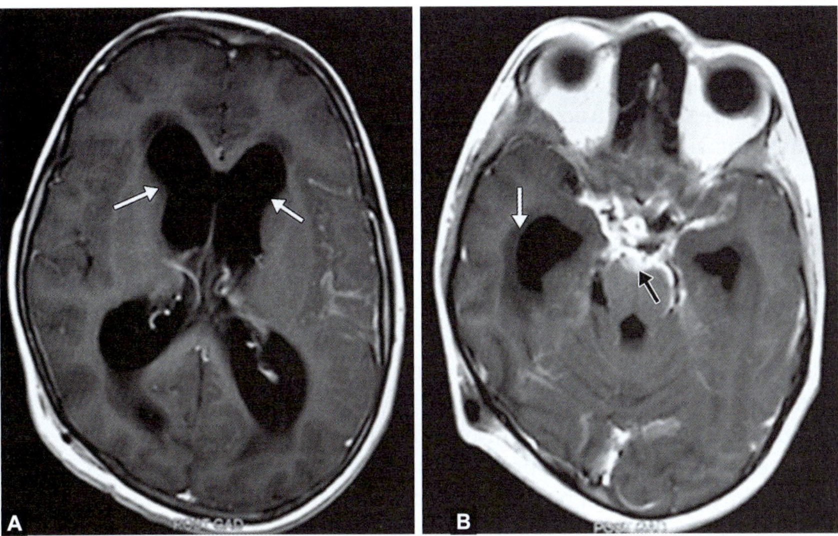

Figs. 21.4A and B: Hydrocephalus: (A) Contrast-enhanced axial T1 images showing dilated bilateral lateral ventricles; (B) Dilated temporal horns *(white arrow)* along with enhancing basal exudates *(black arrow)* suggestive of tubercular meningitis causing hydrocephalus.

Hydrocephalus (Figs. 21.4A and B)

- Hydrocephalus, which translates to "fluid accumulation within the brain," occurs when various factors culminate in the expansion of ventricles, causing compression of brain tissue and surrounding spaces, thereby resulting in elevated intracranial pressure (ICP).
- This imaging findings also having long list of causes (e.g., TBM, brain tumors, Dandy Walker continuum, etc.)
- CT and MRI serve as primary modalities for assessing ventricular size, while ultrasound is preferred in infants with macrocephaly.
- **Enlargement of the anterior and posterior recesses of the third ventricle** is a reliable sign of hydrocephalus due to less resistance from surrounding structures.
- **Commensurate dilation of the temporal horns** with the lateral ventricles is indicative of hydrocephalus and can be observed on coronal T2-weighted images.
- **Reduction of the mamillopontine distance** and **diminution of the ventricular angle** suggest hydrocephalus, as seen on MRI images.
- Hydrocephalus may lead **to periventricular interstitial edema**, which is appreciable on MRI with fluid-attenuated inversion recovery and proton density sequences.
- These imaging findings aid in distinguishing hydrocephalus from other conditions, guiding treatment decisions, and monitoring disease progression.

Child Abuse

- Skeletal surveys are conducted in suspected abuse cases to evaluate and record skeletal injuries. The "babygram" technique, capturing the entire infant in one view, is deemed inadequate due to its lower image quality and the need for varied exposures for different anatomical regions.
- Bone scans are utilized in certain institutions for their capability to identify fractures not visible on radiographs.

- Specific fractures, such as **metaphyseal fractures** (such as **bucket handle** or **corner fractures**) and rib fractures, are highly indicative of non-accidental injuries, particularly in abused infants under 18 months.
- Suspicious features of skull fractures include non-parietal locations, involvement of multiple bones, diastatic sutures, cross-suture patterns, and depressed fractures resembling a signature. Other moderately specific fractures for non-accidental injury include bilateral fractures with differing ages, digital fractures in non-ambulant children, vertebral fractures, spiral humeral fractures, and complex skull fractures.
- **Subdural hemorrhage** is the most common, often located interhemispherically.
- Subarachnoid hemorrhage is also observed.
- Cerebral edema may manifest as focal, multifocal, or diffuse swelling.
- Acute cerebral contusion appears as an ovoid collection of intraparenchymal blood with surrounding edema.
- MR imaging is more sensitive in identifying hematomas of varying ages.
- White matter shearing injuries present as areas of prolonged T1 and T2 signals at the corticomedullary junction, centrum semiovale, and corpus callosum.
- Visceral injuries—trauma to abdominal viscera, accounting for 3% of cases, is the second leading cause of death in child abuse. Causes include crushing blows to the abdomen (e.g., punches, kicks), with victims often older than two years.

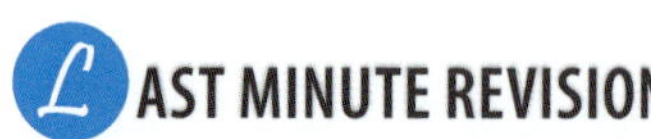

- **MRI is superior** for detailed brain structure, e.g., to see tumor extension, for etiology and stage of infection etc.
- **Ultrasound** is quick and effective for initial screenings and safe for frequent use.
- **CT scans** are reserved for urgent assessments due to quick imaging capabilities but carry radiation risk.
- Medulloblastoma is most prevalent childhood posterior fossa tumors

REVIEW QUESTIONS

Multiple Choice Questions (MCQs)

1. **What is the initial imaging modality typically employed for assessing neonatal brain injuries due to its portability?**
   a. MRI
   b. CT
   c. Ultrasound
   d. X-ray
2. **Which MRI sequence is particularly useful for evaluating brain ischemia and white matter tract integrity in neonates?**
   a. T1-weighted
   b. T2-weighted
   c. Diffusion-weighted imaging (DWI)
   d. Gradient-Echo
3. **What is a major limitation of using CT scans in pediatric patients?**
   a. Time-consuming procedures
   b. High cost of the scans
   c. Radiation exposure
   d. Need for sedation

4. Which condition is MRI particularly sensitive to at 24 hours post-insult due to its ability to detect elevated lactate and reduced N-acetyl-aspartate (NAA)?

a. Prematurity
b. Hypoxic-ischemic encephalopathy (HIE)
c. Intraventricular hemorrhage
d. Periventricular leukomalacia

5. Chiari malformation type II often involves the displacement of which of the following through the foramen magnum?

a. Medulla, fourth ventricle, and cerebellar vermis
b. Only cerebellar tonsils
c. Cerebellum without displacement
d. None of the above

Answer Key

1. c 2. c 3. c 4. b 5. a

SUGGESTED READING

1. Aldinger KA, Lehmann OJ, Hudgins L, et al. FOXC1 is required for normal cerebellar development and is a major contributor to chromosome 6p25.3 Dandy-Walker malformation. Nat Genet. 2009;41(9): 1037-42.
2. Kimura-Hayama ET, Higuera JA, Corona-Cedillo R et al. Neurocysticercosis: radiologic-pathologic correlation. Radiographics. 2010;30(6):1705-19. doi:10.1148/rg.306105522 - Pubmed citation
3. Martinez-Biarge M, Diez-Sebastian J, Kapellou O, et al. Predicting motor outcome and death in term hypoxic-ischemic encephalopathy. Neurology. 2011;76(24):2055-61.
4. Shofty B, Ben-Sira L, Constantini S. Neurofibromatosis 1-associated optic pathway gliomas. Childs Nerv Syst. 2020;36:2351-61. doi: 10.1007/s00381-020-04697-1. [PubMed] [CrossRef] [Google Scholar]
5. Verma R. MRI features of Japanese encephalitis. BMJ Case Rep. 2012;2012:bcr0320126088. [PMC free article] [PubMed] [Google Scholar]

CHAPTER

22

Pediatric Musculoskeletal Imaging

"From first steps to growing pains, pediatric musculoskeletal imaging captures the story of movement, resilience, and repair."

INTRODUCTION

Pediatric musculoskeletal imaging is a specialized branch of radiology focused on diagnosing and managing disorders of the bones, joints, and soft tissues in infants and children. This field addresses the unique challenges and considerations associated with the developing musculoskeletal system of children, which is significantly different from adults due to the presence of growth plates, evolving biomechanics, and varying degrees of ossification. Proper imaging is very crucial not only for accurate diagnosis but also for guiding treatment decisions and monitoring therapeutic outcomes in the pediatric population. There are so many challenges in pediatric imaging that include minimizing radiation exposure, managing patient movement during procedures (often requiring sedation or anesthesia in younger children), and interpreting images in the context of a maturing skeletal system. The primary aim of this chapter is to provide detailed, noninvasive insights into a wide array of congenital, developmental, traumatic, infectious, and neoplastic conditions. Various imaging modalities used in pediatric musculoskeletal system are as follows **(Table 22.1)**.

Table 22.1: Imaging modalities for pediatric musculoskeletal system.

Imaging modality	*Utilities*
Radiographs (X-rays)	Initial evaluation of bone fractures, alignments, and skeletal maturity. Useful for assessing chronic conditions and monitoring progression. Standard modality for most acute injuries
Ultrasound	Ideal for assessing soft tissue structures, such as muscles, tendons, and ligaments. Used for dynamic assessments (e.g., hip movements in developmental dysplasia of the hip). Useful for guiding joint aspiration or injections
Magnetic resonance imaging (MRI)	Provides detailed images of bone marrow, soft tissues, and cartilage. Essential for evaluating complex joint diseases and bone tumors. Preferred for spinal imaging and assessing inflammatory conditions without radiation exposure
Computed tomography (CT)	High-detail imaging of complex bone structures and fractures. Used in surgical planning and when MRI is contraindicated. Superior for evaluating fine bone details and subtle fractures not visible on X-rays
Nuclear medicine	Bone scintigraphy for identifying areas of increased bone activity, suggesting infection or tumor. Used when multifocal bone involvement is suspected, such as in multifocal osteomyelitis or metastatic disease

COMMON PATHOLOGIES

Congenital Variants

Klippel–Feil Syndrome

It is called as congenital brevicollis/cervical assimilation:

- Congenital segmentation defects of the cervical spine
- Reserved for congenital fusions involving more than one motion segment (more than two vertebrae).
- **Classic triad (present in ~50% of cases):** Short webbed neck, low posterior hairline, reduced cervical motion.
- **Most consistent finding:** Limitation of neck motion
- Appearance of no neck with head continuous with shoulders
- Torticollis common, scoliosis present in ~80% of cases
- **Plain film** is first step in investigation
- MRI shows multiple block vertebrae with hypoplastic vertebrae and anterior concavity (wasp-waist sign), small intervertebral disc spaces with potential calcification of the nucleus pulposus.
- Complete assessment of spine and thorax to identify other osseous anomalies, such as hemivertebrae, variable posterior element anomalies (fusion, spina bifida, etc.).

Craniosynostosis

Craniosynostosis is the premature fusion of one or more skull sutures, occurring in about 1 in 2,000 live births. It can be primary (nonsyndromic) or secondary, the latter associated with conditions, such as rickets or thyroid disorders. In craniosynostosis, affected sutures show a straight rather than serrated line, with potential osseous fusion or sclerosis. MRI and CT scans help assess-associated facial and central nervous system abnormalities. Three-dimensional CT imaging can show suture patency and fusion extent. The most common pattern is sagittal suture closure, followed by coronal and lambdoid closures, each resulting in distinct skull deformities. Coronal synostosis leads to a shortened skull, while lambdoid closure flattens one side of the occiput, and metopic closure results in a triangular forehead.

Skeletal Dysplasias

Skeletal dysplasias are a complex and varied group of disorders resulting from faulty development, often caused by specific genetic mutations. Advances in genetic and laboratory studies are improving our understanding, though significant variation remains within these conditions. Most are congenital, but some develop in adolescence or early adulthood. Accurate diagnosis is crucial to rule out serious conditions, such as malignancy or toxicity and to identify and prevent severe complications, such as life-threatening aneurysms in Marfan's syndrome and paralysis from congenital spinal stenosis in achondroplasia.

Achondroplasia

Achondroplasia is an autosomal dominant disorder affecting the growth and maturation of chondroblasts in the epiphyseal regions. It is the most common form of congenital dwarfism.

- Narrowing of the spinal canal is the hallmark of achondroplasia.
- Symmetric shortening of all long bones, with the proximal portions most affected.
- Fingers are all the same length, with separation of the middle and ring fingers (**trident hand**).
- Entire pelvis is small with characteristic **champagne glass appearance (Figs. 22.1A to E)**.

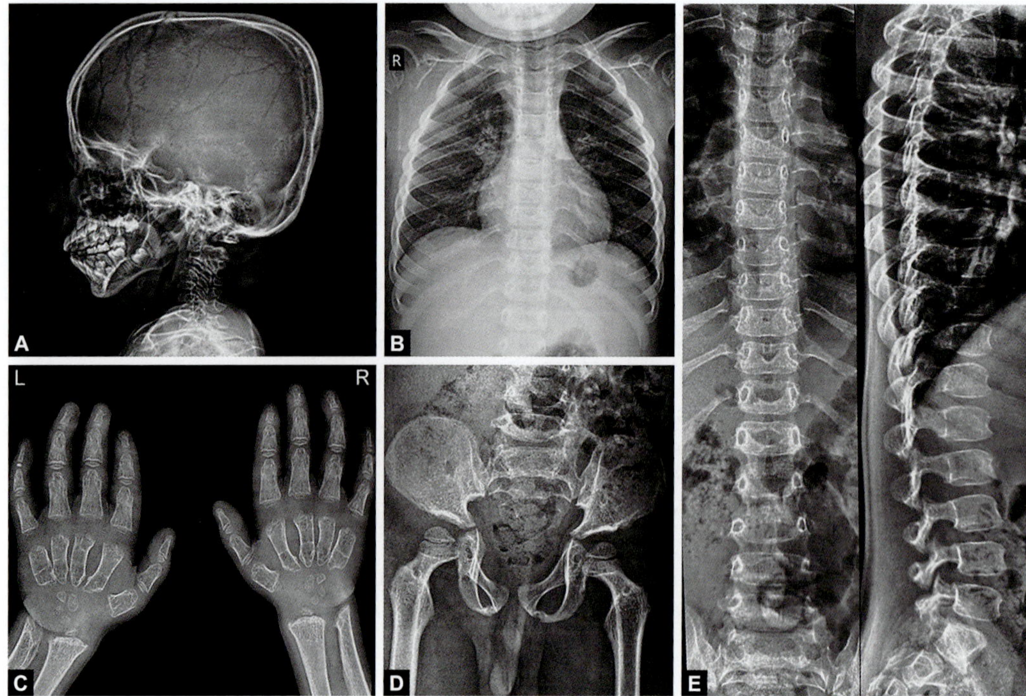

Figs. 22.1A to E: Achondroplasia: (A) The characteristic Wormian bones seen in achondroplasia are not seen in the skull X-ray; (B) Chest X-ray appears unremarkable. Expected findings: Widening of the ribs and anteroposterior narrowing of the ribs; (C) X-ray both hands: Shortening of the metacarpals and the phalanges; (D) X-ray pelvis with both hips: There is flattening of the iliac wings (Mickey Mouse ear appearance). The acetabular roof on the left appears horizontal. Champagne glass configuration of the pelvis is also seen; (E) X-ray whole spine AP/Lateral views: Mild anterior beaking of the vertebral bodies is seen. A differential diagnosis of MPS can be considered.

Marfan's Syndrome

Marfan's syndrome, an autosomal dominant condition, involves elongated tubular bones, ocular issues, and aortic aneurysms.

- **Classic feature of Marfan's syndrome:** Elongation of extremities without increased width.
- Hands and feet exhibit long, slender, gracile tubular bones, termed arachnodactyly or spider-like fingers.

Mucopolysaccharidoses

Mucopolysaccharidosis (MPS) is a group of inheritable lysosomal storage diseases where the buildup of undegraded glycosaminoglycans (GAGs) causes tissue damage. Common symptoms include organomegaly, dysostosis multiplex, mental retardation, and developmental delay. Diagnosis is typically confirmed through enzymatic assays of the defective enzyme in cultured fibroblasts or leukocytes.

- **MPS-I (MPS-I-H):** Hurler's syndrome
- **MPS-II:** Hunter's syndrome
- **MPS-III (subtypes A, B, C, and D):** Sanfilippo's syndrome
- **MPS-IV:** (subtypes A and B) Morquio's syndrome

- **MPS-VI:** Maroteaux-Lamy syndrome
- **MPS-VII:** Sly's syndrome

Osteogenesis Imperfecta

- Generalized inheritable disorder of connective tissue with widespread abnormalities.
- Occurs in about 1/20,000 births.
- Caused by quantitative and qualitative defects in collagen I synthesis.
- Autosomal dominant transmission.

Clinical Features

- **Four major diagnostic criteria:** Osteoporosis with abnormal skeletal fragility, blue sclera, abnormal dentition (dentin genesis imperfecta), and premature otosclerosis.
- Diagnosis confirmed if two criteria are present.
- Severe congenital form characterized by osseous fractures and deformities observable in utero; can lead to death due to intracranial hemorrhage **(Fig. 22.2)**.
- Blue sclerae found in >90% of individuals.
- Important to distinguish from child abuse; DEXA and CT bone density measurements useful in diagnosis.
- Severely affected individuals often have dwarfism due to abnormal growth patterns and severe fractures.

Radiologic Features

- **Cardinal features:** Diffuse decrease in bone density, **pencil-thin cortices**, and multiple fractures.
- **Common radiographic findings:** Transverse fractures, tumoral callus, **Wormian bones**, enlarged sinuses, lucent and thin calvaria, platybasia, basilar impression, kyphoscoliosis, anteriorly wedged or biconcave vertebral bodies, protrusio acetabuli, and shepherd's crook deformity of the proximal femur.
- Differentiating child abuse from osteogenesis imperfecta can generally be accomplished through clinical findings and collagen analysis in challenging cases.

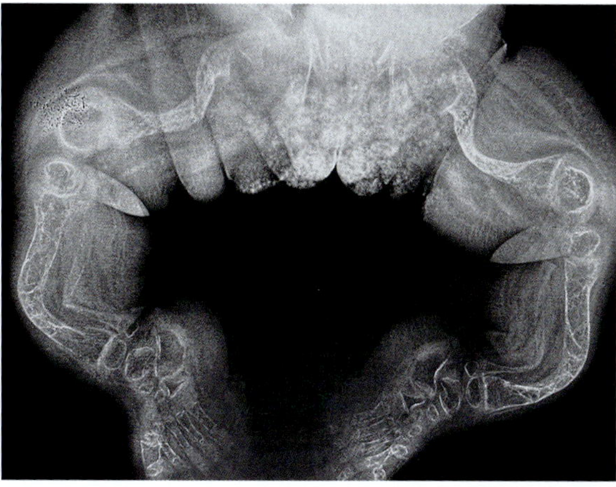

Fig. 22.2: Osteogenesis imperfecta: X-ray both lower limbs AP view: The bone density is reduced with markedly deformed long bones, bowing. Multiple linear densities are seen within the tibia and femur, indicative of multiple fractures. Joint spaces appear normal.

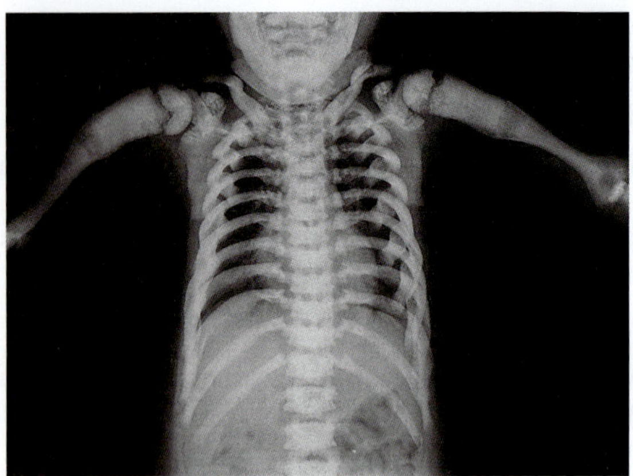

Fig. 22.3: Osteopetrorickets: X-ray chest and upper abdomen showing increased bone density of the humerus, ribs and clavicles. There is widening of the humeral epiphysis seen with fraying. Linear hypoechoic bands are seen in the diaphysis of humerus bilaterally. This needs to be differentiated from osteopetrosis. Osteopetrosis will not show hypoechoic areas within the bone. There will be no fraying of epiphysis in osteopetrosis.

Osteopetrosis

Albers-Schönberg disease, osteosclerosis, osteopetrosis generalisata, osteosclerosis generalisata, **marble bones, chalk bones**.

- Osteopetrosis is a rare hereditary and familial bone abnormality characterized by a lack of resorption of normal primitive osteochondrous tissue.
- Persistence of this tissue inhibits the formation of normal mature adult bone with a medullary canal containing marrow tissue.
- MRI aids in evaluating marrow involvement.
- Failure of remodeling produces flared metaphyses (**Erlenmeyer flask deformity**).
- Bone is radiopaque and hard but brittle, prone to pathologic fractures **(Fig. 22.3)**.
- Diagnosis primarily radiographic, supported by CT.
- Generalized sclerosis of the skeleton with homogeneous increased density, little trabeculation, and no differentiation between cortical and medullary regions.
- **Bone within a bone appearance** (endobones) due to fetal vestiges.
- Long bones have flared and elongated metaphyses; shafts may be widened.
- Spine may show uniformly dense vertebrae or dense bands adjacent to endplates with normal midbody (**sandwich vertebra**).
- **Skull changes:** Calvarial and basilar thickening, sclerosis, poor sinus development, macrocephaly, hydrocephalus, prognathism.

Fracture

Torus Fracture

- Also known as buckling fracture. These are incomplete fractures of long bones caused due to axial loading forces along the long axis of the bones.
- It is characterized by bulging of the cortex without a visible break in the bone cortex.
- The most common joint involved is the distal radial epiphysis.

Greenstick Fracture

Greenstick fractures are incomplete fractures caused due to forces applied to the bone such that there is a bend in the bone on one side and visible break in the cortex on the other side.

Bowing Fracture

Bowing fractures, typically found in pediatric patients, involve incomplete fractures of tubular long bones, particularly the radius and ulna. These fractures often necessitate no intervention as they heal naturally through remodeling. The radius and ulna are frequently affected, with the fibula being another commonly involved bone. When a longitudinal force with an angle is exerted on a bone, it causes bending. Bowing of the bone can be observed on plain radiographs, especially when the view is perpendicular to the direction of bowing. These fractures typically lack a visible fracture line or cortical injury.

Radial Head Subluxation

In the majority of cases involving isolated traumatic radial head dislocation, the dislocation occurs anteriorly. This is most evident in lateral projection, where the radiocapitellar line, drawn along the radial neck, should intersect with the capitellum. Disruption of this alignment indicates radial head dislocation. If the ulna remains intact, it may appear bowed.

Malignancy

Osteogenic sarcoma and Ewing sarcoma represent the primary types of bone tumors prevalent among children and adolescents. These tumors typically manifest more frequently during the second decade of life and exhibit a higher incidence among males.

Osteosarcoma

Conventional radiography remains crucial in diagnosis.

Osteosarcomas are malignant tumors that form in bone tissue, ranking as the second most prevalent primary bone tumor following multiple myeloma, comprising approximately 20% of all primary bone tumors. Among children, they are the most frequently encountered primary bone tumor. These tumors can be categorized into primary and secondary forms, along with various histologic types, with conventional osteosarcoma being the most prevalent.

Radiologic Features

- Medullary and cortical bone destruction **(Fig. 22.4)**
- Aggressive periosteal reaction
- Sunburst pattern
- Codman triangle
- Lamellated (onion skin) reaction, albeit less common
- Presence of soft-tissue mass
- Ossification/calcification of tumor matrix
- Variable appearance, reflecting tumor bone production, calcified matrix, and osteoid.
- Ill-defined "fluffy" or "cloud-like" compared to chondroid lesions.
- Potential for ossified lung and nodal metastases.
- Occasional occurrence of spontaneous pneumothorax in patients with lung metastases.

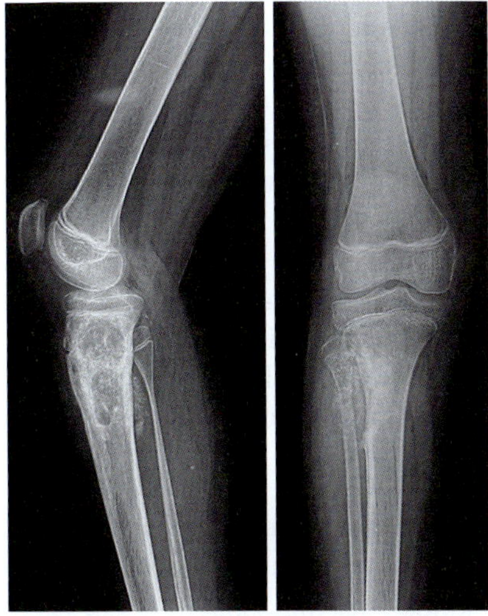

Fig. 22.4: Conventional osteosarcoma: X-ray right knee AP/Lateral views showing two well-defined expansile lytic lesions in the meta-diaphysis of the tibia with surrounding sclerosis. An associated sunburst type of periosteal reaction is seen.

Ewings

Following osteosarcoma, Ewing sarcomas stand as the second most prevalent malignant primary bone tumors in childhood. Typically originating from the medullary cavity and infiltrating the Haversian system, Ewing sarcomas often manifest as **moth-eaten**, penetrative lucent lesions in the diaphyses of long bone of proximal extremities, accompanied by a considerable soft tissue presence and characteristic **onion skin periostitis** (mimicks osteomyelitis).

Childhood Leukemia

- Acute leukemia is the most common malignant childhood disease.
- Together with lymphomas, these account for approximately 40% of malignant childhood diseases.
- Peak incidence is between 2 and 5 years of age.
- The most common form is acute lymphocytic leukemia, usually fatal within 1 year.
- **Diagnosis:** Definitive by bone marrow evaluation; peripheral blood smear may reveal abnormal white blood cell counts and immature cell forms.
- Radiographic osseous changes occur in 50–70% of children with leukemia.
- Conspicuous radiologic features are best visualized in the long bones.

Metabolic Deficiencies

Scurvy

Scurvy, a result of vitamin C deficiency, may manifest radiographically as a scorbutic zone characterized by a radiolucent band beneath the zone of provisional calcification. Subperiosteal hemorrhage, common in scurvy, can cause lifting of the periosteum from the bone, potentially leading to calcification during healing.

Several radiographic signs are indicative of specific bone conditions:

- **Dense zone of provisional calcification (white line of Frenkel):** This sign denotes enhanced density in the metaphyseal zone of calcified cartilage, resulting from delayed conversion to bone.
- **Ring epiphysis (Wimberger's sign):** Characterized by a dense peripheral margin surrounding a more radiolucent central portion in the epiphysis.
- **Pelkan spur:** Bony protrusions at metaphyseal margins extending perpendicular to the shaft axis.
- **Scorbutic zone (Trummer field zone):** A radiolucent band beneath the zone of provisional calcification, indicating disordered osteoid formation.
- **Subperiosteal hemorrhage:** Blood extravasation lifting the periosteum from the bone, often leading to calcification, particularly during the healing process.

Rickets

The most common and nonspecific radiologic finding in patients of rickets is osteopenia. Characteristic changes occur at the open growth plates.

Changes are best seen in those areas showing most active growth.

- Early radiological changes focus on the lower ends of the radius and ulna.
- Anteroposterior views of wrists and knees are key for rickets screening.
- Signs include delayed epiphyseal appearance and widened epiphyseal plates due to excessive uncalcified osteoid accumulation.
- Cupping of the metaphysis occurs as the smooth line of sclerosis disappears, forming an irregular metaphyseal end.

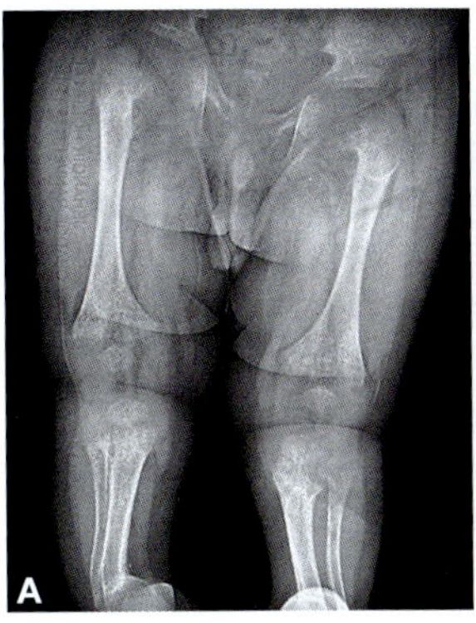
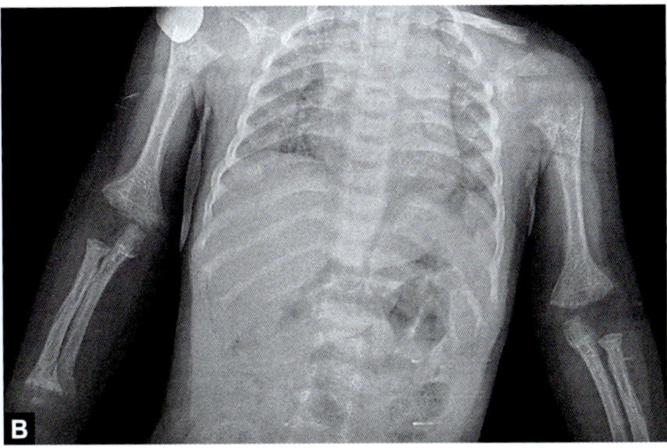

Figs. 22.5A and B: (A) Radiograph of both knees including thighs and proximal legs showing reduced bone density with widening of the femoral, tibial and fibular metaphysis. There is irregularity of the metaphyseal ends, suggestive of fraying (Rickets); (B) X-ray chest with upper limbs also show reduced bone density with metaphyseal widening and fraying of the visualized long bones. Widening of the anterior ends of ribs are widened suggestive of rachitic rosary.

- Splaying of the metaphysis results from pressure by cartilage cells at the growth plate **(Figs. 22.5A and B)**.
- Common bone deformities include knock knees, bowlegs, and coxa vara in older children with rickets.
- **Rachitic rosary:** Widened anterior ends of ribs due to hypertrophy of costochondral junction.
- **Triradiate pelvis:** Protrusion of hip and spine into soft pelvis with protrusio acetabuli.

Hyperparathyroidism

Hyperparathyroidism is marked by excessive production of parathyroid hormone, leading to elevated calcium levels and extensive bone remodeling. Clinical manifestations include hypercalcemia resulting from increased intestinal absorption, bone turnover, and tubular resorption of calcium. Skeletal changes characteristic of hyperparathyroidism include increased resorption of cortical and cancellous bone with substitutive fibrosis, reflecting histological alterations.

- X-ray examination includes lateral skull view, dorsolumbar spine (AP/lateral), hands (AP), pelvis (AP), and region with symptoms.
- Radiographic signs may include irregular diffuse bone rarefaction and a **salt pepper appearance in the skull**, with small pin-sized opaque areas.
- Loss of lamina dura, the thin cortical bone surrounding teeth, is evident in hyperparathyroidism.
- Subperiosteal resorption of phalanges, especially at the lateral clavicle end, is diagnostic for generalized hyperparathyroidism.
- Spine may exhibit central collapse of vertebral bodies and biconvex discs.
- Brown's tumor, resembling an expansile lytic lesion, typically affects the maxilla/mandible.
- Extraosseous features like renal calculi may also be present on radiographs.

Subperiosteal bone resorption, a characteristic feature of hyperparathyroidism, typically affects the radial aspects of the proximal and middle phalanges of the 2nd and 3rd fingers, as well as the medial aspect of the tibia, femur, and humerus. Intracortical resorption manifests as cigar or tunnel-shaped radiolucencies in the cortex, while terminal tuft erosion (**acro-osteolysis**) and a **rugger jersey** spine are also common findings.

Fluorosis

Fluorosis is caused by excessive fluoride intake, often from drinking water with high fluoride levels, particularly prevalent in regions, such as India and parts of Southeast Asia. It leads to excessive calcium deposition in bones and soft tissues, posing a significant public health concern in states, such as Punjab, Andhra Pradesh, and Tamil Nadu.

X-rays of spine, pelvis, and forearms are crucial in suspected fluorosis cases. Radiographic features include:

- **Spine:** Increased density, calcification of posterior longitudinal ligament.
- **Pelvis:** Increased density, calcification of ischiopubic and sacroiliac ligaments.
- **Forearms and legs:** Interosseous membrane calcification.

Perthes (Fig. 22.6)

This condition, known as **osteochondritis (misnomer as cartilage is not affected)** of the femoral head epiphysis, before closure of epiphyseal plate results in partial or complete avascular necrosis and deformity of the femoral head.

Its precise cause is uncertain but is thought to involve recurrent ischemic episodes, possibly triggered by synovitis. Pathologically, it progresses through three stages—synovitis, trabecular necrosis, and healing.

Commonly affecting boys aged 3–12 years due to solitary epiphyseal vessel supply.

Presents with hip pain, often radiating to the knee, accompanied by limping or stiffness, reduced mobility, muscle atrophy; Trendelenburg test positive. Later in life, affected adults may develop secondary degenerative joint disease.

Examination may reveal limited abduction, internal rotation, and shortening. Radiologically, there is epiphyseal collapse and sclerosis with increased hip joint space, often contrasting the minimal symptoms with pronounced X-ray changes. Catterall (1972) categorized it into four groups based on head involvement and described adverse prognostic indicators.

- **Early phase:** Isotopic scans are cold before plain film changes; MRI is excellent for early detection and assess stage of disease.
- Treatment for lateral displacement often involves correctional osteotomy (femoral, iliac) to promote remodeling of cartilage and femoral head.

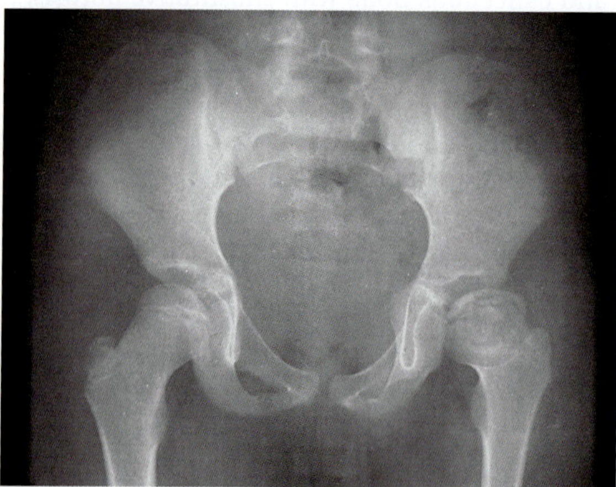

Fig. 22.6: Perthes disease: X-ray PBH showing widening, collapse and flattening of the left femoral epiphysis. The femoral neck shows foreshortening and is widened.

Juvenile Idiopathic Arthritis (JIA)

- Also known as **juvenile rheumatoid arthritis**, is the most common chronic arthritic disease of childhood and corresponds to a group of different subtypes.
- X-ray findings may reveal soft tissue swelling, osteopenia, joint space loss, erosions, growth disturbances, such as epiphyseal overgrowth or "ballooning," and joint subluxation.
- Cervical spine radiographs may show atlantoaxial subluxation, odontoid erosions.
- Regarding the knee, a widened intercondylar notch is a sign associated with juvenile idiopathic arthritis, as well as hemophilic arthropathy and tuberculous arthropathy.

Ankylosing Spondylitis

- Chronic inflammatory disorder affecting articulations, ligaments, and tendons of the spine and pelvis, often leading to complete polyarticular ankylosis.
- Also known as Marie-Strumpell disease, rhizomelic spondylitis, pelvic-spondylitis ossificans.
- Onset typically between ages 15 and 35; predominantly affects males (10:1 ratio).
- Starts at the sacroiliac joints bilaterally, then progressively ascends the spine with skip involvement, especially in the thoracolumbar spine, costal articulations, and cervical spine.
- Symptoms include pain, tenderness, increasing stiffness, and a positive Trendelenburg test.
- **Laboratory findings:** Elevated ESR, mild anemia, positive HLA-B27 and negative rheumatoid arthritis latex (seronegative).
- **Major signs:** Osteoporosis, erosions with surrounding sclerosis, bony ankylosis, and enthesopathy.
- **Sacroiliac joint stages:** Pseudo-widening (stage 1), erosions and sclerosis (stage 2), ankylosis (stage 3).
- **Spine:** Discovertebral junction changes lead to syndesmophyte formation, with initial osteitis causing erosions and anterior squaring, resulting in a **bamboo spine appearance** when multiple segments are involved.

Developmental Dysplasia of the Hip (DDH)

- Describes a spectrum of conditions from irreducible dislocation of the hip at birth to neonatal hip instability. Previously described as congenital hip dislocation and congenital hip dysplasia.

  In children under 1 year, diagnosing a dislocated hip via plain X-rays is challenging due to the non-ossified femoral head epiphysis. Ultrasound examination is valuable for early detection at birth.
- **Known risk factors:** Breech fetal presentation (hip flexion associated with breech presentation can induce DDH by causing psoas shortening and femoral head decentring), oligohydramnios, and firstborn status.
- **Associated abnormalities:** Neuromuscular disorders, congenital torticollis, and skull and foot deformities.
- Increased awareness for early postnatal diagnosis to reverse hip instability and reduce secondary osteoarthritis.
- **Physical examination:** Palpable hip "click" with Ortolani's and Barlow's tests.
- **Effective treatment:** Flexion-abduction bracing techniques (e.g., Pavlik harness).
- Spontaneous improvement after two months is unusual (acetabular growth is dynamic during the first two postnatal months) but influenced by treatment.

- Spica casting may be used if Pavlik harness fails to maintain reduction after four months.
- Best assessed with ultrasound within the first year.
- Plain films show bony changes but not cartilaginous abnormalities in the first 2–3 months.
- Subtle signs on plain films can be evident at six weeks.
- Most useful plain films: from 2 to 8 months.
- **Classic findings:** Absent or small proximal femoral capital epiphysis, lateral displacement of the femur, and shallow acetabulum with increased inclination of the acetabular roof (>30°).
- Disruption of Shenton's line or iliofemoral line indicates superior and lateral subluxation of the femur.
- **Adolescents and adults:** Long-standing dislocation manifests as shallow acetabulum and large, flattened femoral head with superior and lateral displacement.
- **Ultrasound:** Visualizes bony and cartilaginous acetabular margins, cartilaginous femoral head, femoral head coverage by the acetabulum, and hip stability.
- **Critical measurement:** Cartilaginous (β) angle on USG.
- Dynamic hip ultrasound assesses movement, subluxation, and dislocation.
- **Sonographic reassessment:** Every 4–6 weeks for 2–3 months to monitor therapeutic response.
- **CT arthrography:** Used with severe dysplasia when applying a hip spica.
- **Three-dimensional CT:** Useful for subtle adult dysplasia and presurgical planning.
- **MRI:** Increasingly used in adult DDH to assess avascular necrosis and for presurgical planning.

CTEV

The term "clubfoot" encompasses various foot shape abnormalities, but it is commonly associated with the most prevalent congenital deformity, known as Congenital Talipes Equinovarus (CTEV). It affects approximately one in every 1,000 live births.

Assessment requires weight-bearing dorsoplantar and lateral radiographs.

Non-accidental Trauma/Battered Baby Syndrome/Shaken Infant Syndrome

Battered child syndrome, shaken infant syndrome, stress-related infant abuse, and non-accidental trauma are all terms used to describe the constellation of non-accidental injuries observed in infants and young children due to abuse. Shaken infant syndrome is often considered the most apt term to delineate the classic injury pattern. It involves forcefully shaking the child around the chest, causing the extremities and head to flail back and forth in a whiplash motion. This motion leads to intracranial injuries due to severe angular acceleration, deceleration, and direct impact against solid surfaces. Additionally, compression of the chest results in rib fractures, while the whiplash motion of the arms and legs can cause characteristic 'corner' or 'bucket-handle' fractures in the metaphyseal region. Multiple fractures at varying stages of healing; fresh fractures next to callused, deformed bones.

Brodie's Abscess

- Brodie's abscess was first described by Brodie in 1832.
- It is defined as a localized, aborted form of suppurative osteomyelitis.
- Most common in male children.
- *Staphylococcus aureus* is the most common bacterial agent isolated.
- X-ray depicted as an oval, elliptical, or serpiginous radiolucency with a halo or doughnut rim of heavy reactive sclerosis.

LAST MINUTE REVISION

- Pediatric musculoskeletal imaging requires tailored approaches due to growth plates and developing biomechanics.
- **X-rays is the modality used for** Initial evaluation of bone fractures, alignment, skeletal maturity and in almost all pathology.
- Most of the pathology needs either combination of at least two modalities or one modality with strong clinical features for early diagnosis and management.

REVIEW QUESTIONS

Multiple Choice Questions (MCQs)

1. **A 16-year-old child presents with a short neck, low posterior hairline, and limited neck motion. Radiographs show congenital fusion of multiple cervical vertebrae. What is the most likely diagnosis?**
   a. Achondroplasia
   b. Klippel-feil syndrome
   c. Osteogenesis imperfecta
   d. Craniosynostosis
2. **A 3-year-old child presents with bow legs and delayed walking. Radiographs of the wrists and knees show widened epiphyseal plates and cupping of the metaphysis. What is the most likely diagnosis?**
   a. Osteogenesis imperfecta
   b. Scurvy
   c. Rickets
   d. Marfan syndrome
3. **A 7-year-old boy presents with a history of multiple fractures, blue sclerae, and abnormal dentition. Radiographs reveal diffuse osteopenia and thin cortices. What is the most likely diagnosis?**
   a. Achondroplasia
   b. Osteogenesis imperfecta
   c. Marfan syndrome
   d. Ewing sarcoma
4. **A 14-year-old boy presents with chronic hip pain and limited range of motion. Radiographs show a collapsed and sclerotic femoral head. What is the most likely diagnosis?**
   a. Osteosarcoma
   b. Developmental dysplasia of the hip
   c. Perthes disease
   d. Juvenile idiopathic arthritis
5. **A 10-year-old boy presents with a hard, painful mass on the femur. Radiographs show a sunburst pattern and Codman triangle. What is the most likely diagnosis?**
   a. Ewing sarcoma
   b. Osteosarcoma
   c. Osteomyelitis
   d. Achondroplasia
6. **A 5-year-old girl presents with a limp and pain in her knee. Physical examination shows a positive Trendelenburg test. Radiographs reveal lateral displacement of the femur and a shallow acetabulum. What is the most likely diagnosis?**
   a. Osteogenesis imperfecta
   b. Perthes disease
   c. Developmental dysplasia of the hip
   d. Juvenile idiopathic arthritis

Answer Key

1. b 2. c 3. b 4. c 5. b 6. c

SUGGESTED READING

1. Emilio J Clemente, Maria PAG, Jordi CM, Ricardo R. "Ankle and Foot Deformities in Children", Seminars in Musculoskeletal Radiology; 2023.
2. Michael JP. "Rickets and Osteomalacia Are Still Around", Radiologic Clinics of North America; 1991.
3. Pediatric Orthopedic Deformities Volume 1;2016.
4. Richard JM, Thomas DB. "Pediatric Orthopedics", Springer Nature; 1994.
5. Sadashiva GH. "Radiology of Handmirror of Various Systemic Diseases." J Evol Med Dent Sci. 2016.

CHAPTER 23

Cardiovascular Imaging in Pediatric

"In the smallest chambers and narrowest vessels, radiologists find answers that save young hearts."

INTRODUCTION

Imaging plays a crucial role in evaluation of cardiovascular diseases, including congenital heart diseases (CHD) in pediatric population. Congenital heart disease is the most common congenital defect in the live-born children with an estimated incidence of almost one per 100 babies. The spectrum of anomalies ranges from simple isolated defects to complex structural abnormalities. Accurate evaluation by imaging is essential for detailed anatomical delineation and functional assessment for proper management planning. Apart from the congenital heart diseases, other pediatric cardiovascular diseases include acquired myocardial and pericardial diseases, cardiac tumors and vasculitis affecting larger vessels. The primary goal of this chapter is to review the role of imaging in pediatric cardiac diseases, with special focus on congenital heart diseases.

MODALITIES

Chest Radiography

Chest radiography is a quick, readily available, inexpensive investigation, and is often the first-line imaging technique performed in cases of symptoms attributed to cardiothoracic system. It can provide the first clue in unsuspected cardiovascular disease. Apart from the detection, it plays an important role in the post-surgical period and follow-up imaging. Inserted tubes and lines can also be assessed especially in critical care settings. Approach to reading a chest radiograph includes a systematic approach as discussed below. Typically, a frontal chest radiograph is obtained. Sequential assessment of the airway, cardiac silhouette, lung fields, pleural cavity (for effusion or pneumothorax), bony cage and lower abdomen is adopted.

The normal chest radiograph of an infant differs from that of an adult in the following points:

- A cardiothoracic ratio (cardiac width/thoracic width) up to 0.6 is considered normal in infants, while for adults it is up to 0.5.
- The thymus can mimic cardiomegaly and can also be mistaken for a lung pathology, hence the following signs are useful for its identification:
  Thymic sail sign: A triangular opacity on the right of the mediastinum at the apex of the right lung.
  Thymic wave sign: There is indentation of the thymus by the ribs, resulting in a wavy border.
  Thymic notch sign: The inferior margin of the thymus merges with the margin of the cardiac silhouette.
  As the child grows, the radiographic appearance approaches to that of an adult patient.

A. Role of Chest Radiography in Congenital Heart Disease

In addition to adoption of the sequential approach for assessment of chest radiography described above, interpretation of the chest radiograph in a case of suspected congenital heart disease focuses on assessment of the following points:

Assessment of the Pulmonary Vasculature

- Normally, the pulmonary vessels in the upper lung zones are smaller than those in the lower lung zones and the pulmonary vessels show gradual tapering towards the periphery of the lungs.
- An increase in the pulmonary vascularity is called plethora and is suggested when the pulmonary vessels are enlarged, tortuous and extend till peripheral third of the lung.
- Pulmonary plethora is usually seen in large left-to-right shunts, such as atrial and ventricular septal defects or patent ductus arteriosus.
- Decreased blood flow through the pulmonary circulation is called oligemia, where the lungs appear hyperlucent with reduced vascular markings.
- Pulmonary oligemia usually results from right ventricular outflow obstruction and is seen commonly in tetralogy of Fallot (TOF), tricuspid atresia and Ebstein's anomaly.

Assessment of the Cardiac Silhouette

- **Cardiac size:**
  - Cardiomegaly in pediatric patients is a cardiothoracic ratio of more than 0.6.
  - In infants and younger children, a lateral view may be obtained for assessment of the heart size, as it may be obscured by the thymus.
- **Cardiac shape:** The shape of the heart can provide important clues to the underlying disease. The common signs described for variable cardiac shape include:
  - *Shmoo sign:* This refers to the appearance of a prominent, rounded left ventricle and dilated aorta giving the appearance of Shmoo, a fictional cartoon character in the comic strip Li'l Abner, and is indicative of left ventricular enlargement.
  - *Water bottle sign:* It is described as a markedly enlarged cardiac silhouette with sagging appearance of its margins on both sides mimicking an old-fashioned water bottle, and is seen in a case of very large pericardial effusion.
  - Straightening of the left heart border is seen in rheumatic heart disease and mitral stenosis.
- **Position of the heart:**
  - Cardiac malposition—normally, the apex of the heart is directed towards the left, known as levocardia. If the apex of the heart is directed towards the right, it is called as dextrocardia. When the heart lies in the midline without a well-defined apex, it is known as mesocardia.
  - It is important to look at the gastric bubble as well as the shadows of the liver and spleen to determine the situs.
  - Normal positioning of the organs is known as visceral situs solitus. **In situs inversus totalis,** there is inversion of the chest and abdominal organs. The patient has a mirror-image dextrocardia with the gastric bubble and spleen lying on the right side and the liver on the left side.

Classical Signs on Chest X-ray in Various Common Congenital Heart Diseases (Figs. 23.1A to F)

- **Transposition of great arteries (TGA)**—*'egg-on-a-string' appearance*: There is narrowing of the superior mediastinum, enlargement of the cardiac silhouette, abnormal convexity of the right atrial border, and increased vascular flow.

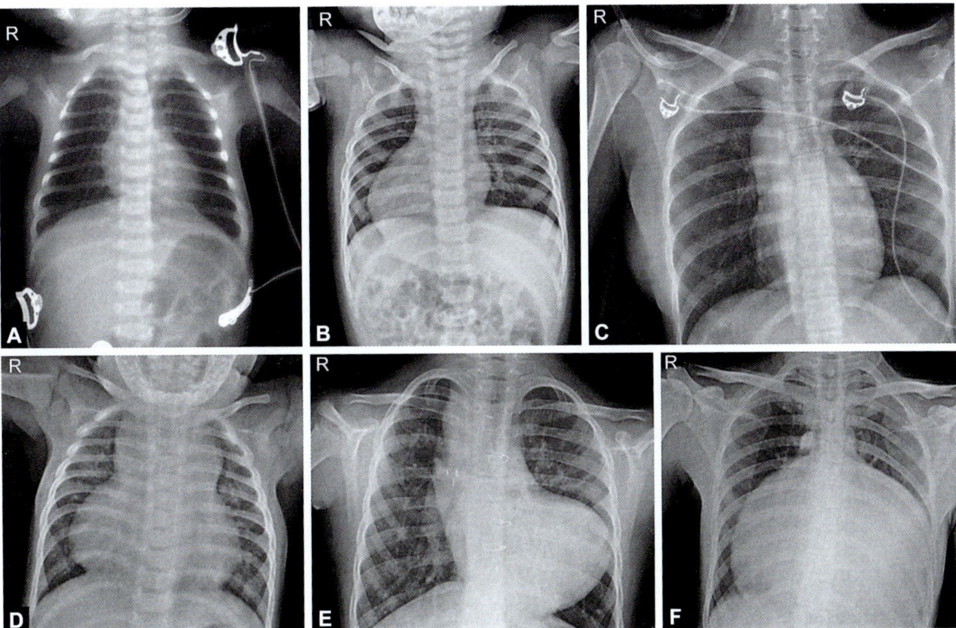

Figs. 23.1A to F: (A) Normal frontal chest radiograph of a child; (B) The cardiac apex is towards the right side—dextrocardia; (C) Aortic knuckle is on the right side—Right-sided aortic arch; (D) 'Snowman or figure of 8' appearance—TAPVC; (E) 'Boot-shaped heart'—TOF; (F) 'Box-shaped heart'—Ebstein's anomaly.

- **Total anomalous pulmonary venous return (TAPVR)**—*'snowman' or 'cottage loaf' appearance or 'figure of 8' sign*: The head of the snowman is formed by the dilated vertical vein on the left, brachiocephalic vein on the top and SVC on right. The body of the snowman is formed by the enlarged right atrium.
- **Partial anomalous pulmonary venous return (PAPVR)**—*'scimitar Sign'*: A prominent curvilinear opacity that extends downward from the right hilum.
- **Tetralogy of Fallot (TOF)**—*'coeur en sabot' appearance or boot-shaped heart*: Upturning of the cardiac apex because of right ventricular hypertrophy.
- **Aortic coarctation**—*figure of three appearance*: The number 3 is formed by dilatation of the left subclavian artery and aorta proximal to the site of coarctation, indentation of the site, and dilatation of the aorta distal to the site. The reverse figure-of-three sign, a mirror image of the number 3, is observed during barium esophagography.
- **Ebstein's anomaly**—*box-shaped heart*: Due to right atrial enlargement. The right atrium may be huge and fill the entire right hemithorax.

B. Chest Radiography in Acquired Cardiac Diseases in Pediatric Population

While the chest radiography plays an important role in evaluation of suspected congenital heart disease, its role in acquired myocardial and pericardial disease remains limited. Pericardial effusion may manifest as money bag appearance, as described above. Dilated pulmonary arteries may be demonstrated in cases of pulmonary arterial hypertension. Valvular calcification may be seen in cases of valvular disease, while pericardial calcification may be seen in cases of constrictive pericarditis. Radiographic appearances in mitral or aortic valve disease is similar to that seen in adults.

Cross-sectional Imaging in Cases of Congenital Heart Disease

A. Echocardiography

It is the first-line imaging modality in evaluation of congenital heart disease. It is easily available, cost effective and radiation free modality. Performed by sector probe of frequency 5 to 8 MHz.

However, it has the following limitations:

- Poor acoustic windows can limit the evaluation, especially in adolescents and those who have undergone prior cardiac surgery.
- Detailed anatomy of the extracardiac vascular structures is better depicted with cross-sectional imaging, such as computed tomography (CT) or magnetic resonance imaging (MRI).
- It is highly operator dependent and subjective modality.

B. Cardiac CT (Figs. 23.2A to F)

Cardiac CT with pulmonary and aortic angiography of thorax is now the work horse for imaging evaluation of congenital heart diseases. The high spatial and temporal resolution with multiplanar and volume rendered post processing techniques allow detailed anatomical depiction of the cardiac anatomy and structural anomalies.

Advantages of CT

- Newer CT machines have rapid examination time, unlike echocardiography and MRI which can take up to 20 minutes and 1–2 hours respectively.

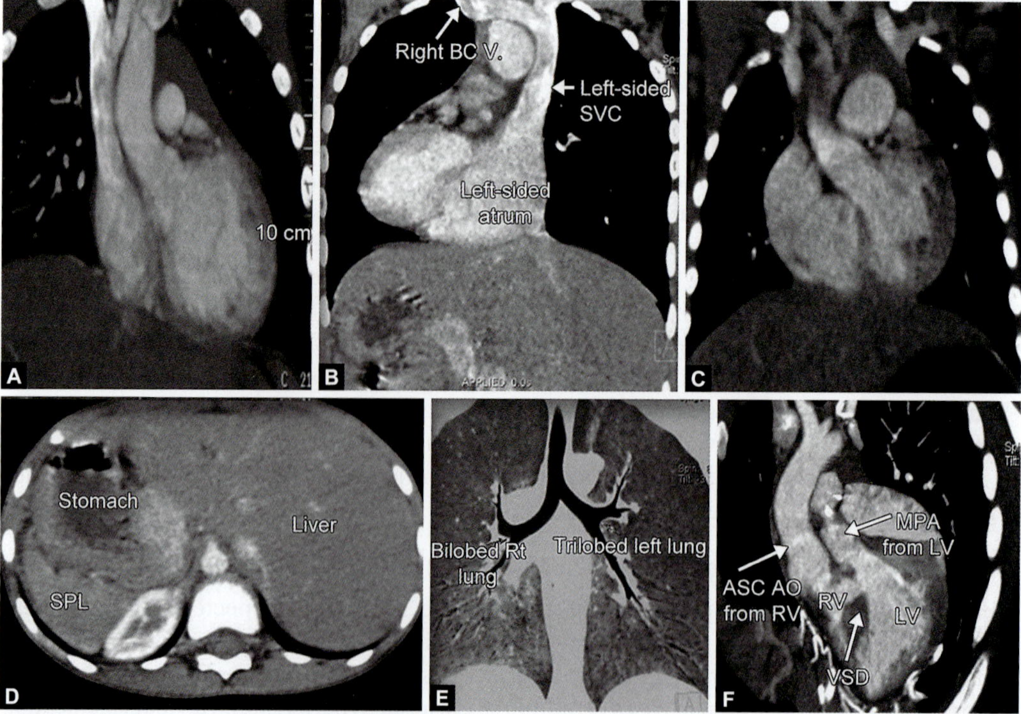

Figs. 23.2A to F: Multidetector computed-tomography angiography images showing the: (A) The normal position of the heart, i.e., levocardia; (B) The cardiac apex is towards the right side, which suggests dextrocardia. Note the left-sided SVC; (C) Mesocardia; (D) Situs inversus; (E) Inversion of the tracheobronchial tree pattern; (F) Transposition of the great arteries. Note the VSD.

- CT is useful in evaluation of extracardiac structures which cannot be visualized on echocardiography, such as distal pulmonary arteries, pulmonary veins, aortic arch and great vessels.
- CT is the best modality for the assessment of the lung fields, airways and bones.
- It is also the modality of choice in patients with metallic stents, conduits, implantable pacemakers and defibrillators, which are contraindications for MRI.
- It is useful for the assessment of suspected vascular rings, suspected coronary artery anomalies and aortopulmonary collaterals.
- CT is also very helpful in the evaluation of post-surgical complications, such as pulmonary embolism, pneumonia, pneumothorax or effusion.
- CT, when compared to MRI, is cheaper and more easily available.
- The data obtained from CT can be reconstructed into multiplanar reformatted (MPR) and 3D reformatted images, which can assist in the accurate measurements of vessel size or diameter.
- 3D printing using CT data for is now being used for preoperative planning of complex CHD.

Disadvantages

- CT exposes the patient to ionizing radiation, which is of concern especially in children.
- Iodinated contrast agents are required, which may be contraindicated in patients with impaired renal function.
- Sedation may be required in those children requiring detailed information about the cardiac or coronary anatomy.

ECG vs non-ECG Gated Scans

ECG gating have reduced artefacts associated with cardiac motion, hence, it is more useful for evaluation of the heart, coronary arteries and great vessels.

Disadvantages of ECG Gating

- Increased radiation dose (up to three times when compared to non-ECG gated scans).
- There is need for good control of the heart rate—if heart rate is more than 100 beats/min then oral propranolol is given (1–2 mg/kg) to control the heart rate.

ALARA stands for "as low as reasonably achievable". ALARA means avoiding any exposure to ionizing radiation, even small doses, that does not have a direct benefit to the patient.

C. Cardiac MRI

Advantages

- MRI provides anatomic and functional assessments, flow measurements and tissue characterization.
- It is the gold-standard investigation for noninvasive cardiac functional assessment, especially in assessment of right ventricular function.
- There is no risk of ionizing radiation exposure.
- It is highly useful in evaluation of cardiac tumors, myocarditis and cardiomyopathies.
- It is also useful for postoperative assessment of the patient.

Disadvantages

- The gantry noise can be loud, which can be frightening for the children.
- MRI requires strict immobilization of the patient, which may be default in younger children.
- MRI is time consuming and requires a long scan time and repeated breath holding.

- Sedation or even general anesthesia with endotracheal intubation may be required.
- The newer generation of vascular stents, coils and implants are no longer a contraindication for MRI. These items are can be either MR Safe, i.e., it does not pose any hazard in all MR environments and MR conditional, i.e., they do not pose any hazard in specific MR environments, e.g., an item may be safe near a 1.5 T magnet but not near a 3 T magnet.
- MR unsafe are those items which are unsafe in all MR environments and include intraocular metal foreign bodies and insulin pumps.

Contrast in MRI

MRI uses gadolinium-based contrast agents (GBCA), which is a rare earth metal chelated to a carrier ligand. The optimal dosage of GBCA in pediatric population is 0.1–0.2 mmol/kg.

Standard sequences used in cardiac MRI:

- **Dark or black blood imaging:** Here, the fast-flowing blood appears dark, hence provide anatomic delineation of blood vessel lumen and cardiac chambers. It is also used to look for myocardial edema. It is a fast sequence, hence minimizes respiratory and cardiac movement artefacts.
- **Bright or white blood imaging:** Here, the blood remains bright and is used for evaluation of vascular flow and cardiac function.
- Late gadolinium enhancement (LGE) is an MRI sequence where the heart is imaged approximately 10 minutes after administration of GBCA. This sequence is used to assess myocardial fibrosis and scar.
- T1 and T2 myocardial mapping are newer techniques being used for noninvasive tissue characterization of the myocardium.
- The main imaging planes used in cardiac MRI are short axis (horizontal 2C), horizontal long axis (4C) and vertical long axis (vertical 2C), which are oblique to one another.
- Both static and CINE images are used.

COMMON CONGENITAL HEART DISEASES

A standardized approach to congenital heart disease is applied which helps in evaluation of various co-existent lesions. Richard Van Praagh from USA and Maria Victoria de la Crux from Mexico first introduced the basic segmental approach to congenital heart diseases based on the topographic arrangements of the atrium, the ventricles, great arteries, and their concordance and discordances. Thus, the morphology of the cardiac components, their connections and relations are analyzed.

The heart is considered to be made of three building blocks, namely the atria, the ventricular mass, and the great arterial trunks, with two junctions between them—the atrioventricular and ventriculoarterial junctions. Each region is partitioned into the left- and right-sided component. The following six points are then studied in assessing the cardiac disease:

1. Determining the visceroatrial situs.
2. Ascertaining atrioventricular junction and the arrangement of AV valves.
3. Determining the orientation of the ventricular loop.
4. Analyzing ventriculoarterial connections.
5. Determining the origin and position of the great vessels.
6. Related intra- and intersegmental abnormalities.

The morphology of each chamber and valve is summarized in **Tables 23.1 and 23.2** respectively below:

Table 23.1: Morphology of heart chamber.

Character	*Right atrium*	*Left atrium*
Appendage	Blunt triangle	Tubular
Appendageal orifice with atrium	Wide	Narrow
Pectinate muscle	Extends up to AV junction	Confined to appendage
Crista terminalis	Present	Absent
Fossa ovalis and limbus	Present	Absent
IVC and coronary sinus	Usually drains into right atrium	—

Table 23.2: Morphology of valve.

Character	*Morphological RV*	*Morphological LV*
Moderator band	Present	Absent
Trabeculations	Coarse and irregular	Thin and fine
Septal surface	Coarse due to attachment of the septal papillary muscle	Smooth
AV valve	Tricuspid	Bicuspid
Septal attachment of AV valve	More apical	More basal
Continuity between AV valve and semilunar valve	Discontinuous by infundibulum	Fibrous, continuity
Septal and parietal band	Present	Smooth superior septal surface

A. Congenital Aortic and Conotruncal Anomalies

Tetralogy of Fallot (TOF)

- TOF is the most common cyanotic congenital heart disease.
- Its components are:
  - Right ventricular outflow tract obstruction (RVOTO).
  - Ventricular septal defect
  - Overriding of the VSD by the aorta
  - Right ventricular hypertrophy
- When TOF is associated with an ASD, it is known as **Pentalogy of Fallot.**
- When the RVOT obstruction is severe, there is a right to left shunting of blood, which results in cyanosis.
- When the RVOT stenosis is mild, cyanosis may not be apparent. This is known as pink tetralogy.
- **Plain radiography of the chest** shows an upturned cardiac apex due to right ventricular hypertrophy which is known as 'wooden shoe or Coeur en Sabot cardiac configuration or boot-shaped left lung field and left CP angle is obscured by heart shadow.'
- The lungs show oligemia due to pulmonary outflow obstruction.

Transposition of Great Arteries (TGA)

- It results from ventriculoarterial discordance, i.e., the aorta arises from the right ventricle and the pulmonary artery arises from the left ventricle.

Table 23.3: Coarctation of aorta.

Preductal	*Postductal*
The narrowing is proximal to the ductus arteriosus	The narrowing is distal to the ductus arteriosus
Presents in infancy	Presents in adulthood
Less common	More common

- It is the second most common cyanotic CHD.
- An isolated TGA is incompatible with life at birth—an additional shunt is mandatory for survival.
- **Plain radiography of the chest** shows an 'egg-on-a-string' appearance due to the narrow pedicle. The full extent of pedicle is best seen on a lateral view.
- Pulmonary plethora is also present.

Truncus Arteriosus (TA)

- TA results from the lack of adequate separation between the aorta and pulmonary trunk, i.e., there is a common vascular trunk with a common valve overriding a VSD.
- After a variable length, the common vascular trunk divides into the aorta and pulmonary arteries.
- The pattern of origin of pulmonary arteries decides the type of TA.
- TA was first classified by Collett and Edwards, which was later modified by Van Praagh.
- On imaging, cardiomegaly and increased pulmonary blood flow is seen. An associated right aortic arch may be seen in 30% of cases.

Coarctation of Aorta

- It is defined as narrowing of the thoracic aorta close to the level of ductus arteriosus insertion.
- It accounts for 4–8% of all CHD and is more common in males with a ratio of 1.5:1.
- It is associated with a bicuspid aortic valve (80% of cases) and VSD (11–18% of cases).
- It is also associated with Turner's syndrome.
- The narrowing of the aorta can be preductal, ductal or postductal **(Table 23.3)**.
- **On chest radiography,** the 'figure of 3 sign may' be seen due to pre- and post-stenotic dilatation of the descending aorta. The proximal bulge represents the dilated aorta and the base of the left subclavian artery, and the distal bulge is consistent with post-stenotic dilation.
- Rib notching is another radiographic finding, usually involving the posterior fourth to eight ribs, and is seen in older patients. It is the result of increased collateral flow through the intercostal arteries.
- CT can provide excellent anatomic detail of the aorta, measurement of the diameter of the coarcted segment, its distance from the ipsilateral subclavian artery as well as other associating aortic and cardiac abnormalities. It also helps in the evaluation of the thoracic collaterals.

B. Vascular Rings and Slings

Vascular ring refers to the encirclement of the trachea and esophagus by the abnormal embryological development of the aortic arch. It may be complete or incomplete ring. The most common type is double aortic arch.

C. Congenital Pulmonary and Systemic Venous Anomalies

Congenital Pulmonary Venous Anomalies

Partial Anomalous Pulmonary Venous Connection (PAPVC)

- PAPVC refers to the drainage of one or more pulmonary veins into the systemic circulation.
- To differentiate it from TAPVC, at least one pulmonary vein must drain normally into the left atrium.
- It accounts for approx. 0.4–0.7% of all cardiac malformations.
- The anomalous drainage is more commonly seen on the right side and the most common form of PAPVC overall is the drainage of the right superior pulmonary vein into the SVC.
- The most common form on the left side is the drainage of the left superior pulmonary vein into the left innominate vein.
- On chest radiography, cardiomegaly is seen with right heart enlargement and pulmonary plethora.
- Cross-sectional imaging is very useful for evaluation of the anomalous vein and identification of any associated ASD.

Scimitar Syndrome

- Scimitar syndrome refers to an anomalous pulmonary vein draining all or part of the right lung and emptying into the IVC either above or below the diaphragm. This anomalous veins parallels the right heart border and resembles a 'scimitar,' which is a curved traditional sword held by Turkish warriors.
- Scimitar syndrome is associated with hypoplasia of the right lung with hypoplastic right pulmonary artery.
- A meandering pulmonary vein (MPV) is a rare pulmonary vascular anomaly characterized by an abnormal course of the pulmonary vein draining into the left atrium. It looks similar to scimitar syndrome hence is also called **pseudoscimitar syndrome**.
- Scimitar syndrome may be associated with **horseshoe lung**, where an isthmus of pulmonary parenchyma extends from the right lung across the midline behind the pericardium and fuses with the left lung.

Total Anomalous Pulmonary Venous Connection (TAPVC)

- TAPVC refers to the drainage of all four of the pulmonary veins to the systemic circulation.
- It accounts for approx. 1–5% of all cardiac malformations.
- There are four types of TAPVC: Supracardiac > Infracardiac > Cardiac > Mixed TAPVC.
- Supracardiac TAPVC:
  - Most common type (accounting for approx. 50% of all cases).
  - All four pulmonary veins join to form a common pulmonary vein posterior to the left atrium → drains into an ascending left vertical vein → which drains into the left innominate vein → right SVC → right atrium.
  - The right heart is dilated due to volume overload.
  - It is associated with an ASD which is the only source of blood flow to the left heart.
  - As described before, the classical frontal radiograph of TAPVC shows the snowman or Figure of '8' appearance.

Congenital Systemic Venous Anomalies

Bilateral SVC

There is persistence of the left SVC. The right SVC drains into the right atrium and the left SVC drains into the right atrium via the coronary sinus which may be dilated. An intercommunicating vein may be present between the two SVCs.

D. Systemic to Pulmonary Arterial Shunts

a. **Atrial septal defect (ASD):**
   - ASD is defined as a defect in the interatrial septum that allows communication between the right and left atria.
   - It is the second most common congenital heart disease (after ventricular septal defect), accounting for 10–13% of all cases. It is more common in women with a M:F ratio of 2:1.
   - It is associated with numerous syndromes, such as Down's syndrome, Ellis-van Creveld syndrome, Lutembacher syndrome and Holt-Oram syndrome.
   - It is usually asymptomatic, detected incidentally in adulthood (by 60 years, almost all the patients will be symptomatic).
   - There are four main types of ASD:
     1. Ostium secundum (most common type, accounting for 70–75% of all ASDs)—here, the defect is seen at the center of the interatrial septum in the region of fossa ovalis.
     2. Ostium primum (second most common type, accounting for 10–15% of all ASDs)—the defect is seen at the anteroinferior end of the interatrial septum near the atrioventricular valves. It occurs due to the failure of fusion between the lower end of septum primum and endocardial cushion. It has a strong association with Trisomy 21.
     3. Sinus venosus ASD (accounts for 10% of all ASDs)
     4. Unroofed coronary sinus (rare-approx. 1% of ASDs)
   - Chest radiography will be normal in small shunts. In larger shunts, there may be enlarged pulmonary arteries, pulmonary plethora and cardiomegaly (due to volume overload resulting in dilated right atrium and right ventricle) will be seen. The aortic knuckle and descending aorta are normal in size, hence appear smaller in comparison.
   - MRI and CT are useful for assessment of the interatrial septum. MRI is also helpful for shunt quantification.

b. **Ventricular septal defect (VSD):**
   - VSD was first identified by Dalrymple in 1847.
   - It is the most common type of congenital heart disease, accounting for 35–40% of all cases. It is slightly more common in women.
   - VSD can be isolated or associated with complex congenital heart disease.
   - The ventricular septum can be divided into the membranous septum (which is smaller and located at the base of heart) and the muscular septum. Difference shown in **Table 23.4**.

Table 23.4: Difference between membranous and muscular type of VSD.

Membranous type of VSD	*Muscular type of VSD*
MC type, accounting for 75–80% of all VSDs	20% of all VSDs
Occurs in the superior part of the interventricular septum, just inferior to the aortic valve	Involves the muscular septum. Small defects close spontaneously. Multiple muscular VSDs may be present, which gives the Swiss cheese appearance to the septum

- Small VSDs will have normal chest radiography. Larger VSDs will show cardiomegaly due to left atrial and left ventricular enlargement), enlarged pulmonary arteries and increased pulmonary blood flow.
- CT and MRI are useful for the noninvasive evaluation of the VSD.

c. **Atrioventricular septal defect (AVSD),** also known as endocardial cushion defect or atrioventricular cushion defect (AVCD).
   - It accounts for 2–7% of CHD.
   - It is associated with Down's syndrome (in 50% of cases), Edwards syndrome (in 25% of cases) and asplenia or Ivemark syndrome.
   - AVSD results from the deficient development of the apical portion of IAS, the basal portion of IVS and the AV valves.
   - AVSD can be complete or incomplete; balanced or unbalanced. In complete AVSD, there is an ostium primum ASD, a perimembranous VSD and a single common AV valve.
   - On chest radiography, there will cardiomegaly due to dilated right atrium and right ventricle and features of pulmonary artery hypertension.
   - On cross-sectional imaging, large defect of the midline heart structures would be seen.

d. **Patent ductus arteriosus (PDA):**
   - PDA occurs due to the failure of closure of ductus arteriosus beyond the neonatal period.
   - It accounts for 10–12% of all CHD and is more common in women with a F:M ratio of 2:1
   - On chest radiography, cardiomegaly is seen (predominantly due to LA and LV enlargement) along with features of pulmonary artery hypertension.
   - Cross-sectional imaging is helpful in measuring the size and diameter of the PDA, to look for any stenosis and any associated anomalies.
   - PDA has been classified by Krichenko based on its appearance on CT angiography.

Miscellaneous

Ebstein's Anomaly

- It is rare, seen in 1 per 20,000 live births and accounts for less than 1% of all CHD.
- It is associated with maternal lithium therapy.
- Ebstein's anomaly is characterized by abnormal development and positioning of the tricuspid valve with downward displacement of the septal and posterior leaflets into right ventricular cavity. This results in atrialization of a portion of the basal right ventricle.
- On chest radiograph, the classic "Box shaped heart" may be seen which is secondary to the hugely dilated RA which may fill the entire right hemithorax.
- The most commonly used classification for Ebstein's anomaly is the Carpentier's classification.

Tricuspid Atresia

- It is a cyanotic CHD characterized by the absence of the tricuspid valve. Hence, there is a lack of direct communication between the right atrium and right ventricle.
- It accounts for 3–4% of all CHD.
- It is almost always associated with an ASD and VSD which leads to mixing of the blood and varying degree of cyanosis.
- The most common classification used was by Tandon and Edwards.
- Chest radiograph may show pulmonary oligemia.
- CT and MRI allows direct visualization of the anomaly and may show a fatty and/or muscular separation of the right atrium from the right ventricle.

Hypoplastic Left Heart Syndrome

- It is characterized by the underdevelopment of the left heart, structures like ascending aorta, arch of aorta, aortic valves, mitral valves and left ventricle.
- It accounts for 2–3% of all CHD.
- It is one of the most common causes for a neonate to present with congestive cardiac failure.
- PDA and ASD are essential for survival.
- Antenatal ultrasound is especially useful for in-utero assessment.
- Chest radiograph will show cardiomegaly due to right heart enlargement with prominent right atrial border. Lung fields will show pulmonary plethora.
- CT will help in direct visualization of the anomaly while MRI helps in dynamic assessment.

Aortic Stenosis (AS)

- Aortic stenosis is the MC valvulopathy and represents approx. 10% of all CHD.
- It has a male predominance.
- Its most commonly associated with William's syndrome (seen in up to 50% of cases).
- Depending on the location the stenosis, AS can valvular (MC), supravalvular (least common) and subvalvular.
- Chest radiograph demonstrates cardiomegaly due to left atrial and left ventricular enlargement.
- Cardiac MRI allows quantification of the ventricular function and evaluation of the myocardium.

Other Pediatric Cardiac Diseases

The spectrum of other non-congenital pediatric cardiac diseases include cardiomyopathies, infective endocarditis, pericarditis, pericardial effusions and cardiac tumors.

Rhabdomyoma is the most common primary cardiac tumor of the childhood, accounting for 60–70% of cases.

The imaging evaluation of these diseases including the imaging findings is similar to that of adult population as is covered in the adult chapter.

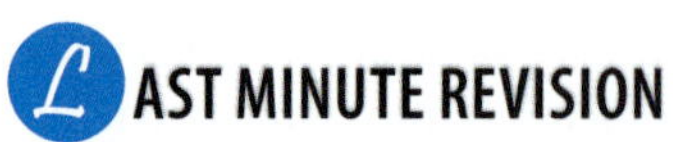

- ♦ Congenital heart disease is the most common congenital defect seen in live born children.
- ♦ Chest radiograph is the first line investigation for evaluation of CHD as it is readily available and inexpensive.
- ♦ A cardiothoracic ratio (cardiac width/thoracic width) is useful for determining cardiomegaly on chest radiograph. A CTR of up to 0.6 is considered normal in infants.
- ♦ An increase in the pulmonary vascularity is called plethora, where the pulmonary vessels are enlarged, tortuous and extend till the periphery of the lung. It is seen in large left-to-right shunts, such as ASD, VSD and PDA.
- ♦ Conversely, a decrease in pulmonary vascularity is called oligemia and is seen in TOF, tricuspid atresia and Ebstein's anomaly.
- ♦ Few classical signs seen on chest radiograph include 'Egg-on-a-string' appearance (TGA), 'snowman' sign (TAPVC), 'coeur en sabot' appearance or boot-shaped heart (TOF), figure of 3 appearance (coarctation of aorta), Box-shaped heart (Ebstein's anomaly).
- ♦ Cardiac CT is the workhorse for evaluation of CHD due to its high spatial and temporal resolution and is very useful for preoperative assessment. However, its limitations include exposure to ionizing radiation and need for iodinated contrast agents.

- Cardiac MRI has the distinct advantage of functional assessment along with no radiation exposure. It is also very useful for postoperative assessment. However, its disadvantages include long scanning time, strict immobilization and need for sedation which may not be suitable in younger patients.
- TOF is the most common cyanotic congenital heart disease and is associated with four components—right ventricular outflow tract obstruction, ventricular septal defect, overriding of the VSD by the aorta and right ventricular hypertrophy.
- TGA is the second most common cyanotic CHD and results from ventriculoarterial discordance, i.e., the aorta arises from the right ventricle and the pulmonary artery arises from the left ventricle.

REVIEW QUESTIONS

Multiple Choice Questions (MCQs)

1. A newborn presents with cyanosis and a chest X-ray showing an "egg-on-a-string" appearance. Which congenital heart disease is most likely?

a. Tetralogy of Fallot
b. Transposition of the great arteries (TGA)
c. Total anomalous pulmonary venous return (TAPVR)
d. Ebstein's anomaly

2. An infant presents with a prominent right atrium and a chest X-ray showing a "box-shaped heart." What is the most likely diagnosis?

a. Tetralogy of Fallot
b. Hypoplastic left heart syndrome
c. Ebstein's anomaly
d. Tricuspid atresia

3. A 6-month-old infant has a chest X-ray showing a "boot-shaped" heart and decreased pulmonary vascularity. What is the most likely diagnosis?

a. Tetralogy of Fallot
b. Transposition of the great arteries
c. Coarctation of the aorta
d. Total anomalous pulmonary venous return

4. A child presents with cyanosis and a chest X-ray showing a "snowman" or "figure of 8" appearance. What congenital heart disease does this suggest?

a. Tetralogy of Fallot
b. Transposition of the great arteries
c. Total anomalous pulmonary venous return (TAPVR)
d. Ebstein's anomaly

5. A 1-year-old child presents with shortness of breath and a chest X-ray revealing a cardiothoracic ratio of 0.6. What is the interpretation of this finding?

a. It is correct
b. It is wrong
c. Sometime correct
d. Sometime wrong

6. A child presents with a history of recurrent chest infections and a chest X-ray showing rib notching. What is the most likely diagnosis?

a. Tetralogy of Fallot
b. Coarctation of the aorta
c. Total anomalous pulmonary venous return
d. Ebstein's anomaly

7. A child presents with shortness of breath and a chest X-ray showing cardiomegaly and increased pulmonary vascular markings. What is the most likely diagnosis?

a. Atrial septal defect (ASD)
b. Tetralogy of Fallot
c. Ebstein's anomaly
d. Tricuspid atresia

Answer Key

1. b 2. c 3. a 4. c 5. a 6. b 7. a

SUGGESTED READING

1. Coley BD. Caffey's Pediatric Diagnostic Imaging, 13th edition.
2. DiGeorge NW, El-Ali AM, White AM, Harris MA, Biko DM. Pediatric Cardiac CT and MRI: Considerations for the General Radiologist. AJR Am J Roentgenol. 2020;215(6):1464-73.
3. Opfer E, Shah S. Advances in Pediatric Cardiovascular Imaging. Mo Med. 2018;115(4):354-60.
4. Rajeshkannan R, Raj V, Viswamitra S. CT and MRI in Congenital Heart Diseases. https://doi.org/10.1007/978-981-15-6755-1

CHAPTER

24

Interventional Radiology in Pediatrics

"With image-guided precision and gentle hands, radiologists perform miracles in miniature."

INTRODUCTION

Interventional radiology (IR) represents a frontier of minimal invasive therapy that plays a crucial role in the management of few specific pediatric diseases. This subspecialty combines the expertise of diagnostic imaging with the precision of surgical techniques to provide targeted treatments with fewer complications and shorter recovery times than traditional surgery. In pediatric patients, IR is invaluable due to its ability to minimize surgical stress and preserve future growth potential.

Pediatric interventional radiology has witnessed rapid advancements and expanded applications across a range of conditions, including vascular malformations, organ obstructions, and fluid collections. This chapter aims to provide a basic overview of pediatric interventional radiology which can be broadly divided into vascular and non-vascular interventions.

Nonvascular Interventions

In pediatric patients, nonvascular interventional radiology plays a critical role in managing gastrointestinal and other abdominal disorders without the need for invasive surgery.

Pancreatic Fluid Collections (PFCs)

Percutaneous drainage of PFCs, such as pseudocysts and walled-off necrosis, is a common nonvascular intervention in pediatric gastroenterology. Utilizing ultrasound or CT guidance, interventional radiologists can precisely place drainage catheters to manage these fluid collections effectively.

Risks and Considerations

While generally safe, these procedures carry potential risks, such as infection, bleeding, and damage to adjacent organs. Pancreatic fistula formation is a specific complication where the connection between the pancreas and the drainage site persists, which might require further intervention.

Percutaneous Transhepatic Biliary Drainage (PTBD)

PTBD is utilized to manage biliary obstructions that can cause significant health issues, including jaundice and liver damage. This technique involves inserting a catheter directly into the bile duct to relieve obstruction.

Risks and Considerations

The procedure may involve complications, such as biliary leaks, infections, or accidental injuries to nearby structures. Additionally, repeated procedures may be necessary if the stent becomes clogged or dislodged.

Gastrointestinal Foreign Body Retrieval

Children often ingest objects that may require non-surgical retrieval. Interventional radiologists can remove these objects using endoscopic techniques under imaging guidance, thus avoiding surgery.

Risks and Considerations

The primary risks include potential perforation of the GI tract and anesthesia-related complications, especially in younger children who may not tolerate awake procedures.

Trauma

Interventional radiology (IR) plays a crucial role in the management of pediatric trauma, offering timely and minimally invasive solutions that are vital in acute care settings. Pediatric trauma can involve multiple organ systems, with injuries ranging from vascular damage and internal bleeding to organ lacerations and bone fractures.

In cases of internal bleeding, **(Figs. 24.1A to C)** IR techniques, such as embolization can be lifesaving. This procedure involves the targeted delivery of embolic agents via catheters to occlude bleeding vessels, effectively controlling hemorrhage without the need for open surgery. This is particularly advantageous in stabilizing patients quickly with less physiological stress and reduced need for blood transfusions.

For traumatic injuries involving the kidneys, spleen, or liver, IR can be employed to manage organ lacerations and arteriovenous fistulas. Techniques like stent or coil embolization help preserve organ function and reduce the risks associated with surgical interventions.

Moreover, in pediatric patients with fractures, IR can assist in minimally invasive bone realignment and stabilization techniques. These procedures, often performed under image guidance, ensure precise alignment and promote faster healing with minimal disruption to the growth plates, which is essential in the pediatric population.

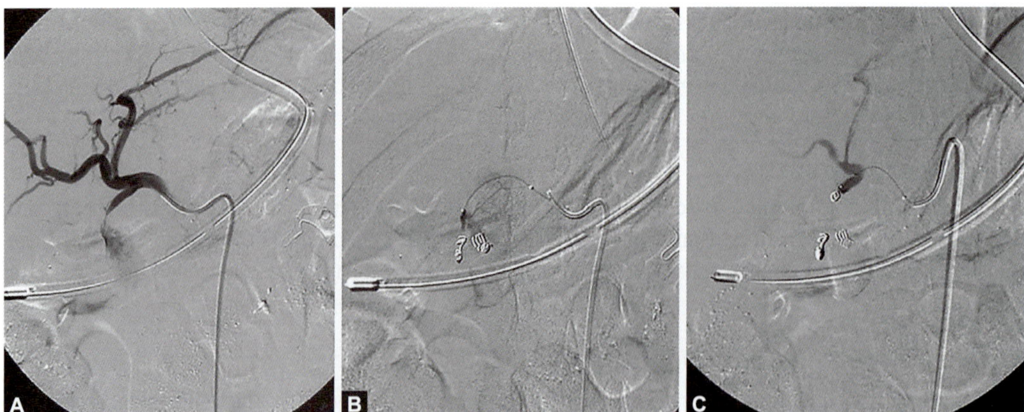

Figs. 24.1A to C: Angioembolization in a 17-year-old female with postcholecystectomy bleed, showing the technique from bleeding site identification to successful embolization.

Pediatric Oncology

In pediatric oncology, interventional radiology offers several minimally invasive procedures that can be pivotal in both diagnosis and treatment:

- **Tumor embolization:** Preoperative embolization of tumors to reduce blood loss during surgery.
- **Biopsies:** Image-guided needle biopsies provide diagnostic tissue samples with minimal discomfort and risk.
- **Port placement:** IR techniques are used to place central venous catheters and ports that facilitate long-term chemotherapy, reducing the need for repeated venipunctures.

These procedures are integrated within a multidisciplinary approach to care, ensuring that each child receives a personalized treatment plan that maximizes efficacy while minimizing physical and psychological burdens.

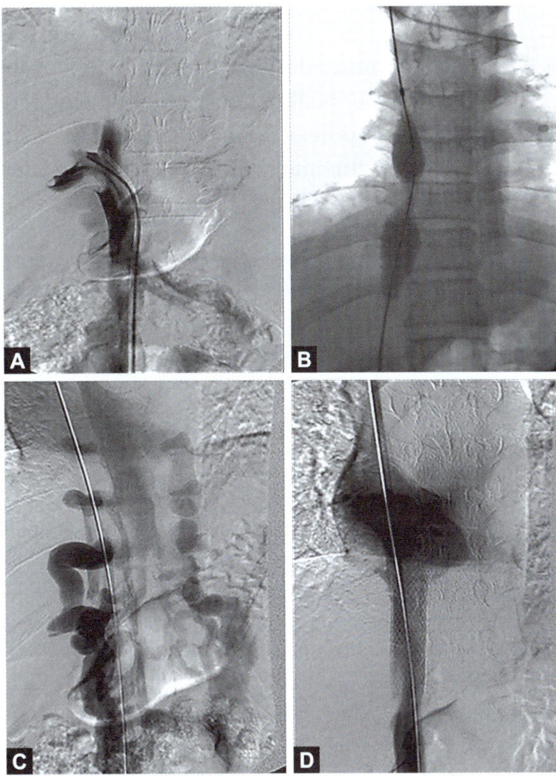

Figs. 24.2A to D: Inferior vena cava stenting in a 15-year-old with Budd-Chiari syndrome, from venogram to stent deployment.

Vascular Interventions

Budd-Chiari Syndrome (Figs. 24.2A to D)

This condition involves obstruction of hepatic veins or the inferior vena cava, which can be effectively managed through angioplasty or stenting, restoring normal blood flow and reducing liver damage.

Angioembolization for Pseudoaneurysms

Used to manage vascular anomalies or bleeding, this procedure involves the targeted placement of materials to seal off abnormal vessels.

RISKS AND SAFETY CONCERNS

Radiation Exposure

One of the significant risks in pediatric IR is radiation exposure. Children are more sensitive to radiation, which can increase the risk of future cancers. Techniques, such as using the lowest possible radiation dose and shielding are critical to minimizing this risk.

Anesthesia Requirements

Many IR procedures in children require sedation or general anesthesia due to the need for stillness and cooperation. Anesthesia risks, particularly in younger or medically complex children, include respiratory issues and reactions to anesthetic agents. Collaboration with pediatric anesthesiologists is essential to mitigate these risks.

POST-PROCEDURE CARE AND MONITORING

After an IR procedure, pediatric patients require careful monitoring to detect and manage potential complications early. The post-procedure care plan should include:

- **Pain management:** Effective strategies to manage pain, which could include pharmaceuticals and holistic approaches, should be tailored to the needs of the child and the specifics of the procedure.
- **Infection prevention:** Guidelines on how to care for entry points or incisions to prevent infection.
- **Activity recommendations:** Clear instructions on any restrictions related to physical activity, to ensure proper healing and prevent dislodgement of any catheters or stents.
- **Follow-up schedule:** A defined schedule for follow-up visits to monitor recovery and evaluate the success of the intervention. Advantages and disadvantages of pediatric interventional radiology shown in **Table 24.1**.

Table 24.1: Advantages and disadvantages of pediatric interventional radiology.

Advantages	*Disadvantages*
Minimally invasive: Less traumatic for the patient, involving smaller incisions, which reduces pain and speeds up recovery	**Radiation exposure:** Despite advances in technology, the exposure to radiation remains a concern, especially in children due to their increased susceptibility to its harmful effects
Reduced hospital stay: Many IR procedures can be performed on an outpatient basis, which minimizes hospital stays and lowers the risk of hospital-acquired infections	**Anesthesia risks:** Procedures often require sedation or general anesthesia, which carries its own risks, particularly in very young or medically fragile children
High Precision: Image-guided techniques allow for targeted treatment, improving the efficacy of interventions and minimizing damage to surrounding tissues	**Limited availability:** Advanced IR services may not be available in all hospitals, particularly in rural or underserved areas, limiting access to essential care
Cost-effective: By reducing the need for extensive surgery and shortening hospital stays, IR can be more cost-effective compared to traditional surgical approaches	**Technical challenges:** Some complex pediatric conditions may pose unique technical challenges due to the smaller size and more delicate nature of children's anatomy

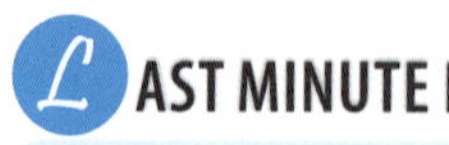

AST MINUTE REVISION

- Pediatric interventional radiology offers a range of minimally invasive procedures that are instrumental in managing complex conditions in children with fewer complications and quicker recovery times than traditional surgery.
- Main disadvantages include radiation exposure and anesthesia.
- Commonly performed procedure includes percutaneous drainage of fluid or cyst and guided biopsy.

REVIEW QUESTIONS

Multiple Choice Questions (MCQs)

1. **A 7-year-old child presents with a history of acute pancreatitis and is now developing symptoms consistent with a pseudocyst. Which of the following is the most appropriate interventional radiology procedure to manage this condition?**
   a. Endoscopic retrograde cholangiopancreatography (ERCP)
   b. Percutaneous drainage under ultrasound or CT guidance
   c. Surgical resection
   d. Observation and repeat imaging
2. **A pediatric patient with jaundice and suspected biliary obstruction is referred to the interventional radiology team. Which procedure is most appropriate for relieving the obstruction?**
   a. Percutaneous transhepatic biliary drainage (PTBD)
   b. Liver biopsy
   c. Laparoscopic cholecystectomy
   d. MRI cholangiopancreatography (MRCP)
3. **Which of the following is an advantage of using interventional radiology (IR) techniques, such as embolization, in the management of pediatric trauma?**
   a. Increased risk of infection
   b. Higher likelihood of blood transfusions
   c. Minimally invasive with reduced physiological stress
   d. Longer recovery time compared to surgery
4. **Which of the following is a significant disadvantage or risk associated with pediatric interventional radiology procedures?**
   a. No need for anesthesia
   b. Radiation exposure and potential long-term effects
   c. Shorter hospital stays
   d. Reduced need for surgery
5. **A 12-year-old child is diagnosed with an arteriovenous malformation (AVM) in the brain, presenting with headaches and seizures. Which interventional radiology procedure is most appropriate to manage this condition?**
   a. Surgical craniotomy
   b. Endovascular embolization
   c. Observation with medication
   d. Stereotactic radiosurgery

Answer Key

1. b 2. a 3. c 4. b 5. b

SUGGESTED READING

1. Nabi Z, Singh JR, Haris A, Shava U, Chavan R, Nageshwar RD. Outcome of radiological interventions in pediatric gastrointestinal diseases: A large tertiary center experience. JGH Open. 2018 27;3(2):140-147. doi: 10.1002/jgh3.12119. PMID: 31061889; PMCID: PMC6487811.
2. Young VA, Thakor AS, Josephs SC. Update on Pediatric Interventional Radiology. Radiographics. 2022;42(6):1580-1597. doi: 10.1148/rg.220019. PMID: 36190845.

UNIT 5

Comprehensive Radiological Review

Unit Outline

CHAPTER

25

Breast Imaging

"Breast imaging is more than detection—it's early intervention, silent strength, and a radiologist's commitment to saving lives with family."

INTRODUCTION

Breast imaging plays a crucial role in the early detection, diagnosis, and management of breast diseases, particularly breast cancer. Two-thirds of breast pathologies are benign in nature, most commonly fibrocystic breast disease followed by fibroadenoma. Breast cancer is globally the most prevalent form of cancer among women. In India, what was the fourth most common type of cancer in the 1990s has risen to the top position? According to Globocan data from 2020, breast cancer represents 13.5% of all cancer cases and 10.6% of all cancer-related deaths in the country. The survival rates for breast cancer patients in India are lower than those in Western countries, attributed to the late stage of the disease at the time of diagnosis, delayed start of definitive treatment, and incomplete or fragmented care.

Imaging plays a crucial role in the early detection of breast cancer and accurate diagnosis of breast conditions. Mammography and ultrasound are the primary methods for evaluation of the breasts diseases, while Magnetic Resonance Imaging (MRI) serves as an important problem-solving tool in cases with indeterminate findings on mammography and/or ultrasound. Digital mammography is regarded as the benchmark for screening breast cancer, boasting an overall sensitivity of 78% and a specificity of 99%. Despite its acclaim, it faces criticism for its purported low sensitivity and specificity in women possessing dense breast tissue. To address this concern, numerous technologies have been suggested to complement full-field digital mammography (FFDM), including digital breast tomosynthesis (DBT) or 3D mammography, breast ultrasound (US), and breast magnetic resonance imaging (MRI). Recently, contrast-enhanced spectral mammography (CESM) has emerged as a novel and clinically valuable technique for evaluating the breast.

IMAGING TECHNIQUES

Mammography

Mammography is a specialized form of imaging that the use specific X-ray tubes equipped with molybdenum or rhodium anodes to generate the low-energy X-rays essential for achieving high tissue contrast. Mammographic examinations performed these days are radiation safe, with the mean glandular radiation dose to the breast being 2 mGy (0.2 rad) per exposure. Limited use in dense breast especially in young, lactating women.

Mammographic Projections

Mammograms are classically displayed in a conventional paired manner, permitting for bilateral comparison. Shows two standard projections mediolateral oblique (MLO) view done with beam angle 30–60 degrees and the craniocaudal (CC) view done with zero degree, with right breast appearing on the left side of the screen and the left breast on the right side.

A correctly positioned CC view should profile the nipple, displaying almost all of the medial tissue and the majority of the lateral tissue, except for the breast's axillary tail. An accurately positioned MLO view should reveal nipple in profile, inframammary fold, and nipple should be align with lower border of pectoralis. Supplementary views, such as exaggerated CC (lateral or medial), true lateral view, cleavage view, spot compression view and magnification views may be taken to answer specific diagnostic problems.

Ultrasonography

Using sound waves, it is the most beneficial and widely used supplementary tool alongside mammography for diagnoses, and guiding biopsies. It is a safe and noninvasive technique, utilizing no radiation. It is conducted using a linear array transducer that has a frequency of at least 10 MHz, as advised by the American College of Radiology (ACR). Transducers with higher frequencies, ranging from 12 to 18 MHz, are optimal for producing high-resolution images. Meanwhile, lower frequencies are used for deep tissue penetration and are recommended for patients with larger breasts.

USG is widely used as an adjunct to mammography to improve lesion detection and characterization. Given that women under 30 years of age have denser breast tissue, which is more sensitive to radiation, ultrasound (US) is the preferred imaging technique for this demographic, as well as for lactating and pregnant women. Limitation includes it is highly operator-dependent, and less ability to detect microcalcifications.

Digital Breast Tomosynthesis (DBT)

Two-dimensional mammography has few limitations, such as anatomical noise caused by the superimposition of normal glandular tissue and pathological changes. This overlap can result in the appearance of false masses or the concealment of actual masses. DBT, also known as three-dimensional mammography, has emerged as a supplementary tool in breast imaging. Essentially, it introduces an additional dimension (tissue depth) to the standard two-dimensional mammogram. DBT operates by capturing multiple projection radiographs of the breast tissue at fixed intervals. These images are then displayed on high-resolution workstations, allowing for the examination of mammography layers one by one.

Limitations: Higher radiation dose compared to standard mammography, increased interpretation time.

Dynamic Contrast-enhanced Breast Magnetic Resonance Imaging (DCE-MRI)

Neo angiogenesis observed in malignant lesions forms the basis for detecting and characterizing breast cancer through MR imaging. In a diagnostic context, it is employed as a problem-solving tool for evaluating breast lesions that are indeterminate by mammography and/or ultrasonography. DCE-MRI for breast cancer diagnosis boasts very high sensitivity but only moderate specificity. The most common approach in DCE-MRI analysis includes assessment of the type of kinetic curve, based on gadolinium contrast agent's washout pattern. These patterns are divided into type I (persistently enhancing or progressive), seen in benign conditions; type II (plateau), suggesting a moderate risk of malignancy; and type III (washout), indicating a high likelihood of malignancy.

For patients already diagnosed with breast cancer, MR imaging is essential for delineating the extent of the disease, screening the contralateral breast, and assessing the response to neoadjuvant chemotherapy or hormonal therapy. Additionally, it is utilized for breast cancer screening in high-risk women.

Limitations: High cost, limited availability, potential for false positives, requires contrast administration.

Contrast-enhanced Spectral Mammography (CESM)

Contrast-enhanced mammography has recently emerged as an alternative to DCE-MRI, potentially expanding access to vascular imaging and lowering the cost of examinations. In CESM, intravenous iodinated contrast agents are utilized to improve the visibility of tumor neovascularity.

NORMAL BREAST ANATOMY

The breast is an apocrine gland composed of adipose tissue, glandular tissue, suspensory Cooper's ligaments, and connective tissues, such as collagen and elastin.

The mammographic appearance of the normal breast depends on the presence of its primary components—fat tissue, which appears radiolucent, and stromal and glandular tissues, which appear radio-opaque. As one ages, the glandular tissue tends to involute, resulting in the majority of the breast tissue presenting with a fatty density.

On ultrasound, starting from the cutaneous surface going deep, four different regions may be identified:

1. **Skin:** Seen as two echogenic lines separated by a hypoechoic line representing the dermis.
2. **Subcutaneous (pre-mammary) region:** It is located between the skin and the mammary fascia and it contains mostly hypoechoic adipose tissue. This region is crossed by thin hyperechoic lines known as Cooper's ligaments which extend from the skin to the glandular region.
3. **Glandular region:** It is located between the pre-mammary region and the retromammary region. The echogenicity of this region varies in relation to the percentages of glandular and adipose tissues. Fat tissue is hypoechoic, while the glandular tissue and stroma are echogenic.
4. **Retromammary region:** It is made from the retromammary fat that is hypoechoic. The pectoralis major muscle is slightly more echogenic than the retromammary fat.

IMAGING APPROACH TO BREAST LESIONS

The American College of Radiology (ACR) has designed BI-RADS (Breast Imaging-Reporting and Data System) to standardize breast imaging reporting and to reduce misunderstanding in breast imaging interpretations. It also facilitates outcome monitoring and quality assessment. The most up-to-date version, the 5th edition, was published in 2013. It introduces a universally accepted lexicon and reporting framework for breast imaging, applicable to mammography, ultrasound, and MRI. The standard terms and definitions utilized in the Atlas have received approval from the ACR Committee on BI-RADS. It is the hope that all professionals involved in breast imaging will embrace and exclusively use these terms, ensuring that reports are clear, succinct, and uniform. In the **Table 25.1**, various mammographic BI-RADS descriptors and their distinctive features are outlined to facilitate understanding.

Table 25.1: ACR BI-RADS atlas fifth edition—mammography lexicon.

Breast composition (in terms of density)	a. Almost entirely fatty b. Scattered areas of fibroglandular density c. Heterogeneously dense breasts, which may obscure small masses d. Extremely dense breasts, which lowers the sensitivity of mammography	
Mass	Shape **(Figs. 25.1A to C)**	• Oval (may include two or three undulations) • Round (spherical, ball-shaped, circular, or globular in shape) • Irregular (neither round nor oval, usually implies a suspicious finding)
	Margin **(Figs. 25.2A to E)**	• Circumscribed—(at least 75% of the margin must be sharply defined) • Obscured—(>25% of the margin is hidden by superimposed or adjacent fibroglandular tissue) • Microlobulated—(short cycle undulations, usually implies a suspicious finding) • Indistinct—(no clear demarcation of the entire or any portion of the margin, from the surrounding tissue) • Spiculated—(characterized by lines radiating from the mass, usually implies a suspicious finding)
	Density **(Figs. 25.3A to C)**	• High • Equal • Low • Fat containing Relative to the expected attenuation of an equal volume of normal fibroglandular tissue
Calcifications	Typically, benign	• Dermal • Vascular • Round (<1.0 mm)/punctate (<0.5 mm) • Rim • Coarse or popcorn • Large rod-like • Dystrophic • Suture • Milk of calcium
	Suspicious morphology **(Figs. 25.4A to E)**	• Amorphous (so small and/or hazy that a specific shape cannot be determined) • Coarse heterogenous (irregular, conspicuous calcifications between 0.5–1 mm) • Fine pleomorphic (usually <0.5 mm with variable size and shape) • Fine linear or fine linear branching
	Distribution **(Figs. 25.5A to E)**	• Diffuse (randomly distributed throughout the breast) • Regional (numerous calcifications that occupy a large portion >2 cm of breast tissue, not conforming to a duct distribution) • Grouped (at least five calcifications are grouped within 1 cm of each other) • Linear (arrayed in a line) • Segmental (in a triangle with apex towards nipple)
Architectural distortion	(Parenchyma is distorted with no definite mass visible)	
Asymmetries	• Asymmetry (area of fibroglandular tissue that is visible on only one mammographic projection) • Global (usually a normal variant and represents a large amount of fibroglandular-density tissue over at least one quadrant) • Focal (small amount of fibroglandular tissue over less than one quadrant). • Developing (focal asymmetry that is new, larger, or more conspicuous than on a previous examination)	
Intramammary lymph node		

Contd...

Contd...

Skin lesion		
Solitary dilated duct		
Associated features	Skin thickening or retraction, nipple retraction, axillary lymphadenopathy	

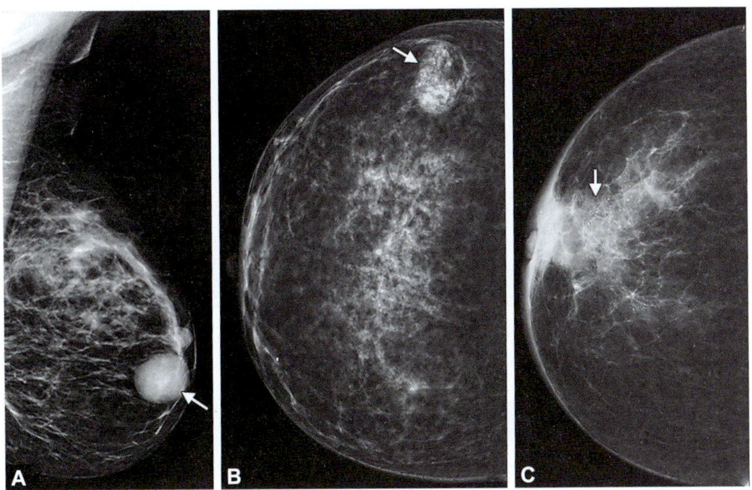

Figs. 25.1A to C: Mammogram shows: (A) Round; (B) Oval; and (C) Irregular shape of lesions (arrow).

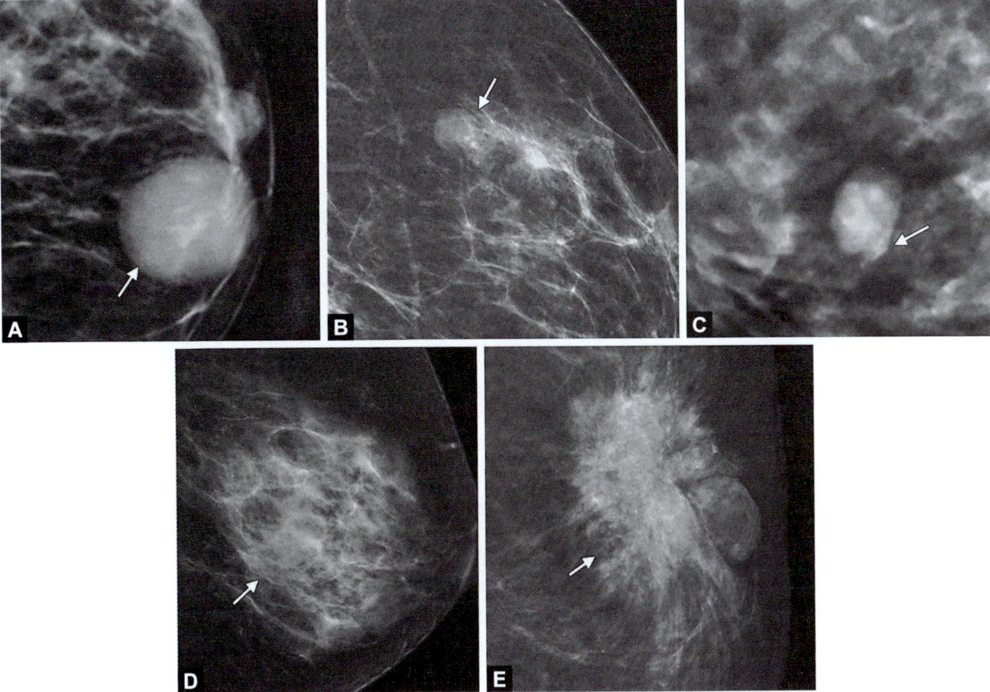

Figs. 25.2A to E: Mammogram shows: (A) Circumscribed; (B) Obscured; (C) Microlobulated; (D) Indistinct; and (E) Spiculated margin of the lesions (arrow).

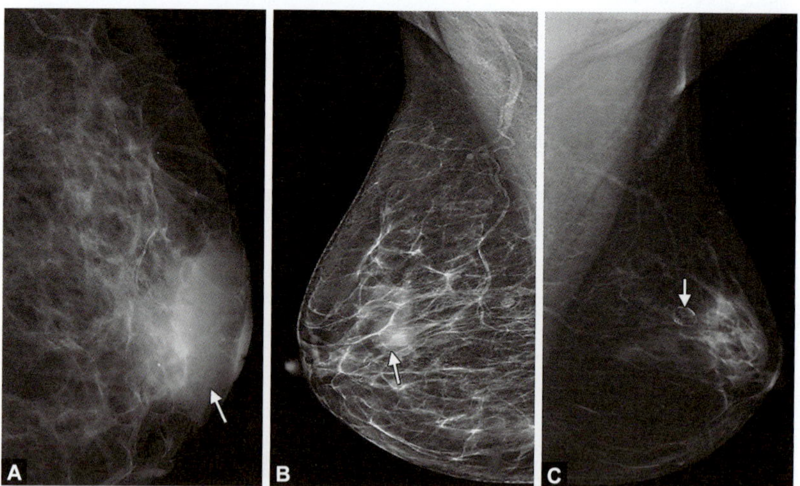

Figs. 25.3A to C: Mammogram shows: (A) High density; (B) Equal density; and (C) Fat containing lesions (arrow).

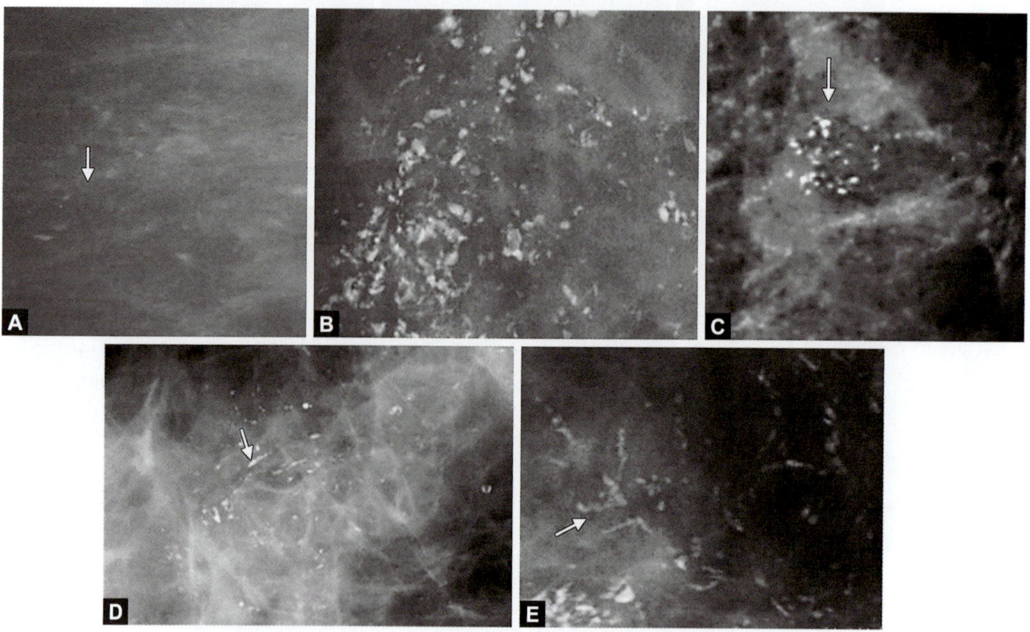

Figs. 25.4A to E: Mammogram shows suspicious morphology: (A) Amorphous; (B) Coarse heterogenous; (C) Fine pleomorphic; (D) Fine linear; and (E) Fine linear branching calcifications (arrow).

After reviewing mammograms, ultrasonography is typically conducted if an abnormality is suspected or identified, to confirm and characterize the nature of the abnormality. Additionally, ultrasonography is used to assess and describe palpable masses and other signs or symptoms related to the breast, particularly in young, lactating, and pregnant women.

The ACR BI-RADS Atlas, similar to the mammographic lexicon, endorses and advocates for the application of different ultrasonographic BI-RADS descriptors and their unique characteristics **(Table 25.2)**.

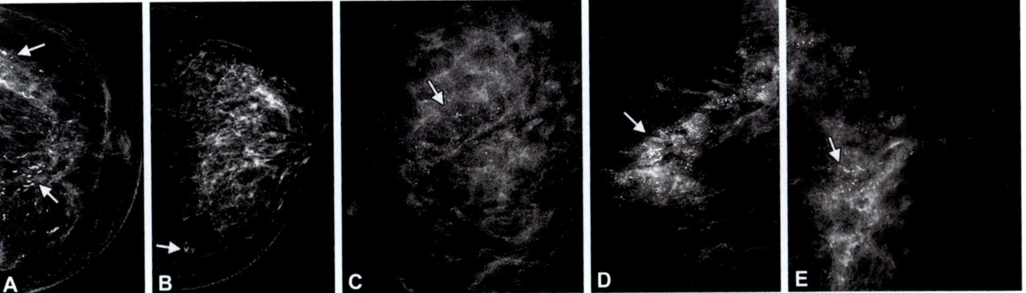

Figs. 25.5A to E: Mammogram shows distribution pattern of calcifications: (A) Diffuse; (B) Grouped; (C) regional; (D) Segmental; and (E) Linear (arrow).

Table 25.2: ACR BI-RADS atlas fifth edition—ultrasound lexicon.

Tissue composition (screening only)	a. Homogeneous background echotexture—fat b. Homogeneous background echotexture—fibroglandular c. Heterogeneous background echotexture	
Masses	Shape **(Figs. 25.6A to H)**	• Oval • Round • Irregular
	Orientation	• Parallel • Not parallel
	Margin **(Figs. 25.6A to H)**	• Circumscribed • Not circumscribed ♦ Indistinct ♦ Angular ♦ Microlobulated ♦ Spiculated
	Echo pattern **(Figs. 25.7A to I)**	• Anechoic • Hyperechoic • Complex cystic and solid • Hypoechoic • Isoechoic • Heterogeneous
	Posterior features **(Figs. 25.7A to I)**	• No posterior features • Enhancement • Shadowing • Combined pattern
Calcifications	• Calcifications in a mass • Calcifications outside of a mass • Intraductal calcifications	
Associated features	Architectural distortion	
	Duct changes	
	Skin changes	• Skin thickening • Skin retraction
	Edema	
	Vascularity	• Absent • Internal vascularity • Vessels in rim
	Elasticity assessment	• Soft • Intermediate • Hard

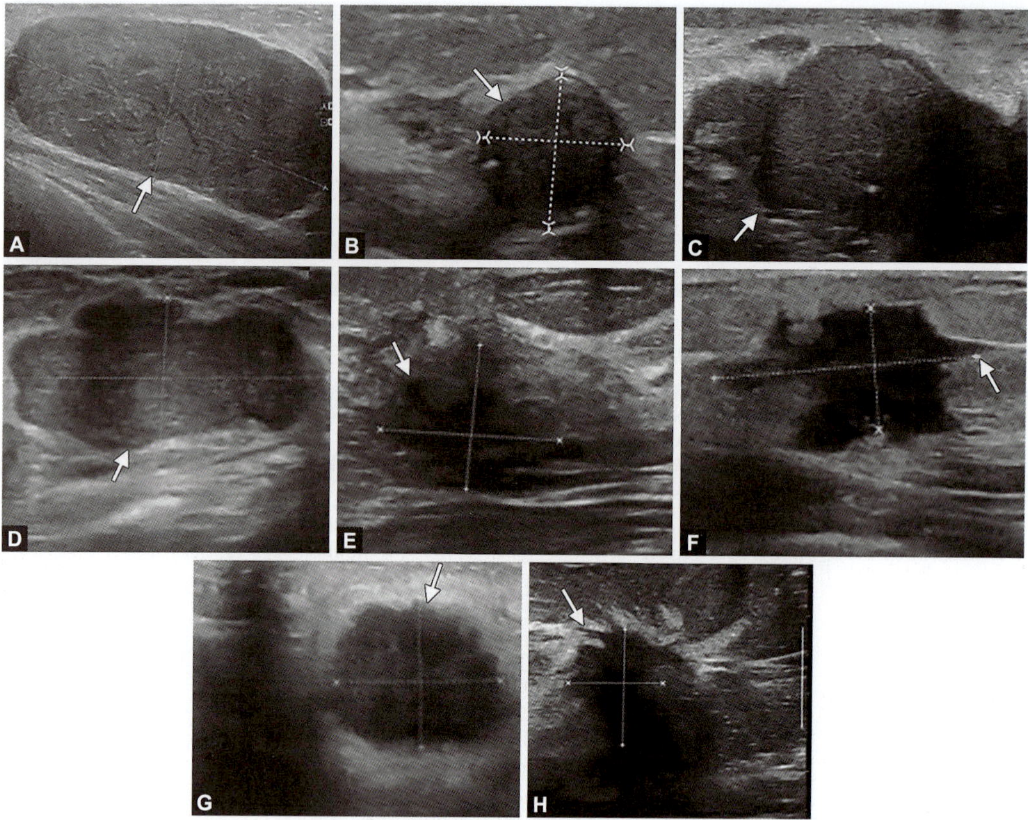

Figs. 25.6A to H: Ultrasound shows variation in shape: (A) An oval fibroadenoma; (B) Round nodule in fibrocystic mastopathy; and (C) Irregular invasive ductal carcinoma. The margins of the lesions are; (D) Circumscribed in a fibroadenoma; and (E) Indistinct; (F) Angular; (G) Microlobulated; and (H) Spiculated in different histopathologically proven cases of invasive ductal carcinoma (No special type) (arrow).

Based on thorough evaluation of mammographic features, (with clinical and ultrasound correlation whenever required), a final assessment category (BI-RADS-1, 2, 3, 4, 5 or 6) should be assigned for each scan. These BI-RADS assessment categories are designed to be concordant with specific management recommendations **(Table 25.3)**.

Table 25.3: ACR BI-RADS atlas fifth edition—assessment categories.

Category	*Management*	*Likelihood of cancer*
Category 0: Incomplete—need additional imaging and/or prior mammograms for comparison	Recall for additional imaging and/or comparison with prior examination	N/A
Category 1: Negative	Routine mammography screening	0%
Category 2: Benign	Routine mammography screening	0%
Category 3: Probably benign	Short-interval (6 month) follow-up or continued surveillance mammography	>0% but ≤2%

Contd...

Contd...

Category	*Management*	*Likelihood of cancer*
Category 4: Suspicious		
Category 4A: Low suspicion for malignancy		>2% to ≤10%
Category 4B: Moderate suspicion for malignancy	Tissue diagnosis	>10% to ≤50%
Category 4C: High suspicion for malignancy		>50% to <95%
Category 5: Highly suggestive of malignancy	Tissue diagnosis	≥95%
Category 6: Known biopsy-proven malignancy	Surgical excision when clinically appropriate	N/A

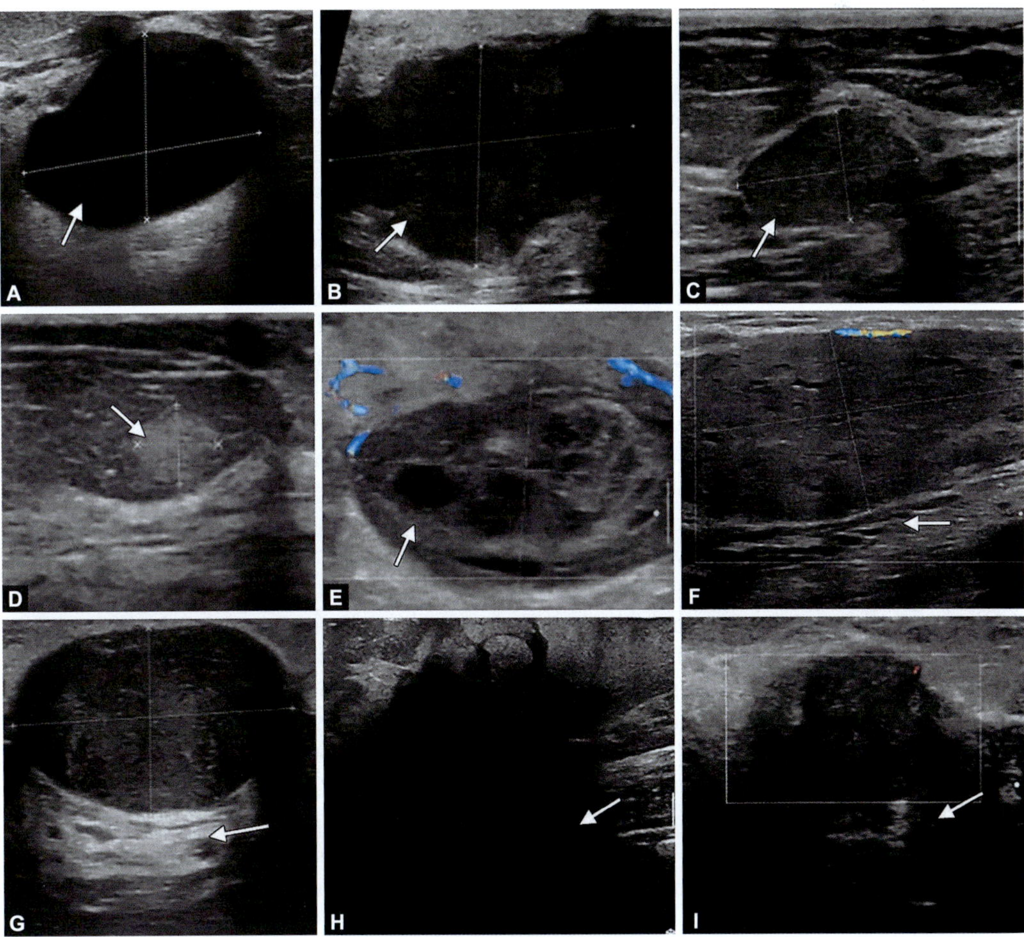

Figs. 25.7A to I: Ultrasound shows variation in echopattern of the lesions: (A) Anechoic simple cyst; (B) Hypoechoic invasive breast cancer; (C) Isoechoic fibroadenoma; (D) Hyperechoic lipoma; and (E) Heterogeneous invasive ductal carcinoma (arrow). Posterior features of the lesions are also shown; (F) No posterior features in a case of phyllodes; (G) Enhancement in a complicated cyst filled with echoes; (H) Shadowing in an invasive lobular carcinoma; and (I) Combined pattern (both shadowing and enhancement in an invasive ductal carcinoma).

Category 1: This category should be used when no specific benign findings are described in the text of the report.

Category 2: This category should be used when at least one finding with characteristically benign appearance is described. The lesions which fall in this category include involuting fibroadenomas, fat-containing lesions [like oil cyst, lipoma, galactocele and mixed-density hamartomas], simple cyst, complicated cyst in setting of multiple cysts, intramammary lymph nodes, vascular and multiple large, rod-like calcifications, and architectural distortion clearly related to prior surgery.

Category 3: It should be used for noncalcified circumscribed solid mass (usually a fibroadenoma), focal asymmetry which becomes less dense on spot compression view, and a solitary group of punctate calcifications that have likelihoods of malignancy in the defined (≤2%) probably-benign range. This category is suitable for USG findings that strongly indicate the presence of a typical fibroadenoma, an isolated complicated cyst, and clustered microcysts. For category three assessments, the initial short-term follow-up interval for the concerned breast typically spans six months. If stability is confirmed at this six month check, the assessment should once again be classified as category three, accompanied by a management suggestion for another short-interval follow-up examination after six-months, this time including both breasts. Should stability be maintained at this subsequent short-interval follow-up, the examination is reassessed as category 3. However, the recommended follow-up interval is usually extended to 1 year at this point.

Category 4: This category is designated for observations that lack the typical characteristics of malignancy yet exhibit enough suspicion to warrant a biopsy recommendation. This category is further segmented into 4A, 4B, and 4C, with the aim of highlighting specific probabilities of malignancy within this category, thereby enabling the patient and their clinician to decide the next plan of action.

Category 4A: This category may be applied to findings that require intervention but have a low likelihood of being malignant. It is unlikely that a malignant finding will be identified. Following a benign percutaneous tissue diagnosis, it is appropriate to suggest a six-month or routine follow up. This category is appropriate for cases including partially circumscribed and partially obscured masses with ultrasonography characteristics indicative of an (atypical) fibroadenoma, as well as palpable, isolated, complex cysts, and probable abscesses.

Category 4B: This category encompasses lesions that moderately raise suspicion for malignancy. Lesions classified in this category necessitate meticulous correlation between radiologic and pathologic findings following a percutaneous tissue diagnosis. Should the results be benign, the subsequent follow-up will hinge on their concordance. Assigning this category is advised in instances featuring grouped amorphous or fine pleomorphic calcifications, as well as nondescript solid masses with unclear boundaries.

Category 4C: This category encompasses observations that are highly suspicious for malignancy, yet not strongly indicative of it, as seen in category 5. Mammograms demonstrating a new cluster of fine linear calcifications or a new, vague, irregular solitary mass should be classified under this category.

Category 5: The probability of cancer is 95% or higher; therefore, the use of this assessment category should be limited to classic examples of malignancy. The current rationale for employing a category five assessment is to pinpoint lesions, where any noncancerous percutaneous tissue diagnosis is immediately deemed inconsistent, leading to the suggestion for a repeat biopsy (usually surgical). This category is designated for characteristics, such as a spiculated, irregular

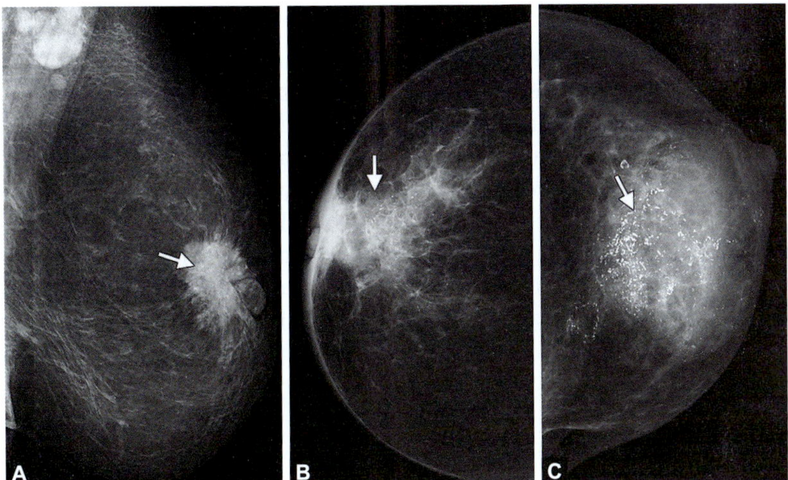

Figs. 25.8A to C: Mammogram of three different patients show irregular, high density lesions with microcalcifications; and (A) Spiculated; (B) Indistinct; and (C) Obscured margins. These lesions were categorized as BI-RADS 5 and trucut biopsy confirmed infiltrating ductal carcinoma.

dense mass, a segmental or linear pattern of fine linear calcifications, and an irregular spiculated mass accompanied by pleomorphic calcifications **(Figs. 25.8A to C)**.

IMAGING FEATURES OF COMMON BREAST PATHOLOGIES

Breast Cyst

Breast cysts are one of the most commonly encountered clinical entity, seen in women of all age but are most frequently found in those aged between 30 and 50. Mostly they are discovered incidentally during screening mammograms or may manifest with a palpable lump. In mammograms, a cystic lesion is identified as a mass that is round, oval, or lobulated circumscribed masses. However, margin can become obscured or indistinct due to the superimposition of the fibroglandular tissue or due to the presence of peri cystic fibrosis. Since mammography alone cannot definitively diagnose a cyst, additional mammographic views, such as spot-compression view and ultrasound become essential. Based on ultrasound features cysts are further subdivided into: Simple cyst, Clustered microcyst (separated by thin septa <0.5 mm), complicated cyst (acute fat necrosis, hematoma, filariasis, cysticercosis and frank abscess), complex cyst (Wall & septa > 0.5 mm) and cystic-solid mass (intracystic man or solid masses with cystic areas).

Fibroadenoma

Fibroadenoma is the most prevalent solid breast lesion, typically affecting women aged between 10 and 40 years. It also stands as the most common solid benign breast lesion. It usually presents as a mobile palpable lump. On mammograms, fibroadenomas exhibit a range of appearances from oval, circumscribed, isodense masses to macrolobulated lesions with obscured margins. In older patients, particularly those who are postmenopausal, involuting fibroadenomas may include calcifications, often presenting the characteristic, "popcorn calcification" look. On ultrasound, fibroadenomas generally present as round or oval, well-circumscribed, homogeneous masses that are hypoechoic or isoechoic and hypovascular, with varying posterior acoustic characteristics. Occasionally, a thin echogenic rim (pseudocapsule) might be observed.

Phyllodes

Phyllodes tumor, previously referred to as cystosarcoma phyllodes, is rare fibroepithelial tumor found in the breast. These tumors typically manifest as painless, large, and rapidly expanding masses, sharing clinical and imaging characteristics with fibroadenomas. The common mammographic presentation of phyllodes tumor is a well-defined round or oval mass. Unlike fibroadenomas, phyllodes tumors usually do not occur in multiple instances or bilaterally. Moreover, while fibroadenomas often show typical popcorn calcifications, phyllodes tumors generally do not exhibit calcification. On ultrasound, phyllodes tumors present as solid, well-circumscribed masses with heterogeneous echogenicity **(Fig. 25.7F)**. They can appear with single or multiple, round, or cleft-like cystic spaces and display posterior acoustic enhancement. The solid components of these tumors typically show vascularization.

Breast Abscess

Abscesses can develop from infections in the subareolar ducts and/or existing galactoceles (puerperal mastitis), or from the rupture of cysts or ectatic ducts. They are categorized into lactational and nonlactational abscesses, with lactational ones being more prevalent. Typically, patients present with a painful, tender lump. Overlying skin may appear erythematous and thickened. In a typical clinical scenario, ultrasonography is the imaging investigation of choice. Classical USG features include multiloculated hypoechoic collection with posterior acoustic enhancement and an echogenic, vascular rim. If the clinical presentation is not typical, especially in nonlactating women, mammography is recommended to exclude the possibility of malignancy. Mammographic appearance is often variable and nonspecific. Mammography may demonstrate asymmetric density, mass or distortion associated with skin thickening. USG may demonstrate multiple intercommunicating hypoechoic masses with collection pockets and adjacent echogenic inflamed fat. Sometimes, these tracts may reach up to the skin surface and form a discharging sinus.

Hamartoma

Breast hamartoma, also referred to as fibroadenolipoma, is an uncommon, slowly growing benign lesion. It is typically observed in middle-aged women who are over 35 years of age. Breast hamartomas are usually asymptomatic, though some may present as a painless soft lump in the breast or unilateral breast enlargement without a palpable mass. In mammography, they are characterized by a classic "breast within a breast" appearance, which includes a well-circumscribed, round or oval mixed-density solid mass. This mass contains both fat and fibroglandular elements and is surrounded by a thin pseudocapsule. Ultrasound imaging shows a range from a well-encapsulated and well-circumscribed isoechoic solid mass that is mildly heterogeneous (featuring both hyperechoic and hypoechoic components) to an ill-defined mass resembling normal breast tissue. The margins of these masses are often difficult to delineate. They may also exhibit intralesional microcalcification.

Ductal Carcinoma in situ (DCIS)

DCIS of the breast represents neoplastic lesions, typically localized to the breast ducts with no evidence of invasion beyond the basement membrane. The mammographic features of DCIS vary, with microcalcifications being the most frequent, appearing in 50–75% of cases. The types of calcifications associated with DCIS include amorphous, coarse heterogenous, fine pleomorphic, and fine linear type **(Figs. 25.4A to E)**. Distribution in linear or segmental patterns are particularly indicative of DCIS **(Figs. 25.5A to E)**. On USG, a micro-lobulated, hypoechoic mass that extends along the ducts is the most common feature.

Dynamic contrast-enhanced MRI of the breast complements mammography in identifying DCIS since it can reveal enhancements in both calcified and noncalcified areas of intraductal carcinoma. It enables precise extent delineation thereby enhancing the effectiveness of treatment and prognosis. On MRI, DCIS usually presents as an area of nonmass enhancement of clumped or clustered ring pattern, typically in a segmental or linear distribution. Conducting an image-guided core needle biopsy from the suspicious area yields a histological diagnosis.

Breast Cancer

Breast cancer usually presents as a painless, palpable, hard, immobile mass. Mammography is usually the first-line imaging investigation performed. Typical mammographic features include irregular shape, indistinct or spiculated margins, high density of the lesions, with/without calcifications **(Figs. 25.8A to C)**. Typical ultrasound features include irregular, hypoechoic, nonparallel lesion with angular or spiculated or indistinct margins **(Figs. 25.6E to H)**. "Invasive breast carcinoma (IBC) of no special type (NST)" is the most common type found in approximately 75–80% of the cases.

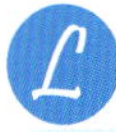

AST MINUTE REVISION

- Breast cancer is globally the most prevalent form of cancer among women.
- Digital mammography is universally accepted modality for screening of breast cancer, boasting an overall sensitivity of 78% and a specificity of 99%.
- USG is the first-line investigation in young, pregnant and lactating women.
- Magnetic resonance imaging serves as an important problem-solving tool in cases with indeterminate findings on mammography and/or ultrasound.
- DCE-MRI analysis is based on the assessment of the type of kinetic curve, depending upon gadolinium contrast agent's washout pattern.
- Contrast-enhanced mammography has recently emerged as an alternative to DCE-MRI, offering the benefits of lower cost, ease of performance, and reduced time consumption.
- The recently ACR-BI-RADS Atlas 5th edition has introduced and recommends the usage of a universally accepted lexicon and reporting framework for breast imaging, applicable to mammography, ultrasound, and MRI.
- ACR-BI-RADS Atlas also recommends categorization of breast lesions into final assessment categories to standardize breast imaging reporting and to reduce misunderstanding in breast imaging interpretations.
- Ductography is contrast procedure for intraductal lesion.
- CT has limited role in breast imaging, done to rule out bony metastasis in breast malignancy.

REVIEW QUESTIONS

Multiple Choice Questions (MCQs)

1. **A 56-year-old lady presents with a painless, palpable lump. First imaging investigation that should be performed in this case is:**

   a. Ultrasound
   b. Mammography
   c. Contrast MRI
   d. Digital breast tomosynthesis

2. **A lactating mother presents with painful, tender mass for one week. Imaging modality of choice in this case is:**
   a. Ultrasound
   b. Mammography
   c. Contrast MRI
   d. Digital breast tomosynthesis
3. **Which of the following is not included among the suspicious morphology calcifications?**
   a. Coarse heterogenous
   b. Popcorn
   c. Fine pleomorphic
   d. Amorphous
4. **A 28-year-old female presents with a palpable mobile lump. Ultrasound shows an oval, circumscribed, homogenous, hypoechoic, parallel lesion with thin echogenic capsule. Most accurate BI-RADS assessment category and most probable diagnosis is:**
   a. BI-RADS 3 (Fibroadenoma)
   b. BI-RADS 2 (Fibroadenoma)
   c. BI-RADS 4a (Fibroadenoma)
   d. BI-RADS 3 (Lipoma)
5. **Which of the following mammographic descriptor if present, can assign a BI-RADS category 5 to a breast lesion:**
   a. Irregular shape
   b. High density with microcalcification
   c. Spiculation
   d. Combination of all of the above

Answer Key

1. b 2. a 3. b 4. a 5. d

SUGGESTED READING

1. D'Orsi CJ, Sickles, EA, Mendelson EB, Morris EA. ACR BI-RADS Atlas: Breast Imaging Reporting and Data System. American College of Radiology, Reston, VA, USA; 2013.
2. Lazarus E, Mainiero MB, Schepps B, Koelliker SL, Livingston LS. BI-RADS lexicon for US and mammography: interobserver variability and positive predictive value. Radiology. 2006;239(2):385-91. doi: 10.1148/radiol.2392042127. Epub 2006 Mar 28. PMID: 16569780.
3. Sung H, Ferlay J, Siegel RL, Laversanne M, Soerjomataram I, Jemal A, Bray F. Global Cancer Statistics 2020: GLOBOCAN Estimates of Incidence and Mortality Worldwide for 36 Cancers in 185 Countries. CA Cancer J Clin. 2021;71:209-49.

CHAPTER

26 Imaging in Joint Disease

"Every joint tells a story of wear, injury, or inflammation—and radiology gives it a voice."

INTRODUCTION

A joint is any place in the body where two bones meet. Joints are crucial in the body as they allow for movement and structural support. The classification of joints based on histology or function is an important concept in anatomy. The histological classification categorizes joints based on the primary connective tissue present, including fibrous, cartilaginous, or synovial joints. Meanwhile, functional classification is based on the range of motion permitted by the joint.

There are three main functional types of joints:

1. **Synarthrosis:** These are immovable joints that provide structural support.
2. **Amphiarthrosis:** Slightly moveable joints that offer a balance between motion and stability.
3. **Diarthrosis:** Freely moveable joints that allow for a wide range of movements.

It is interesting to note that the two classification systems align: synarthroses are typically fibrous joints, amphiarthroses are often cartilaginous joints, and diarthroses are commonly synovial joints.

Furthermore, synovial joints, which are diarthroses, are subcategorized into **(Fig. 26.1)** condyloid, hinge, ball and socket, plane, and saddle joints, each with its own distinct characteristics and range of motion.

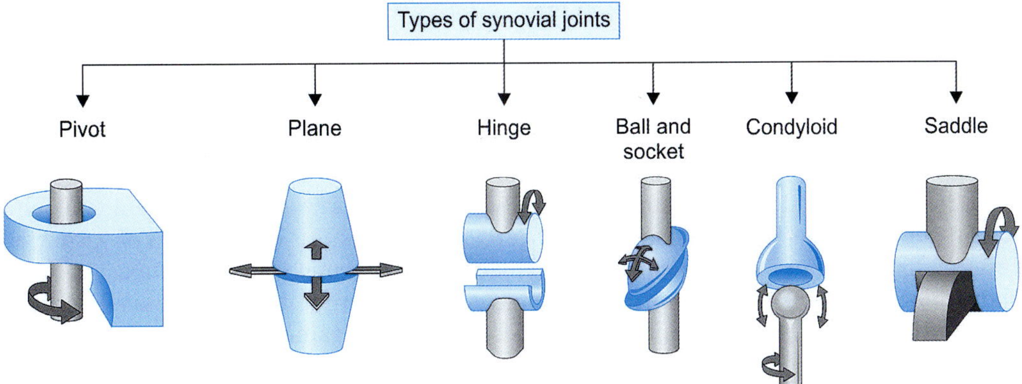

Fig. 26.1: Types of synovial joints.

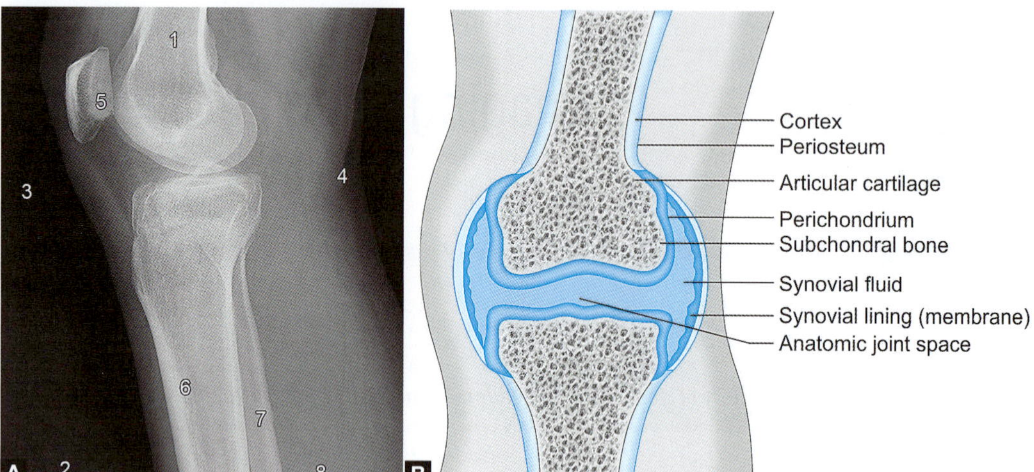

Figs. 26.2A and B: (A) Shows X-ray knee joint lateral view depicting proximal/femur (1), distal/tibia-fibula (2), anterior (3), posterior (4), patella (5), Tibia (6), fibula (7) and soft tissue leg (8); (B) Anatomy of synovial joint.

Anatomy of a synovial joint is described in **Figs. 26.2A and B**. The true or diarthrodial joint consists of cartilage covering the articular ends of the bones forming the joint; the articular capsule, which is reinforced by ligamentous structures and the joint space, which is lined with synovial membrane and filled with synovial fluid.

The factors affecting joints are anatomical/physiological that can be related to developmental/congenital, trauma, infection/inflammation, degeneration or tumors. The pattern of involvement of the different component of joints may point towards specific etiology/prognosis. The aim of this chapter is to provide an overview of the imaging features of the joint related pathology with a focus to optimize the evaluation.

IMAGING MODALITY

In the current era of multiple imaging modalities, choosing the appropriate modality for a precise indication is of the utmost importance. Each imaging modality has its advantages and is useful in the appropriate setting. It is important to be familiar with the views and the techniques that best demonstrate the suspected abnormality.

A. Radiography

X-ray is the first investigation to be performed for evaluation of joint pathology. The skeletal radiography series requires a minimal of two orthogonal views with each view including two adjacent joints if possible. Additional views may be taken for better analysis, such as oblique views for better visualization of superimposed structures, stress views for ligament tear/joint stability, or weightbearing views for joint space/cartilage thickness evaluation. For suspected cases of disruption of the ulnar collateral ligament of the first metacarpophalangeal joint, an abduction-stress film of the thumb may be obtained. In the lower extremity, stress views of the knee and ankle joints are occasionally obtained for evaluating ligament injuries of knee causing knee instability.

The role of radiograph in cortical bone pathologies is of paramount importance in depicting fractures, periosteal reactions and new bone formation.

For evaluation of bone tumors, a plain radiograph is the most helpful tool for evaluating the lesion morphology, matrix, margins and pattern of bone destruction, and should always be used as the first-choice imaging modality.

For assessment of arthritis, X-rays depicts erosion and sclerosis, joint space changes (reflects cartilage thickness and synovial lined space) and periarticular soft tissue pathologies like calcification, air-fluid level, fat fluid level, air, etc. Various bony deformities depicted on X-ray may be highly suggestive towards a particular diagnosis.

Recommended X-ray positioning:

- **Hand:** AP and Ball catcher view
- **Elbow:** AP and lateral views
- **Shoulder:** AP view in internal and external rotation and oblique view for joint
- **Hip:** AP with internal rotation and frog leg view
- **Knee:** Knee bilateral knee AP view, Lateral view, Intercondylar view, Skyline view, Rosenberg view
- **Ankle:** AP, lateral and oblique view
- **SI joint:** Pelvis AP (Oblique view)
- **Spine:** AP and lateral views

B. Computerized Tomographic Scan

The role of CT in joint disorders lies in its ability to image cortical and trabecular bone, especially in trauma; bone density quantification with quantitative CT and material decomposition analysis using Dual Energy CT (DECT).

In cases of trauma, CT allows the use of thin slice imaging within shortest possible scanning times, reduces motion artifacts even in noncompliant patients to generate high-quality real-time volumetric data. It is routinely used in spinal fractures for assessing posterior elements. Complex fractures like shoulder, scapula, elbow, wrist, tibial plateau, ankle and calcaneum highly demands CT scan due to its multiplanar reconstructions and 3D volume rendered images.

CT is useful in osteomyelitis and soft tissue infections. Sclerosis surrounding Brodie's abscess is well demarcated using CT. Chronic osteomyelitic changes of sequestrum and cortical tunneling are also well delineated on CT. CT is valuable for tumor imaging in conditions like documentation of nidus in osteoid osteoma; diagnosis and guided intervention for biopsy/ treatment (ablation).

Quantitative CT is useful in measuring bone mineral density and diagnosing osteopenia. Material decomposition analysis using DECT maps, substances of known attenuation like calcium, uric acid etc., is having clinical applications in evaluation of gout. DECT data yields color-coded cross-sectional images, clearly depicting the foci of accumulation of urate crystals. The major disadvantage of CT is its high radiation dose and poor bone marrow evaluation and soft tissue resolution.

C. Magnetic Resonance Imaging

MRI has excellent soft tissue resolution with lack of ionizing radiation and multiplanar imaging capabilities. MRI offers detailed visualization of cartilage, ligaments, tendons and is superior to other imaging modalities in assessing bone marrow, synovial hypertrophy, extent of tumor involvement in malignancies, and periarticular erosions. Imaging of fibrocartilaginous structures, such as the meniscus of the knee, the labrum of the shoulder and the triangular fibrocartilage complex of the wrist, can be demonstrated with spin-echo (SE) and GRE sequences. Hyaline cartilage is routinely evaluated on fat-suppressed 3D spoiled T1-GRE sequences for thinning, areas of altered signal, erosion of deep cartilage loss extending to bone, as well as intermediate fat saturated images.

D. Ultrasonography

With wide availability and recent improvements in technology coupled with portability, low cost, and safety, ultrasound is one of the first-choice imaging investigations for the evaluation of musculoskeletal diseases. It can be employed in inflammatory and noninflammatory pathologies, imaging of nerves, tendons, ligaments and joint effusions. It is particularly useful in synovitis, enthesitis, picking up early erosions and assessing vascularity. Apart from this, it has a role in providing diagnostic and therapeutic interventions. There are limitations to ultrasonography like operator dependence and poor visualization beyond bony cortex and deeper structures.

COMMON PATHOLOGY

Joint Trauma

Evaluation of traumatic injury to joint needs evaluation by radiograph for instability by alignment, stress view to see the ligament laxity, decubitus view to document lipohemarthrosis as an indirect sign of intraarticular cortical breech or displaced fat pad as an indirect sign of effusion/hemarthrosis. CT scans and MRI are also used for evaluation in suspected cases of bone injury and ligament/cartilage injury respectively.

The physeal plate is often involved in traumatic pediatric injuries. Up to one-third of all pediatric fractures involving long bones will involve the physis. These fractures carry added significance because involvement of the "growth plate" may lead to arrested development of the affected limb. The standard classification for physeal fractures was set forth by Salter and Harris.

Injury to joint can be osseous or nonosseous (include capsule, ligamentous and tendon). Nonosseous injury usually led to chronic morbidity to patient, So radiologist play vital role not only in acute diagnosis of fractures but is the only channel to clearly depict cause of symptoms in old trauma too, e.g., injured labrum, an important stabilizer of shoulder joint if allowed for large range of motion is vulnerable to injury and chronic instability.

The elbow joint is the second most commonly dislocated joint after the shoulder. Dislocations can be either simple or complex, based on the presence or absence of associated fracture, respectively.

Magnetic resonance imaging **(Figs. 26.3A to D)** plays a vital role in the identification of ACL/PCL/meniscal tears and associated injuries. Signs of tear include increased signal intensity with partial or complete interruption of the ligament fibers, altered contour, avulsed bony fragment, bone contusions, etc.

Depending on the etiopathogenesis, meniscal tears can be broadly categorized into traumatic and degenerative tears. The major criteria for a meniscal tear on MRI include the presence of high signal within the meniscal substance and abnormal morphology of the meniscus.

Arthritis

Arthritis is a group of disorders presenting clinically with joint swelling or limitation of motion of joint accompanied by pain and/or tenderness. There is a wide spectrum of disease presentation with significant overlap among them. The arthropathies can be degenerative, inflammatory, infective, connective tissue-associated, metabolic and endocrine-related. The key to evaluation is to have an organized approach which includes regional and global joint assessment to identify

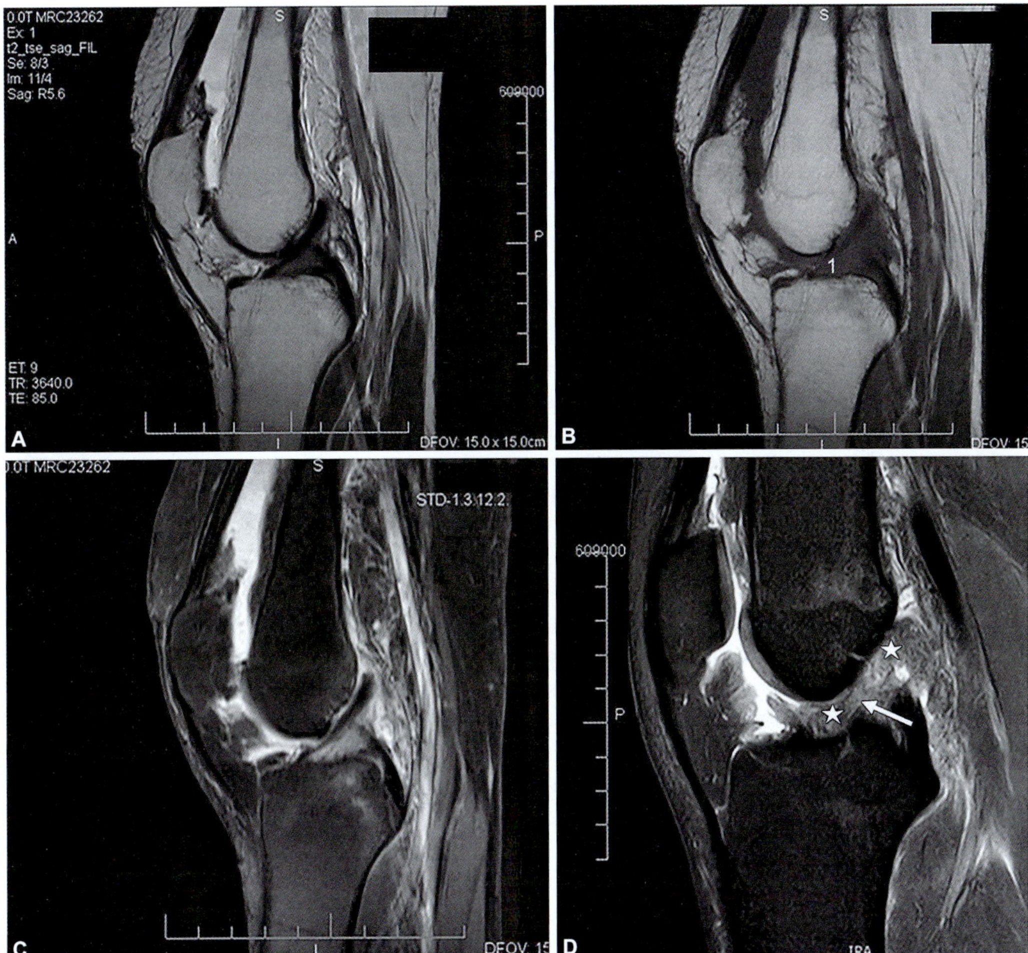

Figs. 26.3A to D: MRI images of the knee. (A) Sagittal T2 weighted showing hypointense cruciate ligament (normal) and hyperintense joint effusion; (B) Sagittal T1 shows hypointense joint fluid; (C) PD Sagittal shows partial tear of PCL and bone contusion; (D) Sagittal STIR shows ACL tear.

the clues for diagnosis. Almost all arthritic processes have a preferential joint distribution, as well as a specific radiological pattern within a joint.

The algorithm on radiograph is evaluation of joint space narrowing followed by evaluation if the joint process is inflammatory or degenerative. While an inflammatory condition is suggested by osteopenia and soft tissue swelling, it is the presence of bone erosions that is the characteristic finding. Early erosions will appear as discontinuities of the thin, white, subchondral bone plate or more commonly the joint margins (bare areas). In contrast, a degenerative cause of joint space narrowing is characterized by osteophytes, bone sclerosis, subchondral cysts, or geodes, asymmetric joint space narrowing, and lack of inflammatory features such as bone erosions.

Degenerative Joint Disease/Osteoarthritis (OA)

Osteoarthritis can be primary and secondary. Primary OA is a familial arthritis that affects middle-aged females almost exclusively in the hands and rarely foot. Secondary OA is due to other diseases leading to cartilage damage, as in trauma, synovitis, crystal deposition, infection, etc. Bone density is maintained with an exception in erosive arthritis. A degenerative process is suspected when joint space narrowing, osteophyte formation, bone sclerosis, and subchondral cysts are seen in the absence of inflammatory changes. Joints commonly affected are the hip, knee, first metatarsophalangeal (MTP) joint, distal interphalangeal (DIP) joint of the hand, base of thumb, cervical and lumbosacral spine. Magnetic resonance imaging (MRI) has allowed a comprehensive evaluation of articular disease, increasing the detection of early cartilage involvement, edema in soft tissue and bone marrow. The changes of degenerative joint disease is more marked in joints that has acquired extra load or activity due to erect postures like knee, hip and first carpometacarpal joint (pincer grip).

Osteoarthritis is the most common arthritis of the knee. As the cartilage is lost, there is subchondral sclerosis and osteophyte formation and cystic changes. Pieces of bone or cartilage break off and form loose bodies of different sizes.

Degenerative changes in the spine are most commonly seen in the lower cervical, dorsolumbar and lower lumbar vertebrae which are the most affected segments due to erect posture. The changes are seen as loss of joint space, subchondral sclerosis, marginal osteophytosis and vacuum phenomena.

Rheumatoid Arthritis

Rheumatoid arthritis (RA) is the most common autoimmune chronic inflammatory arthritis of unknown etiology. RA is characterized by symmetric small joint polyarthritis with significant functional disability. The diagnosis of RA is considered in cases presenting with small joint polyarthritis (three or more joints) with associated imaging findings of inflammatory erosive arthritis and/or presence of rheumatoid factor with classical joint involvement especially metacarpophalangeal and metatarsophalangeal joints.

It is symmetrical arthritis of primarily the appendicular skeleton, sparing the axial skeleton except for the cervical spine and at times SI joint. Structural changes in bone are usually a late feature and are well picked up on radiographs. However, ultrasound (US) and magnetic resonance imaging (MRI) are able to pick up inflammatory changes early on in the disease process and is important to arrest the disease process/activity before irreversible structural changes occur.

Imaging assessment of the wrist is the single most important tool in the assessment of RA. The involvement of the wrist is characteristic with the involvement of flexor tendon tenosynovitis with trigger as frequent accompaniment. Erosion of MCP is usually seen on the radial side. Swan-neck, Boutonniere, Hitchhiker and Z-line deformities are characteristically seen with RA.

Seronegative Spondyloarthropathies

Seronegative spondyloarthropathy (SpA) comprises a group of interrelated chronic inflammatory rheumatic diseases which share overlapping clinical features. These patients are negative for rheumatoid factor and show familial clustering with a strong association with Human Leukocyte Antigen-B27 (HLA-B27) gene. These diseases include ankylosing spondylitis (AS), psoriatic arthritis (PsA) with spondylitis, arthritis/spondylitis related to chronic inflammatory bowel disease (AIBD) or enteropathic arthritis (EA), reactive arthritis (ReA) and undifferentiated spondyloarthritis (uSpA). SpA being a chronic disease with debilitating outcome; early diagnosis and therapeutic interventions are crucial to modify disease progression. Various classification criteria have been advocated for diagnosing SpA, the most recent classification criteria being the assessment in SpondyloArthritis International Society (ASAS) criteria. Depending on their clinical presentation, SpA is broadly divided into two subtypes: axial spondyloarthropathy (axSpA) and peripheral spondyloarthropathy (pSpA), with some overlap between these two subtypes. Diagnostic criteria for ax-SpA has been formulated by ASAS to include an imaging arm and a clinical arm. Radiography is the first-line imaging modality for diagnosis. The sacroiliac joints are the most important joints to image because the disease nearly always starts in this location. Early radiographic findings are predominant on the iliac side of the cartilage with erosion of subchondral bone, indistinctness of articular margins, variable adjacent osteoporosis, surrounding reactive sclerosis and in advanced cases intraarticular ankylosis. Since X-rays are insensitive for the detection of early disease, if these are normal, MR imaging of the sacroiliac joints is recommended.

On MRI, imaging findings may be described as active inflammatory or chronic structural changes. Active inflammatory lesions are bone marrow edema (osteitis), synovitis, capsulitis and enthesitis. Chronic or structural lesions are well seen on T1-weighted images and include subchondral sclerosis, erosions, periarticular fat deposits and ankylosis.

- **Ankylosing spondylitis:** Sacroiliac joint involvement is usually bilateral, symmetric and precedes spinal involvement. Spinal involvement causes erosions (the 'Romanus lesion') which develop at the sites of attachment of annulus fibrosis to the anterior corner of vertebral endplates. It also produces the 'shiny corner sign which signifies progressively increasing sclerosis at focal areas of osteitis. Thick continuous syndesmophytes produce the 'bamboo spine' with bone proliferation producing a squared appearance. There is ossification of posterior interspinous ligament called the 'dagger sign', on AP views of the lumbar spine. These ligamentous ossifications are prone to fracture on trivial trauma creating emergencies that is better evaluated by CT scan.
- **Psoriatic arthritis:** PsA typically affects people between 30 and 50 years of age, equally distributed among men and women. However, the subtype showing spinal involvement occurs more frequently in men. It produces dactylitis, deformity of fingers, pencil-in-cup deformity, destructive changes—subchondral cysts and erosions (commonly in DIP joints of hand, foot and IP joint of big toe), bone proliferation, periosteositis, ankylosis and enthesopathy.
- **Reactive arthritis:** Reactive arthritis is an inflammatory arthritis manifesting after days to weeks following a gastrointestinal or genitourinary infection. The classic triad of arthritis, urethritis and conjunctivitis is described but is not always present. Imaging features are similar to those of psoriatic arthritis and the differentiation is mostly based on clinical history.
- **Enteropathic arthritis:** Occurs in patients with inflammatory bowel diseases (IBDs) and other gastrointestinal diseases, such as Whipple disease (WD), celiac disease (CD) and intestinal bypass surgery.
- Undifferentiated spondyloarthritis.

Infective Arthritis

Infective arthritis is a serious condition that should be diagnosed early before irreversible joint damage occurs. Young children and older patients are particularly prone to joint infection. The knee and hip joints are most affected. In <10% of patients, more than one joint is affected though, unlike inflammatory arthritis, symmetrical disease is rare.

Radiographs are typically normal at presentation except for showing soft tissue thickening around the joint ± and a discrete effusion. About one-tenth of children with septic arthritis will have adjacent osteomyelitis, and in these patients, radiographic features of osteomyelitis (focal osteolysis, periosteal new bone formation) are common. Ultrasound or MRI should be performed as soon as possible in patients with suspected acute or subacute septic arthritis. On MR imaging, severe diffuse synovial thickening, bony erosions, relative absence of subchondral bone marrow edema, and the presence of extraarticular smooth-walled abscesses favor a tuberculous arthritis, whilst more pronounced subchondral bone marrow edema and no extraarticular abscesses favor pyogenic arthritis. Ultrasound at an early stage will usually show a moderate to severe joint effusion with mild synovial proliferation though rarely only a small amount of joint fluid will be present and it can be used for guiding aspiration.

Crystal Associated Arthritis

The crystal deposition disorders include gout, calcium pyrophosphate dihydrate (CPPD) deposition disease (pseudogout), hydroxyapatite deposition disease (HADD), hemochromatosis, and ochronosis. The use of polarizing light microscopy and dual-energy CT scan techniques has made the identification of various crystals in synovial fluid and tissue samples possible. The most common is gout classically present acutely with involvement of the first MTP joint is commonly seen in middle-aged. However, in elderly the first presentation may be in hand, at a site of osteoarthritis (OA). Deposition of monosodium urate in soft tissue presents as tophaceous gout, causing slow erosion of underlying bone, usually away from joint, with a sclerotic border. Joint space is characteristically preserved and in advance cases, only a ghost outline of the joint space is observed. This preservation of cortical outline in the joint exclude infection.

Masses and Tumors of the Joints

Synovial tumors arise from the synovium, though may, at presentation, appear either articular or periarticular in location, and also comprise a diverse range of pathologies. These tumors are classified by their predominant tissue type. For example, giant cell tumor of tendon sheath and pigmented villonodular synovitis are classified as fibrohistiocytic tumors, while synovial chondromatosis is classified as a chondrogenic tumor.

Benign Tumors

Synovial Hemangioma

It is a rare benign tumor that is essentially a synovial vascular malformation rather than a hemangioma. It usually occurs in children and young adults. The knee is the commonest affected location and, in particular, Hoffa fat pad region.

Lipoma Arborescence

It is a rare tumor-like lesion of the synovium characterized by frond-like fatty masses arising from the synovial fat. The commonest affected joint is the knee, preferentially in the suprapatellar pouch. Radiographs may demonstrate a soft tissue swelling. Ultrasound can demonstrate a joint effusion with an intraarticular frond-like hyperechoic fatty mass. The typical MRI features comprise a frond-like synovial proliferation which is of fat signal on all sequences.

Synovial Chondromatosis

It can be primary and secondary. In the initial phase, radiographs may show an intraarticular soft tissue mass with or without chondroid type of calcifications. MRI appearance is variable and depends on the relative preponderance of synovial proliferation, loose bodies formation, and extent of calcification or ossification. The most frequent pattern is one of predominantly unmineralized nodules that demonstrate typical chondroid signal characteristics: intermediate to low signal on T1, high signal on T2, blooming artifact on GRE.

PVNS

Pigmented villonodular synovitis is a benign tumor classified as a fibrohistiocytic tumor by WHO characterized by synovial proliferation having diffuse and focal forms. In the diffuse form of PVNS which is four times more common, the synovial masses extend along the synovium and can reach a large size. Radiographs can show a soft tissue mass which may be dense due to the presence of hemosiderin. On MRI, one can appreciate synovial thickening of the synovium and joint capsule which may have 'finger like' projections. On T1- and T2-weighted sequences, the lesions are usually lower signal intensity than skeletal muscle with blooming artifacts on GRE due to hemosiderin.

Malignant Tumors

- **Synovial chondrosarcoma:** Synovial chondrosarcoma is a rare tumor. The majority of cases arise from malignant conversion of long-standing, preexisting primary synovial (osteo) chondromatosis. MRI will show a large lobulated intraarticular mass with chondroid calcification. This mass will be hypointense to isointense to skeletal muscle on T1 weighting and hyperintense on fluid sensitive sequences. Calcifications will be low-signal intensity on all sequences. They may be infiltrative destruction of adjacent bone which may show an aggressive periosteal reaction.
- **Synovial sarcoma:** It is a misnomer, and it is not arising from the joint. It gets its name from the fact that these lesions are commonly located in an articular or periarticular location, and histologically, the cells can resemble developing synovium. Radiographs are nonspecific but can show a periarticular soft tissue mass if the lesion is large or superficial. Calcifications will be seen in 20–30%. MRI is the imaging modality of choice for local staging.

Evaluation of Prosthesis (Fig. 26.4)

Evaluation of joint prostheses is crucial for assessing the positioning, integrity, and function of the prosthetic components, as well as identifying any complications. Plain radiography is the most commonly used imaging modality for evaluating joint prostheses. It provides detailed

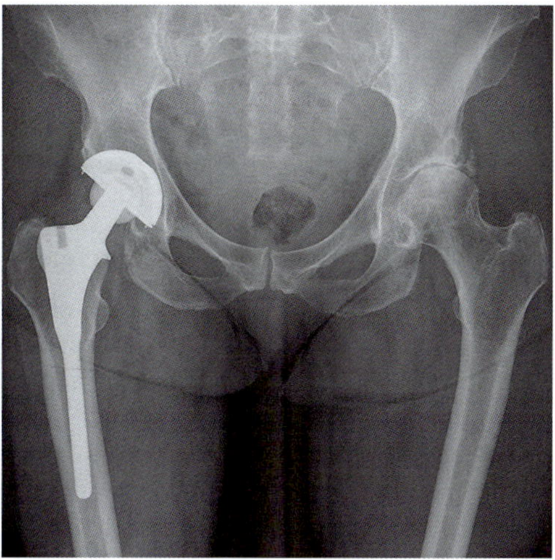

Fig. 26.4: Hip prosthesis.

information on the alignment, positioning, and integrity of the prosthetic components. CT scans (3D reconstruction) offer detailed cross-sectional images and are particularly useful for evaluating the integrity of the prosthetic components and surrounding bone (subtle fractures, bone-implant interface). MRI is less commonly used due to metal artifacts but can be valuable for evaluating the soft tissues around the prosthesis.

Ultrasound is useful for evaluating the soft tissues surrounding the prosthesis, especially for detecting fluid collections, bursitis, or tendinopathies.

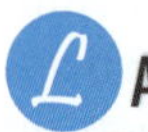

AST MINUTE REVISION

- Radiographs provide initial assessment and diagnosis, CT scans offer high-resolution anatomical details, MRI is excellent in soft tissue and bone marrow evaluation, and ultrasound aids in real-time imaging and guiding interventions.
- Joint space narrowing, osteophyte formation, subchondral sclerosis, and subchondral cysts are radiological features of osteoarthritis.
- Symmetrical joint space narrowing, periarticular osteopenia, marginal erosions, and soft tissue swelling are characteristic features of rheumatoid arthritis.
- Bilateral sacroiliitis, syndesmophytes, bamboo spine (vertebral body squaring), and ossification of spinal ligaments are common findings in ankylosing spondylitis.

REVIEW QUESTIONS

Multiple Choice Questions (MCQs)

1. **A 55-year-old woman presents with chronic knee pain and stiffness. X-rays show joint space narrowing, osteophytes, and subchondral sclerosis. What is the most likely diagnosis?**
   a. Rheumatoid arthritis
   b. Osteoarthritis
   c. Gout
   d. Septic arthritis
2. **A 45-year-old man presents with pain and swelling in the metatarsophalangeal joint of the big toe. X-rays reveal joint space preservation with punched-out erosions and overhanging edges. What is the most likely diagnosis?**
   a. Psoriatic arthritis
   b. Rheumatoid arthritis
   c. Gout
   d. Ankylosing spondylitis
3. **A 30-year-old woman presents with symmetrical swelling and pain in the small joints of her hands and feet. X-rays show periarticular osteopenia, joint space narrowing, and marginal erosions. What is the most likely diagnosis?**
   a. Osteoarthritis
   b. Septic arthritis
   c. Rheumatoid arthritis
   d. Pigmented villonodular synovitis
4. **A 40-year-old man presents with lower back pain and stiffness. X-rays reveal bilateral sacroiliitis and syndesmophytes, with vertebral body squaring. What is the most likely diagnosis?**
   a. Ankylosing spondylitis
   b. Osteoarthritis
   c. Psoriatic arthritis
   d. Gout

5. A 35-year-old woman presents with pain and swelling in her knee. MRI shows a joint effusion, synovial thickening, and low signal intensity on both T1 and T2-weighted images with blooming on GRE sequences. What is the most likely diagnosis?

a. Osteoarthritis
b. Pigmented villonodular synovitis (PVNS)
c. Rheumatoid arthritis
d. Gout

Answer Key

1. b 2. c 3. c 4. a 5. b

SUGGESTED READING

1. Chauhan K, Jandu JS, Brent LH, Al-Dhahir MA. Rheumatoid Arthritis. 2023 May 25. In: StatPearls [Internet]. Treasure Island (FL): StatPearls Publishing; 2024 Jan–. PMID: 28723028.
2. Juneja P, Munjal A, Hubbard JB. Anatomy, Joints. 2024 Apr 21. In: StatPearls [Internet]. Treasure Island (FL): StatPearls Publishing; 2024 Jan–. PMID: 29939670.
3. Sen R, Hurley JA. Osteoarthritis. [Updated 2023 Feb 20]. In: StatPearls [Internet]. Treasure Island (FL): StatPearls Publishing; 2024 Jan.

CHAPTER

27 Gastrointestinal Tract Imaging

"From gut feelings to guided findings, radiology plays a vital role in digestive health."

INTRODUCTION

Gastrointestinal diseases are common and lead to significant hospital workload. Apart from clinical, endoscopic, and laboratory evaluation, radiological evaluation forms core of comprehensive work-up in management of gastrointestinal diseases. The most important aspect of radiology is confirming or excluding suspected diagnosis, providing alternative diagnosis and also defining extent of disease if already detected. In large number of cases, disease extent is defined precisely by radiological investigations.

Initially only planar or projectional imaging modalities were available such as X-ray and fluoroscopy. Introduction of cross-sectional imaging modalities such as ultrasound, CT and MRI revolutionized entire radiology practice leading to better diagnosis and wider spectrum of disease being diagnosed and managed.

IMAGING MODALITIES

Radiography

Plain radiography, commonly called X-ray, has been oldest imaging method for patients presenting with acute abdominal complaints such as abdominal distension. It can be done in erect or supine position. Abdominal radiography can reveal dilated bowel loops suggesting bowel obstruction. It can also reveal air in peritoneal cavity (pneumoperitoneum) or retroperitoneal space (pneumoretroperitoneum) which can result from bowel perforation. Pneumoperitoneum is classically seen as air/gas under diaphragm, on X-ray abdomen performed in erect position. Similarly, in cases of bowel obstruction multiple air-fluid levels can be seen within dilated bowel loops **(Figs. 27.1A and B)**. Apart from these two major kind of findings it can also reveal various calcifications such as randomly distributed calcified mesenteric nodes, calcified GB stones in right hypochondrium, pancreatic calcifications along course of pancreas usually in cases of chronic calcific pancreatitis, calculi along outline of kidneys, ureters and urinary bladder. Overall sensitivity of radiography is low in evaluation of abdominal diseases; however, it is still commonly performed to look for pneumoperitoneum or bowel obstruction. It is also done to look for position of post-op abdominal drains or catheters and stents.

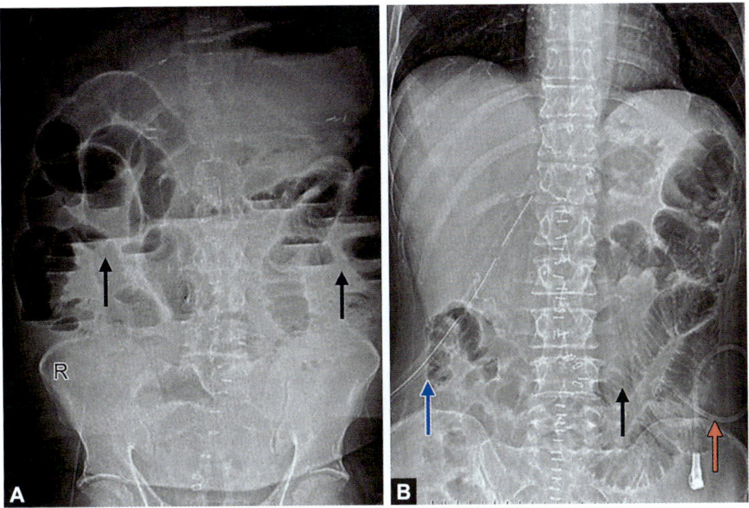

Figs. 27.1A and B: (A) Abdominal radiograph taken in erect position showing dilated small bowel lops with multiple air-fluid levels (black arrows) suggestive of bowel obstruction; (B) Abdominal radiograph taken in supine position showing post-op ileus with few prominent air-filled jejunal loops (black arrow); also surgical drain on right side (blue arrow) and feeding jejunostomy tube on left side (red arrow).

Fluoroscopy

It is low-dose continuous X-ray examination done for few seconds to minutes, usually in pulsed manner to reduce radiation dose. It is kind of functional evaluation of gastrointestinal tract. Traditionally, it has been performed using barium sulfate suspension as positive luminal contrast agent, except for conditions where bowel perforation is suspected. Iodinated water soluble contrast is used where bowel perforation/leakage is suspected or to look for patency of post-op bowel segment (loopogram). Different studies are used for different parts of GI tract, i.e., barium swallow for esophagus, barium meal for stomach, barium meal follow through and enteroclysis for small bowel, and barium enema for large bowel. If with positive oral contrast, air is also used it is referred as double contrast barium study such as double contrast barium enema (DCBE). Double contrast studies are performed to look for fine mucosal details, whereas more commonly performed single contrast studies give details about gross luminal outline/patency and bowel transit time. Barium swallow is usually done in cases of difficulty in swallowing, i.e., dysphagia **(Figs. 27.2A and B)**, while barium meal

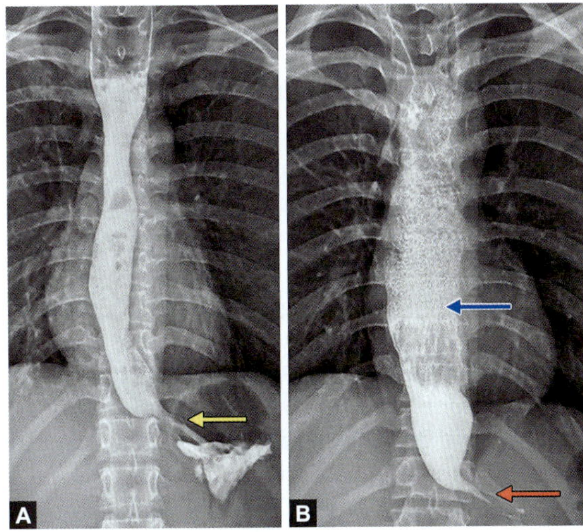

Figs. 27.2A and B: (A) Barium swallow showing normal outline of gastroesophageal junction (yellow arrow); (B) Smooth gradually narrowed GE junction (rat tail appearance; red arrow) with dilated esophagus (blue arrow) in a patient with achalasia cardia.

is performed in cases with suspected peptic ulcer disease/gastric ulcer or chronic gastritis. Gastric ulcers can be benign as well as malignant. Barium meal follow through or enteroclysis is usually indicated in cases of recurrent vomiting, suspected bowel strictures/obstruction, altered bowel habits and recurrent gastrointestinal bleeding. Suspected malrotation is another common indication for small bowel follow through. In cases where bowel perforation, post-op leak, or fistula is suspected water soluble iodinated contrast agent is used in abdominal region.

However, with introduction of CT and further advances in CT technology, number of barium studies have gone down.

Ultrasound

Most commonly used type of ultrasound techniques are B-mode grayscale and color Doppler ultrasound. As far as role of ultrasound is considered in evaluation of GI tract it has limited but important applications, more so in pediatric patient. This modality is easily available, relatively inexpensive and free of radiation risk. It can easily reveal dilated bowel loops and bowel peristalsis (differentiate mechanical and functional obstruction). Thickened bowel loops of different etiologies can be picked up. Acute appendicitis is one of the most common diseases diagnosed on ultrasound as thickened aperistaltic blind ending bowel segment in right iliac fossa. Intussusception is another entity, especially in children, commonly diagnosed in ultrasound. Bowel ascariasis is also readily detected on ultrasound. Other bowel or omentomesenteric pathologies such diverticulitis, omental fat inflammation, epiploic appendicitis, mass lesion can be also suspected and advised for further evaluation. Addition of color Doppler mode may help in further diagnostic yield by revealing vascularity changes in suspected area. Patency of main mesenteric vessels, such as celiac trunk, SMA, SMV and portal vein can be assessed. SMA-SMV relationship is altered in patients with bowel malrotation or volvulus. Mesenteric nodes are easily detected on ultrasound. If patient is of thin or average body built, retroperitoneal nodes (paraaortic, paracaval) can be also detected. Abdominal ultrasound readily detects findings which may be due to bowel disease or other causes. These may include free fluid in peritoneal cavity (ascites) or localized fluid collections or abscesses.

However, there are certain limiting factors for ultrasound. Obesity interferes with transmission of ultrasound waves through tissues and thus leads to suboptimal evaluation. Presence of excessive bowel gases also limits diagnostic yield of ultrasound.

Note: On ultrasonography, abnormalities can be termed as anechoic (appearing dark), hypoechoic (varying grayscale) or hyperechoic (bright).

Computed Tomography (Fig. 27.3)

CT has revolutionized imaging of gastrointestinal diseases, number of requests for fluoroscopic studies are decreasing day by day. It is a cross sectional imaging modality and gives direct evidence of abnormalities or diseases however, fluoroscopy and endoscopic studies give idea of luminal changes or inner lining changes but no definite information about what is going around bowel wall can be inferred. Currently available CT scans readily depict luminal, mural and perienteric, pericolonic or distant extraintestinal changes in scanned area such as lymphadenopathy, ascites, fluid collections, vascular changes, metastasis etc. CT can be used without intravenous (IV) contrast (non-contrast CT) or with intravenous contrast, (CECT) using water soluble iodinated contrast. It can be single portal venous phase study or it can be multiphasic CECT study requiring image acquisition in arterial, portal venous phase and venous phase. CT enterography is CECT abdomen acquired after distending small bowel with neutral oral contrast such as plain drinking water or water mixed with hygroscopic agent such

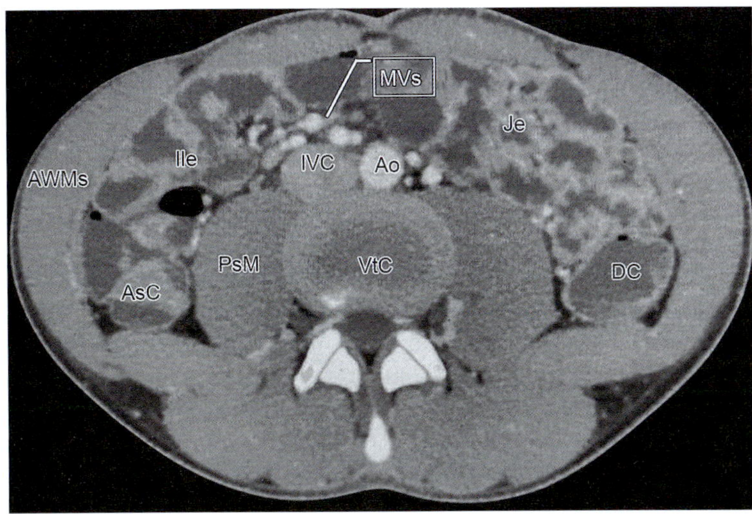

Fig. 27.3: Axial CT section through mid abdomen showing large bowel segments—ascending colon (AsC) and descending colon (DC) in peripheral flank regions, and small bowel loops—jejunum (Je) and ileum (Ile) in central abdomen.

(MVs: Mesenteric vessels; Ao: Abdominal Aorta; IVC: Inferior Vena Cava; VtC: vertebral column at disc level; PsM: Psoas Muscle; AWMs: Abdominal wall muscles).

as polyethylene glycol **(Figs. 27.3 and 27.4)**. CT colonography is obtained after distending large bowel with air insufflate per rectum. It helps in detection of small lesions as well as provide complete colonic examination in cases where obstructive lesions preclude colonoscopy. CT colonography can be done with or without IV contrast.

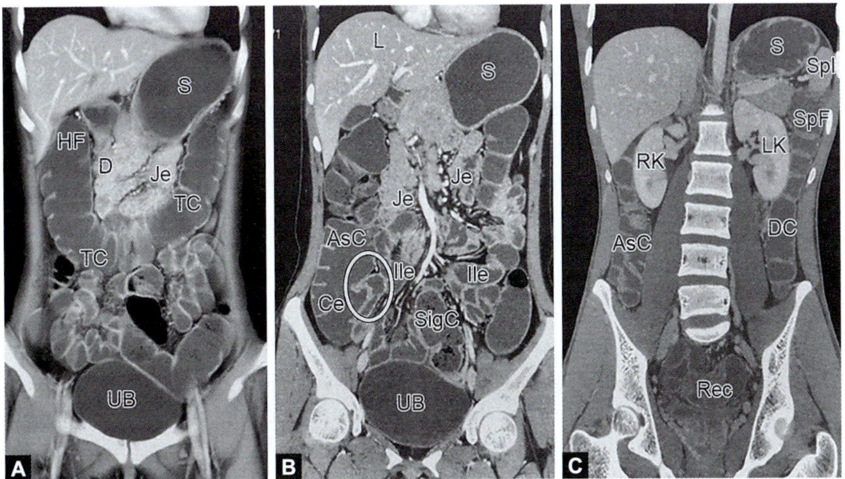

Figs. 27.4A to C: Coronal reformatted images (A-C, anterior to posterior) from CT enterography study depicting different bowel segments with other landmarks/organs.

(L: liver; S: stomach; D: duodenum; Je: jejunum; Ile: ileum; IC junction encircled; Ce: cecum; AsC: ascending colon; HF: hepatic flexure; TC: transverse colon; SpF: splenic flexure; DC: descending colon; SigC: sigmoid colon; Rec: rectum; RK and LK: right and left kidney respectively; UB: urinary bladder).

On CT, bowel diseases most commonly manifest as wall thickening of different types depending on etiologies ranging from inflammatory-infective to neoplastic diseases. Bowel thickening may or may not be accompanied by luminal narrowing. Neoplastic etiologies can also cause polypoid lesions or mass replacing bowel wall. Cause and level of bowel obstruction can be readily identified with CT, as are perienteric or pericolonic extension of disease.

Post-contrast enhancement pattern of bowel wall also helps in characterizing disease process. Increased enhancement of bowel wall can be seen in inflammatory as well as neoplastic disease. Lack of enhancement is feature of bowel ischemia which may result from vascular occlusion.

Lymphadenopathy, mesenteric or retroperitoneal can be easily detected and characterized by CT. Enlarged lymph nodes can be characterized in terms of fatty hilum, calcification, necrosis and enhancement pattern. Loss of fatty hilum is a nonspecific feature; however an enlarged non-necrotic rounded node with loss of fatty hilum is suspicious of malignant etiology, whereas enlarged oval node with maintained fatty hilum is more suggestive of benign etiology. Necrotic nodes can be seen in both infective etiologies (most common cause TB) and malignant etiology. Enlarged homogeneous non-necrotic noncalcified nodes with variably effaced fatty hilum are characteristic of lymphoproliferative disease or lymphoma. Calcification can be seen in lymphomatous nodes after treatment.

Ascites is important accompanying feature of bowel diseases. It's extent is well delineated by CT. It can be accompanied by peritoneal thickening suggesting peritonitis or neoplastic spread which can be more conclusively defined using other imaging criteria (pattern and enhancement of thickening), clinical presentation and cytological analysis.

Bowel disease can be also complicated by entities such as sinus/fistula and bowel perforation. These are most frequently due to TB, inflammatory bowel disease (Crohn's Disease), post-op, post-trauma or cancer. Post-op anastomotic site leakage can be readily detected on CT using water soluble luminal contrast agent (iodinated contrast).

Pneumoperitoneum or bowel obstruction are better defined on CT. Main added advantage of CT over plain radiography in this context is identification of site and cause of bowel perforation or obstruction.

Nowadays, CT scan has become indispensable part of management of wide spectrum of diseases including abdominal/gastrointestinal diseases. Currently, is not possible to imagine optimal management of various diseases whether infection or cancer, without CT scan. CECT is an integral part of staging of various cancers.

Note: Term "density" is CT descriptor. Abnormalities can be termed hypodense, hyperdense or isodense as compared to reference tissue or adjoining normal tissue.

Magnetic Resonance Imaging

Being a comprehensive imaging modality devoid of radiation risk is biggest advantage of MRI. MRI has limited role in evaluation of bowel diseases, partly due to intraluminal contents/air, motion artifacts and bowel peristalsis. These limitations are less in evaluation of pelvic bowel diseases such as evaluation of perianal fistula or diseases of defecation. MR enterography is study performed for evaluation of small bowel diseases. It is done after distending small bowel with plain water or hygroscopic water drink such as polyethylene glycol solution. An intravenous agent such as buscopan may be given to reduce bowel peristalsis and thus associated artifacts. It is most frequently used for evaluation and follow-up of inflammatory bowel diseases especially Crohn's disease. MR fistulogram used for detection of perianal fistulas and further characterization as simple or complex perianal fistulas which define treatment strategies. MR defecography is study done to look for problems of defecation such as chronic constipation or pelvic organ/rectal prolapse. In MRI, signal intensity parameter is used to define changes in organs, i.e., hypointense, hyperintense or isointense. T1-weighted, T2 weighted and post-contrast T1 are most basic sequences of MRI. These sequences along with their modifications and other advanced sequences such as diffusion-weighted imaging and perfusion imaging are used in evaluation.

Catheter Angiography/Digital Subtraction Angiography

These are vascular fluoroscopic studies performed after taking vascular access via common femoral or radial artery, access needles, catheter and guidewires. After gaining access, specific vessel (e.g., Celiac, SMA or IMA in cases with GI bleed or mesenteric ischemia) is cannulated and angiography is performed using water soluble iodinated contrast. Attempts are made to localize abnormalities such as leakage of contrast, abnormal vascularity or vessel stenosis. Since noninvasive modality such as CT angiography has become available, catheter angiography, being an invasive method, is less frequently used solely for diagnostic applications especially in abdominal or other non-neurological indications. Most of the times it is used as part of therapeutic procedure such as embolization or angioplasty.

Nuclear Medicine Studies

Tc-99m labeled red blood cell (RBC) scintigraphy has been used localization of source of occult gastrointestinal bleed. FDG-PET alone or combined with CT (PET-CT) is commonly used in staging and follow-up of cancer. Somatostatin Receptor Scintigraphy also known as DOTANOC (68Ga-DOTA-Nal3) or Octreotide scan is used for detection of neuroendocrine tumors/carcinoid, which may occur at various sites including bowel loops or mesentery.

COMMON DISEASES OF GIT

Disorders of Motility/Peristalsis

One of prime functions of gastrointestinal tract is to allow passage of ingested contents through its various segments (oral cavity to oro-/hypopharynx, esophagus, stomach, small and large bowel) for digestion, absorption, assimilation of contents and finally allow expulsion of residual contents via anal canal.

This transit of luminal contents is facilitated by intramural neural plexuses, integrity of muscularis propria, and luminal integrity/patency. Disease affecting any of these contributors will negatively affect bowel motility and transit of luminal contents.

Primary Motility Disorders

These result from functional disturbances (esophageal spasm-uncoordinated peristalsis) or structural dysfunction of intramural neural plexuses (achalasia cardia and Hirschsprung's disease resulting from hypoplasia or aplasia of intramural plexus); or muscle layer weakness (scleroderma—a connective tissue disorder).

Secondary Motility Disorders

These result from lesions destroying intramural plexus or affecting its gross morphology (outline and luminal integrity), or course and position of bowel segments. All of the acquired diseases of bowel to some extent affect bowel motility. However, clinically significant motility disturbances result from when the lesion is causing fixed luminal narrowing/stricture formation. Mild bowel thickening or small polypoid lesion is unlikely to cause any significant motility disturbance.

Ileus is motility disorder which may result from acute inflammatory changes or prolonged immobilization of patient, and is not secondary to mechanical obstruction.

Barium fluoroscopic studies are still used in patients suspected of motility diseases, except cases of severe small/large bowel obstruction. Barium swallow study is commonly performed in cases of dysphagia, with timed barium swallow study dedicated for evaluation motility disorders such as achalasia cardia. Barium meal follow through study helps in assessing time taken in transit of contents form stomach through small bowel to ileocecal junction. In motility disorders other tests are also used such as colonic transit time study and gut manometry.

Disorders of Position and Formation

These include abnormal positions of bowel loops in abdomen-pelvic region, most common being malrotation of bowel loops. In complete malrotation duodenum does not cross midline, DJ junction lies on right side and IC junction may be seen on left side of abdomen. Malrotation predisposes to small bowel/mid gut volvulus presenting as bowel obstruction. Reversal in position of bowel segments can be also part of situs inversus totalis; however, here bowel segments are not malrotated, rather transposed.

Disorders of formation included abnormally formed or undeveloped segment of gastrointestinal tract. These included esophageal atresia with or without TEF, microgastria, small bowel atresia and microcolon.

Other congenital anomalies included idiopathic hypertrophic pyloric stenosis and duodenal webs. These both conditions present as upper GI obstruction.

Disorders of position and formation are readily detected on contrast/barium fluoroscopic studies and computed tomography; can be also detected on MR enterography. Ultrasound is imaging modality of choice in patients suspected of idiopathic hypertrophic pyloric stenosis.

Inflammatory-Infective Diseases

Inflammatory diseases of GI tract can be due to infections (tubercular and nontubercular infective enterocolitis) or noninfective conditions (Crohn's disease, ulcerative colitis). In both groups, there is variable degree of thickening of bowel segments with maintained layered architecture of bowel wall (mucosa, submucosa, muscularis and serosal layer) in uncomplicated cases. In complicated cases, there may be loss of normal layered architecture, bowel 'stricture and perforation. Imaging features overlap, and many times it may be difficult to differentiate infective from noninfective inflammatory thickening of bowel loops. **(Figs. 27.5 and 27.6)** Associated necrotic lymphadenopathy is characteristic of tuberculosis, and it helps to differentiate it from Crohn's Disease.

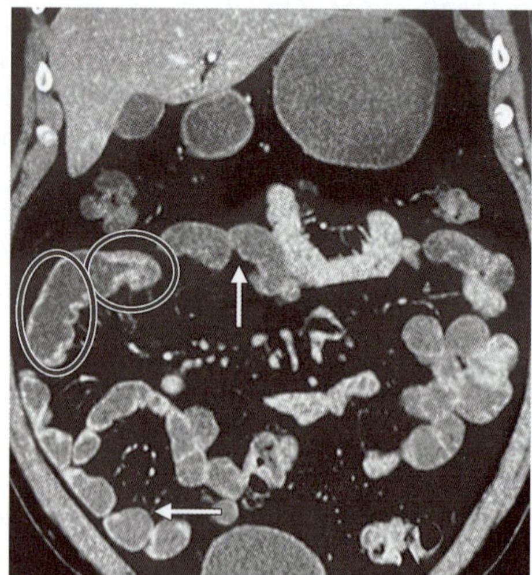

Fig. 27.5: Coronal reformatted image from CECT abdomen study showing mild variably thickened enhancing ileal segment (encircled) possibly due to inflammatory etiology. Normal ileal segments can be appreciated in vicinity (white arrows).

Appendicitis is characterized by thickened blind ending bowel segment extending from cecum in right iliac fossa.

These diseases can be suspected and diagnosed on ultrasound, however CECT or CT enterography

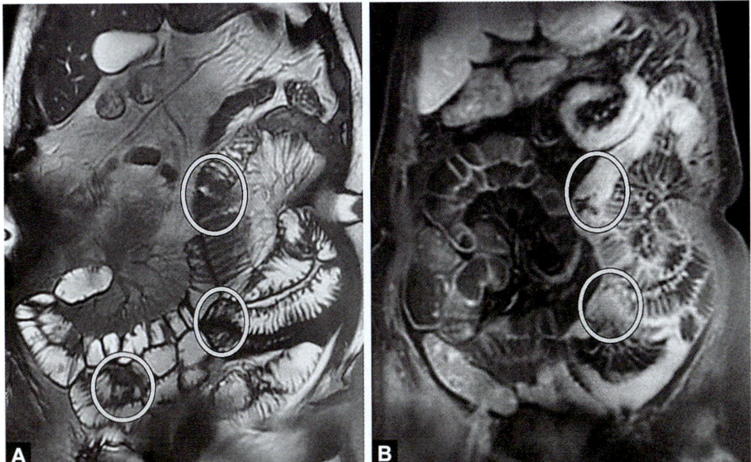

Figs. 27.6A and B: MR enterography study: coronal T2W/FIESTA. (A) and post-contrast T1; (B) Images showing multifocal short segment thickening of jejunal and ileal segments (encircled) in a probable case of Crohn's disease. Enhancement of thickened segments can be appreciated on one of given representative post-contrast T1 images (B).

provides most comprehensive evaluation and serves as problem-solving tool in difficult cases. Similarly, optimally done MR enterography is almost as good as CT enterography but availability, cost and artifacts are limiting factors.

Neoplastic Disease

Neoplastic lesions of gastrointestinal tract can be seen as asymmetric mural thickening, mass replacing part of gut wall or intraluminal polyps. **(Figs. 27.7A and B)** All these morphological types in advanced stage lead to altered bowel habits, bowel obstruction and bleeding. Various types of malignant tumors of gastrointestinal tract are adenocarcinoma, neuroendocrine tumors/carcinoid and lymphoma. In early stages, differentiation from infective-inflammatory pathologies may be difficult alone on imaging studies. Benign neoplasms are uncommon, most common of these being submucosal lipoma and leiomyoma.

Vascular Lesions: Ischemia

Mesenteric arterial or venous occlusion due to thromboembolic diseases lead to bowel ischemia and abdominal pain. CT Angiography with enterography is imaging modality of choice in these cases. Thickened nonenhancing bowel loops indicate nonviable segment requiring surgery. Vascular malformations such as AV malformations, telangiectasias and varices lead to bleeding, while lymphangiectasias lead to malabsorption syndrome. These can be also detected on CT angiography with enterography.

Bowel Obstruction

Mechanical bowel obstruction results from narrowing of bowel lumen. This luminal narrowing may result from varied causes such as infective-inflammatory diseases, mass lesions, adhesions or malrotation. Bowel obstruction can be detected on plain radiograph of abdomen (erect and supine position). Abdominal radiograph will show dilated bowel loops, with radiograph taken in erect position also showing air fluid levels. Contrast enhanced CT or CT enterography helps in define exact level of bowel obstruction and possible cause of obstruction. Contrast fluoroscopic

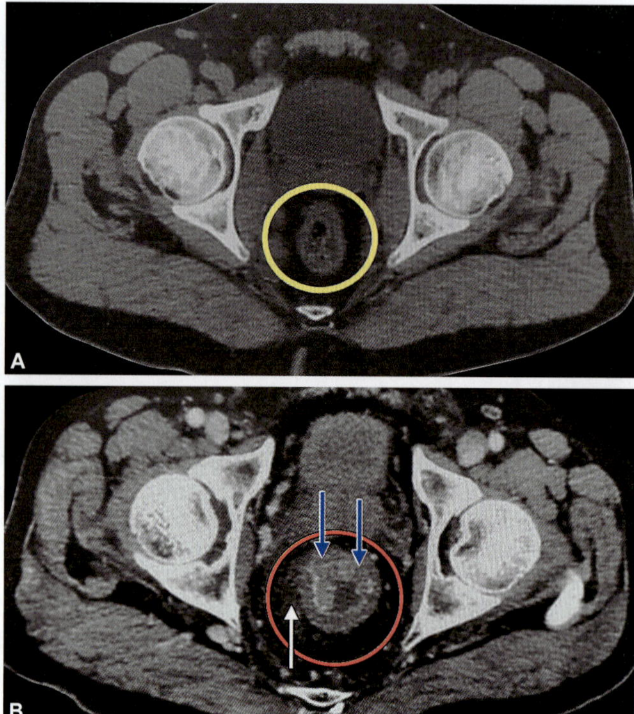

Figs. 27.7A and B: Axial CECT images through lower pelvis showing (A) Normal lower rectum with clear perirectal fat [encircled in yellow]; and (B) Asymmetrically thickened enhancing rectal wall [blue arrows] with perirectal/mesorectal fat stranding [white arrow] in case of carcinoma rectum (encircled in red).

studies of can also detect level of obstruction however, should be avoided if bowel obstruction is severe. In cases of suspected bowel obstruction, if contrast fluoroscopic study is to be performed it should be performed with diluted water soluble iodinated contrast and not barium sulfate suspension. Overall, CECT (enterography or colonography protocol as required) is imaging modality of choice in patients with bowel obstruction.

Malabsorption Syndrome

Impaired absorptive function of bowel may result from any disease affecting luminal or mural integrity of bowel. If the disease is focal, malabsorption may not be clinically significant. However, if disease is involving long segment of bowel it would cause clinically significant malabsorption which might manifest as weight loss and chronic diarrhea. Apart from common infective-inflammatory diseases (various forms chronic enterocolitis), other causes of malabsorption syndrome primarily affecting bowel wall include celiac sprue, Whipple disease and intestinal lymphangiectasia. Lack of enzymes may also lead to malabsorption syndrome such as seen in patients with chronic pancreatic insufficiency.

Contrast fluoroscopic studies such as barium meal follow through or barium enteroclysis still hold importance in evaluation of malabsorption syndrome. Certain findings such as diffuse effacement of small bowel mucosal folds, flattening and irregularity of mucosal folds, visualization of jejunum like mucosal folds in ileum, and flocculation of barium contrast are characteristic of malabsorption syndrome, though nonspecific. Further evaluation with CT enterography may help in defining the cause. Often, in addition to imaging other clinical and laboratory tests are required to establish the cause of malabsorption syndrome.

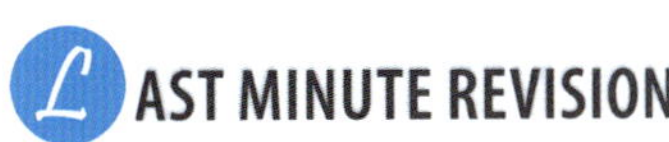

- Plain radiography is essential for initial evaluation in acute abdominal conditions such as bowel obstruction and pneumoperitoneum.
- Fluoroscopy is utilized for dynamic functional evaluation of the gastrointestinal tract using barium or iodinated contrast.
- Ultrasound is particularly useful in pediatric patients and for conditions like acute appendicitis, intussusception, and detecting thickened bowel loops.
- Computed tomography (CT) is go-to modality for comprehensive evaluation of abdominal and gastrointestinal diseases. CT can identify bowel wall thickening, obstruction, perforation, and detect associated lymphadenopathy and ascites. It is also crucial for staging cancers and detecting metastasis.
- MR enterography is used for inflammatory bowel diseases like Crohn's disease, and MR defecography for evaluating pelvic floor disorders.

REVIEW QUESTIONS

Multiple Choice Questions (MCQs)

1. **Following used in evaluation of motility disorder:**
   a. Gut manometry
   b. Barium swallow
   c. Barium meal follow through
   d. All of above
2. **Imaging modality of choice in patients with small bowel obstruction:**
   a. CECT abdomen/CT enterography
   b. MR enterography
   c. Barium meal follow through
   d. Barium enteroclysis
3. **True about tuberculosis and Crohn's disease of GI tract:**
   a. IC junction involvement is not seen in Crohn's disease
   b. Necrotic lymphadenopathy is a common feature of Crohn's disease
   c. Tubercular enteritis can be easily differentiated from Crohn's enteritis using MR enterography
   d. Contrast enhancement pattern of bowel may help in determining disease activity in enteritis.
4. **Features of Malabsorption syndrome:**
   a. Jejunization of ileal loops
   b. Flattened mucosal folds
   c. Flocculation of barium contrast
   d. All of above
5. **True about bowel perforation:**
   a. Pneumoperitoneum on abdominal radiograph
   b. CT can help define level of bowel perforation using diluted water-soluble iodinated contrast as oral contrast
   c. Cause of bowel perforation can be identified on CECT
   d. All of above

Answer Key

1. d 2. a 3. d 4. d 5. d

SUGGESTED READING

1. Guglielmo FF, Anupindi SA, Fletcher JG, Al-Hawary MM, Dillman JR, Grand DJ, et al. Small Bowel Crohn Disease at CT and MR Enterography: Imaging Atlas and Glossary of Terms. Radiographics. 2020;40(2):354-375.
2. Joshi AR, Basantani AS, Patel TC. Role of CT and MRI in Abdominal Tuberculosis. Curr Radiol Rep. 2014; 2:66.
3. Macari M, Balthazar EJ. CT of bowel wall thickening: significance and pitfalls of interpretation. AJR Am J Roentgenol. 2001;176(5):1105-16.
4. Richard M. Gore, Marc S. Levine. Textbook of Gastrointestinal Radiology, 5th edition. Elsevier; 2021.
5. Shalom NE, Gong GX, Auster M. Fluoroscopy: An essential diagnostic modality in the age of high-resolution cross-sectional imaging. World J Radiol. 2020;12(10):213-230.

CHAPTER

28 Hepatobiliary and Pancreatic Imaging

"In the complexity of hepatobiliary imaging, radiologists bring direction, diagnosis, and decisions to the forefront."

LIVER

EMBRYOLOGY

The liver is formed from an endodermal bud, which arises from ventral aspect of gut at the junction of the foregut and midgut. Then this bud expands within the ventral mesogastrium and proceeds through it into the septum transversum. Its size gets increased and divided into two parts larger cranial part called as pars hepatica (which forms liver) and pars cystica (which forms gallbladder and cystic duct). Pars hepatica gets divided into two parts right and left, each of which forms one lobe of the liver.

Endodermal cell of hepatic bud give rise to bile capillaries and liver parenchyma, capsule and fibrous tissue are formed by mesoderm of septum transversum.

ANATOMY

The liver is the largest gland of body situated in the right upper quadrant occupying the whole right hypochondrium, greater part of epigastrium, and extends into left hypochondrium. It lies mostly under costal cartilages and ribs just below diaphragm. The upper boundary extends to the xiphisternal joint level. Its distinct lower edge intersects the midline at the transpyloric plane level. It is a wedge-shaped, four-sided pyramid with two surfaces, diaphragmatic and visceral surfaces and one inferior border. The visceral surface is covered by the peritoneum except at the fossa for gallbladder and the porta hepatis **(Fig. 28.1)**.

Blood Supply

The liver receives oxygenated arterial blood from the hepatic artery (20%) and nutrient-rich venous blood from the portal vein (80%). In a typical adult lying down, approximately one-third of the cardiac output flows through the liver.

Hepatic Segments

Based on the intrahepatic distribution of the hepatic artery, portal vein, and biliary ducts, the liver can be categorized into right and left functional lobes. The right lobe further divides into anterior and posterior segments, while the left lobe divides into medial and lateral segments. Each segment further divides into upper and lower parts, resulting in a total of eight segments **(Fig. 28.2)**.

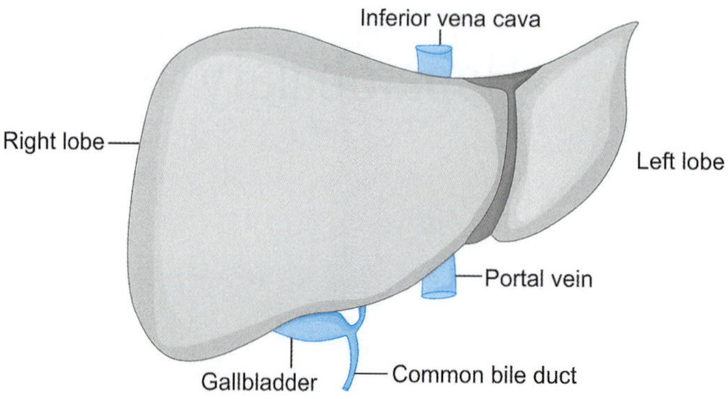

Fig. 28.1: Anatomical lobes of liver.

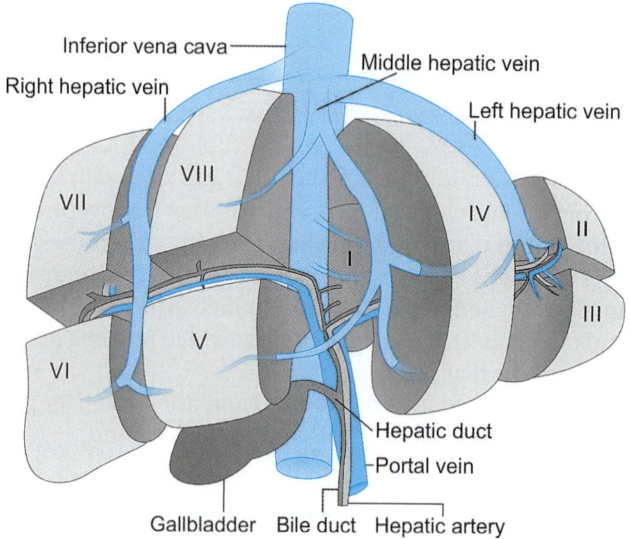

Fig. 28.2: Functional segments of liver.

BILIARY APPARATUS

Biliary apparatus **(Fig. 28.3)** consists of right and left hepatic duct (HD), Common hepatic duct (CHD), Gallbladder (GB), Cystic duct, Bile duct (CBD). Both right and left hepatic ducts emerge at the porta hepatis from both right and left lobes of the liver. They join to form common hepatic duct near the right end of porta hepatis, it is 3 cm long and goes downward and join to cystic duct to form bile duct at an acute angle.

Gallbladder is reservoir of bile situated in fossa of inferior surface of right lobe. It is pear-shaped and divided into three parts, fundus, body and neck. **Fundus** can be seen beyond inferior border of the liver and entirely surrounded by the peritoneum. **Body** lies in the fossa for the gallbladder on the inferior surface of liver. Upper end of body is narrow and continue as neck of gallbladder which is devoid of peritoneum. **Neck** lies at the right end of the porta hepatis. The posteromedial wall of the neck is dilated outward to form pouch called Hartmann's pouch (which is gallstone prone).

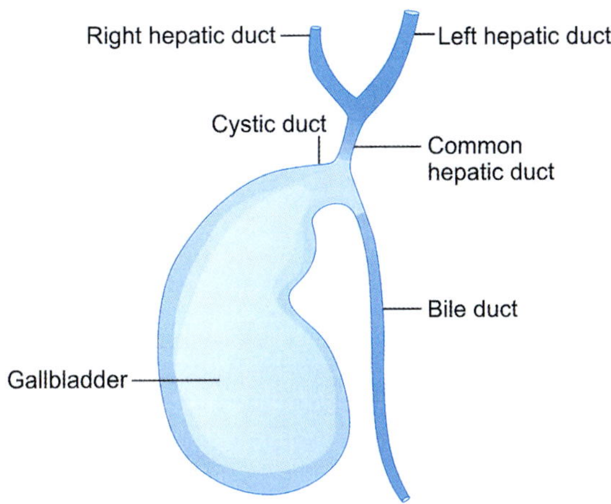

Fig. 28.3: Anatomy of biliary apparatus.

Cystic duct is 3–4 cm long, arises from neck of gallbladder, runs downward, posteriorly and to the left and finally join common hepatic duct at acute angle and forms common bile duct.

Bile duct is 8 cm long and diameter is 6 mm. At the middle of left side of second part of duodenum, it comes in contact with pancreatic duct and accompanies it through the wall of duodenum, and opens at ampulla of Vater.

PANCREAS

EMBRYOLOGY

The pancreas develops from two endodermal buds: dorsal and ventral. The ventral bud arises near the hepatic bud, while the dorsal bud emerges from the gut's dorsal aspect. As the duodenal loop shifts, their positions change, resulting in their fusion to form the pancreas. The ventral bud forms the lower part of the head and the uncinate process, while the dorsal bud forms the upper part of the head, body, and tail.

ANATOMY

The pancreas is a soft, elongated gland with lobulated structure. It secretes pancreatic juice (exocrine function) and hormones insulin and glucagon (endocrine function). It is positioned horizontally on the posterior abdominal wall in the epigastric and left hypochondriac regions. It extends diagonally from the duodenal concavity to the spleen's hilum, aligning with the T12–L3 vertebrae level **(Fig. 28.4)**.

Blood Supply

Arteria pancreatica magna and arteria caudae pancreatis (pancreatic branches of splenic artery).

IMAGING TECHNIQUES

Radiologically, liver is imaged by a variety of techniques ranging from conventional plain radiograph, cholangiography, ultrasound, radionuclide scanning, computed tomography (CT) and magnetic resonance imaging (MRI), positron emission tomography (PET) and certain diagnostic angiographic methods.

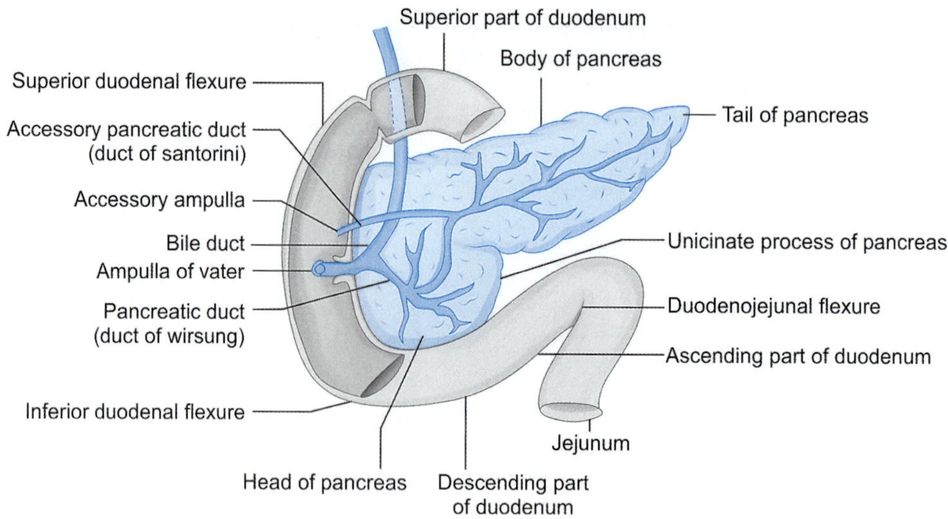

Fig. 28.4: Anatomy of pancreas.

Plain Radiograph

It is often performed as a first line investigation in any patient who presents with abdominal pain. This has superseded by ultrasound with ease of performance and wide availability. Plain radiograph helps us to identify abnormal calcification or air in the biliary tree region. Enlargement of the liver can often be made out on plain radiographs as well.

Although majority of the gall stones are radiolucent, but approximately 20–30% of the gall stones give radiopacities and can be identified on plain X-ray. They often show intervening gas containing fissures in between (Mercedes Benz sign). Mulberry stones which are denser contains predominantly calcium carbonate.

Limy bile is another entity which can be identified as dense bile on X-ray which is predominantly seen in intensive care unit patients who are on parenteral nutrition. Rarely the gallbladder wall may undergo calcification pertaining to chronic inflammatory changes leading to porcelain gallbladder, which predisposes to malignant change.

Diabetics and immunocompromised patients can develop emphysematous cholecystitis which appears as rim of radiolucency surrounding gallbladder on plain radiograph. Apart from that, any old healed granulomatous lesion, hydatid cyst, chronic liver abscess, certain tumoral calcifications can be seen in right hypochondrium.

Calcification in the epigastric region can help us to delineate chronic pancreatitis in alcoholics.

Contrast Radiography

There are certain indirect methods through which the hepatobiliary system can be identified with radiopaque contrast like, oral cholecystography, percutaneous cholecystography, intravenous cholecystography (less commonly done due to advanced techniques like MRCP, CT), special T tube cholangiography (done postsurgery like choledocholithotomy) and endoscopic retrograde cholangiopancreatography.

Oral cholecystography is performed by administration of an oral dye sodium or calcium ipodate which is then absorbed from the gut and then reaches the liver through the portal system and then it is excreted through bile back into the bowel and the enterohepatic circulation continues. Thereafter, X-rays are taken to view the biliary system. Non-visualization of the gallbladder can be due to acute cholecystitis. It is to be kept in mind that any abnormality in above process and malabsorption will lead to wrong findings.

Similarly, percutaneous cholecystography is performed using dye (Ioglycamide) which is administered into the biliary tree using the fine gauge Chiba needle (20–22 G) under fluoroscopic or ultrasound guidance and then X-rays are taken, it can help us to identify the cause and level of biliary obstruction, patency of biliary systems after certain surgeries like Roux-en-Y, hepatojejunostomy, portoenterostomy. The level of biliary leaks can be identified along with the biliary-enteric or biliary-cutaneous fistulas. Lastly, it can help us to delineate whole of the biliary anatomy so certain interventional procedures like PTBD (percutaneous transhepatic biliary drainage) can be performed.

ERCP has an advantage of being a therapeutic procedure along with a diagnostic one and can be performed endoscopically, it carries an additional advantage of visualization of the pancreatic ductal system along with the biliary tree. ERCP is widely done to diagnose choledocholithiasis along with removal of stones by sphincterotomy. The disadvantage of ERCP is that it cannot be performed if the patient has undergone hepatojejunostomy or there is duodenal obstruction secondary to carcinoma head of pancreas.

Ultrasound

It is routinely performed for liver and pancreatic diseases as it does not carry any radiation harm, is widely available and cheap. Ultrasound is one the primary investigations in settings of acute pain abdomen. It is performed using a 3–5 MHz transducer in both the subcostal and intercostal planes to scan the full volume of the organ. Normal liver parenchyma appears as solid homogenous echotexture with short dots or lines within because of the portal and biliary radicals.

Along with B-mode scanning, color Doppler is also performed to visualize the blood-flow in the hepatic and portal radicals. Color Doppler study also finds its use in identifying the vascular supply to the tumor in cases of hepatic masses.

Nowadays, normal ultrasound is also coupled with the use of ultrasound contrast media (Sonovue/Levovist) which consist of microbubbles and result in the increased backscatter of blood which can help in the assessment of tumor vascularity. Ultrasound also helps us to identify the composition of the lesion (solid or cystic), areas of calcification, heterogeneity and posterior acoustic enhancement or shadowing. In the recent times, intraoperative ultrasound has also come into play with the use of ultrasound in operation theaters for the transplant surgeries in which any presence of collateral vessels on ultrasound should be accurately documented to give an overview of complete vascular anatomy so that surgeon can anastomose vessels accurately, also vessel patency can be easily assessed postoperatively.

USG elastography helps to assess liver stiffness and fat quantification which aids in early diagnosis of liver parenchymal changes in fatty liver.

Computed Tomography

Multidetector CT (MDCT) represents a breakthrough in CT technology. It has transformed CT from a transaxial cross-sectional technique into a true 3D imaging modality that allows for arbitrary cut planes as well as excellent 3D displays of the data volume. Multislice CT scanners provide a huge gain in performance that can be used to reduce scan time, to reduce section collimation, or to increase scan length substantially. The use of iodinated contrast media has also improved the sensitivity and specificity of the CT in identifying the pathologies. There is a set protocol of triple phase contrast assessment of liver SOLs which includes arterial (15–30 seconds post bolus trigger), portal venous (60–75 seconds postinjection) and delayed phase (2–5 minutes) of the contrast excretion and simultaneous assessment of the lesion. The portal vein accounts for ~75–80% of the liver's blood supply with the remainder from the hepatic artery, so late arterial phase is required for the best enhancement of the parenchyma.

Periampullary region could also be well evaluated for any mass or any ongoing chronic inflammatory process. The difference in the Hounsfield units (HU) of the various tissues can help in characterizing the components within the lesion and thus better diagnostic accuracy can be established.

Magnetic Resonance Imaging

Abdominal MRI is limited because of two major factors, i.e., motion artifacts from respiration and peristalsis. However, due to advent of breath hold imaging techniques has largely overcome the former problem. A basic liver examination will require T1 and T2 W images. Flow and pulsation artifacts can be reduced by using motion compensation, (e.g., gradient moment nulling) or presaturation bands above and below the liver. A phased array body coil should be used to improve images.

Fat suppression imaging techniques are also used so as to allow increased dynamic range of signals from the tissue of interest, so that liver lesion contrast and gadolinium enhancement effects are magnified.

Most of the patients presenting to us nowadays have fatty liver and chemical shift imaging can help us to quantify with the combination of in-phase and out-phase GRE (gradient echo sequences) images. Water and fat signals are additive in in-phase images and tend to cancel out each other in out-phase images.

Gadolinium enhancement images are taken by dynamic GRE T1 images following intravenous injection of gadolinium chelate agent and helps in characterizing a liver lesion. A hybrid technique using a time-of-flight (TOF) MR angiography (MRA) method with gadolinium enhancement may have further advantages. Certain contrast agents have their excretion from hepatobiliary route, like, gadobenate dimeglumine, gadoxetic acid and magnafodipir. Superparamagnetic iron oxide (SPIO) particles are selectively taken up by reticuloendothelial cells in liver, spleen and bone marrow and help us to diagnose by markedly decreasing the T2* values.

Magnetic resonance cholangiopancreatography (MRCP) is another method of demonstration the biliary and pancreatic ducts by MRI which uses heavily T2 W images to visualize the biliary tree. Gastric and duodenal contents should be excluded from the imaging volume as far as possible. Any strictures, abnormal dilatations and calculi can be easily identified within these ducts, also abnormal pancreatobiliary confluence and variant anatomy could be studied.

Magnetic resonance elastography (MRE) is a noninvasive imaging technique that has become increasingly important in the assessment of liver disease, particularly in the staging of liver fibrosis and to assess disease progression or regression in response to treatment but its high cost, technical limitation (iron overload) and limited availability restrict its clinical use.

Angiography (DSA)

Although with the advent of CT and MR angiographic techniques, the role of direct hepatic angiography has largely been reduced. It is used in the preoperative assessment of the patency of the hepatic and portal veins. After delivering the contrast into the vessel of interest, X-ray images are taken. Any variant anatomy can be identified and be taken into consideration. It helps us to plan the access point and plan the path of radioembolization and is performed approximately 1–3 weeks prior to radioembolization.

Radionuclide Imaging Techniques

Hepatocytes in the liver parenchyma are crucial cells which synthesize and excrete a variety of substances in the body. Kupffer cells in the liver parenchyma have reticuloendothelial system. Radiopharmaceuticals based on iminodiacetic acid (IDA) are readily taken up by normal functioning hepatocytes and are excreted unchanged in bile and thus help us to study liver function. Beside this number of Tc^{99m}-labeled tracers are used to evaluate the functions of the hepatocytes and Kupffer cells.

Positron emission tomography (PET) is based on identification of molecular biologic changes, as tumors are metabolically distinct from normal tissue, their detectability on PET may be independent of their structural changes, although for anatomical localization, PET is often paired with low dose computed tomography (CT) as a hybrid anatomical and metabolic imaging technique. Because PET tracers have little if any pharmacologic side effects, PET can safely provide biologic information about hepatobiliary and pancreatic tumors without the complications associated with other diagnostic interventions. Neuroendocrine tumors of the pancreas can be identified using somatostatin-receptor scintigraphy (SRS) and octreotide scans.

Interventional Techniques

In recent times there has been a marked increase in the number of interventions done by interventional radiologists, since most of the procedures are day care and there is no large surgical cuts and stitches involved, patients are favoring these therapeutic methods. Certain palliative measures like percutaneous transhepatic biliary drainage (PTBD) procedures have found to be effective in improving the quality of life of patients with high staged, nonresectable tumors. In this interventional procedure, access is being made to the right or left hepatic drainage system using a thin gauge Chiba/lumbar puncture needle and hydrophilic guidewires are then used to sustain the access site and then under fluoroscopic guidance drainage catheter is placed into the biliary system for the external or external-internal drainage of bile. It helps the patients to get relieved of their cholangitis due to prolonged stasis of bile, hence improving patient outcome.

COMMON ANATOMICAL VARIANTS AND CONGENITAL ANOMALIES

Agenesis and Hypoplasia of the Hepatic Lobe or Segment

Agenesis is a complete absence of hepatic lobe or segment whereas in hypoplasia size of the hepatic lobe or segment is small which is otherwise normal. Most commonly involved segments are the anterior segment of right lobe and medial segment (segment IV). In case of agenesis, there is absence of lobar or segmental vessel whereas in case of acquired atrophy (due to cirrhosis, biliary obstruction, postsurgical resection, etc.), one of these structures is detected. Diagnosed by CECT.

Reidel's Lobe

Reidel's lobe is downward tongue like projection from anterior aspect of the right hepatic lobe. It is one of the causes of right sided abdominal palpable masses and may cause acute or intermittent abdominal pain if it is complicated by torsion. Diagnosis is done on USG.

Biliary Anatomic Variants

The right posterior duct is most anomalous insertion site. The anomalous right posterior duct drains into left hepatic duct before its confluence with the right anterior duct, known as ***Crossover anomaly***.

The ***trifurcation or triple confluence*** is another common variant of the biliary system characterized by simultaneous emptying of the right posterior duct, right anterior duct and left hepatic duct in common hepatic duct to form a trifurcation.

The ***low insertion of cystic duct*** in which the cystic duct fuses with the distal third of the extrahepatic bile duct, is the most common variant of cystic duct anomaly.

The ***medial cystic duct insertion*** is characterized by cystic duct draining into the left side of common hepatic duct.

All these are diagnosed, on the basis of MRCP.

Choledochal Cyst

It is rare cystic dilatation of biliary tree. More in common in females. Choledochal cyst is usually diagnosed in children with the classical triad of obstructive jaundice, right upper quadrant pain and palpable mass. In adults the most common symptom is chronic relapsing cholangitis and jaundice. Choledochal cysts are frequently associated with cholangiocarcinoma and gallbladder carcinoma.

Todani Classification of Choledochal Cyst (Figs. 28.5A to F)

- **Type I:** Fusiform dilatation of the common bile duct (most common)
- **Type II:** Localized diverticulum originating from common bile duct or common hepatic duct
- **Type III:** Also known as choledochocele, is protrusion of focally dilated intramural segment of the distal common bile duct into the duodenum.

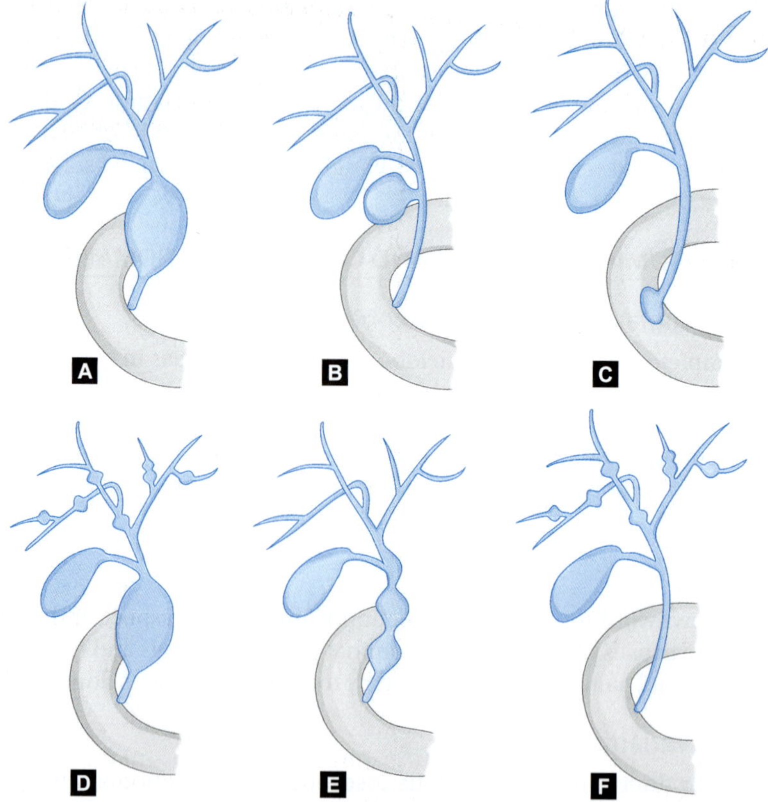

Figs. 28.5A to F: Illustration of Todani classification of choledochal cyst.

- **Type IVa:** Saccular dilatation involving both common bile duct and intrahepatic bile ducts.
- **Type IVb:** Multiple cystic dilatations involving only extrahepatic bile duct
- **Type V:** Cystic dilatation of intrahepatic bile ducts only (Carolis disease)

Phrygian Cap

It is the most common abnormality of gallbladder shape and presents as a fold or septum between the body and fundus of gallbladder **(Fig. 28.6)**.

The ***gallbladder may be intrahepatic*** in which it is attached to the liver by short portal veins and bile ducts (of Luschka).

Agenesis of gallbladder occurs due to a defect in the development of gallbladder bud that arises from caudal portion of the hepatic bud.

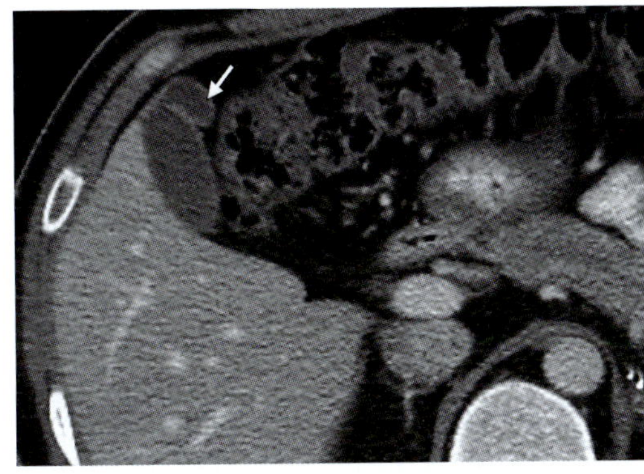

Fig. 28.6: Phrygian cap of the gallbladder.

Pancreas Divisum

It is the most common congenital anomaly of pancreatic ductal system and is characterized by failure of fusion of ventral and dorsal pancreatic ducts during embryological development. The majority of pancreatic secretions empty into minor papilla through duct of Santorini whereas duct of Wirsung and common bile duct drain normally into major papilla **(Fig. 28.7)**.

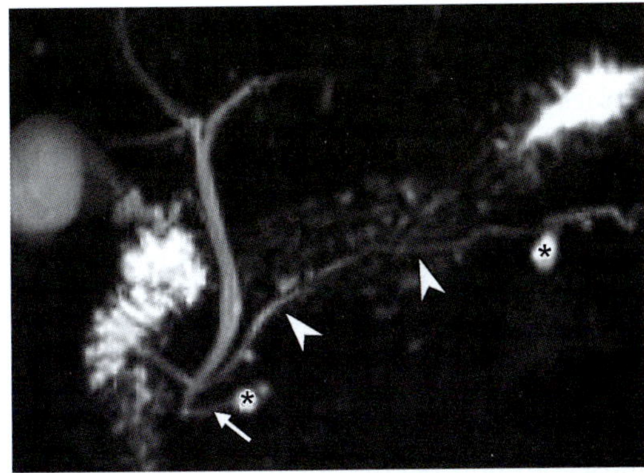

Fig. 28.7: MRCP shows that dorsal pancreatic duct (arrowheads) continues with the duct of Santorini, which drains in the minor papilla and the distal CBD joins the duct of Wirsung (arrow) and drains into major papilla.

Annular Pancreas

It is a rare congenital anomaly in which a band of pancreatic tissue encircles the second part of duodenum either completely or incompletely. It typically presents in neonates with gastrointestinal or bile duct obstruction in association with pancreatitis. Typical radiologic sign of ***"Double bubble" appearance is seen on radiograph***.

BENIGN HEPATOBILIARY DISEASES

Fatty Liver

Fatty liver comprises a variety of conditions including simple hepatic steatosis and steatohepatitis of various causes such as toxic, ischemic and metabolic liver injuries. On ultrasound, normal liver parenchyma shows almost similar echogenicity as renal cortex whereas in fatty liver the echogenicity is increased.

On CT, fatty liver shows decreased attenuation than spleen whereas normal liver parenchyma shows higher attenuation than that of spleen. On MRI chemical shift imaging is done to detect small amount of fatty infiltration of liver parenchyma by providing in-phase and opposed-phase imaging. Normal liver shows higher signal intensity on both in-phase and opposed phase images than that of spleen whereas in fatty liver there is a significant signal drop on opposed phase image than on in-phase image.

Hepatitis

Hepatitis is defined as inflammation of liver parenchyma caused by viral, fungal, bacterial and exogenous toxic agents.

In *acute* ***hepatitis*** imaging is done to exclude other underlying diseases such as biliary obstruction, focal liver lesions or chronic liver disease. On ultrasound, normal findings are more frequently encountered but in severe acute hepatitis liver and spleen may be enlarged and the liver parenchymal echogenicity may decrease than renal echogenicity and portal venule may be prominent due to parenchymal edema. The gallbladder wall may also appear edematous.

In ***chronic hepatitis*** liver shows increased and coarse parenchymal echogenicity with loss of mural definition of portal veins on ultrasound.

Liver Cirrhosis

Liver cirrhosis is the terminal stage of chronic liver disease, which is characterized by fibrosis and multiple regenerative and dysplastic nodules. There is nodularity of liver surface and atrophy of right lobe and quadrate lobe and enlargement of left lateral segment and caudate lobe. Consequently, portal hypertension develops, and main portal vein diameter exceeds 13 mm. Portal hypertension leads to splenomegaly, ascites and bowel wall edema. Multiple paraesophageal, left gastric, gastrorenal, splenorenal, paraumbilical, mesenteric portosystemic collaterals are also noted.

Alcoholic Liver Disease

It is a spectrum which consists of fatty liver, alcoholic hepatitis and cirrhosis. Liver may be enlarged in early disease, and it becomes atrophic as cirrhosis progresses.

Pyogenic Liver Abscess

Pyogenic/bacterial liver abscess can develop via five routes: (1) ***Biliary route*** which is the most common, occurs due to ascending cholangitis from biliary obstruction. (2) ***Portal venous route,*** due to pylephlebitis from appendicitis, diverticulitis and inflammatory bowel disease. (3) ***Hepatic arterial route*** from septicemia. (4) ***Direct extension*** from contiguous organ infection. (5) ***Traumatic route*** from blunt or penetrating injuries. *Escherichia coli* is most common organism. On imaging in early stages, the abscess has an ill-defined margin and usually appear as a cluster of small microabscesses that coalesce focally. During evolution the abscess cavity appears as unilocular or multilocular cystic lesion filled with thick and purulent material and lined by fibrous tissue. On CT "cluster *sign"* is seen in which small abscesses appear to cluster and coalesce into a single large abscess cavity and "Double *target sign"* which represents hypodense central abscess cavity surrounded by an inner hyperdense ring and an outer hypodense zone **(Fig. 28.8)**.

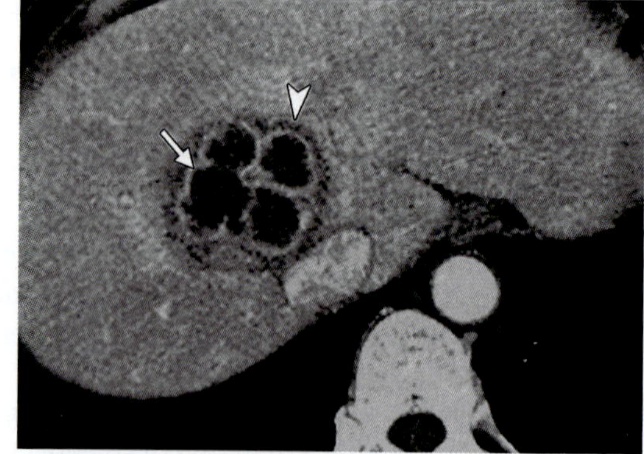

Fig. 28.8: Pyogenic hepatic abscess with double target sign.

Hydatid Disease

Hydatid disease is caused by *Echinococcus granulosus* or less commonly by *Echinococcus multilocularis.* They are usually asymptomatic or may cause abdominal pain, hepatosplenomegaly and jaundice when large.

On abdominal radiograph it may present as ring like or curvilinear calcification. On ultrasound hydatid cyst may appear as (1) a multiseptated cyst with daughter cyst and echogenic debris between the cyst (2) a cyst with a floating detached endocyst membrane visible as wavy bands the "water lily sign". On CT, hydatid cyst appears as well-defined unilocular or multilocular cysts with discernible walls.

Note: Shift "Gallstones, Cholecystitis, Primary Sclerosing Cholangitis, and Pancreatitis" here, before 'Tumors' heading.

Gallstones (Cholelithiasis)

Investigation of choice for gallstones is ultrasound as only 15–20% of stones are radiopaque. On ultrasound, they appear as highly reflective echogenic focus within gallbladder lumen with posterior acoustic shadowing. Gravity dependent movement is often seen with a change of patient position the "rolling stone sign". On plain radiograph they may be lamellated, may have a faceted outline or may show *Mercedes-Benz sign.*

Cholecystitis

Cholecystitis is inflammation of gallbladder which may be acute or chronic.

Acute calculus cholecystitis indicates obstruction by gallstones. Ultrasound is the preferred initial modality of investigation. The most sensitive ultrasound finding is the presence of cholelithiasis in combination with *sonographic Murphy sign.* Both gallbladder wall thickening (>3 mm) and pericholecystic fluid are secondary findings.

Chronic cholecystitis results due to wall damage by repeated attacks of inflammation, usually caused by gallstone and manifests as thickened wall and luminal contraction by fibrosis and scarring.

Primary Sclerosing Cholangitis (PSC)

Primary sclerosing cholangitis is chronic cholestatic liver disease of unknown cause characterized by inflammation, fibrosis and destruction of intrahepatic and extrahepatic bile ducts. PSC is commonly associated with inflammatory bowel disease particularly ulcerative colitis. On direct cholangiography, multiple segmental strictures involving both intra and extrahepatic bile ducts are the characteristic finding of PSC, and alternating strictures and dilatation result in the "beaded appearance".

Pancreatitis

Pancreatitis is classified into acute and chronic pancreatitis according to clinical, morphologic and histologic criteria. Groove pancreatitis and autoimmune pancreatitis are uncommon forms of acute pancreatitis.

Acute Pancreatitis

Acute pancreatitis is an acute inflammatory disease of pancreas. In adults, gallstones and chronic alcohol consumption are the most common causes.

The diagnosis of acute pancreatitis is based on two of the following three features: (1) abdominal pain consistent with acute pancreatitis (acute onset of a persistent, severe, epigastric pain often radiating to the back), (2) serum lipase activity (or amylase activity) at least three times greater than the upper limit of normal and (3) characteristic imaging findings of acute pancreatitis.

Atlanta classification of acute pancreatitis

Types of pancreatitis	*Interstitial edematous pancreatitis (IEP)*	*Necrotizing pancreatitis*
Definition	Acute inflammation of the pancreatic parenchyma and peripancreatic tissues due to inflammatory edema	Inflammation associated with pancreatic parenchymal necrosis and/or peripancreatic necrosis
Contrast-enhanced CT criteria	Homogeneous pancreatic parenchyma enhancement and/or mild haziness of stranding in peripancreatic tissue and no findings of peripancreatic necrosis	Lack of pancreatic parenchymal enhancement and/or presence of peripancreatic necrosis like acute necrotic collection and walled-off necrosis

Classification of pancreatic and peripancreatic collections in acute pancreatitis

Types of collection	*Types of pancreatitis*	*Time*	*Location*	*Density and morphology*	*Presence of definable wall*
Acute peripancreatic fluid collection **(Fig. 28.9)**	Interstitial edematous pancreatitis	≤4 weeks	Adjacent to pancreas, no intrapancreatic extension	Homogenous fluid density No non-liquid component No definite wall	No
Pancreatic pseudocyst	Interstitial edematous pancreatitis	≥4 weeks	Adjacent or distant to pancreas	Homogeneous fluid density No non-liquid component Well-enhanced wall	Yes
Acute necrotic collection	Necrotizing pancreatitis	≤4 weeks	Intrapancreatic and/or extra pancreatic	Heterogeneous and non-liquid density of varying degrees No definite wall	No
Walled-off necrosis	Necrotizing pancreatitis	≥4 weeks	Intrapancreatic and/or extra pancreatic	Heterogeneous with liquid and non-liquid density with varying degree of loculations Well-enhanced wall	Yes

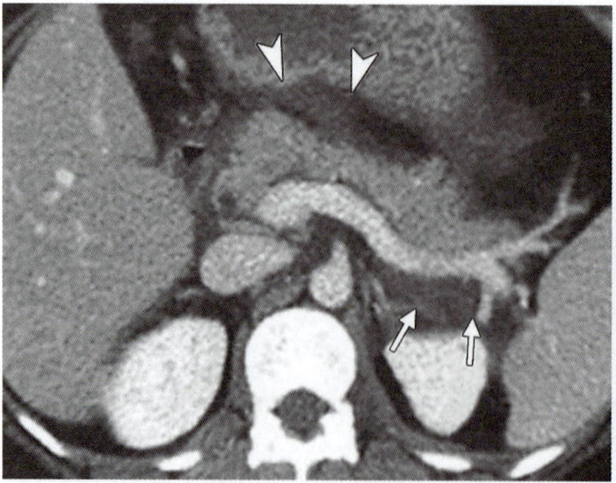

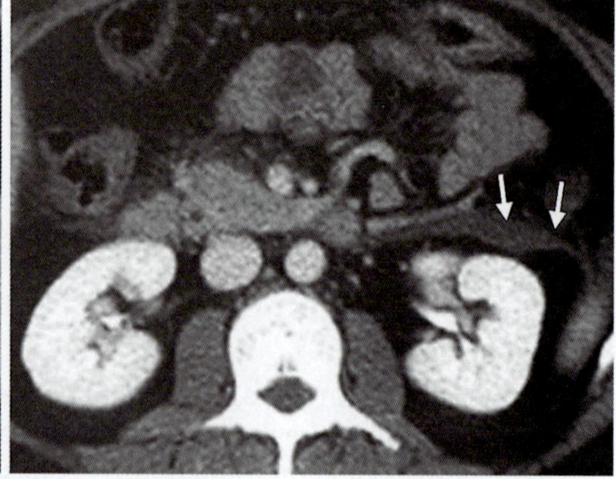

Fig. 28.9: Acute interstitial pancreatitis with peripancreatic fluid collection-CECT demonstrates homogeneous enhancement of pancreas with peripancreatic fluid collection in lesser sac.

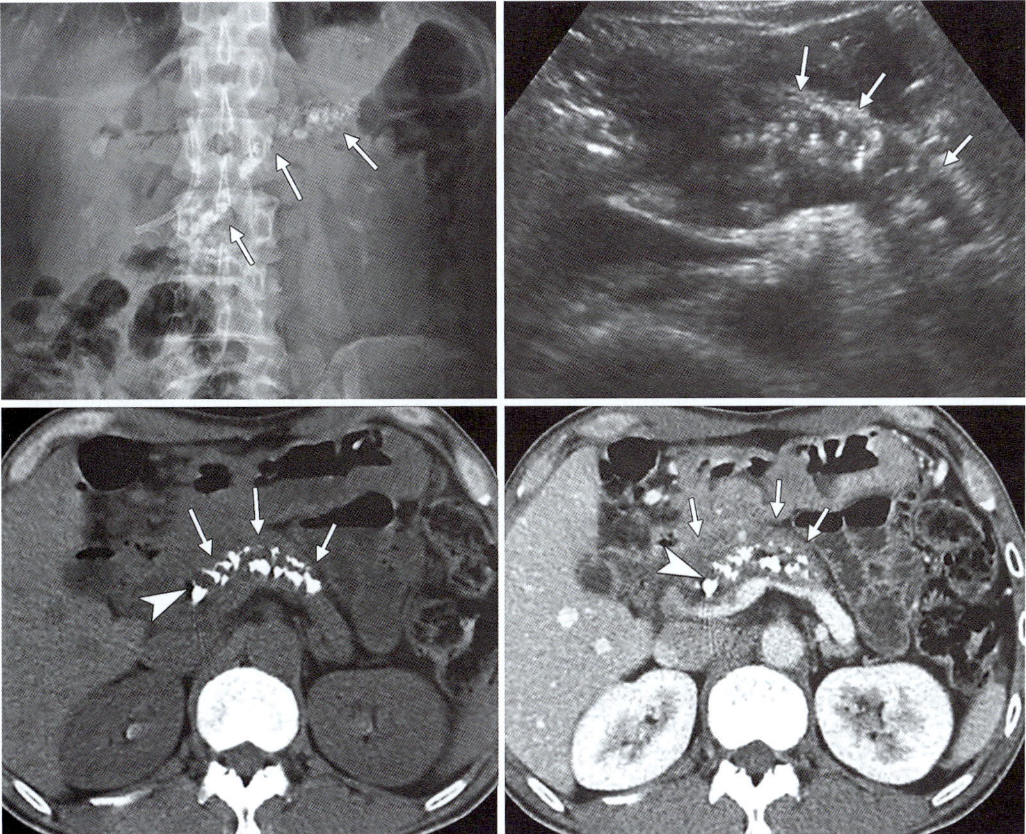

Fig. 28.10: Chronic pancreatitis: Atrophic pancreas with dilated main pancreatic duct and parenchymal as well as intraductal calcification as seen on abdominal radiograph, ultrasound, NCCT and CECT scan.

Chronic Pancreatitis

Chronic pancreatitis is defined as a progressive inflammatory disorder in which pancreatic parenchyma is destroyed and replaced by fibrous tissue, eventually leading to permanent impairment of endocrine and exocrine functions. Abdominal pain is the most common clinical symptom, and patients can also present with local complications such as pseudocysts, obstruction of adjacent organs or vascular thrombosis.

On abdominal radiography, pancreatic calcification can be found in 30–70% of the patients. On CECT imaging features of chronic pancreatitis include, parenchymal and intraductal calcification and alteration in size of the pancreas. On MRI early findings of chronic pancreatitis include loss of T1W hyperintensity, decreased and delayed contrast enhancement and dilated side branches. Late findings include parenchymal atrophy, pseudocyst formation and dilatation and beading of the pancreatic duct with intraductal calcification to give "chain of lakes "appearance **(Fig. 28.10)**.

TUMORS

Hemangioma

Hemangioma is the most common benign tumor of the liver. On ultrasound they appear as uniform hyperechogenicity, well-defined margin and posterior echo enhancement.

On color Doppler ultrasound, vascular signals are absent. Characteristic enhancement pattern of hemangioma includes nodular enhancement at the periphery of the lesion in the arterial phase and subsequent centripetal filling followed by sustained enhancement on contrast-enhanced ultrasound, CT, and MRI.

Focal Nodular Hyperplasia (FNH)

It is a benign tumor composed of non-neoplastic hepatocytes that is associated with a central fibrous scar. On CECT FNH shows enhancement in the arterial phase with a central non nonenhancing scar which shows enhancement on delayed phase.

Hepatocellular Adenoma (HCA)

It is an uncommon benign tumor associated with the usage of oral contraceptive agents. Hepatocellular adenoma may present as a palpable mass or pain in the right upper quadrant, rarely patient may present with acute shock due to the tendency of the tumor to rupture and cause hemoperitoneum. On CECT they show enhancement on arterial phase and become isodense to liver parenchyma on portal venous phase.

Hepatocellular Carcinoma (HCC)

Hepatocellular carcinoma is the fifth most common tumor in the world and the strongest predisposing factor for developing hepatocellular carcinoma is cirrhosis. HCC is a malignant neoplasm composed of cells with hepatocellular differentiation. Imaging features on CT and MRI are (1) contrast enhancement during hepatic arterial phase and washout during the later portal venous and equilibrium phase, (2) capsular rim enhancement on portal venous and delayed phase images, (3) hyperintensity on T2W images, (4) corona enhancement on arterial or portal venous phase images, (5) hypointensity on hepatobiliary phase after administration of hepatobiliary contrast agent, and (6) restricted diffusion on DWI.

Fibrolamellar Variant of HCC

Fibrolamellar variant of HCC is not associated with hepatitis or cirrhosis and occurs in young adults. On non-contrast CT the tumor is hypodense as compared to adjacent liver parenchyma. Fibrolamellar HCC is characterized by intratumoral calcification, central scar and pseudo capsule which are visible on CT. On CECT it shows heterogeneous enhancement.

Angiosarcoma

Angiosarcoma is the most common mesenchymal tumor of the liver and is a malignant spindle cell tumor of endothelial lining cell origin. It occurs in adult male with a history of radiation exposure and exposure to chemical agents such as vinyl chloride, thorium oxide and arsenicals, etc. On ultrasound angiosarcoma appear as either solitary or multiple hyperechoic masses. On non-contrast CT, they appear as low attenuating lesions with internal high attenuating areas of hemorrhage.

Hepatic Metastasis

Liver is the most commonly involved organ by metastasis and hepatic metastasis are the most common malignant tumor of the liver without cirrhosis. Liver has dual blood supply (hepatic arteries and portal veins) and therefore liver is most commonly involved organ by metastases. They have variable appearance, like hyperechoic (e.g., in colonic cancer), hypoechoic (in breast and lung), etc.

Cholangiocarcinoma

Cholangiocarcinoma is a malignant tumor arising from bile duct epithelium and is classified into intrahepatic, hilar (Klatskin tumor), and extrahepatic according to the location in biliary tree. Cholangiocarcinoma is associated with liver fluke infestation (clonorchiasis), recurrent pyogenic cholangitis (hepatolithiasis) and chronic hepatitis B and C.

Cholangiocarcinoma is classified according to morphology and growth pattern as the periductal infiltrative type, mass-forming type and intraduct growing type.

Cystic Neoplasms of Pancreas

Serous Cystadenoma

It is a benign tumor and known as grandmother lesion as they are most common in the sixth decade. It usually involves head of pancreas and has a lobulated microcystic or honeycomb like appearance with central scar and calcification. There is no communication between cysts and pancreatic duct.

Mucinous Cystic Neoplasm

It is a premalignant lesion and may transform into cystadenocarcinoma. They are also known as mother lesion as are typically seen in fourth-fifth decade. Mucinous cystadenomas usually involve tail and body of pancreas and are macrocystic with thick wall septations and peripheral calcifications.

Ductal Adenocarcinoma of Pancreas

Pancreatic ductal adenocarcinoma is the most common type of malignant pancreatic neoplasms. Most commonly occurs in elderly male. Ductal carcinoma appears as a solid mass without necrosis or hemorrhage and on dynamic contrast enhanced CT appears hypoattenuating as compared to normal pancreas. Ductal carcinoma involving the head of pancreas may cause dilatation of both the bile duct and pancreatic duct known as the **Double Duct Sign** with atrophy of upstream pancreas whereas tumors involving the body of pancreas cause upstream pancreatic duct dilatation with atrophy of the pancreas.

On MRI ductal adenocarcinoma appears hypointense as compared to normal pancreas on conventional and fat suppressed T1W images while the signal intensity varies on T2W images depending on the degree of desmoplastic reaction, hemorrhage, necrosis and associated inflammatory changes. On dynamic gadolinium enhanced MRI, the tumor appears non enhancing relative to the normally enhancing pancreas.

LAST MINUTE REVISION

- **Ultrasound** is the first-line investigation for liver and gallbladder diseases due to its noninvasive nature and lack of radiation.
- Triple-phase CT (arterial, portal venous, and delayed phases) enhances sensitivity and specificity in diagnosing focal liver lesions.
- MRCP (Magnetic resonance cholangiopancreatography) is excellent for noninvasive visualization of the biliary and pancreatic ducts.
- ERCP combines diagnostic and therapeutic capabilities, useful for stone removal and stenting in biliary obstructions.

REVIEW QUESTIONS

Multiple Choice Questions (MCQs)

1. **A 45-year-old male presents with acute right upper quadrant pain and jaundice. Ultrasound reveals a distended gallbladder with thickened walls and pericholecystic fluid. Which imaging modality is most appropriate for further evaluation and possible intervention?**
   a. Plain radiography
   b. Computed tomography (CT)
   c. Endoscopic retrograde cholangiopancreatography (ERCP)
   d. Magnetic resonance imaging (MRI)
2. **A 60-year-old female with a history of chronic pancreatitis presents with epigastric pain and weight loss. What imaging modality is best for evaluating pancreatic calcifications and assessing the pancreatic duct?**
   a. Plain radiography
   b. Ultrasound
   c. Computed tomography (CT)
   d. Magnetic resonance cholangiopancreatography (MRCP)
3. **A 35-year-old patient with suspected liver cirrhosis needs an assessment of liver stiffness and fat quantification. Which imaging modality should be used?**
   a. Plain radiography
   b. Ultrasound elastography
   c. Computed tomography (CT)
   d. Magnetic resonance imaging (MRI)
4. **A patient presents with jaundice, and ultrasound shows dilated intrahepatic bile ducts. What is the next best imaging modality to evaluate the biliary tree non-invasively?**
   a. Plain radiography
   b. Endoscopic retrograde cholangiopancreatography (ERCP)
   c. Magnetic resonance cholangiopancreatography (MRCP)
   d. Computed tomography (CT)
5. **A 50-year-old male with a history of alcohol abuse presents with chronic abdominal pain. CT shows calcifications in the pancreatic region. What is the most likely diagnosis?**
   a. Acute pancreatitis
   b. Chronic pancreatitis
   c. Pancreatic cancer
   d. Gallstones

Answer Key

1. c 2. c 3. b 4. c 5. b

SUGGESTED READING

1. Chaurasia BD. BD Chaurasia's Human Anatomy Vol-2 Regional and Applied Dissection & Clinical Lower Limb Abdomen and Pelvis, 9th edition. Extra Biliary Apparatus. 2023;336.
2. Choi JI, Choi BI. Other Malignant Tumors of the Liver. In: Choi BI (Ed). Radiology Illustrated: Hepatobiliary and Pancreatic Radiology. 2014;169.
3. Kim SY. Pancreatitis. In: Choi BI (Ed). Radiology Illustrated: Hepatobiliary and Pancreatic Radiology. 2014;587.
4. Lee YJ, Kim YH. Focal Hepatic Infections. In: Choi BI (Ed). Radiology Illustrated: Hepatobiliary and Pancreatic Radiology. 2014;233.
5. Singh I. Human embryology, 13th edition. Liver and Biliary Apparatus. 2022;190.

CHAPTER 29

Imaging in Urinary Tract and Male Reproductive System

"In urogenital imaging, radiologists navigate complexity with clarity—because every detail matters in preserving function and dignity."

INTRODUCTION

Imaging plays a pivotal role in the comprehensive evaluation and management of disorders affecting the urinary tract. From routine screenings to complex diagnostic dilemmas, the ability to visualize and assess the kidneys, ureters, bladder, and associated structures is essential in clinical practice. Various imaging modalities offer distinct advantages, ranging from noninvasive assessments with ultrasound to detailed anatomical and functional insights provided by computed tomography (CT) and magnetic resonance imaging (MRI). The urinary tract comprises of kidneys, ureters, urinary bladder and urethra is susceptible to a wide array of conditions, including congenital anomalies, stones, infections, tumors, and trauma. Each of these conditions requires precise imaging techniques tailored to the clinical scenario, guiding therapeutic decisions and optimizing patient outcomes. Imaging not only aids in the initial diagnosis but also serves as a crucial tool for monitoring disease progression, treatment response, and postoperative surveillance.

In this chapter, we explore the spectrum of imaging modalities employed in urinary tract evaluation, emphasizing their unique strengths and applications.

By integrating imaging findings with clinical assessments, we navigate the complexities of urinary tract pathology, ensuring timely and informed therapeutic interventions. This chapter aims to provide a comprehensive overview of how imaging contributes to the holistic management of urinary tract disorders, underscoring its indispensable role in modern medical practice.

EMBRYOLOGY AND ANATOMY

Urogenital ridge give rise to pronephros, mesonephros and metanephros. Pronephros regresses by around 4th week. Mesonephros forms the ureteric bud, from which develops the collecting system (distal convoluted tubules, major and minor calyces, renal pelvis and ureters). Metanephros forms the metanephric blastema, which form the excretory system (glomeruli, Bowmans capsule, proximal and distal convoluted tubules). Urinary bladder and urethra develops from cloaca. Initially kidneys are located in pelvis and ascends later to its final position. It has renal cortex and medulla.

Kidney is retroperitoneal structure, located in renal fossa in lumbar region, with right kidney located slightly lower than left, around 12th rib, between T12 to L4 vertebrae. Kidneys are directed obliquely with superior pole more medial and posterior, than inferior pole. Average length of kidneys: 9 to 13 cm. Average renal parenchymal thickness at poles: 3 to 3.5 cm, and at interpolar region: 2 to 2.5 cm.

Renal arteries originate from the abdominal aorta; in 30% of individuals, an accessory renal artery is present. It divides into segmental branches, interlobar, arcuate, and interlobular arteries.

Veins lie anterior to the renal arteries; the left renal vein is longer and passes between the aorta and superior mesenteric artery.

IMAGING MODALITIES (TABLE 29.1)

X-ray KUB (Kidney, Ureter, Urinary Bladder)

Taken in supine position in full inspiration. During full inspiration, diaphragm contracts and pushes the kidney downwards, and entire KUB region can be visualized on single film. Rays are directed anteroposteriorly with centering at Iliac crest. Exposure factor: 70–80 kVp, 30–40 mAs.

Helps in detection of radio-opaque density along the urinary tract. Thus, aids in detecting renal and ureteric calculi, renal medullary sponge kidney, vesical calculi and urinary bladder schistosomiasis.

Table 29.1: Comparative overview of various imaging modalities used in urinary tract.

Imaging modality	*Description*	*Advantages*	*Disadvantages*
Computed tomography (CT)	Utilizes X-rays to create detailed cross-sectional images of the urinary tract	Excellent spatial resolution, rapid imaging, widespread availability	Ionizing radiation exposure, contrast-induced nephropathy risk, higher cost
Magnetic resonance imaging (MRI)	Uses magnetic fields and radio waves to generate high-resolution images of the urinary tract	Superior soft tissue contrast, multiplanar imaging capability, no ionizing radiation	Longer acquisition time, limited availability, contraindicated in certain patients (e.g., with metallic implants)
Ultrasound (US)	Employs sound waves to visualize the urinary tract in real-time	Noninvasive, lack of ionizing radiation, widely available, cost-effective	Operator-dependent, limited penetration in obese patients, may have suboptimal visualization of deep structures
Intravenous pyelography (IVP)	Involves intravenous injection of contrast dye followed by X-ray imaging to visualize the urinary tract	Provides dynamic images of the renal collecting system and ureters	Invasive, exposure to ionizing radiation and contrast dye, limited sensitivity in detecting small lesions
Voiding cystourethrogram (VCUG)	A fluoroscopic study involving contrast dye injection into the bladder, to assess reflux	Gold standard for diagnosing vesicoureteral reflux, assesses bladder function	Invasive, exposure to ionizing radiation and contrast dye may be uncomfortable for patient
Positron emission tomography-computed tomography (PET-CT)	Combines metabolic PET imaging with anatomical CT imaging, for comprehensive evaluation	Detects metastases and evaluates treatment response	Expensive, limited availability, exposure to ionizing radiation, may require contrast administration

IVP

X-ray examination that uses iodinated contrast media injected intravenously, to visualize kidney, ureters and urinary bladder. Nowadays, this procedure is done under fluoroscopy.

Helps in detection of renal size and contour, mass lesion (as filling defect), renal scarring, renal papillary necrosis, hydroureteronephrosis, ureteric narrowing, anatomic variants like horseshoe kidney, duplex collecting system, retroperitoneal fibrosis (medial deviation of ureters), renal function, calculi and bladder diverticulum.

Procedure: Patient should be fasting for 5–6 hours prior to investigation. Laxatives can be taken to reduce obscuration of urinary tract by bowel loops. EGFR of patient should be calculated. IVP shouldn't be done if EGFR is below 30. IVP can't be done if kidney is nonfunctioning, as there will not be any uptake, and renal tracts will not be visualized. Urinary bladder should be empty before the procedure.

Patients should be lying in supine position. Scout view should be taken to look for any calculi. Then bolus injection of nonionic iodinated contrast media should be given. Iodinated contrast flows through renal vasculature, and is filtered into the collecting system, highlighting the anatomic structures on X-ray image. After injecting contrast media, immediate AP radiograph should be taken to see nephrogram. Contrast material will then start appearing in pelvicalyceal system. Another film should be taken after 5 minutes postinjection. Thereafter, abdominal compression should be applied for 10 minutes, and radiograph should be taken in early bladder filling phase. Immediately after release of compression, KUB radiograph should be obtained. Postvoid film should be taken to see significant residual urine. Parenchymal breaking and double contour can be seen in case of neoplasm, clubbing of calyces can be seen in chronic obstruction, static column of contrast suggests chronic obstruction, cobra head appearance can be seen in case of ureterocele.

MCU

Diagnostic procedure for evaluation of structure and function of urinary bladder, and urethra **(Fig. 29.1)**.

Indications: Vesicoureteral reflux (VUR), PUV, urinary bladder diverticulum, urethral stricture, urethral diverticulum.

Procedure: Done under fluoroscopic guidance. Bladder should be empty before the procedure. Foleys catheter is inserted into urinary bladder for filling contrast. Scout film is taken first to look for any calcification. Bladder volume is calculated according to age. Bladder is filled with nonionic iodinated contrast media, according to volume calculated through foleys catheter. Intermittent fluoroscopy images are taken to look for any reflux. When the bladder is full, right and left posterior oblique films pelvis AP with KUB are taken. Then, another film is taken when the patient is micturating.

- Post void film also taken for residual urine
- Procedure shouldn't be done in case of urinary tract infection

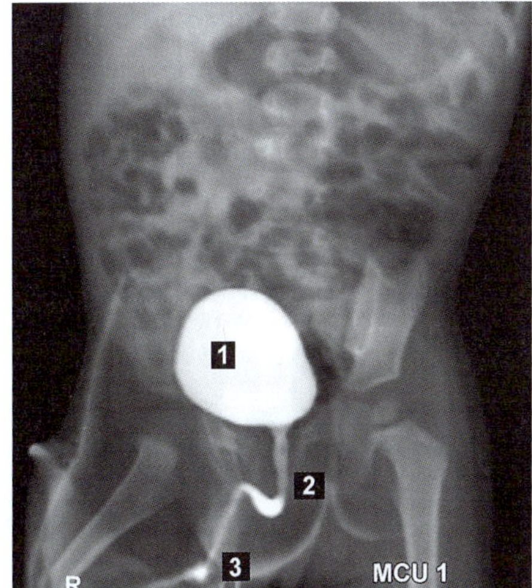

Fig. 29.1: Micturating cystourethrography (MCU). (1) Urinary bladder; (2) Posterior urethra; (3) Anterior urethra.

RGU

Diagnostic procedure of choice for evaluation of urethra.

Indication: Traumatic urethral injuries, urethral strictures, fistulas and diverticulum.

Procedure: Under aseptic precautions, foleys catheter or nasogastric tube is inserted into penile urethra. Patient lies in supine 45° position, with mild traction on penis, so that it lies laterally over thigh. Then iodinated contrast media is injected under fluoroscopic guidance.

USG

It is the 1st imaging modality to be performed in case of flank pain. It is noninvasive, radiation free and easily available modality. Renal cortex appears isoechoic to liver parenchyma, and medulla appears hypoechoic. Major and minor calyces lie between the hyperechoic fat of renal pelvis.

Indication: Renal calculi, hydronephrosis, renal tumors, renal parenchymal disease, cystic renal disease, renal abscess, bladder diverticulum, cystitis, bladder carcinoma, posterior urethral valve. Renal calculi, hydronephrosis, renal tumors, renal parenchymal disease, cystic renal disease, renal abscess, bladder diverticulum, cystitis, bladder carcinoma, posterior urethral valve.

Procedure: Done using curvilinear probe (1–5 MHz). Patients will be in supine, and lateral decubitus position. Kidneys are examined in longitudinal and transverse planes. Color Doppler and spectral Doppler are performed to look for renal perfusion, and peak systolic velocity. Pulsatility index and resistive index can also be measured. These indices help in diagnosis of renovascular hypertension.

Renal Doppler (Table 29.2)

Evaluate renal vascular conditions using Doppler ultrasound.

It is noninvasive, low cost, generally well-tolerated. But it is highly operator-dependent, time-consuming, with challenging interpretation. Limitations are obesity, overlying bowel gas, aberrant anatomy, cardiac/aortic pulsations, very difficult in critically ill patients.

Indication

- **Native renal arteries:** Hypertension (renovascular), follow-up of known disease, abdominal/ flank bruit, vascular pathology evaluation, etc.
- **Transplant renal arteries:** Baseline screening, postbiopsy complications, evaluation of vascular patency, assessment of lymphoproliferative diseases.

Normal waveform of the main renal artery shows rapid upstroke in systole with notch (hump) and a low resistance waveform with continuous forward flow throughout the cardiac cycle. The normal peak systolic velocity of the main renal artery is less than 180 cm/s. The resistive

Table 29.2: Renal Doppler-equipment and technique.

Parameter	*Details*
Equipment	Duplex scanning with 2D B-mode imaging, color Doppler, power Doppler, and spectral Doppler
Probe selection	3.5–5 MHz curvilinear transducer for adults; 6–12 MHz linear transducer for pediatric or thin patients
Preparation	NPO for 8 hours (except transplant exams); Simethicone may be administered to reduce gas artifacts
Imaging technique	Begin with B-mode imaging, evaluate with color (at origin, main artery, segmental at poles) and spectral Doppler, measure peak systolic velocity (PSV) and resistive index (RI)

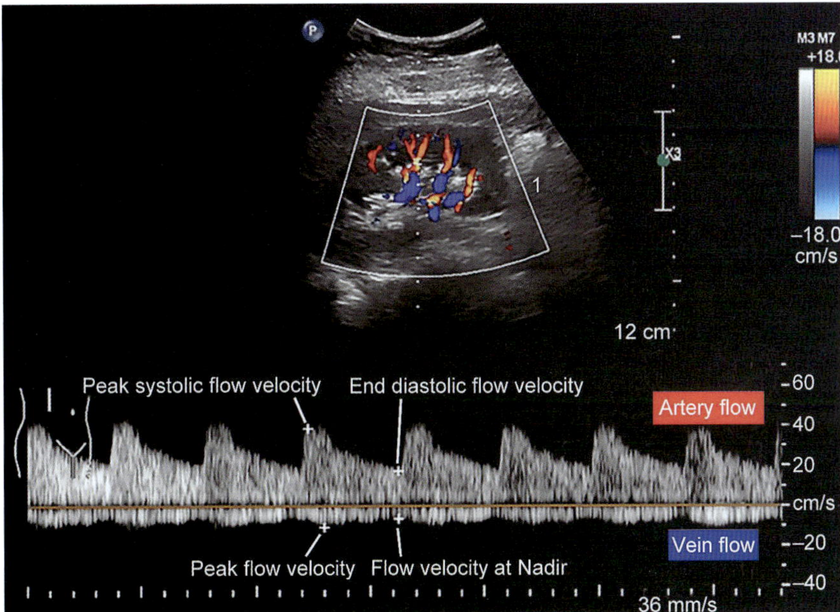

Fig. 29.2: Shows color Doppler image of kidney with pulse wave of renal segmental artery depicting PSV as peak systolic flow velocity and diastolic velocity.

index is less than 0.70 **(Fig. 29.2)**. Common pathologies evaluated by renal Doppler shown in **Table 29.3**.

CT

Non-contrast CT is done to look for renal calculi and renal concretions. Contrast enhanced CT or CT urography (split bolus or three phase study) is done to look for functioning of kidneys, renal abscess, renal cyst, tumors, angiomyolipoma **(Fig. 29.3)**.

Table 29.3: Common pathologies evaluated by renal Doppler.

Pathology	*Details*
Renal artery stenosis (RAS)	Direct signs: PSV >200 cm/s, renal/aortic PSV ratio >3.5:1, poststenotic turbulence Indirect signs: Parvus-tardus waveform, AI <3 m/s, AT >70 msec, PI >0.7
Renal artery thrombosis	Absence of flow, abnormal waveform, possible renal enlargement and heterogeneity
Renal vein thrombosis (RVT)	Partial occlusion: Filling defects in Doppler Complete obstruction: Absence of flow, reversal of diastolic flow
Pseudoaneurysm/ arteriovenous fistula	PSA: "Yin-yang" sign on color Doppler, "to-and-fro" flow on spectral Doppler. AVF: Arterialized venous flow

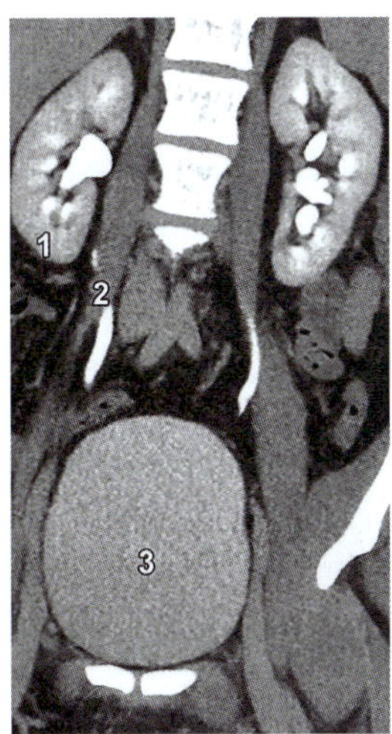

Fig. 29.3: Shows CT urography with contrast excretion in Kidney collecting system (1) ureter (2), and also reaches urinary bladder (3).

Technique

For contrast scan, EGFR is calculated. Contrast is given only if EGFR is more than 40 mL/min/1.73 m^2. First non-contrast scan is taken from diaphragm to pubic symphysis. Then, corticomedullary phase is taken, 25–30 seconds after injecting nonionic iodinated contrast media (100–150 mL of 300 mgI/mL at 2–4 mL/s). After 90–100 seconds, nephrographic phase is taken. Then, after 5–10 minutes, excretory phase is taken.

On non-contrast scans, Hounsfield unit of calculi can be calculated, which helps in predicting the type of stone. If HU is less than 500, then uric acid stone is considered; and if HU is more than 500, then calcium stone will be considered. Type of stone helps in deciding the appropriate treatments like ESWL (extracorporeal shock wave lithotripsy), PCNL (percutaneous nephrolithotomy), ureteroscopic lithotripsy, and medical expulsive treatment. More energy is needed for fragmentation in ESWL, in case of high HU. Success of ESWL decreases with increasing HU.

There should be synchronous uptake, and excretion by both kidneys. In case of non-functioning kidney, there will not be any uptake for kidneys. Cortical cysts are well-delineated on contrast scan. Bosniak classification is given for renal cyst. This classification depends on Hounsfield unit of cyst, thickness and number of cyst and wall thickness of cyst. In case of angiomyolipoma, fat attenuation content is seen within the lesion, which have HU of –10. If enhancement is more than 20 HU, then there is higher probability of malignancy. Ureteric and urinary bladder tumors are more appreciable in excretory phase images and appear as filling defect.

CT renal angiography is a vital tool in the diagnosis and management of renal vascular conditions. Its ability to produce detailed images of the renal arteries and veins makes it indispensable in both clinical and surgical settings, particularly in the evaluation of renal artery stenosis, kidney donor suitability, and post-transplant vascular complications.

Dual energy CT (DECT): It is an emerging technology that uses two different spectra of photon energy. By using this technology, different attenuation images can be created, by using single exposure to patient. It also helps in reduction of dose to patient, and helps in detecting the nature of renal calculus, by using different attenuation properties of calculi, which helps in deciding the management of renal calculus.

Magnetic Resonance Imaging (MRI)

It is an imaging modality that uses protons in our body to create different images. T1, T2, FLAIR, and DWI are main sequences that help in detection of various pathologies.

On T2-weighted image, fluid appears bright. So, renal pelvi-calyceal system, ureters and urinary bladder show bright lumen on T2-weighted image. Any filling defect on T2-weighted imaging, suggests pathology. It can be due to calculus or tumor.

T1-weighted imaging is better to reveal anatomy, and T2 weighted imaging for pathology. Generally, most of tissue appears hyper on T2, and hypo on T1-weighted sequence. Fat, calcium, melanin, and contrast appears hyper on T1 weighted image.

MRI also plays a crucial role in evaluation of prostate cancer.

COMMON PATHOLOGIES

Urinary Tract Infections

Common are pyelonephritis, xanthogranulomatous pyelonephritis, emphysematous pyelonephritis, cystitis, tuberculosis, and schistosomiasis.

On plain radiography: Lucencies around renal shadow or around urinary bladder suggest emphysematous pyelonephritis or emphysematous cystitis. Staghorn calculus that appears as branching radio-opacity can be seen in case of xanthogranulomatous pyelonephritis.

On USG: Debris or thickening can be seen in pelvicalyceal system, reduced renal vascularity on color Doppler in case of pyelonephritis, few floating or dependent echoes in case of cystitis, thickening of wall of urinary bladder in case of chronic cystitis. Normal wall thickness is less than 3 mm in well-distended bladder and less than 6 mm in case of partially distended urinary bladder. Altered areas of renal echogenicity (focal or segmental hypoechoic areas) suggest renal infection. Distorted renal outline with staghorn calculus suggest xanthogranulomatous pyelonephritis.

CT: Perirenal fat stranding suggests pyelonephritis. In xanthogranulomatous pyelonephritis, there is presence of staghorn calculus with distorted renal outline. Pelvis will be contracted with dilatation of pelvicalyceal system, giving bear paw appearance. Presence of air within or around the kidneys suggest emphysematous pyelonephritis and in urinary bladder suggest emphysematous cystitis.

Calculus

Calculi are common cause of flank pain. Types of calculi are as follows—calcium oxalate/ phosphate (MC), uric acid, cystine and struvite.

On plain radiography: Calculi appear radioopaque in region of renal shadow. Uric acid calculi and medications calculi are not visible on radiograph.

IVP: Appears as filling defect in the urinary tract.

USG: Appears as echogenic foci, giving posterior acoustic shadowing. On color Doppler, twinkling artifacts will be seen. Calculi can be seen in pelvicalyceal system, ureters, VUJ, urinary bladder and urethra. Large calculi can cause obstruction and result in hydroureteronephrosis.

CT: They appear hyperdense on NCCT, with HU of 100–200 in case of uric acid and cystine calculi, and 500–600 HU in case of calcium stone. Calculi are seen as filling defect on excretory phase.

DECT: Used to know the components of calculus, depending on the attenuation of calculi, on two different kVp.

Hydroureteronephrosis

Dilatation of pelvicalyceal system and ureter occurs due to any obstruction along the urinary tract. It can be due to calculi, stricture, PUJ obstruction, bladder outlet obstruction, and vesicoureteral reflux.

On plain radiography: Generally, not diagnosed on plain radiograph. Enlarged renal shadow can be seen in some cases. Radio-opaque calculi are seen, which are cause of hydroureteronephrosis.

IVP: Dilation of pelvicalyceal system, ureter and blunting of calyces are seen.

USG: There will be dilation of pelvicalyceal system and ureters. In case of pyonephrosis, echogenic debris are seen in dilated pelvicalyceal system.

CT: On CT, cause of hydronephrosis can be confirmed. Functioning of kidney can also be evaluated by assessing renal uptake, and excretion of contrast.

Grading of Hydronephrosis (Table 29.4)

On the basis of blunting of pelvicalyceal system, and on basis of thinning of renal parenchyma.

Table 29.4: Grading of hydronephrosis.

Grade	*Type*	*Findings*
0	No dilatation	Calyceal walls opposed to each other, no dilatation
1	Mild	Dilatation of renal pelvis, without calyceal dilatation; no parenchymal atrophy
2	Mild	Mild dilatation of renal pelvis and calyces; pelvicalyceal pattern retained; no parenchymal atrophy
3	Moderate	Moderate dilatation of renal pelvis and calyces; blunting of fornices, flattening of papillae; mild cortical thinning may be seen
4	Severe	Gross dilatation of renal pelvis and calyces; ballooning appearance; loss of borders between pelvis and calyces; renal atrophy with cortical thinning

Renal Parenchymal Disease

It is damage of renal parenchyma with decrease in renal function. Common in patients with diabetes mellitus and hypertension.

USG findings include decrease in length of kidneys, cortical thickness can be reduced (<6 mm), increase cortical echogenicity, loss of corticomedullary differentiation, cortical irregularity, decreased vascularity on color Doppler.

CT: In known patient of chronic kidney disease, contrast scan shouldn't be done, as kidneys are not able to excrete the contrast, and this can further damage the kidneys. Contrast scan should be followed by dialysis in patient with chronic kidney disease. There will be a decrease in length of kidneys, along with decrease in uptake and excretion of contrast.

Renal Cortical Cyst

These are well defined cystic lesions in renal cortex. Can be confused with renal abscess, focal pyelectasis, or renal cell carcinoma. There are many cysts in autosomal dominant polycystic kidney disease/autosomal recessive polycystic kidney disease. Renal cyst are also common in patient on dialysis.

USG: Appear as well-defined anechoic lesion. Based on complexity of cyst, we can see internal echoes and septa.

CT: Modality of choice for classification of cyst. Appear as well defined, hypodense lesion. Bosniak classification is given based on septa, and HU of cyst.

Horseshoe Kidney

Most common fusion anomaly of kidney. Horseshoe kidney is a congenital condition where the kidneys fuse together at lower poles during fetal development, forming a U-shaped structure resembling a horseshoe. Patient with horseshoe kidney are susceptible for having renal calculi, and transitional cell carcinoma. Imaging plays a crucial role in diagnosing and evaluating horseshoe kidney.

USG: This is often the initial imaging modality used, due to its accessibility, lack of ionizing radiation, and cost-effectiveness. Ultrasound can visualize the characteristic U-shaped configuration of the kidneys, and their abnormal position. It can also detect associated anomalies such as hydronephrosis, renal calculi, or renal tumors.

CT/MRI: Provides detailed cross-sectional images of the kidneys, allowing for precise visualization of horseshoe kidney, and its vascular anatomy. It is particularly useful for evaluating associated complications such as renal stones, tumors, or obstruction. CT urography can also assess the renal collecting system and ureters, for any anomalies, or obstruction.

IVP: Although less commonly used nowadays, IVP shows fusion of kidneys, and any associated urinary tract abnormality.

Renal scintigraphy: This nuclear medicine imaging technique involves the injection of a radioactive tracer, which is taken up by the kidneys, and emits gamma rays. Renal scintigraphy can assess renal function, drainage, and perfusion. It is particularly useful for evaluation of renal function in horseshoe kidneys and for detecting any obstructive anomalies.

Imaging of horseshoe kidney aims to not only confirm the diagnosis but also to evaluate associated anomalies, assess renal function and vascular supply, and guide treatment decisions. The choice of imaging modality depends on various factors such as the clinical indication, availability, patient characteristics, and specific questions to be answered.

Ectopic Kidney

A rare congenital anomaly, occurring when one or both kidneys fail to ascend to their normal position in the retroperitoneum during embryonic development. Instead, they are found at abnormal locations within abdomen or pelvis. In crossed fused renal ectopia, both kidneys are on same side and are fused.

USG: Ultrasound is often the first-line imaging modality for assessing ectopic kidneys. It can visualize the abnormal location of the kidneys, and assess their size, shape, and parenchymal echogenicity. USG is particularly useful for detecting associated anomalies such as hydronephrosis, renal cysts, or renal calculi.

CT/MRI: Provides detailed cross-sectional images of abdomen and pelvis, allowing for precise localization and characterization of ectopic kidneys. It can delineate the relationship of ectopic kidneys with adjacent structures, assess vascular anatomy, and detect complications such as hydronephrosis, renal masses, or urinary tract obstruction. CT urography may be performed to evaluate the renal collecting system and ureters for any anomalies or obstruction.

IVP: Although less commonly used today, it visualizes the renal collecting system, ureters, and bladder. It can demonstrate the ectopic location of the kidneys and any associated urinary tract abnormalities, such as ureteral obstruction or reflux.

Duplex Pelvicalyceal System

Also known as duplicated collecting system, it is a congenital anomaly characterized by presence of two separate renal pelvis and ureters, draining a single kidney. This condition can be unilateral or bilateral and is often associated with other renal anomalies.

Weigert-Meyer law, also known as law of ureteral duplication, is a principle that describes the relationship between the ureters, in cases of duplicated pelvicalyceal systems.

According to Weigert-Meyer law:

- **Upper pole ureter:** The ureter that arises from the upper moiety (the superior renal pelvis) of a duplicated kidney, typically inserts into the bladder more caudally and medially, compared to the ureter from the lower moiety (the inferior renal pelvis) or even ectopic insertion.
- **Lower pole ureter:** Conversely, the ureter from the lower moiety usually inserts into the bladder more cranially and laterally, compared to the ureter from the upper moiety.

Clinical implications of the Weigert-Meyer law include:

- **Vesicoureteral reflux (VUR):** The differing insertion sites of the duplicated ureters can influence the likelihood and severity of VUR. The lower pole ureter, with its more cranial and lateral insertion, is more prone to reflux and associated complications, such as urinary tract infection and renal damage.
- **Obstructive uropathy:** Anomalies such as ureteropelvic junction obstruction or ureterovesical junction obstruction, may occur more commonly in one of the duplicated ureters, often the upper pole ureter, due to its more tortuous course and smaller calibre.
- **Surgical consideration:** In cases where surgical intervention is necessary, understanding the course and insertion sites of the duplicated ureters is crucial for planning procedures such as ureteral reimplantation or reconstructive surgery, to correct associated anomalies or reflux.

USG: It can visualize the duplicated renal pelvis and ureters, assess the renal parenchyma, and detect associated anomalies such as hydronephrosis, ureteral obstruction, or renal calculi.

IVP: It is particularly useful for delineating the anatomy of a duplex pelvicalyceal system, demonstrating the presence of two separate renal pelvises and ureters, and assessing the degree of ureteral obstruction or reflux.

CT/MRI: Provides detailed cross-sectional images of the kidneys, ureters, and bladder, allowing for precise visualization and characterization of a duplex pelvicalyceal system. It can accurately delineate the anatomy of the duplicated collecting system, assess renal function, and detect associated complications such as ureteropelvic junction obstruction, ureteral duplication anomalies, or renal calculi and guides surgical planning if needed.

Voiding Cystourethrography (VCUG)

VCUG is performed to evaluate the lower urinary tract, particularly in cases of suspected vesicoureteral reflux (VUR), associated with a duplex pelvicalyceal system. It involves the instillation of contrast into the bladder, followed by fluoroscopic imaging during voiding to assess the presence and severity of VUR, and its impact on the upper urinary tract.

Vesicoureteral Reflux (VUR)

It is a condition where urine flows backward from the bladder into one or both ureters and sometimes up to the kidneys. This condition is common in children and can lead to urinary tract infections and kidney damage, if left untreated.

Grading is typically based on the extent and duration of reflux observed during imaging studies, such as voiding cystourethrogram (VCUG). The International Reflux Study Committee (IRSC) classification system is widely used for grading VUR, and it consists of five grades:

1. **Grade I:** Reflux into the ureter without dilatation of the collecting system (mild reflux). Grade I reflux is characterized by a small amount of contrast material flowing back into the ureter during voiding, without significant dilation of the renal pelvis or calyces. This grade is often considered clinically insignificant and may resolve spontaneously without intervention.
2. **Grade II:** Reflux into the ureter and collecting system (mild to moderate reflux) without dilatation. While still considered low-grade, Grade II reflux may increase the risk of urinary tract infections and renal scarring, especially if it is bilateral or associated with recurrent infections.
3. **Grade III:** Reflux into the ureter with mild dilatation of the collecting system (moderate reflux). Grade III reflux is characterized by reflux into the ureter with mild dilatation of the renal pelvis and calyces. This grade of reflux poses a higher risk of renal damage and is often associated with recurrent urinary tract infections.

4. **Grade IV:** Reflux into the ureter with moderate dilatation of the collecting system (moderate to severe reflux), indicating significant urinary stasis and a high risk of renal scarring and complications. Surgical intervention may be considered for Grade IV reflux to prevent long-term sequelae.
5. **Grade V:** Gross reflux with severe dilatation of the collecting system and tortuous ureter (severe reflux). Grade V reflux is the most severe form, characterized by the gross reflux of contrast material into the ureter and collecting system, often with marked dilatation of the renal pelvis and calyces. Grade V reflux poses the highest risk of renal damage and may require prompt surgical intervention to prevent irreversible renal injury.

VCUG: VCUG is the gold standard for diagnosing VUR. VCUG allows visualization of the contrast material flowing backward from the bladder into the ureters and kidneys during voiding, helping to identify the presence, severity, and pattern of VUR.

USG: While it may not directly visualize VUR, ultrasound can detect associated findings such as hydronephrosis, renal scarring, or dilatation of the renal pelvis and ureters, which may suggest the presence of VUR.

Nuclear medicine scans: Nuclear medicine scans such as dimercaptosuccinic acid (DMSA) scan and technetium-99m mercaptoacetyltriglycine (MAG3) scan are used to assess renal function and detect renal scarring, which are common consequences of severe or recurrent VUR. While these scans do not directly visualize VUR, they provide valuable information about renal anatomy and function.

CT: Reserved for cases if some abnormalities or complications are suspected.

MRI: MRI may be utilized in select cases to evaluate VUR, especially when detailed anatomical information is needed or when assessing for associated abnormalities. MR urography, which involves the use of contrast agents, can provide high-resolution images of the urinary tract without ionizing radiation, making it suitable for pediatric patients or individuals with contraindications to CT or VCUG.

Urinary Tract Carcinoma

Imaging plays a crucial role in detection, staging, and management of urinary tract carcinomas, which include cancers of kidneys, ureters, bladder, and urethra. Imaging of urinary tract carcinomas aims to detect and characterize lesions, assess the extent of disease, determine the presence of lymph node involvement or distant metastases, guide treatment planning, and monitor treatment response.

CT: CT scan is one of the primary imaging modalities for evaluating urinary tract carcinoma. CT urography can detect abnormalities such as masses, hydronephrosis, lymphadenopathy, and distant metastases. Contrast-enhanced CT scans are particularly valuable for assessing tumor vascularity and staging.

MRI: It is particularly useful for evaluating renal masses as well as for assessing tumor invasion into adjacent structures such as the renal sinus, perinephric fat, or renal veins. MRI can also visualize the extent of bladder tumors and assess for local invasion into the bladder wall or adjacent organs. Dynamic contrast-enhanced MRI may provide additional information on tumor perfusion and vascularity.

USG: It can detect renal masses, hydronephrosis, and bladder wall thickening, although it may have limitations in assessing deeper structures or small lesions. Doppler ultrasound can assess tumor vascularity and distinguish solid masses from cystic lesions.

PET-CT: It combines functional metabolic information from PET with anatomical detail from CT scans. It is valuable for detecting metastatic disease and assessing the extent of tumor spread beyond the primary site. PET-CT can help identify distant metastases in lymph nodes, bones, or other organs, guiding treatment decisions and prognosis.

Cystoscopy: Cystoscopy is an essential diagnostic tool for evaluating bladder tumors. It involves the insertion of a flexible or rigid scope into the bladder via the urethra, allowing direct visualization of the bladder mucosa. Cystoscopy enables the identification, biopsy, and staging of bladder tumors, as well as assessment of tumor resectability and response to treatment.

IVP: It can detect filling defects, ureteral obstruction, and bladder abnormalities, but it has largely been replaced by CT urography and MRI due to their superior imaging capabilities.

IMAGING IN MALE REPRODUCTIVE SYSTEM

INTRODUCTION

Imaging of the male reproductive system is a critical component in the evaluation of various conditions affecting male fertility, sexual function, and other urogenital disorders. Various imaging modalities are used depending on the clinical scenario, each providing specific information about different anatomical structures and pathologies. Before understanding utilities of various modalities embryologic origin of male genitalia **(Table 29.5)** makes the anomalies easy to understand. Modalities with its clinical uses, advantages, and disadvantages related to male reproductive system shown in **Table 29.6**.

Table 29.5: Embryologic origin of male reproductive organs.

Embryologic origin	*Developmental stage*	*Abnormal development*	*Clinical consequences*
Bipotential gonad/genital ridge	Differentiation into testes under SRY gene influence	**Gonadal dysgenesis**	Ambiguous genitalia, infertility, increased risk of gonadal tumors
	—	**Klinefelter syndrome 47XXY**	Small testes, gynecomastia, infertility, hypogonadism
Wolffian ducts	Development into epididymis, vas deferens, seminal vesicles under testosterone influence	**Vas deferens agenesis**	Infertility, absence of vas deferens, often associated with cystic fibrosis
Müllerian ducts (= Paramesonephric ducts - develops into fallopian tubes, uterus and upper 1/3 of vagina in female)	Regression due to anti-Müllerian hormone (AMH)	**Persistent Müllerian duct syndrome**	Presence of uterus and fallopian tubes in a genetically male individual, leading to possible infertility
Genital tubercle	Elongation to form the penis under DHT influence	**Hypospadias**	Abnormal placement of urethral opening, difficulties with urination and sexual function
Urogenital folds	Fusion to form penile urethra	**Hypospadias**	Same as above

Contd...

Contd...

Embryologic origin	*Developmental stage*	*Abnormal development*	*Clinical consequences*
Labioscrotal swellings	Fusion to form scrotum	**Hypospadias or undescended testes**	Incomplete scrotal fusion or undescended testes, increased risk of infertility, and testicular cancer
Testes	Descent through inguinal canal into scrotum	**Cryptorchidism (undescended testes)**	Increased risk of infertility, testicular torsion, and testicular cancer
Testosterone/DHT production	Androgen production critical for male genital development	**Androgen insensitivity syndrome (AIS)**	Complete AIS: Female external genitalia in a genetically male individual; Partial AIS: Ambiguous genitalia
Steroid hormone synthesis	Balanced production of adrenal and gonadal hormones	**Congenital adrenal hyperplasia (CAH)**	Virilization of external genitalia in females, early virilization in males, possible salt-wasting crisis
Leydig and Sertoli cells	Leydig cells produce testosterone; Sertoli cells produce AMH	**Testicular dysgenesis syndrome (TDS)**	Reduced sperm quality, increased risk of testicular cancer, hypospadias, infertility

Table 29.6: Modalities with its clinical uses, advantages, and disadvantages related to male reproductive system.

Imaging modality	*Clinical uses*	*Advantages*	*Disadvantages*
Ultrasound	**Scrotal ultrasound:** Testicular torsion, epididymoorchitis, varicocele, hydrocele, testicular tumors **Transrectal ultrasound (TRUS):** Prostate evaluation (prostatitis, BPH), prostate biopsy	• Noninvasive • High-resolution images • Real-time imaging • No radiation exposure • Widely available	• Operator-dependent • Limited penetration depth (especially in obese patients) • Less effective for deep pelvic structures
Magnetic resonance imaging (MRI)	**Prostate MRI:** Prostate cancer detection, staging, and monitoring **Scrotal MRI:** Characterization of testicular masses **Penile MRI:** Evaluation of penile abnormalities	• Superior soft-tissue contrast • Detailed anatomical information • Multiparametric capabilities (e.g., mpMRI for prostate)	• High cost • Limited availability • Longer scan times • Potential for claustrophobia in patients • Contraindicated with certain implants
Computed tomography (CT)	**CT scan:** Staging of malignancies, detection of lymph node involvement, metastatic disease assessment **CT urography:** Evaluation of urinary tract, seminal vesicles	• Fast imaging • Excellent for staging cancers and assessing metastatic spread • Good anatomical detail	• Ionizing radiation exposure • Less effective for soft tissue contrast compared to MRI • Limited use for specific reproductive structures

Contd...

Contd...

Imaging modality	*Clinical uses*	*Advantages*	*Disadvantages*
X-Ray and fluoroscopy	**Retrograde urethrography/ VCUG:** Evaluation of urethral strictures, trauma, postoperative complications	• Real-time imaging • Detailed evaluation of urethral anatomy • Useful for dynamic studies	• Ionizing radiation exposure • Invasive procedure (requires catheterization and contrast injection)
Nuclear medicine	**Bone scintigraphy:** Detection of bone metastases, particularly in prostate cancer	• Highly sensitive for detecting bone metastases • Can assess the entire skeleton in one scan	• Ionizing radiation exposure • Limited anatomical detail • Less specific (false positives can occur)
Doppler imaging	**Penile Doppler ultrasound:** Assessment of erectile dysfunction, vascular causes	• Noninvasive • Real-time evaluation of blood flow • Can quantify blood flow velocities	• Operator-dependent • Limited by patient anatomy (e.g., obesity)
Elastography	**Prostate elastography:** Differentiation of benign and malignant prostate lesions	• Noninvasive • Provides additional information on tissue stiffness • Complements traditional ultrasound	• Operator-dependent • Limited availability • Relatively new technique with less widespread adoption
PET-CT/MRI	**Prostate cancer imaging:** Evaluation of metastatic disease, recurrent cancer	• Combines metabolic and anatomical imaging • High sensitivity and specificity for detecting cancer recurrence or metastases	• Very high cost • Limited availability • Exposure to ionizing radiation (in PET-CT)

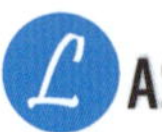

AST MINUTE REVISION

- Ultrasound serves as a versatile tool for initial screening, monitoring renal function, and detecting bladder pathology.
- CT scans offer detailed cross-sectional images, allowing for precise assessment of renal masses, urinary tract obstruction, and metastatic disease.
- MRI provides excellent soft tissue contrast and is particularly valuable for evaluating renal masses and for assessing tumor invasion into adjacent structures.
- Cystoscopy offers direct visualization of the bladder mucosa, facilitating the diagnosis and staging of bladder tumors.
- Contrast-enhanced CT and dynamic MRI sequences, enable clinicians to make informed decisions regarding treatment strategies, including surgery, chemotherapy, and radiation therapy.
- Modalities also play a crucial role in guiding minimally invasive interventions, such as percutaneous nephrostomy tube placement, ureteral stent placement, and image-guided biopsies.

REVIEW QUESTIONS

Multiple Choice Questions (MCQs)

1. **A 55-year-old male presents with sudden onset of severe flank pain and hematuria. Which imaging modality is most appropriate for best evaluation of suspected renal colic?**
   a. Plain abdominal X-ray
   b. Ultrasonography (USG)
   c. Non-contrast CT scan
   d. Intravenous pyelogram (IVP)
2. **A 30-year-old female with a history of recurrent urinary tract infections presents with dysuria and frequency. Which imaging modality is preferred to evaluate for underlying structural abnormalities?**
   a. Plain abdominal X-ray
   b. Voiding cystourethrography (VCUG)
   c. MRI of the pelvis
   d. Ultrasonography (USG)
3. **A 70-year-old male presents with difficulty urinating and elevated prostate-specific antigen (PSA) levels. Which imaging modality should be used to evaluate the prostate gland?**
   a. Plain abdominal X-ray
   b. Transrectal ultrasonography (TRUS)
   c. Non-contrast CT scan
   d. Voiding cystourethrography (VCUG)
4. **A 25-year-old male presents with scrotal pain and swelling. Which imaging modality is most appropriate for initial evaluation of suspected testicular torsion?**
   a. Plain abdominal X-ray
   b. Ultrasonography (USG) with Doppler
   c. MRI of the scrotum
   d. Non-contrast CT scan
5. **A 45-year-old female presents with painless gross hematuria. Which imaging modality should be considered first to evaluate for potential bladder pathology?**
   a. Plain abdominal X-ray
   b. Non-contrast CT scan
   c. Radionuclide study
   d. Ultrasound
6. **Which of the following conditions is most likely to occur due to a failure in the descent of the testes during the embryologic development of the male reproductive system?**
   a. Hypospadias
   b. Cryptorchidism
   c. Androgen insensitivity syndrome (AIS)
   d. Persistent Müllerian duct syndrome (PMDS)

Answer Key

1. c 2. d 3. b 4. b 5. d 6. b

SUGGESTED READING

1. Lotfollahzadeh S, Leslie SW, Aeddula NR. Vesicoureteral reflux. [Updated 2024 Apr 30]. In: StatPearls [Internet]. Treasure Island (FL): StatPearls Publishing; 2024. Available from: https://www.ncbi.nlm.nih.gov/books/NBK537282/
2. Sigmon DF, Shikhman R, Nielson JL. Renal cyst (archived). In: StatPearls [Internet]. Treasure Island (FL): StatPearls Publishing; 2024. PMID: 29261909. Available from: https://www.ncbi.nlm.nih.gov/books/NBK459349/
3. Thotakura R, Anjum F. Hydronephrosis, hydroureter. In: StatPearls [Internet]. Treasure Island (FL): StatPearls Publishing; 2023. Available from: https://www.ncbi.nlm.nih.gov/books/NBK557865/
4. Trunz LM, Balasubramanya R. Doppler renal assessment, protocols, and interpretation. [Updated 2023 Jun 5]. In: StatPearls [Internet]. Treasure Island (FL): StatPearls Publishing; 2024. Available from: https://www.ncbi.nlm.nih.gov/books/NBK572135/

CHAPTER

30 Radiology in Geriatric Patients

"In geriatric imaging, wisdom meets compassion—radiologists honor a lifetime by ensuring comfort and clarity in every scan."

INTRODUCTION

Geriatric imaging is an essential facet of radiology that focuses on the diagnostic evaluation and therapeutic monitoring of diseases prevalent in the elderly population. It plays a pivotal role in the comprehensive care of the aging population. As the global demographic shifts towards an increased elderly population, the role of imaging in the screening, diagnosis, management, and treatment of conditions commonly associated with aging becomes increasingly crucial.

The approach to geriatric imaging must consider the physical and cognitive limitations of elderly patients like reduced mobility or hearing and vision impairments and multimorbidity that can decide how imaging procedures should be performed. There is also a greater emphasis on minimizing exposure to radiation and invasive procedures, reflecting the principles of geriatric medicine, which prioritize patient comfort and quality of life. Effective geriatric care often involves a multidisciplinary team approach, integrating insights from radiologists, geriatricians, surgeons, and other specialists. This collaboration ensures that imaging strategies are aligned with the overall health status and treatment goals of the elderly patients.

Renal function declines with age, increasing the risk of contrast-induced nephropathy in geriatric patients undergoing contrast-enhanced imaging studies. Careful assessment of renal function and judicious use of contrast agents are necessary to minimize adverse effects.

Elderly patients often present with complex medical histories and multiple comorbidities, making the interpretation of imaging studies more challenging and critical. Normal anatomical and physiological changes in aging is important in geriatric population to differentiate normal aging from the pathological disease process.

INDICATION OF GERIATRIC IMAGING

- **Osteoporosis**: Dual-energy X-ray absorptiometry (DEXA) scans are the gold standard for measuring bone mineral density to assess the risk of fractures.
- **Osteoarthritis**: X-rays and MRI are extensively used to visualize joint degradation and inflammation.
- **Cardiovascular diseases**: Echocardiograms, CT angiography, and cardiac MRI help in assessing heart function and detecting vascular diseases.
- **Neurological disorders**: MRI and CT scans are crucial for diagnoses and disease progression in stroke, dementia, and other neurodegenerative disorders such as Alzheimer's disease.

- **Cancers**: Depending on the type and location of the cancer, CT scans, MRIs, PET scans, and ultrasounds are utilized for both diagnosis and monitoring.
- Geriatric trauma

IMAGING OF GERIATRIC BRAIN

Common Age-related Changes in Geriatric Brain

- **Brain atrophy**: Geriatric patients commonly exhibit age-related brain atrophy, characterized by ventricular enlargement, cortical thinning, and hippocampal volume loss. Understanding these changes is crucial for distinguishing normal aging from pathological conditions such as neurodegenerative diseases.
- **White matter changes**: White matter hyperintensities seen on MRI are prevalent in geriatric populations and may indicate underlying small vessel disease, cerebral microangiopathy, or chronic ischemic changes, contributing to cognitive decline and vascular dementia.
- **Vascular changes**: Age-related alterations in vascular structure and function, including arterial stiffness, atherosclerosis, and decreased cerebral perfusion, increase the risk of cerebrovascular events such as stroke and transient ischemic attacks in geriatric patients.

Neurodegenerative Diseases in Geriatric Patients

Neurodegenerative diseases are a group of disorders characterized by progressive degeneration of the nervous system, leading to debilitating symptoms and functional impairment. As medical professionals, understanding these conditions is essential for providing effective care to geriatric patients.

Common Neurodegenerative Diseases

- **Alzheimer's disease (AD):** AD is the most prevalent cause of dementia in the elderly population. It is characterized by the accumulation of amyloid plaques and neurofibrillary tangles in the brain, resulting in memory loss, cognitive decline, and behavioral changes.
- **Parkinson's disease (PD):** PD is a movement disorder caused by the loss of dopamine-producing neurons in the brain. Its cardinal features include tremors, bradykinesia, rigidity, and postural instability, affecting mobility and quality of life.

Neurovascular Emergency in Geriatric Patients

Geriatric patients are at increased risk of neurovascular emergencies due to factors such as hypertension, diabetes, atrial fibrillation, and atherosclerosis. Stroke incidence rises exponentially with age, with the majority of cases occurring in individuals over 65 years old.

Common clinical presentation includes: Ischemic stroke, Hemorrhagic stroke, Transient ischemic attack.

Diagnostic Evaluation

Neuroimaging

Non-contrast CT scan **(Figs. 30.1A and B)** is the initial imaging modality to differentiate between ischemic and hemorrhagic strokes and exclude alternative diagnoses.

Vascular Imaging

Assessment of the cerebrovascular anatomy using techniques like CT angiography or magnetic resonance angiography helps identify underlying stenosis, occlusions, or aneurysms requiring specific interventions.

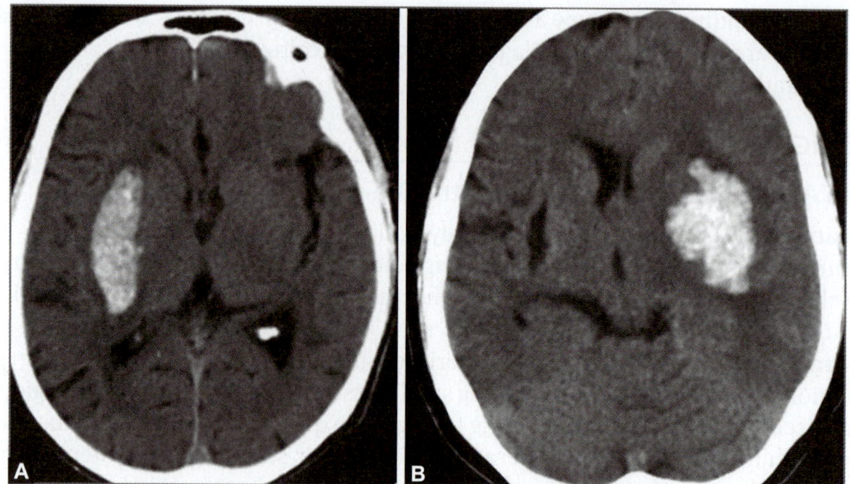

Figs. 30.1A and B: Non-contrast CT scan of the brain: Image A in a 65-year-old male patient with CVA showed acute right basal ganglionic hemorrhage. Image B in a 67-year-old male patient showed CT low-dense chronic hemorrhagic stroke in the right basal ganglia with acute hemorrhagic stroke in the left basal ganglia.

Management Strategies

Acute stroke treatment—time-sensitive interventions such as intravenous thrombolysis with tissue plasminogen activator (tPA) and mechanical thrombectomy are effective in restoring blood-flow to ischemic brain tissue, improving outcomes in eligible patients.

IMAGING HEART DISEASES IN GERIATRIC PATIENTS

Imaging plays a crucial role in the diagnosis, risk stratification, and management of cardiovascular diseases in geriatric patients.

Imaging Modalities

Echocardiography

Transthoracic echocardiography (TTE) and transesophageal echocardiography (TEE) are essential for assessing cardiac structure and function, valvular abnormalities, and hemodynamics in geriatric patients. Doppler imaging provides valuable information on blood flow patterns and cardiac performance.

Cardiac Magnetic Resonance Imaging (MRI) (Figs. 30.2A to C)

Cardiac MRI offers high spatial resolution and tissue characterization capabilities, allowing for detailed evaluation of myocardial viability, fibrosis, and perfusion defects in geriatric patients with ischemic and nonischemic cardiomyopathies.

Cardiac Computed Tomography (CT)

Cardiac CT imaging provides excellent visualization of coronary anatomy, plaque burden, and calcification, facilitating noninvasive assessment of coronary artery disease (CAD), coronary artery anomalies, and structural heart abnormalities in geriatric populations.

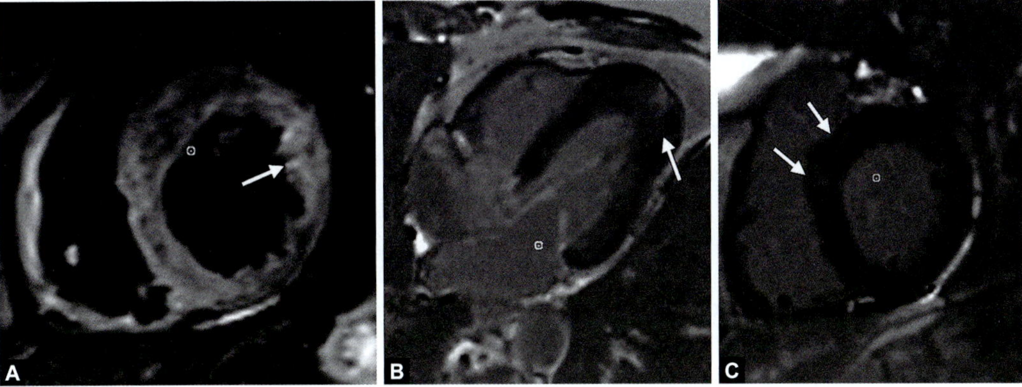

Figs. 30.2A to C: A 72-year-old male presented with chest pain. Cardiac MRI (CMR) reveals hypertensive thickening of the LV walls and IVS (arrow in image A). Post-contrast LGE images show late gadolinium patchy subendocardial enhancement in the LV apex and anterior IVS, representing chronic ischemic infarction with scar formation.

Molecular Imaging

Molecular imaging modalities such as positron emission tomography (PET) and single-photon emission computed tomography (SPECT) enable noninvasive detection of myocardial perfusion, metabolism, and inflammation, offering valuable prognostic information and guiding targeted therapies in geriatric patients with heart diseases.

Challenges in Geriatric Cardiac Imaging

- **Age-related changes**: Physiological changes associated with aging, including vascular stiffness, myocardial fibrosis, and decreased myocardial reserve, may affect imaging interpretation and diagnostic accuracy in geriatric patients with heart diseases.
- **Comorbidities:** Geriatric patients often present with multiple comorbidities such as hypertension, diabetes, and chronic kidney disease, which may influence imaging findings, treatment decisions, and prognosis in cardiovascular diseases.

Clinical Applications

CAD Evaluation

Noninvasive imaging modalities such as cardiac CT angiography and stress echocardiography are valuable for assessing coronary artery anatomy, stenosis severity, and myocardial ischemia in geriatric patients with suspected or known CAD.

Valvular Heart Disease

Echocardiography remains the primary imaging modality for diagnosing and monitoring valvular heart diseases such as aortic stenosis, mitral regurgitation, and aortic regurgitation in geriatric populations, guiding surgical interventions and transcatheter valve therapies.

Heart Failure

Echocardiography, cardiac MRI, and nuclear imaging techniques play essential roles in evaluating left ventricular function, myocardial viability, and myocardial perfusion defects in geriatric patients with heart failure, guiding medical therapy and device implantation decisions.

IMAGING VASCULAR DISEASES IN GERIATRICS

Vascular diseases represent a significant health burden in geriatric patients, contributing to morbidity and mortality worldwide. Imaging plays a pivotal role in the diagnosis, characterization, and management of vascular conditions in the elderly population.

Imaging Modalities

Duplex Ultrasonography

Duplex ultrasonography combines B-mode imaging with Doppler ultrasound to evaluate vascular anatomy, blood-flow velocities, and vascular pathology in geriatric patients. It is widely used for assessing peripheral artery disease (PAD), carotid artery stenosis, and deep vein thrombosis (DVT) in clinical practice.

Computed Tomography Angiography (CTA)

CTA provides high-resolution imaging of the arterial and venous vasculature, allowing for accurate delineation of vascular anatomy, detection of stenosis or occlusions, and assessment of collateral circulation in geriatric patients with atherosclerotic disease, aneurysms, or vascular trauma.

Magnetic Resonance Angiography (MRA)

MRA offers noninvasive visualization of vascular structures using magnetic resonance imaging techniques, with advantages such as multiplanar imaging, tissue contrast, and lack of ionizing radiation. It is particularly valuable for evaluating cerebral, thoracic, and peripheral vascular diseases in geriatric populations.

Clinical Applications in Geriatric Vascular Imaging

Peripheral Artery Disease (PAD)

Imaging modalities such as duplex ultrasonography, CTA, and MRA are essential for diagnosing PAD, assessing disease severity, and guiding revascularization procedures in geriatric patients with lower extremity claudication or critical limb ischemia.

Carotid Artery Disease

Carotid artery duplex ultrasonography and CTA/MRA are valuable for detecting carotid artery stenosis, determining plaque morphology, and stratifying stroke risk in geriatric patients, informing decisions regarding medical therapy or carotid endarterectomy or stenting in asymptomatic or symptomatic individuals.

Venous Thromboembolism (VTE)

Ultrasonography remains the imaging modality of choice for diagnosing DVT and evaluating venous thromboembolism in geriatric patients.

IMAGING RESPIRATORY DISEASES IN GERIATRICS

Respiratory diseases are common in geriatric patients and can significantly impact quality of life and mortality.

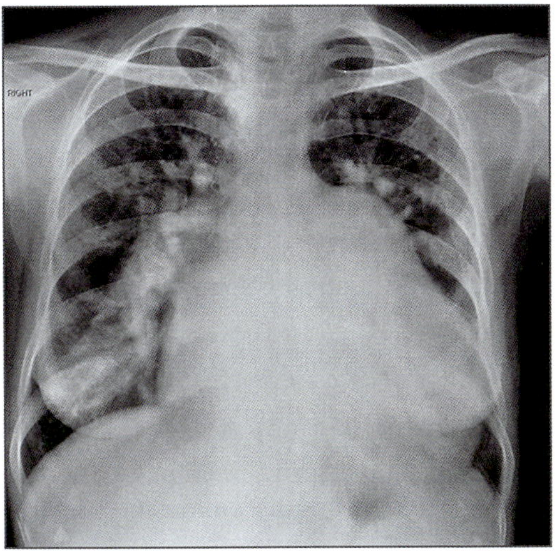

Fig. 30.3: 66-year-old female with pulmonary arterial hypertension with dilated central pulmonary arteries with peripheral pruning.

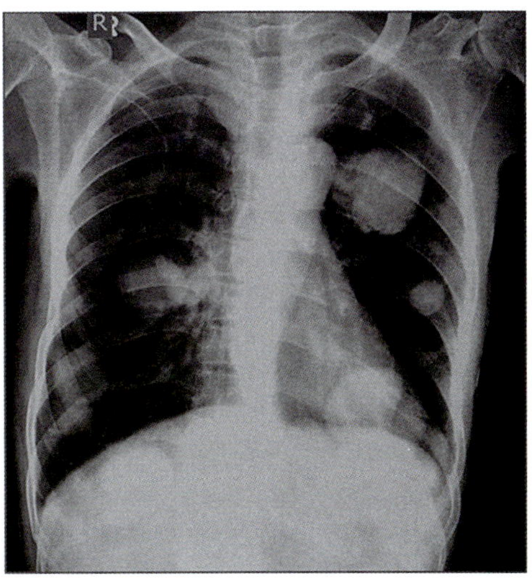

Fig. 30.4: 69-year-male with canon ball metastases in bilateral lung fields.

Imaging Modalities

Includes Chest X-ray and CT.

Note: PFTs (Pulmonary function tests) complement imaging studies by assessing lung function, respiratory mechanics, and gas exchange parameters in geriatric patients with respiratory diseases, aiding in diagnosis, severity staging, and treatment monitoring.

Clinical Applications (Figs. 30.3 and 30.4)

Chronic Obstructive Pulmonary Disease (COPD)

Imaging modalities such as CXR and CT are valuable for diagnosing COPD, assessing disease severity, evaluating pulmonary complications (e.g., emphysema, bronchiectasis), and guiding treatment strategies (e.g., bronchodilators, oxygen therapy) in geriatric patients.

Interstitial Lung Disease (ILD)

High-resolution chest CT is the imaging modality of choice for diagnosing and characterizing ILD subtypes (e.g., idiopathic pulmonary fibrosis, hypersensitivity pneumonitis) in geriatric patients, aiding in differential diagnosis, prognostication, and treatment planning.

Lung Cancer Screening

Low-dose chest CT screening is recommended for early detection of lung cancer in high-risk geriatric patients (e.g., heavy smokers, age 55–80 years), allowing for timely diagnosis, curative-intent treatment, and improved survival outcomes in selected individuals.

IMAGING OF GASTROINTESTINAL TRACT DISEASES IN GERIATRICS

As the population ages, the prevalence of gastrointestinal (GI) diseases among geriatric individuals increases, necessitating tailored approaches to diagnostic imaging.

Imaging Modalities

Radiography and CT.

Magnetic Resonance Imaging (MRI)

MRI is suitable for assessing hepatobiliary disorders, pancreatic tumors, and pelvic floor dysfunction in geriatric individuals.

Note: Endoscopic procedures such as upper endoscopy and colonoscopy are essential for diagnosing and managing GI diseases such as esophageal strictures, colorectal polyps, and gastrointestinal bleeding in older adults.

Advancements in Imaging Technology

Virtual Colonoscopy

CT colonography provides a less invasive option for colorectal cancer screening in geriatric patients, offering high sensitivity for detecting polyps while minimizing discomfort and sedation risks.

Magnetic Resonance Enterography (MRE)

MRE is preferred over CT enterography for evaluating small bowel disorders in elderly patients.

Contrast-enhanced Ultrasound (CEUS)

CEUS is increasingly used for liver imaging in geriatric patients.

Clinical Applications

Inflammatory Bowel Disease (IBD)

Imaging plays a crucial role in assessing disease activity, complications, and treatment response in geriatric patients with IBD, guiding therapeutic decisions and minimizing the risk of complications.

Gastrointestinal Bleeding

Multimodal imaging approaches, including CT angiography and nuclear medicine studies, help localize and characterize sources of GI bleeding in elderly individuals, facilitating prompt intervention and reducing morbidity **(Fig. 30.5)**.

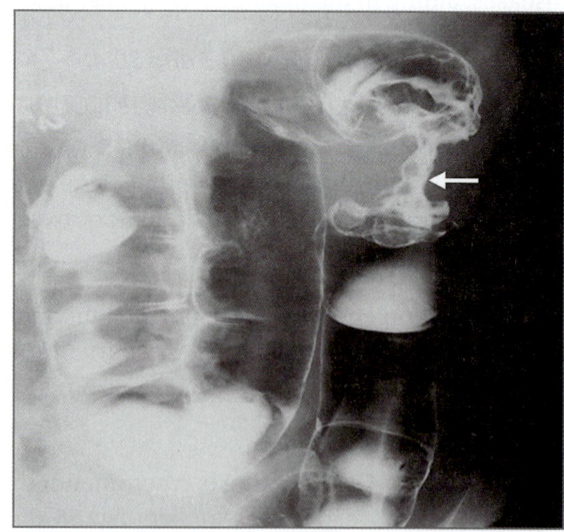

Fig. 30.5: 72-year-old male with rectal bleeding. Double-contrast barium enema showed annular growth in the descending colon.

Hepatobiliary Disorders

MRI is preferred for hepatobiliary imaging in geriatric patients, providing comprehensive evaluation of liver lesions, biliary obstruction, and pancreatic pathology without nephrotoxicity concerns.

IMAGING OF UROLOGIC DISEASES IN GERIATRICS

Ultrasound Imaging

Ultrasound serves as a frontline imaging modality for evaluating urologic diseases especially prostatic enlargement with the amount of post-void residual urine, due to its noninvasive nature and absence of ionizing radiation, making it particularly suitable for geriatric patients. In renal pathologies, ultrasound aids in detecting hydronephrosis, renal masses, and evaluating bladder wall thickness.

CT, MRI and Nuclear medicine also aids in diagnosing and staging urologic diseases.

OSTEOARTHRITIS/DEGENERATIVE IN GERIATRIC PATIENTS

Osteoarthritis (OA) is a prevalent musculoskeletal disorder characterized by progressive joint degeneration, predominantly affecting geriatric individuals. Radiological imaging plays a crucial role in diagnosing OA, assessing disease severity, and guiding therapeutic interventions.

Osteoporosis is one of the leading causes of benign vertebral collapse in elderly patients who were sometimes presented with variable degrees of myelopathy.

Imaging Modalities

Includes X-ray, MRI, CT and USG.

Osteoporosis is a condition characterized by low bone mass and structural deterioration of bone tissue, leading to an increased risk of fractures, particularly in older adults. Geriatric patients, generally defined as those aged 65 years and older, are especially prone to osteoporotic changes due to several age-related factors. Here are the key considerations:

1. **Bone density loss**: With age, bone density naturally decreases. This loss accelerates in women after menopause due to reduced estrogen levels. In men, declining testosterone levels also contribute to bone loss. Lower bone density predisposes geriatric patients to osteoporosis.
2. **Changes in bone architecture**: Aging affects the microarchitecture of bones, making them weaker and more susceptible to fractures **(Fig. 30.6)**.
3. **Nutritional factors**: Poor nutrition or inadequate intake of calcium and vitamin D can contribute to osteoporosis.
4. **Hormonal changes**: Declining levels of estrogen and testosterone in women and men, respectively, affect bone density and strength.
5. **Lifestyle factors**: Sedentary lifestyle, lack of weight-bearing exercise, and smoking can exacerbate bone loss in older adults.
6. **Chronic conditions and medications**: Certain chronic conditions like rheumatoid arthritis, chronic kidney disease, cancer treatment and gastrointestinal disorders can affect bone health.
7. **Fall risk**: Osteoporosis increases the risk of fractures, particularly in geriatric patients who are more prone to falls due to factors like decreased balance, muscle strength, and coordination. Fractures can further reduce mobility and quality of life in older adults **(Figs. 30.7A to C)**.

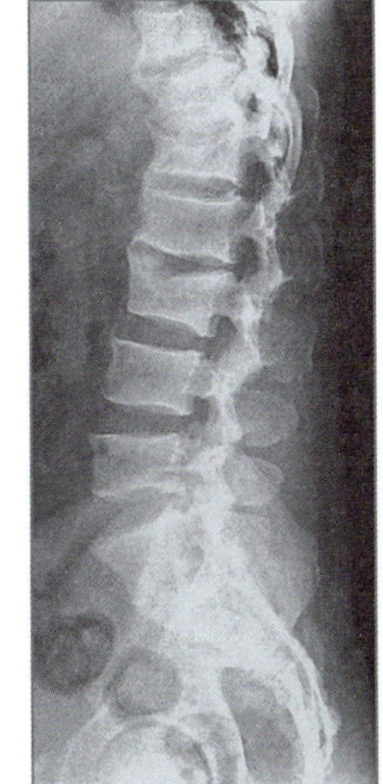

Fig. 30.6: 73-year-old male patient, the lateral view of plain radiograph shows osteoporotic collapse of the multiple lower dorsal and lumbar vertebrae.

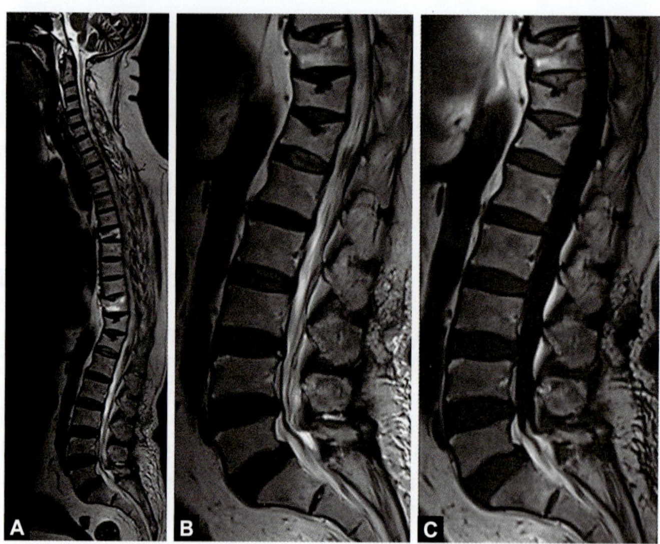

Figs. 30.7A to C: 64-year-female patient, sagittal T2 and T1 W images show the osteoporotic collapse of the multiple lower dorsal vertebrae.

IMAGING IN MYELOID AND LYMPHOID DISEASES

Myeloid and lymphoid diseases encompass a spectrum of hematologic malignancies and disorders that pose diagnostic and management challenges, particularly in geriatric patients.

X-ray imaging: Conventional radiography is often the initial imaging modality employed in the evaluation of skeletal manifestations of hematologic disorders, such as lytic bone lesions in multiple myeloma or osteosclerotic lesions in chronic myeloid leukemia **(Figs. 30.8A and B)**.

Computed tomography (CT): CT imaging offers detailed anatomical assessment and is widely utilized for staging and monitoring of myeloid and lymphoid diseases. In lymphoma, CT helps delineate the extent of disease involvement in lymph nodes, spleen, and extra nodal sites.

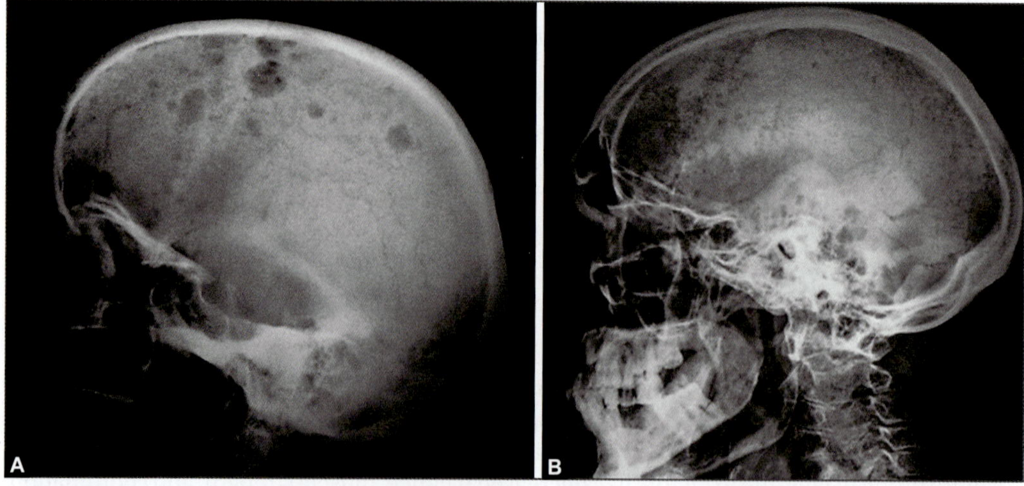

Figs. 30.8A and B: Image A shows variable sizes of osteolytic lesions of skull metastases and Image B shows smaller permeable osteolytic lesions of multiple myeloma.

Magnetic resonance imaging (MRI): MRI provides superior soft tissue contrast and is particularly useful for assessing central nervous system involvement in myeloid and lymphoid diseases, including leukemic infiltration or lymphomatous masses. In myeloma, MRI with diffusion-weighted imaging aids in detecting marrow involvement and evaluating for complications such as spinal cord compression or vertebral fractures.

Positron emission tomography-computed tomography (PET-CT): PET-CT is a powerful tool for assessing metabolic activity and disease extent in lymphoid malignancies, aiding in staging, treatment response assessment, and surveillance. In myeloid disorders, PET-CT may be utilized to detect extramedullary disease involvement or assess for transformation to secondary malignancies.

Bone scintigraphy: Bone scintigraphy is valuable for detecting skeletal involvement in hematologic malignancies, particularly in myeloma and lymphoma.

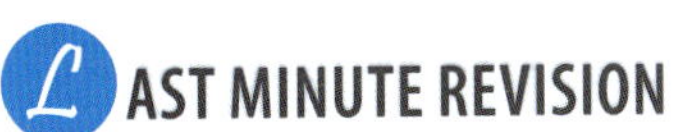

LAST MINUTE REVISION

- The elderly are more susceptible to the harmful effects of radiation. Hence, it's crucial to prioritize imaging modalities with lower radiation exposure, such as ultrasound and MRI.
- Imaging in geriatric patients should not only focus on diagnosing diseases but also on assessing functional capabilities and guiding treatment plans to improve quality of life.
- Multidisciplinary collaboration is effective in geriatric imaging which involves close collaboration with geriatricians, radiologists, and other healthcare providers to create individualized care plans.
- Preventive screening through appropriate imaging can detect early signs of common geriatric conditions, such as osteoporosis, cardiovascular diseases, and cancers, leading to timely intervention.
- Noninvasive techniques are preferred as it can reduce the risk of complications and improve diagnostic accuracy in the elderly population.

REVIEW QUESTIONS

Multiple Choice Questions (MCQs)

1. Which imaging modality is commonly used for the initial evaluation of suspected fractures in geriatric patients?

a. Magnetic resonance imaging (MRI)
b. Computed tomography (CT)
c. Ultrasonography (US)
d. X-ray radiography

2. What imaging technique is utilized to assess osteoporosis and bone mineral density in geriatric patients?

a. MRI
b. Dual-energy X-ray absorptiometry (DEXA)
c. Fluoroscopy
d. Positron Emission Tomography (PET)

3. Which imaging modality serves as the gold standard for evaluating cerebral atrophy and vascular dementia in geriatric patients?

a. CT scan
b. X-ray
c. MRI
d. PET scan

4. What imaging technique is employed for evaluating gastrointestinal bleeding in geriatric patients, allowing both diagnostic and therapeutic interventions?

a. X-ray
b. MRI
c. CT angiography
d. Ultrasound

5. **What is the preferred imaging modality for evaluating suspected deep vein thrombosis (DVT) in geriatric patients?**
   a. X-ray
   b. MRI
   c. CT scan
   d. Doppler ultrasound
6. **Which imaging technique is used for evaluating suspected abdominal aortic dissection in geriatric patients?**
   a. X-ray
   b. MRI
   c. CT scan
   d. Ultrasound

Answer Key

1. d 2. b 3. c 4. c 5. d 6. c

SUGGESTED READING

1. Porter JL, Varacallo M. Osteoporosis. 2023. In: StatPearls [Internet]. Treasure Island (FL): StatPearls Publishing; 2024. PMID: 28722930.
2. Van den Wyngaert T, Strobel K, Kampen WU, Kuwert T, van der Bruggen W, Mohan HK, et al. The EANM practice guidelines for bone scintigraphy. Eur J Nucl Med Mol Imaging. 2016;43(9):1723-38. doi: 10.1007/s00259-016-3415-4. Epub 2016 Jun 4. PMID: 27262701; PMCID: PMC4932135.

CHAPTER

31 Oncological Imaging

"In oncological imaging, every shadow is a clue, every scan a chance—to detect early, guide therapy, and fight with vision."

INTRODUCTION

Steady and rapid advances in imaging in the last few decades have changed oncological disease management today with a pivotal role played by the radiologist. The most significant advance has been multi-parametric imaging which provides both anatomical and functional information to the physician to optimize management. This functional information is available not only through Nuclear Medicine (PET scan) but also with advanced MRI functional techniques. In order to play a more meaningful role, the radiologist needs to be familiar not only with the imaging technique, its strengths and limitations, but also with the issues of clinical concern. Equipped with the knowledge of the disease and with judicious use of new technology, the radiologist can help provide answers concerning diagnosis, response assessment, prognosis and recurrence.

BRAIN NEOPLASMS

Imaging plays an important role in the evaluation of brain neoplasms, in regard to assessment of location, extent and characterization of intracranial tumors, and its post-treatment follow-up. The following are clinical settings in which imaging for brain neoplasm (particularly gliomas) is done:

- Initial diagnostic workup
- Imaging for surgical planning
- For follow up

The initial imaging modality is largely dependent on availability. Initial imaging is usually Computed Tomography (CT) or Magnetic Resonance Imaging (MRI) which identifies an intracranial tumor, to define the number of SOL, location in terms of lobe, parenchyma, intra or extra-axial; extent (adjacent structures, midline shift) and characterization of the lesion in terms of fat/hemorrhage/calcification/enhancement/edema/necrosis/solid or cystic on T1, T2 and DW.

When an initial non-contrast imaging demonstrates an intra-axial or extra-axial space-occupying lesion, the use of intravenous contrast medium is mandatory for defining the extent and characterization of the intracranial space-occupying lesion. It can also be used for planning of surgical approaches and intraoperative navigation.

MRI is a modality of choice for detection of brain neoplasms because of its excellent soft tissue contrast and resolution and it also provides functional information. Advanced MR imaging techniques (physiology-based) like diffusion weighted imaging (DWI), MR spectroscopy (MRS) and MR perfusion scans improve sensitivity and specificity of tumor diagnosis. But it is contraindicated in patients with cardiac pacemakers, aneurysm clips, cochlear implants and intraorbital metallic foreign bodies **(Fig. 31.1)**.

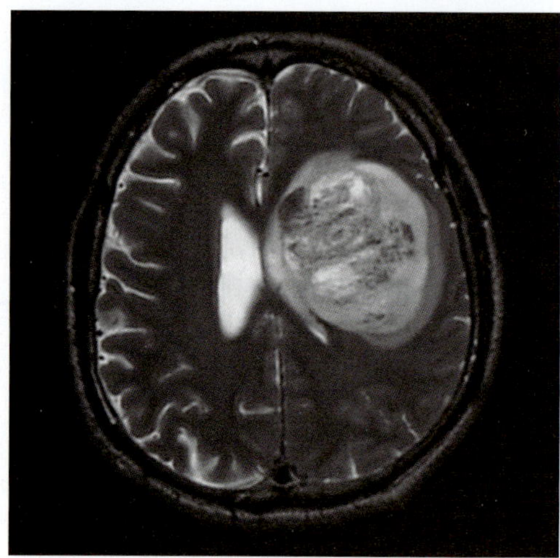

Fig. 31.1: MRI of a large infiltrative brain glioma showing mass effect.

Follow-up imaging: MRI is an ideal modality for follow-up imaging (one of sequence should be a 3D sequence to allow for assessment of post-resection residual tumor volume), to assess response, to distinguish response from pseudo-response, to detect any findings of recurrence and also to distinguish tumor progression from pseudo-progression.

HEAD AND NECK CANCER

Head and neck cancer usually refers to squamous cell cancer (SCC) of the upper aerodigestive tract that comprises primarily of oral, pharyngeal cancers and laryngeal cancers.

The multidimensional role of imaging in the evaluation of head and neck cancers is as follows:

- Accurate staging (as clinical examination is unable to assess the deep extent of disease).
- Assessing therapeutic options (surgery, chemotherapy or radiotherapy, single modality or multimodality).
- To guide biopsies
- To evaluate treatment response and post-treatment surveillance and distinguishing post-treatment changes from recurrence.

Imaging Methods

The imaging methods that have a role in the evaluation of head and neck cancers are contrast enhanced CT, contrast enhanced MRI, ultrasonography and PETCT scanning. Multidetector CT (MDCT) scanners have widely replaced conventional and helical CT scanners. Sixteen or higher section MDCT scanners provide high-resolution isotropic reformations with clarity. In general, MRI is preferred in the suprahyoid neck and CT is preferred in the infrahyoid neck. MRI is superior for evaluating skull base marrow invasion, perineural spread, dural invasion, cavernous sinus invasion and retropharyngeal adenopathy. In the oral cavity, the tumor–tongue contrast is best studied on contrast-enhanced MRI **(Fig. 31.2)**.

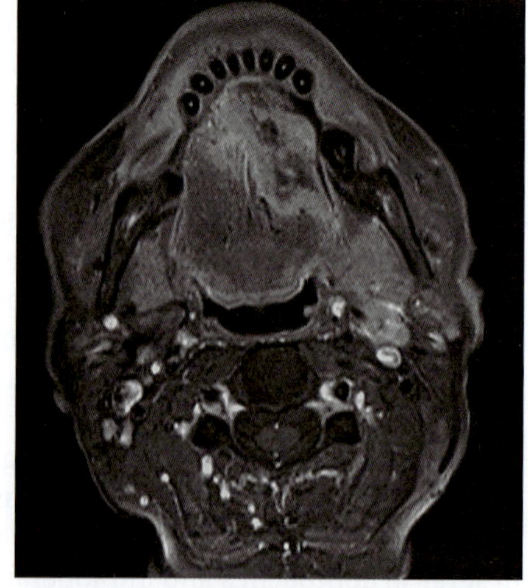

Fig. 31.2: Case of carcinoma anterior 2/3rd left tongue.

Information from imaging familiarity with the T-staging of cancers in various head neck regions helps the radiologist provide a complete report to

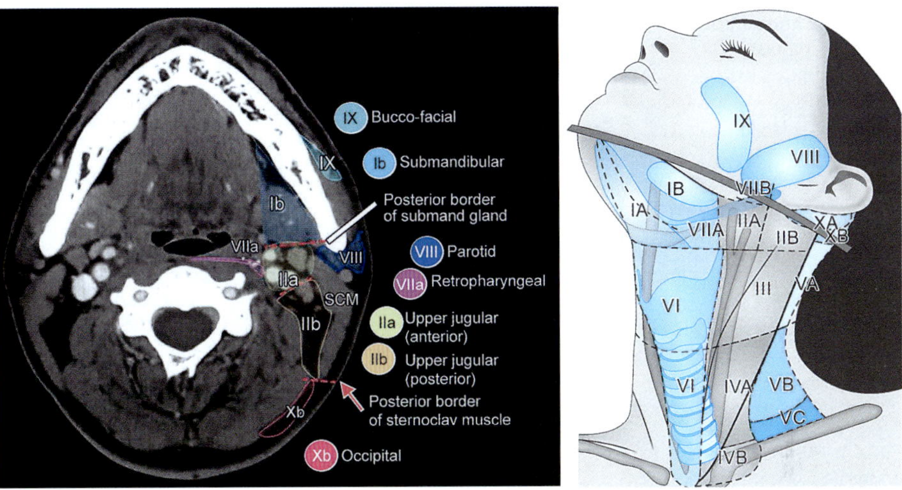

Fig. 31.3: Levels of cervical lymph node and their radiological depiction on axial CT scan.

the clinician. Levels of cervical lymph node and their radiological depiction on axial CT scan shown in **Figure 31.3**.

Retinoblastoma

Retinoblastomas are the most common intraocular neoplasm found in childhood and with modern treatment modalities, are in most cases curable.

On imaging, they are generally characterized by a heterogeneous retinal mass with calcifications, necrotic components, and increased vascularization on Doppler ultrasound/ enhancement on CT/MRI.

CT

It must be emphasized that CT scan is not recommended in the study of children with suspected or known retinoblastoma. Therefore, MRI must be always preferred, because CT scan use may result in an increased risk of secondary malignancies related to radiation exposure. Moreover, high-doses of radiation are especially harmful to this group of patients with heritable and germline retinoblastoma (**Fig. 31.4**).

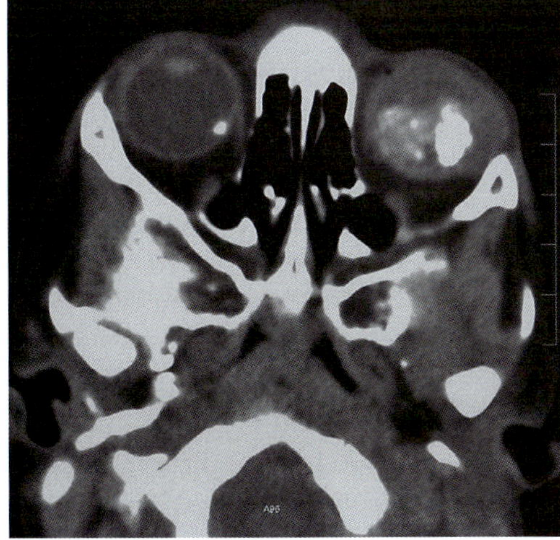

Fig. 31.4: Single axial image from a CT of the orbits demonstrating bilateral intraocular calcified masses, larger on the left, consistent with bilateral retinoblastoma.

MRI

MRI is the modality of choice for pretreatment staging on retinoblastoma.

MRI is often used in searching for optic nerve involvement, extraocular extension, and the possibility of a concomitant primitive neuroectodermal tumor (trilateral retinoblastoma with pineoblastoma).

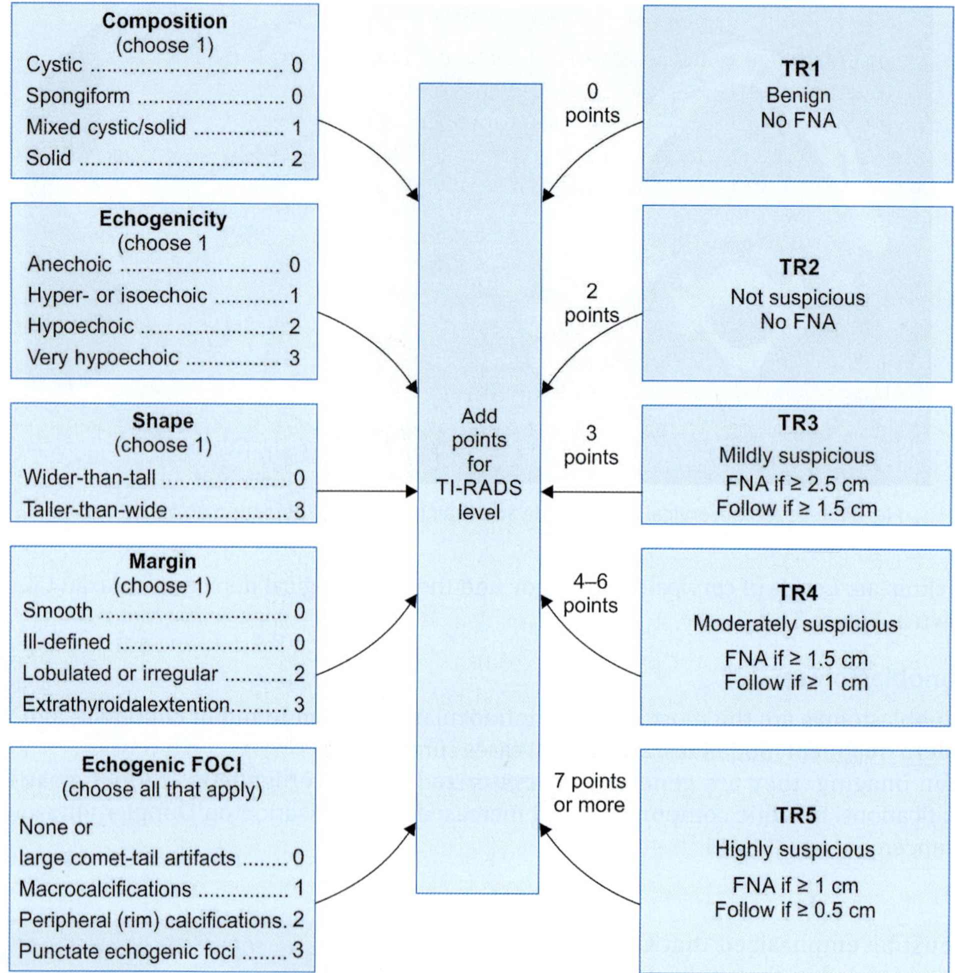

Fig. 31.5: ACR TI-RADS reporting system for thyroid nodules.

Thyroid Malignancy

ACR TI-RADS **(Fig. 31.5)** is a reporting system for thyroid nodules on ultrasound.

This uses a standardized scoring system for reports providing users with recommendations for when to use fine needles aspiration (FNA) or ultrasound follow-up of suspicious nodules, and when to safely leave alone nodules that are benign/not suspicious.

BREAST CANCER

Role of Mammography

Screening reduces breast cancer mortality by 15% (irrespective of age at which screening is started).

Role of Ultrasonography

There is no role of ultrasound alone in screening for breast cancer. A combination of mammography and ultrasound for screening of breast cancer has shown increased detection rate (improved sensitivity).

Role of Breast Imaging in a Newly Diagnosed Case of Breast Cancer

Digital mammography, which is considered the gold standard, along with breast ultrasonography are employed as routine imaging modalities. Breast MRI is used in conjunction with mammography as a problem-solving tool. (Already discussed in chapter 25)

Guided procedure (either by USG or mammography) includes FNA or core needle biopsy or vacuum assisted biopsy (minimally invasive for large sample) and wire localization (for nonpalpable lesion).

LUNG CANCER

- Lung cancer is the most common cancer and a leading cause of cancer-related death.
- In India, approximately 93,000 new lung cancer cases are reported each year.
- Chest radiograph is often an initial investigation; it is universally available and is inexpensive and quite accurate however, it is not helpful in picking up early disease.
- CT is used to map the complete extent of disease and is also useful for CT-guided biopsies. The wide availability of multidetector computed tomography (MDCT), has made it the imaging technique of choice **(Fig. 31.6)**.
- PET CT provides information of metabolic activity of lung-nodes or masses which helps to know the nature of lesion as benign or malignant.
- MRI can be used when CT or PET-CT are inconclusive.

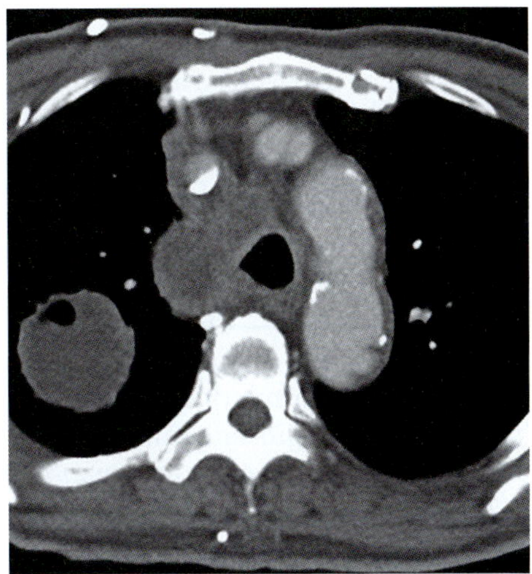

Fig. 31.6: Shows a large soft tissue mass on right side with irregular margins suggestive of bronchogenic carcinoma, along with right hilar lymph node.

A solitary pulmonary nodule (SPN) is defined as a single intraparenchymal lesion <3 cm in size and not associated with atelectasis or lymphadenopathy. A lesion >3 cm in diameter is called a mass. This distinction is made because lesions >3 cm are usually malignant, while smaller lesions can be either benign or malignant.

HEPATOCELLULAR CARCINOMA

Imaging of the liver is performed either to rule out metastasis in patient with known primary or in patients with cirrhosis and/or risk factors for developing hepatocellular carcinoma.

Imaging of liver is performed not only to detect disease but to characterize liver lesions to distinguish liver cancer from other benign focal lesions of the liver.

If CT/MRI scan of the liver is performed for characterization of lesion/s or for staging of liver lesions. The imaging needs to be performed in arterial, portovenous and equilibrium phase following intravenous administration of contrast, this should be preceded by non-contrast scan of the liver. **(Triple phase CT)**. Beside diagnosis, radiologists play vital role in loco-regional therapies like Radiofrequency ablation, Transarterial chemoembolization, PTBD etc.

RENAL-CELL-CARCINOMA

The imaging modality of choice for evaluation of renal-cell-carcinoma is computed tomography with a dedicated renal contrast protocol that allows detection, staging (extent and morphology of the lesion, the nodal status, evaluation of the extrarenal spread, evaluation of renal vein and inferior vena cava) and surgical planning.

Multiphase imaging is a must for optimal evaluation of renal masses. It also provides information of the contralateral kidney and metastases in the abdominal region and CT of the thorax is used for pulmonary metastatic evaluation. Imaging (commonly USG) is used to classify renal lesions as solid or cystic. For solid renal mass, the most important criteria in differentiating a malignant lesion is the presence of enhancement.

Magnetic resonance imaging (MRI) is used as a problem-solving tool. If CT scan findings are indeterminate and when use of iodinated contrast is precluded, due to history of allergy or prior reaction to iodinated contrast medium, in pregnant patients and in patients with renal failure.

CT is frequently used to both diagnose and stage renal cell carcinomas. Approximately 30% demonstrate some calcification. Renal cell carcinoma typically causes hypervascular metastases, best appreciated on arterial phase imaging of the upper abdomen **(Fig. 31.7)**.

PROSTATE CANCER

It is the most common malignancy among men. Local staging (T-staging) of prostate cancer is based on multiparametric magnetic resonance (MR) imaging. The role of magnetic resonance imaging (MRI) in prostate cancer is for assessing the extent of disease than for diagnosing the primary disease. For example, organ-confined disease on MRI may imply that the patient can be benefited from surgery (prostatectomy). MRI proves to be accurate than either digital rectal examination (DRE) or transrectal ultrasound (TRUS) and TRUS guided biopsy, in preoperative anatomical localization of Ca prostate.

Prostate imaging-reporting and data system (PI-RADS) is a structured reporting scheme for multiparametric prostate. A PI-RADS score is given to assess the probability of the lesion being malignant.

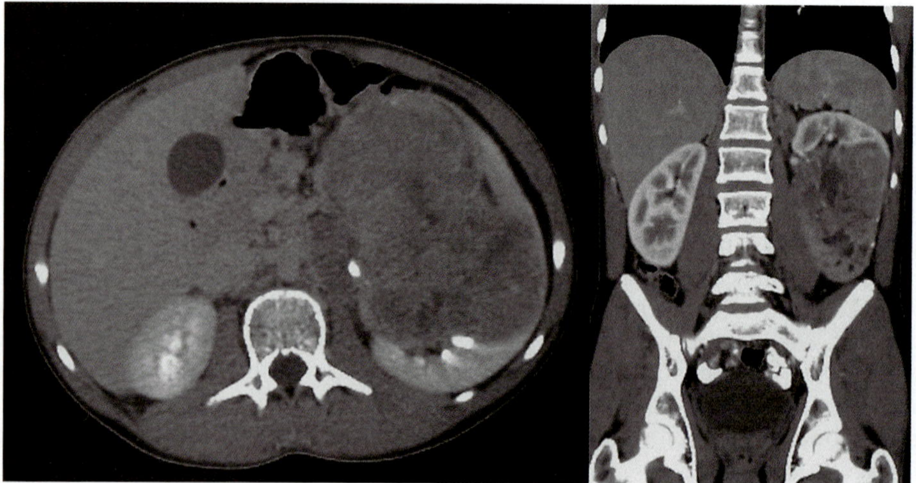

Fig. 31.7: Left renal lower zonal large exophytic soft tissue mass lesion. The mass appears heterogeneous with internal cystic areas of breaking down and heterogeneous post-contrast enhancement.

- **PI-RADS 1:** Very low (clinically significant cancer is highly unlikely to be present)
- **PI-RADS 2:** Low (clinically significant cancer is unlikely to be present)
- **PI-RADS 3:** Intermediate (the presence of clinically significant cancer is equivocal)
- **PI-RADS 4:** High (clinically significant cancer is likely to be present)
- **PI-RADS 5:** Very high (clinically significant cancer is highly likely to be present)
- **PI-RADS X:** Component of exam technically inadequate or not performed

BOWEL CANCER

It is a common malignancy that results in significant morbidity and mortality. Abdominal computed tomography (CT) is valuable in planning surgery for bowel cancer because it can demonstrate regional extension of tumor as well as adenopathy and distant metastases. At CT, colon cancer typically appears as a discrete soft-tissue mass that narrows the colonic lumen.

Currently, rectal MRI plays a key role in the pre- and post-treatment evaluation of **rectal cancer**. In primary staging, rectal MRI helps the radiologist:

- Describe the tumor location and morphology.
- Provide its T (tumor) and N (lymph node) categories.

ENDOMETRIAL AND CERVICAL CANCER

Magnetic resonance imaging (MRI) has become the most efficient technique in the management of women with gynecological cancer **(Fig. 31.8)**.

In endometrial cancer, MRI is dependable in identifying myometrial and cervical invasion and extrauterine disease, thereby informing preoperative surgical planning and giving exact staging **(Fig. 31.9)**.

In cervical cancer, MRI plays a pivotal role in distinguishing early from advanced disease, thereby stratifying patients for surgery and chemoradiation. Diagnosis is initially made at histology in both cancers. Imaging is an important tool for clinical and surgical evaluation. Transvaginal ultrasound (TVUS) is the initial imaging modality for both cancers.

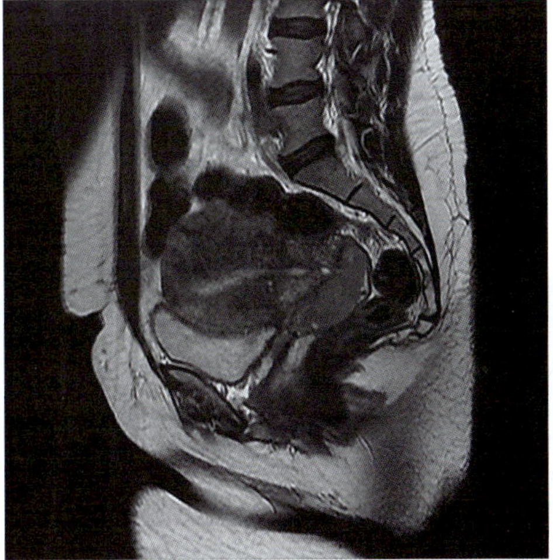

Fig. 31.8: Carcinoma cervix on MRI.

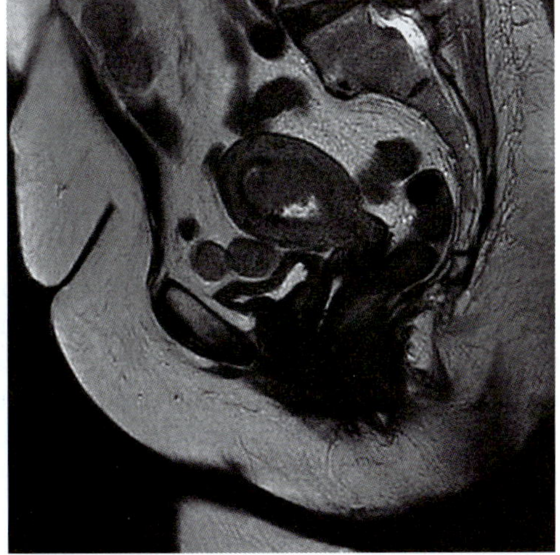

Fig. 31.9: Carcinoma endometrium on MRI.

Table 31.1: Key features of pediatric abdominal tumors.

Neuroblastoma	• Malaise, pain, and abdominal mass; opsoclonus myoclonus syndrome or metastatic disease • US inhomogeneous and echogenic, with bright calcifications • VMA and HVA levels in the urine
Nephroblastoma	• The most common renal tumor in children • Distended painless abdomen, sometimes hematuria or hypertension • US claw sign, small tumors will move synchronous with the kidney
Hodgkin lymphoma	• Cervical lymph node enlargement, and mediastinal masses • Rarely confined to the abdomen
Non-Hodgkin	• Para-aortic and mesenteric nodes • Spleen involvement
Leukemia	• May be present with abdominal involvement, mostly kidneys
Hepatocellular carcinoma	• Uncommon malignant liver tumor in teenagers • Abdominal mass, jaundice, pain, AFP high
Germ cell tumor	• Usually in testis or ovary but many present as abdominal tumor. High AFP, beta-HCG and CA-125

IMAGING OF COMMON EXTRACRANIAL SOLID TUMORS IN CHILDREN

The common pediatric neoplasms are hematolymphoid malignancies followed by solid tumors like brain neoplasms, neuroblastoma, hepatoblastoma, Wilms tumor, rhabdomyosarcoma, etc. Imaging plays an important role in diagnosis, staging, risk stratification, response evaluation and follow-up of most of the pediatric solid tumors. **Key features of pediatric abdominal tumors shown in Table 31.1.**

BONE TUMORS

There are a large number of bone tumors with varied radiological appearances. The most important determinators in the analysis of a bone tumor are:

1. Morphology in terms of matrix; lytic/sclerotic; single/multiple
2. Age of patient in terms of before or after epiphyseal fusion
3. Location of tumor in terms of axial/peripheral skeleton; flat/long bone; diaphyseal/epiphyseal/metaphyseal; cortical/medullary
4. Association with periosteal reaction/soft tissue
5. Combined with all above bone tumors are broadly divided into aggressive and nonaggressive tumors

PANCREATIC CANCER

Most common type is adenocarcinomas commonly located within the head (65%), 15% in the corpus and 10% in the tail. The remaining 10% being multifocal or diffuse. Tumors of the head are usually present earlier due to obstructive jaundice. Other common tumors are neuroendocrine tumor. Insulinomas are a type of pancreatic neuroendocrine tumor (PNET), typically small, benign, and hypervascular, producing insulin and causing hypoglycemia. Accurate localization using CT, MRI, or EUS is crucial for effective surgical management.

Somatostatin receptor scintigraphy is commonly used for gastrointestinal and pancreatic neuroendocrine tumors, (gastrinomas, glucagonomas, VIPomas, and somatostatinoma) as well as carcinoid tumors.

NUCLEAR MEDICINE FOR DIAGNOSIS AND TREATMENT

Nuclear medicine is a subspecialty of radiology, a field of medicine that uses a trace amount of radioactive substances for the diagnosis and treatment of many health conditions such as certain types of cancer. (As discussed in chapter 36)

AST MINUTE REVISION

- Imaging is used for not only for diagnosis and interventions, but can also used in screening, such as mammography for breast cancer and low-dose CT for lung cancer.
- X-ray is especially used for initial assessment of bone involvement and lung metastasis.
- Main role of ultrasound is to assess abdominal organs, thyroid, breast, and testicular cancers.
- CT and MRI are used for staging and extent of malignancy.

REVIEW QUESTIONS

Multiple Choice Questions (MCQs)

1. **The investigation of choice for staging carcinoma rectum is:**
   a. CT scan
   b. PET scan
   c. MRI
   d. Transrectal ultrasound (TRUS)
2. **For screening of breast cancer, the modality of choice is:**
   a. Ultrasound
   b. Mammography
   c. PET scan
   d. Clinical examination
3. **The subspecialty of medicine involving the use of radioactive substances for diagnosis and treatment is known as:**
   a. Radiotherapy
   b. Nuclear medicine
   c. Radiodiagnosis
   d. Theranostic
4. **For characterization of liver lesion and to differentiate cancerous to noncancerous liver lesions, the ideal investigation is:**
   a. Ultrasound
   b. Single-phase CT scan
   c. Triple-phase CT scan
   d. Scintigraphy
5. **For local staging of prostate cancer, the ideal imaging is:**
   a. Transrectal ultrasound (TRUS)
   b. Contrast-enhanced CT scan
   c. Normal MRI
   d. Multiparametric MRI

Answer Key

1. c 2. b 3. b 4. c 5. d

SUGGESTED READING

1. Beyer T, Bidaut L, Dickson J, Kachelriess M, Kiessling F, Leitgeb R, et al. What scans we will read: Imaging instrumentation trends in clinical oncology. Cancer Imaging. 2020;20:1-38.
2. Mainenti P, Stanzione A, Guarino S, Romeo V, Ugga L, Romano F, Storto G, Maurea S, Brunetti A. Colorectal cancer: Parametric evaluation of morphological, functional, and molecular tomographic imaging. World J Gastroenterol. 2019;25:5233-5256.

3. Ronot M, Clift AK, Vilgrain V, Frilling A. Functional imaging in liver tumors. J Hepatol. 2016;65:1017-1030.
4. Vaidya T, Agrawal A, Mahajan A, Thakur MH, Mahajan A, Aggarwal A. The Continuing Evolution of Molecular Functional Imaging in Clinical Oncology: The Road to Precision Medicine and Radiogenomics (Part II). Mol Diagn Ther. 2018;23:27-51.
5. Vaidya T, Agrawal A, Mahajan S, Thakur MH, Mahajan A. The Continuing Evolution of Molecular Functional Imaging in Clinical Oncology: The Road to Precision Medicine and Radiogenomics (Part I). Mol Diagn Ther. 2018;23:1-26.

CHAPTER

32 Cardiovascular Imaging in Adult

"In adult cardiac imaging, radiologists become the heart's translator—reading every beat, blockage, and breakthrough."

INTRODUCTION

Cardiac imaging is pivotal for the early detection and diagnosis of heart diseases, which are leading causes of morbidity and mortality worldwide. Effective imaging allows for the visualization of anatomical structures and functional parameters, which are essential for understanding the extent of disease, planning interventions, and assessing the efficacy of treatments. Though it is immensely beneficial, it comes with challenges such as the potential risks from radiation exposure with certain modalities, the need for contrast agents that might cause allergic reactions or nephrotoxicity, and the high cost and technical expertise required for some advanced imaging techniques. Therefore, the choice of imaging technique **(Table 32.1)** is carefully considered based on the clinical question, patient characteristics, and the inherent risks and benefits of each modality.

Chest PA is the basic modality to assess cardiac size, contour of borders, to see chamber enlargement and associated structures. Other modalities are as follows:

Table 32.1: Cardiovascular imaging techniques.

Imaging modality	*Primary utilities*
Echocardiography	• First-line tool for evaluating heart structure and function • Assesses ventricular function, valvular diseases, and pericardial conditions • Allows real-time visualization of heart motion • Can be enhanced with Doppler and contrast for better flow visualization
Cardiac MRI	• Provides detailed images of the heart's structure and function without radiation • Excellent for tissue characterization, assessing myocardial scarring, fibrosis, and viability • Used in complex congenital heart disease and cardiomyopathies
Cardiac CT	• Ideal for high-resolution imaging of coronary arteries • Used to assess coronary artery disease and calcifications • Valuable for planning surgical and interventional procedures • Can visualize cardiac anatomy and pulmonary vasculature
Nuclear imaging	• SPECT and PET scans measure myocardial blood flow and metabolic activity • Useful for detecting ischemia and viability of the myocardium • Assesses cardiac function and ejection fraction • Useful in evaluation of heart failure and other functional disorders

Contd...

Contd...

Imaging modality	*Primary utilities*
Cardiac catheterization and coronary angiography	• Invasive but provides detailed imaging of coronary arteries • Measures intracardiac pressure and oxygen levels • Enables interventions like angioplasty and stenting • Gold standard for diagnosing coronary artery disease
Electrophysiological studies (EPS)	• Maps electrical activity and diagnoses arrhythmias • Guides procedures for arrhythmia treatment, such as ablations • Assesses risk and severity of arrhythmias
Advanced and emerging technologies	• 4D Flow MRI tracks real-time blood flow dynamics • Hybrid Imaging (e.g., PET/CT, PET/MRI) combines structural and functional insights. • AI in imaging enhances precision in acquisition and interpretation of images

Cardiovascular diseases are very vast, though for imaging purposes can be divided (Table 32.2) as follows:

Table 32.2: Radiological tools for cardiac disease category.

Cardiac disease category	*Radiological tools*
Coronary artery disease (CAD)	• **Cardiac CT:** Especially for coronary artery assessment and calcium scoring • **Coronary angiography:** Gold standard for detailed visualization of coronary arteries • **Nuclear imaging:** For assessing myocardial perfusion and ischemia
Valvular heart disease	• **Echocardiography:** Primary tool for assessing valve structure and function, including regurgitation and stenosis • **Cardiac MRI:** For detailed evaluation of valve anatomy and quantification of flow
Cardiomyopathies	• **Cardiac MRI:** Best for tissue characterization and assessing myocardial fibrosis • **Echocardiography:** For evaluating ventricular size, function, and wall motion abnormalities • **Nuclear imaging:** For functional assessment and viability studies
Heart failure	• **Echocardiography:** For evaluating cardiac function, ejection fraction, and diastolic function • **Cardiac MRI:** For detailed volumetric and functional analysis • **Nuclear imaging:** For ejection fraction and wall motion assessment
Congenital heart disease	• **Cardiac MRI:** For detailed anatomic and functional assessment • **Cardiac CT:** For complex anatomy visualization, especially in adult congenital heart disease • **Echocardiography:** For initial diagnosis and functional assessment
Pericardial diseases	• **Cardiac MRI:** Superior for characterizing pericardial thickness and inflammation • **Echocardiography:** For detecting pericardial effusion and constriction • **CT:** For detailed assessment of calcification and pericardial anatomy
Aortic diseases	• **Cardiac CT:** Preferred for evaluating aortic aneurysms, dissection, and other pathologies • **MRI:** For detailed assessment of aortic pathology without radiation • **Echocardiography:** For initial assessment of aortic root and ascending aorta
Pulmonary hypertension	• **Echocardiography:** For initial screening and assessment of right ventricular function • **Cardiac MRI:** For quantifying right ventricular volumes and pressures • **CT:** For evaluating pulmonary arteries and to rule out thromboembolic disease

After understanding the utilities of various modalities in relation of common cardiac diseases, vast uses of common modalities like radiography, CT, MRI can be understand in terms of common diseases.

RADIOGRAPHIC FEATURES OF COMMON DISEASES

The following figures demonstrates normal related structures on a chest X-ray.

Normal posteroanterior (left) and lateral (right) chest radiographs are shown in **Figures 32.1A to C**.

A systematic approach to standard chest radiography provides valuable insights into any heart disease that includes:

Thoracic Wall

Includes integrity of bony cage, soft tissue, rib or sternal deformities or sternal wire sutures that indicates history of prior surgeries.

Pulmonary Vasculature

- It should be studied to see the type of abnormality (i.e., pulmonary arterial overcirculation vs. pulmonary venous hypertension), severity of abnormality and, symmetry or asymmetry of the abnormality.
- **Abnormality type** in acquired cardiac disease is usually PVH (Pulmonary Venous Hypertension).
  Signs of PVH: Equalization or larger caliber of the upper lobar as compared to the lower lobar vessels; prominent interstitial markings with Kerley's A and B lines; indistinct pulmonary vascular and/or hilar vessel margins; and alveolar filling.

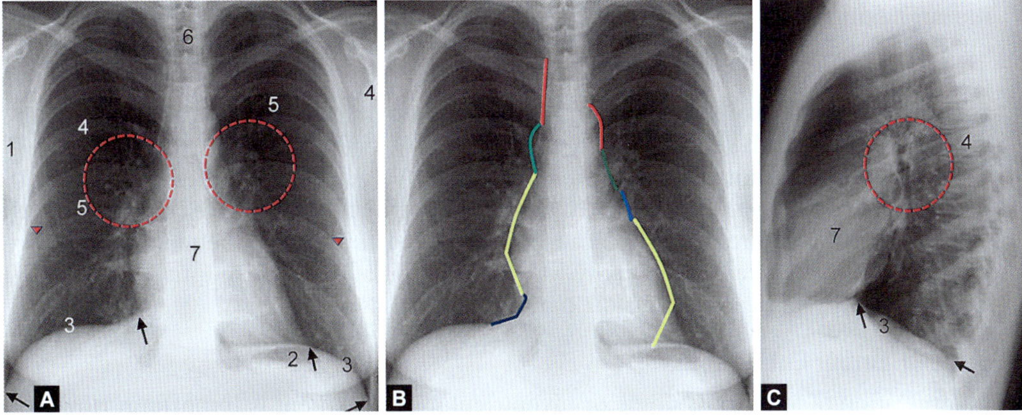

Figs. 32.1A to C: (A) Normal chest radiograph frontal (PA view) with adequate exposure and depth of inspiration. A systematic approach should be adapted for reviewing the radiograph with evaluation of following landmarks; (1) Soft tissue (2) stomach bubble; (3) Diaphragm; (4) Bones; (5) lung fields; (6) Trachea; (7) Cardiac silhouette; arrow laterally–costophrenic angle; arrow medially-cardiophrenic angle; arrowhead-pleura; circle-hilum. (B) Normal chest radiograph frontal (PA view) with adequate exposure and depth of inspiration depicting the structures forming the cardiac silhouette; Right border SVC (green), Right atrium (yellow), IVC (blue); Left-aortic knuckle (red), pulmonary bay (green), left auricle (blue), left ventricle (yellow). In case of dilated ascending aorta, a part of the right heart border may be contributed by it. (C) Lateral chest radiograph showing the normal structures visible on lateral view. Red-colored margin on the right side denotes position of innominate vein.

Table 32.3: Severity of PVH.

Grade I (vascular redistribution)	• Equalized upper and lower lobar vessels • Larger upper lobar vessels
Grade II (interstitial edema)	• Kerleys A or B lines • Prominent interstitial markings • Peribronchial cuffing • Loss of hilar angle with hilar enlargement • Subpleural edema • Indistinct right descending pulmonary artery
Grade III (alveolar pulmonary edema)	Hilar, lower lobar or generalized alveolar airspace opacities

Long standing case of PVH may cause ossific nodule formation which are small bony metaplasia within the lungs.

- **Severity of PVH** can be divided into three grades **(Table 32.3)**:
- **Symmetry or asymmetry of the abnormality:** Most frequent cause of asymmetric abnormality is gravitational as patients tend to sleep on their right side.

Note: Noncardiogenic edema is pulmonary edema that occur without any cardiac disease. Occurs due to damage to the alveolar-capillary membrane → leak of fluid into the lung. **Common** causes are drugs, drowning, asphyxia, high altitude, noxious gases like smoke, ARDS, blood transfusion reactions and some poisons.

Heart Size

Cardiac silhouette:

- **Cardiothoracic ratio:** The ratio taken of the maximum transverse diameter of the heart to the largest internal diameter of the chest wall taken just above the dome of the diaphragm on a PA chest film
- An adult heart is enlarged if it measures >0.5 (>50%).
- For neonates, a ratio of up to 60% is considered normal, while for infants, a ratio of up to 55% is considered within the normal range.
- Common causes of normal cardiac silhouette are: Valvular stenosis (aortic or mitral), pulmonary artery hypertension, hypertrophic cardiomyopathy, restrictive cardiomyopathy, acute myocardial infarction. While causes of enlarged cardiac silhouette are: congestive heart failure-related cardiomyopathy, valvular regurgitation, high-output states, dilated cardiomyopathy, pericardial effusion, paracardiac masses.

Specific Chamber Enlargement

- Identification of left atrial, single or biventricular enlargement is important. However, sometimes it is difficult.
- The radiographic signs observed with enlargement of each of the cardiac chambers are given below.

Left Atrial Enlargement (Commonly Denotes Mitral Valve Involvement)

1. Right retrocardiac double density sign.
2. Enlarged left atrial appendage seen as a bulge along the left cardiac silhouette just below pulmonary artery segment.

Note: Bulge above left bronchus is likely from enlarged main pulmonary artery, (e.g., PAH, pulmonary regurgitation, excess pulmonary flow), while the bulge below or same level is likely due to left atrial appendage enlargement.

3. Splaying of the carina with horizontally orientated left bronchus.

Right Atrial Enlargement (Commonly Denotes Tricuspid Valve Involvement)

1. Lateral bulging of the right heart border.
2. Elongated right heart border.

Left Ventricular Enlargement

1. On PA view, left and downward displacement of the apex
2. Lateral view shows posteriorly displaced cardiac shadow. The **Hoffman-Rigler sign** is measured 2.0 cm above the intersection of the diaphragm and the inferior vena cava. An enlarged LV will have posterior border more than 1.8 cm behind the inferior vena cava shadow.

Right Ventricular Enlargement

1. RV enlargement on PA view causes only leftward or sometimes upward shift of apex.
2. Lateral view shows obliterated retrosternal space. RV is enlarged if right heart border occupies > 1/3rd of sternal length.

Importance of Radiography in Heart Diseases

Clues Regarding Valvular Evaluation is to Look for:

1. **Left atrial enlargement:** Mitral valve
2. **Ascending aortic enlargement:** Aortic valve
3. **Right atrial enlargement:** Tricuspid valve.

Normal Sized Heart or Mild Cardiomegaly

- **Two reasons:** Pressure overload (hypertension, aortic stenosis, or mitral stenosis) or reduced LV compliance (hypertrophic cardiomyopathy, restrictive cardiomyopathy, and constrictive pericardial disease).
- If LA enlarged with normal heart → mitral stenosis
- If aorta is enlarged with normal heart → aortic stenosis.
- If no single chamber enlargement can be found then there may be reduced LV compliance due to causes as mentioned above.

Dilated Enlarged Heart

- **Reasons:** Volume overload lesion (valvular regurgitation) or myocardial failure or pericardial effusion.
- If LA enlarged with dilated heart → mitral regurgitation
- If aorta is enlarged with dilated heart → aortic regurgitation.
- If RA is enlarged with dilated heart → tricuspid regurgitation.
- If no single chamber enlargement can be found then there may be congestive (dilated) cardiomyopathy or pericardial effusion.

RADIOGRAPHS IN SPECIFIC CARDIAC DISEASE (FIGS. 32.2A TO H) (TABLES 32.4 AND 32.5)

Hypertension

Pressure overload lesion, normal heart size, enlarged aorta (entire aorta, not just ascending as in aortic stenosis).

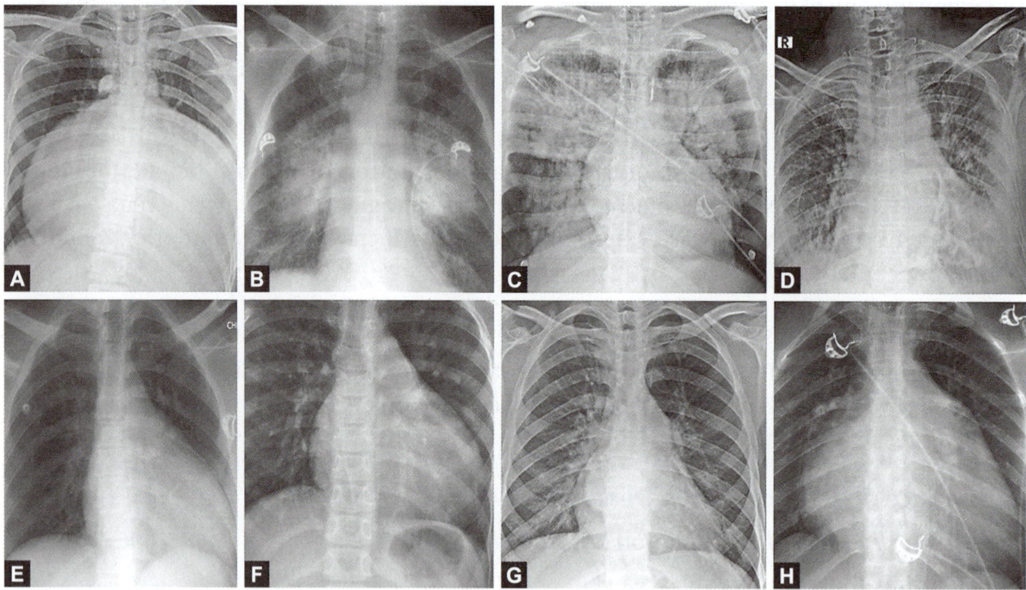

Figs. 32.2A to H: Chest radiograph frontal (PA view) with commonly encountered pathologies: (A) Pericardial effusion; (B) Noncardiogenic pulmonary edema; (C) Cardiogenic pulmonary edema; (D) Cardiogenic pulmonary edema; (E) Cardiomegaly with left ventricle type apex; (F) Cardiomegaly with right ventricle type apex; (G) Dilated left atrium with normal cardiac size (mitral stenosis); (H) Dilated left atrium with cardiomegaly and changes of pulmonary arterial hypertension (mitral regurgitation with mitral stenosis).

Table 32.4: Aortic valvular pathology.

Aortic stenosis (Pressure overload disease)	*Aortic insufficiency/regurgitation*
LV size relatively normal on chest radiograph due to concentric hypertrophy	Dilated LV with shifted LV apex towards left
Aortic valve calcification (+/–) and poststenotic aortic dilatation	

Table 32.5: Mitral valvular pathology.

Mitral stenosis (Pressure overload disease)	*Mitral insufficiency/regurgitation (volume overload)*
LA dilated—double density sign on radiograph	LA dilated—double density sign on radiograph
LV normal	LV dilated
Marked signs of pulmonary venous congestions like hilar enlargement, Kerley B lines and effusion	Relatively mild signs
Signs of pulmonary artery hypertension—enlarged pulmonary arteries	Relatively mild signs

Hypertrophic Cardiomyopathy

- The overall heart size is generally normal (in around 50%).
- Sometimes may cause PVH and sometimes associated with mitral regurgitation causing LA enlargement.

Restrictive Cardiomyopathy

- Idiopathic or infiltrative like sarcoidosis, hemochromatosis, and amyloidosis.
- Early phase, cardiac size is within normal limits.
- Reduced LV compliance → PVH and LA enlargement (may mimics mitral stenosis on radiograph).
- Cardiomegaly in end stage.

Acute Myocardial Infarction

- 50% → Normal heart size on chest x-ray.
- Rest of the 50% cases → Normal heart size with PVH or pulmonary edema.
- Early phase, cardiac size is within normal limits.
- Radiography can help in evaluating acute MI complications like cardiac rupture; pericardial effusion; LV aneurysm, both true and false; papillary muscle rupture and intractable congestive heart failure.
- Dressler's syndrome, one of the complication of MI, occurs in few weeks to months. Autoimmune response to antigens leading to pericardial and pleural effusions with resultant increase in cardiac size.

Congestive or Dilated Cardiomyopathy

- Some degree of PVH and substantial cardiomegaly.
- Marked enlarged heart with no typical chamber enlargement may raise a suspicion for congestive/dilated cardiomyopathy or pericardial effusion.
- Most commonly seen in ischemic heart disease.

Pericardial Effusion

- Clue is the presence of marked cardiomegaly with absent signs of PVH or pulmonary edema.
- Pericardial effusions can be caused by infections like viral and tubercular, uremia or rheumatological diseases, traumatic hemorrhage like aortic dissection and postirradiation changes.
- Xray signs:
  - A "tent" like appearance.
  - Water bottle appearance.
  - Widened carina without LA enlargement.
  - Obscured left cardiac border
  - Significant enlargement of the cardiac silhouette with narrowing of the retrosternal space on lateral radiograph.
- Larger effusions can cause pericardial tamponade with resultant decreased cardiac output which may cause decrease in pulmonary vascular markings and a prominent SVC.

Prosthetic Valve Location on Chest X-ray

It is sometimes difficult to correctly identify the prosthetic valve on a chest radiograph due to fault techniques.

The positioning of the cardiac valves is most accurately identified on a lateral radiograph. A line is traced from the carina to the apex of the heart. The pulmonary and aortic valves are positioned above this line, while the tricuspid and mitral valves are located below it.

Another method to refine the localization of prosthetic valves is by drawing a second line perpendicular to the patient's upright position, dividing the cardiac silhouette in half. The aortic valve appears in the upper quadrant, the mitral in the lower quadrant, and the tricuspid in the anterior quadrant.

ECHO

Echocardiography is a cornerstone in the noninvasive evaluation of cardiac structures, utilizing ultrasound technology to provide real-time images and functional data of the heart **(Table 32.6)**. Initially developed as motion-based (M-mode) echocardiography by Inge Edler in 1953, the field has since evolved to include the widely used two-dimensional (2D) echocardiography,

Table 32.6: Characteristics of ECHO.

Type of ECHO	*Indications*	*Advantages*	*Disadvantages*
Transthoracic echocardiography (TTE) uses phased array sector probe 1.5–5 MHz (It is most widely used technique for ECHO, done in left lateral position)	• Evaluation of suspected heart failure, dyspnea, chest pain	• Noninvasive • Widely available • Provides real-time images	• Image quality may be limited by patient's body habitus (e.g., obesity, lung disease) • Limited views of posterior heart structures
Transesophageal echocardiography (TEE) Uses sector probe 3–7 MHz	• Suspected valvular disease • Infective endocarditis • Intraoperative monitoring	• Superior image quality of posterior heart structures • Less interference from chest wall structures	• Invasive • Requires sedation or anesthesia • Risk of esophageal injury or bleeding
Stress echocardiography	• Suspected coronary artery disease • Preoperative assessment • Ischemia evaluation	• Noninvasive • Can assess functional response to stress • Detects ischemia in real-time	• May require pharmacological agents • Limited use in patients unable to exercise
3D echocardiography	• Complex congenital heart disease • Presurgical planning • Valve assessment	• Provides detailed spatial relationships • Enhanced visualization of cardiac structures	• Requires specialized equipment • Higher cost
Intracardiac echocardiography (ICE) • Miniature phased array probe • Frequency: Typically, 5–10 MHz	• Guiding transcatheter procedures • Intracardiac interventions	• High-resolution images from within the heart • Avoids need for general anesthesia	• Invasive • Requires venous access • Higher cost and technical complexity
Contrast echocardiography	• Suspected pulmonary embolism • Cardioembolic stroke evaluation	• Enhances visualization of cardiac structures • Useful in detecting shunts or thrombi	• Requires administration of contrast agents • Potential allergic reactions or side effects

(Table 32.7) and further advancements like Doppler echocardiography, transesophageal echocardiography (TEE), and three-dimensional (3D) echocardiography. **Echocardiographic findings of pathology are shown in Table 32.8.**

Table 32.7: Various views in ECHO.

Echocardiographic view	*Structures/aspects to evaluate*
Parasternal long axis (PLAX)	• Left ventricle size and function • Left atrium • Mitral valve motion and structure • Aortic valve and aortic root • Right ventricular outflow tract (RVOT)
Parasternal short axis (PSAX)	• Left ventricle cross-section • Papillary muscles • Mitral valve leaflets • Aortic valve cusps • Right ventricular size and function
Apical four-chamber	• Right and left atrial size • Right and left ventricular size and function • Tricuspid and mitral valve function • Detection of right heart strain (e.g., pulmonary embolism)
Apical two-chamber	• Left atrium • Left ventricle • Mitral valve function • Assessment of regional wall motion abnormalities (e.g., myocardial infarction)
Subxiphoid (subcostal) commonly done by curvilinear convex probe	• All four heart chambers • Inferior vena cava (IVC) compressibility (for volume status) • Pericardial effusion • Left lobe of the liver
Apical three-chamber (apical long axis)	• Left ventricular outflow tract (LVOT) • Mitral valve function • Aortic valve function • Left atrium and ventricle
Suprasternal	• Aortic arch • Great vessels (e.g., innominate artery, left common carotid artery, left subclavian artery) • Evaluation of coarctation of the aorta

Table 32.8: Echocardiographic findings of pathology.

Pathology	*Echocardiographic findings*
Congestive heart failure (CHF)	• Reduced ejection fraction (EF) • Dilated ventricles • Diastolic dysfunction • Enlarged atria • Mitral or tricuspid regurgitation
Myocardial infarction (MI)	• Regional wall motion abnormalities • Reduced EF • Ventricular aneurysm • Thrombus formation in the ventricle
Hypertrophic cardiomyopathy (HCM)	• Asymmetric left ventricular hypertrophy • Thickened interventricular septum • Systolic anterior motion of the mitral valve • Left ventricular outflow tract (LVOT) obstruction
Aortic stenosis	• Thickened, calcified aortic valve leaflets • Reduced aortic valve area • Increased transvalvular pressure gradient • Left ventricular hypertrophy
Mitral regurgitation	• Mitral valve prolapse or flail leaflet • Dilated left atrium • Regurgitant jet in the left atrium • Enlarged left ventricle (in chronic cases)
Aortic regurgitation	• Diastolic flow reversal in the descending aorta • Dilated left ventricle • Thickened aortic valve leaflets • Increased LV end-diastolic volume
Pulmonary embolism (PE)	• Right ventricular dilatation • Right heart strain • McConnell's sign (RV free wall hypokinesis with apical sparing) • Dilated pulmonary artery
Pericardial effusion	• Echo-free space surrounding the heart • Compression of cardiac chambers (tamponade physiology) • Collapsed right atrium and right ventricle during diastole
Atrial septal defect (ASD)	• Left-to-right shunt at the atrial level • Enlarged right atrium and ventricle • Dilated pulmonary arteries • Paradoxical septal motion
Infective endocarditis	• Vegetations on valve leaflets • Valve leaflet perforation • Regurgitant jets • Possible abscess formation or pseudoaneurysm

CORONARY CT ANGIOGRAM (FIGS. 32.3A TO H)

Coronary Artery Anatomy

Coronary Artery Origin

Typically, two coronary arteries originate from the proximal aorta at the sinuses of Valsalva.

Aortic valve is tricuspid: Hence three coronary sinuses-cusps are seen. These are:

1. **Right coronary sinus:** Origin of right coronary artery
2. **Left coronary sinus:** Origin of left main coronary artery
3. **Noncoronary sinus:** No arterial origin.

Branches of left main coronary artery (LCA/LMCA): *Includes: Left anterior descending artery (LAD), left circumflex artery (LCx), Ramus intermedius artery (RI).*
Branches of right coronary artery (RCA): *Includes: Conus artery, Sinoatrial nodal artery, Acute marginal branches, Inferior interventricular artery, Posterior left ventricular branch (PLV)*

Supply

- **LAD**: Supplies anterolateral myocardium and apex and anterior two-thirds of the interventricular septum
- **LCx**: Lateral and posterolateral walls of the left ventricle.
- **RCA**: SA and AV nodes, RV free wall and inferior wall and LV inferior wall.

Determination of Dominance

Right dominant circulation (80%), left dominant circulation (15%) and co-dominant circulation (5%)

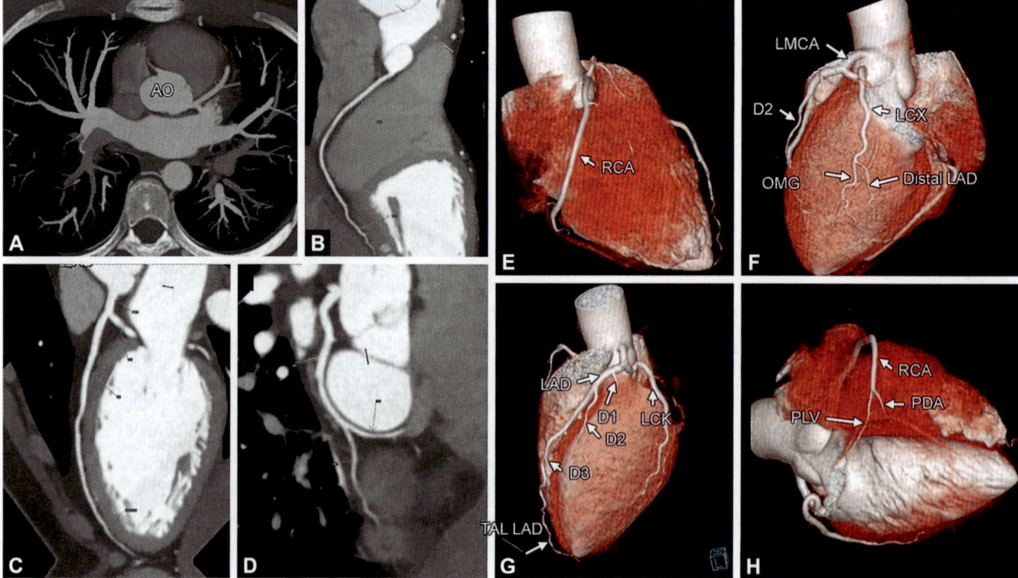

Figs. 32.3A to H: Multi-detector computed-tomography coronary angiography images with normal coronary artery origin, course and termination: (A) Normal origin from respective coronary cusp; (B) Curved reformat of right coronary artery; (C) Curved reformat of left anterior descending artery; (D) Curved reformat of left circumflex artery; (E, F, G, H) Volume rendered images showing the course of coronary arteries.

Systematic and Comprehensive Approach for Coronary Angiography Study

Calcium scoring on plain scan → evaluation of the coronary arteries via contrast enhanced ECG gated scan → other cardiac and extracardiac findings.

Calcium score: Follows the Agatston score protocol, in which any pixel within the coronary arterial tree with a density higher than 130 HU is considered as containing calcium. Results are in Agatston score which is most widely used, calcium volume, or volume score.

The relative risk of coronary related deaths in those with higher than 160 calcium score to that with 160 or less calcium score is approximately 4.2. It should be noted that zero calcium score implying no calcific plaques does not exclude soft plaque, however their likelihood of causing significant luminal stenosis is very low. The negative predictive value for calcium scoring is very high, with an estimated risk of 0.1% per year of developing a major cardiovascular event in 2–5 years.

Cardiac Findings

It should be read under the following points:

1. Size and function of the cardiac chambers
2. Prospectively gated cardiac study (1–2 mSv radiation exposure): Chamber enlargement and myocardial hypertrophy
3. Retrospectively gated cardiac study (10–12 mSv radiation exposure): Ejection fractions, end diastolic, end-systolic, and stroke volume indexes.
4. Wall thinning or aneurysm
5. Thrombus or mass.
6. Valvular thickening, abscess, calcifications or prolapse.

Extracardiac Findings

Great mediastinal vessels, airways, lungs, chest wall, and superior abdomen can be studied.

Note: Two surgeries are mainly done for coronary artery disease.

1. Stent placement in native coronary arteries.
2. **Coronary artery bypass grafts:** Internal thoracic artery (internal mammary artery), radial artery or saphenous vein graft from ascending aorta anastomosing with coronary artery.

CARDIAC MRI (FIGS. 32.4A TO H)

Cardiac MRI utilizes segmented steady-state free precession (SSFP) and gradient echo cine sequences to produce high-resolution dynamic images of the heart.

SSFP, known as a "white blood" sequence, offers superior contrast between myocardium and blood pool, making it ideal for cardiac MRI due to its high temporal resolution and excellent contrast.

Cine MRI enables quantitative evaluation of cardiac morphology and function, with real-time images facilitating subjective analysis in suboptimal gating.

Tissue characterization is commonly accomplished using double or triple inversion fast spin echo sequences.

Contrast-enhanced perfusion MRI is conducted before and after vasodilator stress to assess myocardial perfusion. Normal myocardium shows enhancement, while areas with reduced perfusion appear relatively less enhanced.

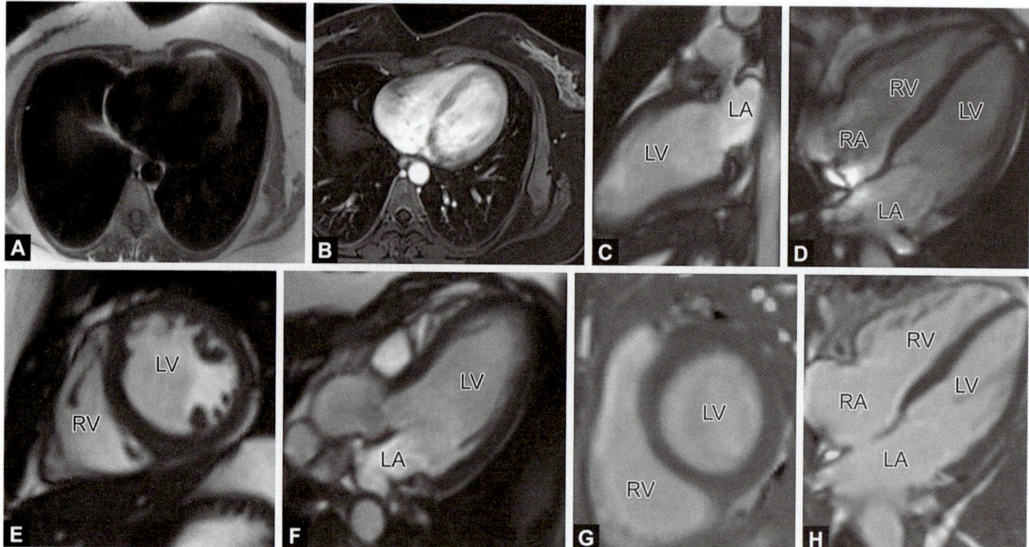

Figs. 32.4A to H: Normal-cardiac MRI: (A) T2W black-blood image true axial plane; (B) Post-contrast T1W true axial plane; (C) White-blood image 2-chamber (TRUFI sequence); (D) White-blood image 4-chamber (TRUFI sequence); (E) White-blood image short axis (TRUFI sequence); (F) White-blood image 3-chamber (TRUFI sequence); (G) Late gadolinium enhancement (15 minutes), PSIR sequence, short axis; (H) Late gadolinium enhancement (15 minutes), PSIR sequence, 4-chamber.

Delayed enhancement is typically due to prior infarction (either sub-endocardial or transmural) but may also indicate nonischemic causes, depending on the enhancement pattern, (e.g. Epicardial delayed enhancement seen in myocarditis).

Note: Stress MRI—pharmacologic stress, usually by infusion of dobutamine, given to look for regional contraction abnormality as a functional indicator for significant stenosis in coronary arteries, as flow may increase three to five times in a normal calibered coronary artery whereas in the significant stenotic artery, flow cannot increase to the appropriate level which results in regional myocardial contractile dysfunction.

COMMON DISEASES

Acute Aorta

Aorta, the largest artery in the body, arises from the left ventricle. It has three segments:

1. **The ascending aorta,** a short segment that gives rise to the left and right coronary arteries supplying the myocardium.
2. **The arch of the aorta,** which curves posteriorly and gives off branches—the brachiocephalic trunk, left common carotid artery, and left subclavian artery.
3. **The descending aorta,** which further divides into the thoracic aorta supplying organs in the chest and the abdominal aorta, providing oxygen-rich blood to organs below the diaphragm, including the digestive tract and lower extremities.

Acute aorta includes acute symptomatic aortic pathology like trauma or rupture, and acute aortic syndromes-intramural hematoma, penetrating aortic ulcer, and aortic dissection.

Traumatic Aortic Injury

- Occur predominantly due to deceleration trauma like fall from height or motor vehicle accidents.
- Most common place of injury is the isthmus of aorta where it is tethered by the ligamentum arteriosum.
- CECT aortogram is the modality of choice now and has mostly replaced catheter angiogram.
- Direct signs includes pseudoaneurysm, intimal flap irregularities, contrast extravasation, while indirect sign is mediastinal hematomas.

Acute Aortic Syndromes (Figs. 32.5A to H)

- **Aortic dissection:** Tear in the intima, where high-pressure blood penetrates and enlarges the intima. Risk factor is hypertension in old age and connective tissue disorder in young.
- The **Stanford classification system**, categorize into: Types A (ascending aorta) and B (non-ascending).
- **Differentiating the true and false channels are shown in Table 32.9.**

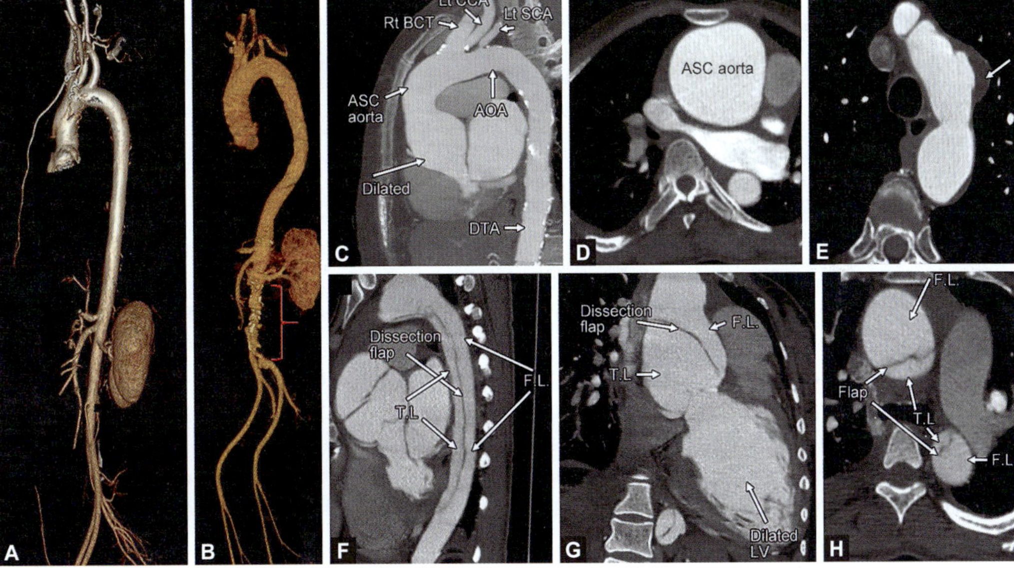

Figs. 32.5A to H: Multidetector computed-tomography angiography images with common aortic pathologies: (A) Normal aortogram; (B) Aortitis involving the abdominal aorta with luminal irregularities (bracket); (C) Ascending aorta aneurysm; (D) Ascending aorta aneurysm; (E) Penetrating aortic ulcer; (F, G, H) Type A aortic dissection. Note the features of false and true lumen.

Table 32.9: True and false lumen.

True lumen	*False lumen*
Smaller lumen	Larger lumen
Round or oval	Crescentic
Outer wall calcifications-specific	Cobweb sign (remnants of torn media)
Thrombus rare	Common
Central	Peripheral
Early brighter enhancement	Late or absent enhancement

- **Intramural hematoma:** Blood accumulation within the aortic wall, without intimal tear likely from ruptured small vessels within the wall. No false channel is formed like dissection. Commonly seen long-term sequelae of IMH is aneurysm. High-density crescent-shaped along the aortic wall is noted which is appreciated best on plain CT.
- **Penetrating aortic ulcer:** Ulcer-like lesions from the intima, penetrating the vessel wall and increase risk of dissection or rupture.
- CECT aortogram angiography is imaging modality of choice.
- Treatment for acute aortic syndrome depends on its location:
  - *Ascending aorta:* Often requires surgery.
  - *Descending aorta:* Usually managed medically with blood pressure control.

Mycotic pseudoaneurysms means aortic wall infection by septic emboli from catheters, intravenous drug use, prosthetic valve infection, or from infected atherosclerotic plaque.

(**Note:** It is important to know the difference between true and pseudo/false aneurysm. In this case, a PAU causes a pseudoaneurysm where its wall is only lined by tunica adventitia. However, a true aneurysm will always have all the three layers as its wall).

Aortic Aneurysms and Aortitis

Aortic Aneurysms

Normal diameters: Sinus of Valsalva 3.3 ± 0.4 cm; mid-ascending aorta 3.0 ± 0.4 cm; proximal descending aorta 2.4 ± 0.4 cm

>4 cm—dilatation

>5 cm—aneurysm or 1.5 times of normal diameter

True aneurysms:

- Fusiform in shape. Mostly result from atherosclerosis.
- **Other causes include:** Hypertension, connective tissue disorders such as Marfan's syndrome, vasculitis and valve-related aortic disease.
- Management depends on symptoms, size, and growth rate of aneurysm.
- Aortic diameters are very important. Elective surgery is generally recommended at ascending aorta is > 5.5 cm and when descending aorta is <6 cm.
- Sometimes surgery is done even at smaller aortic diameters in special conditions like in Marfans syndrome (at 4.5–5 cm) or bicuspid aortic valve (at 4.5 cm) due to increased risk of aortic complication.
  (Marfan's syndrome characteristically shows aneurysmal dilatation of the aortic root like a tulip bulb, referred as annuloaortic ectasia).
- If there is a rupture, imaging shows a periaortic or mediastinal hematoma. Early-contained rupture may show a "draped aorta" sign, i.e., indistinctness of the posterior aortic wall or close alignment of the posterior wall with the adjacent vertebral bodies.
- Treatment complications include rupture, dissection, infection, endoleak (may occur when blood flows within the excluded aneurysmal sac) and paraplegia due to artery of Adamkiewicz occlusion.

Aortitis

- Defined as inflamed aortic wall or its major arteries.
- **Imaging**: Wall thickening, luminal narrowing and irregularity, and aneurysmal dilatation.

- **Complications**: Stenosis, dissection or rupture.
- MRI contrast/FDG PET can better identify active inflammation
- **Common causes** of noninfectious arteritis:
  - Giant cell arteritis (most common autoimmune condition associated with aortitis, most commonly involves thoracic aorta, presents with an aneurysm)
  - Takayasu's arteritis (large vessel vasculitis, affects aorta and its arterial branches subclavian artery > carotids > vertebral artery; the coronaries or even the pulmonary circulation)
  - Systemic disease related aortic inflammation.
- **Treatment** is mostly through steroids. Stenosis and aneurysms require surgery.

Infective Endocarditis

- Infection of the endocardium affecting valve leaflets, chordae tendineae, and also the prosthetic valves and implanted devices.
- Vegetation is the pathologic for infective endocarditis. It appears as mobile or fixed, irregular mass along the endocardium. Sometimes, these vegetation breaks into fragments and can embolize, causing pneumonia or stroke.
- Plain radiographic findings are nonspecific and may show changes of pneumonia or septic pulmonary emboli or end stage congestive heart failure due to valve dysfunction.
- Primary imaging modality is Echocardiography which may help identify vegetations along the valve with other ancillary findings like stenosis, dehiscence of prosthetic valve, pseudoaneurysm or abscess.
- CT shows hypoattenuating filling defects surrounded by contrast.
- It has high morbidity and mortality, even after diagnosis and treatment with complications. Treatment includes either antibiotic or surgery.

Myocarditis

- Myocarditis is usually caused by viral infections like cytomegalovirus and coxsackie B virus, parvovirus and human herpes virus.
- Diagnosis confirmed by endomyocardial biopsy, which typically shows interstitial edema, lymphocyte infiltration, and necrosis of myocytes.
- Interstitial edema may cause increased T2-weighted signals and delayed enhancement which are nonspecific.
- In Lyme disease (spirochete Borrelia burgdorferi) cardiac involvement is infrequent and may show signs of myopericarditis.
- Chagas' disease (protozoan Trypanosoma cruzi) acute, intermediate, and chronic phases. Cardiac involvement is most frequent in chronic phase with typical LV apical aneurysm.

Acute Pericarditis

- Inflammation of the pericardium from various causes like infections (viral, bacterial, fungal, TB), acute MI, acute myocarditis, neoplastic etiology (lymphoma, lung Ca, breast Ca, leukemia), radiation, collagen vascular disease (like SLE), sarcoidosis, systemic diseases (like amyloid), drug reaction, postmyocardial infarction, trauma or idiopathic.
- Viral is the most frequent cause.
- Imaging shows effusion and thickened pericardium (>4 mm).

Constrictive Pericarditis

- There is progressive pericardial fibrosis hampering dilatation during diastole.
- Nonspecific reaction to infectious pericarditis, connective tissue disease, neoplasm, trauma, long-term renal dialysis, cardiac surgery, and radiation therapy.
- In western countries it is most commonly due to cardiac surgery whereas tuberculous pericarditis is the most common cause of constrictive pericarditis in developing countries.
- Sometimes there are concomitant calcifications.
- Four different presentations: Acute inflammatory, effusive-constrictive, adhesive, and chronic fibrous.

To differentiate clinically between constrictive pericarditis and restrictive cardiomyopathy is difficult because both present with diastolic failure.

- Constrictive pericarditis is surgically treated with a good prognosis, while restrictive cardiomyopathy medically treated with a poor outcome.
- One key differentiating point is pericardial thickness (≥4 mm). Second, often there are pericardial calcifications- a feature of constrictive pericarditis.
- Presence of adhesions between pericardial layers, tubelike configuration of ventricles, enlargement of atrium, and dilated vena cave.
- MRI may show ventricular septal motion toward the left ventricle in early diastole due to characteristic increased ventricular interdependence present in constrictive pericarditis.

Pericardial Cysts and Diverticula

- Developmental abnormalities.
- Most of the pericardial cysts develop in the cardiophrenic region more commonly on the right side.
- Cysts mostly do not communicate with the pericardium whereas a diverticulum shows a communication.

Myxoma

- Most common benign cardiac tumor.
- M/c location: LA (75%) and RA (20%).
- Usually spherical but may vary due to its gelatinous consistency.
- Typically attached by a narrow pedicle to the area of the fossa ovalis.
- A wide mural attachment is more likely seen with malignant tumors.
- May grow through a patent foramen ovale and extend in both atria- which is called a "dumbbell" appearance.
- Can prolapse through the funnel of the atrioventricular valve or into the ventricle during diastole.

Rhabdomyoma

- Most common cardiac tumor in children (~40% of cardiac tumor).
- Has association with tuberous sclerosis.
- Are frequently multiple.
- Have intramural location and involve the ventricles.
- Larger tumors distort myocardium, may bulge into the cavity or may also cause bulge in epicardial contour of the heart.
- Signal intensity is similar to myocardium on MRI.
- Shows hyperenhancement after contrast administration.

Table 32.10: Differentiation between tumor and blood clot.

Tumor	*Thrombus*
Medium signal on T1 and high signal on T2	Variable signal depending on age
Early contrast enhancement	No early contrast enhancement
Usually, higher T2 signal than myocardium and skeletal muscle	Lower signal
Inversion delay in delayed myocardial enhancement, higher signal than myocardium	Inversion delay in delayed myocardial enhancement, lower signal than myocardium

Differentiation between tumor and blood clot shown in **Table 32.10**.

Malignant Cardiac Tumors

Characteristics of Malignant Cardiac Tumor

Involves more than one cardiac chamber or its vessel, Extension into pulmonary vessels, vena cava or aorta. Wide base attachment, Intramural and intracavity components, Necrosis, Extension outside cardiac chamber, Hemorrhagic pericardial effusion and Metastasis.

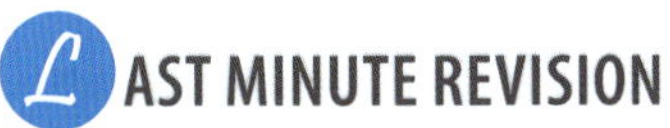

- **Echocardiography** is the first-line for assessing heart structure, function, and valvular diseases. Doppler enhanced the blood flow visualization.
- **Cardiac MRI** is excellent for detailed structural and functional imaging without radiation. Ideal for tissue characterization, including myocardial scarring and fibrosis.
- **Cardiac CT** provides high-resolution imaging of coronary arteries, essential for evaluating coronary artery disease and planning interventions.
- In adults on chest X-ray PA view, Cardiothoracic ratio >50% suggest cardiomegaly.

REVIEW QUESTIONS

Multiple Choice Questions (MCQs)

1. **Which imaging modality is the first-line tool for evaluating heart structure, function, and valvular diseases?**
   a. Cardiac MRI
   b. Echocardiography
   c. Cardiac CT
   d. Nuclear Imaging
2. **A patient with a history of hypertension presents with chest pain. A CT scan shows an intimal flap and two distinct lumens within the aorta. What is the most likely diagnosis?**
   a. Aortic aneurysm
   b. Aortic dissection
   c. Intramural hematoma
   d. Penetrating atherosclerotic ulcer
3. **Which imaging modality is ideal for assessing myocardial viability and ischemia using metabolic activity measurements?**
   a. Echocardiography
   b. Cardiac CT
   c. Nuclear Imaging
   d. Cardiac MRI

4. A 50-year-old patient presents with symptoms of heart failure. An echocardiogram shows an enlarged left atrium and left ventricle with signs of regurgitation. What is the most likely underlying valvular disease?

a. Mitral stenosis
b. Aortic stenosis
c. Mitral regurgitation
d. Tricuspid regurgitation

5. Which of the following is a typical finding on a chest X-ray for a patient with chronic mitral stenosis?

a. Enlarged left ventricle
b. Enlarged left atrium
c. Enlarged right ventricle
d. Enlarged pulmonary arteries

6. What is the primary imaging modality for diagnosing pericardial effusion?

a. Cardiac MRI
b. Echocardiography
c. Cardiac CT
d. Nuclear imaging

Answer Key

1. b 2. b 3. c 4. c 5. b 6. b

SUGGESTED READING

1. Amin H, Siddiqui WJ. Cardiomegaly. [Updated 2022 Nov 20]. In: StatPearls [Internet]. Treasure Island (FL): StatPearls Publishing; 2024 Jan.
2. Busse A, Cantré D, Beller E, Streckenbach F, Öner A, Ince H, Weber MA, Meinel FG. Cardiac CT: why, when, and how: Update 2019. Radiologe. 2019 Dec;59(Suppl 1):1-9. English. doi: 10.1007/s00117-019-0530-9. PMID: 31062037.
3. Omerovic S, Jain A. Echocardiogram. [Updated 2023 Jul 24]. In: StatPearls [Internet]. Treasure Island (FL): StatPearls Publishing; 2024 Jan.
4. Rajiah PS, François CJ, Leiner T. Cardiac MRI: State of the Art. Radiology. 2023;307(3):e223008. doi: 10.1148/radiol.223008. Epub 2023 Apr 11. PMID: 37039684.

UNIT 6

Emergency Radiology

Unit Outline

CHAPTER

33 Imaging in Trauma

"Trauma doesn't wait—and neither do radiologists. One image can mean the difference between chaos and control."

INTRODUCTION

Trauma remains a significant public health challenge globally, particularly as the leading cause of mortality among individuals aged 20–40. This age group experiences a disproportionately high number of deaths from trauma, highlighting the critical need for effective emergency medical responses, where imaging plays a pivotal role. Each year, trauma and injuries claim nearly six million lives worldwide, accounting for about 10% of global mortality. Among these fatalities, brain injury is frequently the most common finding, underscoring the importance of prompt and precise imaging.

Imaging technologies are essential in the acute management of trauma patients, providing crucial diagnostic information that guides therapeutic decisions. As trauma can involve complex injuries across various body systems from skeletal fractures to internal organ damage the appropriate application of imaging modalities like X-rays, CT scans, MRI, and ultrasound is vital. These technologies not only facilitate rapid diagnosis but also help in monitoring the progress of recovery and planning further treatment steps.

This chapter will explore the key imaging techniques used in trauma care, emphasizing their strategic applications during initial evaluations and ongoing management. We will discuss the use of imaging in both primary and secondary trauma surveys and examine specific challenges and innovations in the field.

PRINCIPLES OF IMAGING IN TRAUMA

Imaging in trauma is a critical component of modern emergency medicine, providing essential information that guides the rapid assessment and management of injured patients. Understanding the fundamental principles of various imaging modalities is vital for making informed decisions in trauma care.

Selection and Application

Advanced trauma life support (ATLS) guidelines recommend a systematic approach to imaging in trauma care, starting with a primary survey that includes radiographs and ultrasound, followed by more detailed imaging based on the patient's stability and injury severity. Imaging protocols need to be adaptable and tailored to the specific resources and expertise available at each center.

Technological Considerations

Advancements in imaging technology have significantly improved the speed and resolution of trauma imaging. Portable devices and improvements in software allow for quicker diagnoses directly at the patient's bedside or in the emergency department. However, these advancements come with challenges, such as the need for specialized training and concerns about radiation exposure, especially with CT scans.

Basic Concepts and Modalities (Table 33.1)

Radiography (X-ray)

X-rays are the most commonly used imaging modality in trauma settings due to their availability and speed. They are particularly effective for assessing bony structures and detecting fractures and dislocations. X-rays can also be used to evaluate the chest for pneumothoraxes or hemothorax **(Fig. 33.1)**.

Fig. 33.1: Shows multiple rib fractures with hemothorax and ICD tube in situ left side.

Computed Tomography (CT)

CT scans offer detailed images and are superior for diagnosing complex bone fractures, internal injuries, and vascular abnormalities. They are fast and can be performed on unstable patients, providing a comprehensive overview of injuries to the head, spine, chest, abdomen, and pelvis.

Magnetic Resonance Imaging (MRI)

MRI is limited in acute trauma settings but is invaluable for detailed assessment of brain, spinal cord injuries and can be crucial in non-acute settings for diagnosing soft tissue and vascular injuries.

Ultrasound

Ultrasound is a portable, noninvasive, and dynamic imaging technique that is ideal for evaluating abdominal trauma, cardiac motion, and fluid status in real-time. The focused assessment with sonography in trauma (FAST) exam is a specific protocol used to quickly identify free fluid in the peritoneal, pericardial, or pleural spaces.

Table 33.1: Key imaging modalities in trauma care.

Modality	*Primary uses*	*Advantages*	*Limitations*
X-ray	Fractures, chest trauma	Quick, widely available	Limited soft tissue detail
CT scan	Head, chest, abdomen, spine, complex fractures	Comprehensive, fast, high detail	Higher radiation exposure
MRI	Brain, spinal cord, soft tissue	Excellent soft tissue contrast	Time-consuming, less available
Ultrasound	Abdominal trauma, cardiac evaluation	Portable, no radiation, real-time	Operator dependent, limited scope

Interventional Radiology (IR)

IR plays a vital role in managing hemodynamically unstable patients by providing minimally invasive procedures that stabilize patients enough for further diagnostic evaluations or surgeries.

Approach to a Trauma Patient: Radiological Perspective

In trauma care, the structured approach of primary and secondary surveys ensures the prioritization of life-saving interventions and the thorough identification of all significant injuries. Imaging plays a crucial role in both phases, helping to rapidly diagnose conditions that require immediate or subsequent management.

Imaging in the Primary Survey

The primary survey focuses on identifying life-threatening conditions and stabilizing the patient according to the airway, breathing, circulation, disability, exposure (ABCDE) protocol. Here's how imaging integrates:

X-rays and Ultrasound: Focused Assessment with Sonography for Trauma (FAST)

The FAST scan **(Table 33.2)** is a rapid bedside ultrasound examination used primarily in the initial evaluation of trauma patients. It's designed to quickly identify the presence of free intraperitoneal or pericardial fluid (usually blood) in patients with suspected blunt or penetrating trauma. The primary goal of the FAST scan is to help determine whether a patient needs urgent surgical intervention for internal bleeding. **Chest X-rays** are used to check for pneumothorax, hemothorax, or major bony injuries. **Pelvic X-rays** help detect fractures, which can be sources of significant hemorrhage.

Computed Tomography (CT)

While CT scans provide detailed images, they are generally avoided in the initial primary survey due to the need for patient stabilization and the risks associated with moving a critically

Table 33.2: Tips of FAST scan.

Key Components of the FAST scan

The FAST scan traditionally evaluates four specific areas of the body:

1. **Pericardial area:** To check for fluid accumulation around the heart which might indicate a cardiac tamponade.
2. **Right upper quadrant:** To assess for fluid between the liver and kidney (hepatorenal recess), which can suggest bleeding from liver injuries.
3. **Left upper quadrant:** To look at the space between the spleen and kidney (splenorenal recess) for potential splenic bleeding.
4. **Pelvis:** To evaluate the rectovesical (in males) and rectouterine (in females) spaces for free fluid.

Advantages of the FAST scan

- **Speed and efficiency**: The FAST scan can be performed rapidly, often within minutes, making it highly valuable in the acute setting where time is critical.
- **Noninvasive**: As a sonographic procedure, it does not expose the patient to radiation, making it repeatable if necessary.
- **Diagnostic aid**: While it does not replace CT (computed tomography) for detail and specificity, a FAST scan can quickly aid in the decision to perform urgent surgical intervention, thus potentially saving lives in critical scenarios.

Limitations

- **Sensitivity and specificity**: The FAST scan's effectiveness can be limited by the operator's experience, the patient's body habitus, and the nature of the injuries. Small amounts of fluid may be missed, and it does not provide detailed information about organ injuries.
- **Scope**: It assesses only for free fluid; it is not designed to identify the source of bleeding or to evaluate the integrity of abdominal organs beyond the presence of fluid.

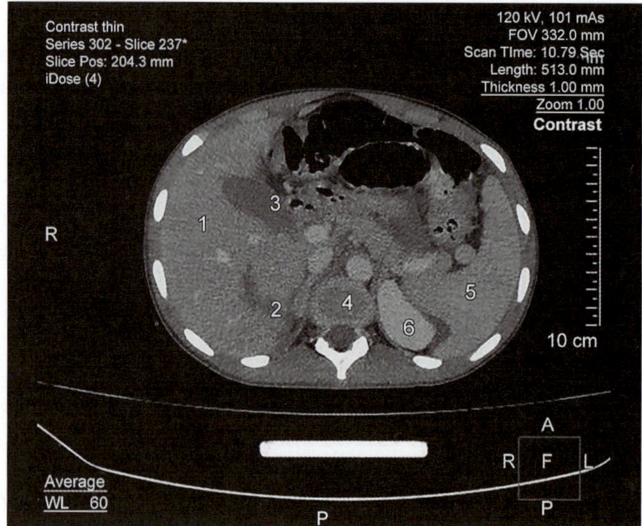

Fig. 33.2: CECT abdomen in patient of abdominal trauma showing normal liver enhancement: (1) with nonenhancing linear hypodensity; (2) Hepatic injury grade I. Other normal structures include; (3) Gallbladder; (4) Vertebrae; (5) Spleen; (6) Left kidney.

unstable patient. However, in cases where external injuries are not evident and the patient is hemodynamically unstable, a CT scan with contrast may be necessary to assess for potential vascular injuries and other nonvisible conditions **(Fig. 33.2)**.

Imaging in the Secondary Survey

After addressing life-threatening conditions and stabilizing the patient, the secondary survey involves a comprehensive evaluation to identify all significant injuries.

CT Scans: Whole Body CT (WBCT)

Known as a "pan-scan," it is increasingly used in the secondary survey for its comprehensive and rapid assessment capabilities, allowing for the detection of injuries that may not be clinically apparent. Radiation exposure is a particular risk in whole body CT and many studies advocated selective CT over whole body CT.

Selective CT: Focuses on specific areas of concern identified during the primary survey or based on clinical suspicions.

MRI

Used for detailed evaluation of suspected spinal cord injuries or complex brain injuries, MRI is typically reserved for stabilized patients due to its time-consuming nature.

Extended FAST (E-FAST)

The FAST scan has also been extended to include evaluation of the thorax for pneumothorax (E-FAST), increasing its utility in trauma assessments by allowing clinicians to also quickly identify potential life-threatening chest injuries.

Imaging in the Tertiary Survey

Imaging plays a crucial role in the tertiary survey by providing detailed visualization of injuries that might not have been fully assessed or were initially obscured by the patient's critical condition. Here are common imaging modalities used during the tertiary survey:

- **MRI:** MRI is particularly useful for detailed evaluation of soft tissue, spinal, and brain injuries. It can help identify subtle fractures, ligamentous injuries, or small areas of brain contusion that were not visible on initial CT scans.
- **Repeated or additional CT scans:** Further CT scans may be ordered to assess areas that were either not fully evaluated previously or where new symptoms suggest hidden injuries.
- **Ultrasound:** Follow-up ultrasound may be used to monitor the evolution of fluid collections, check for the development of thrombosis in vascular injuries, and assess the integrity of surgical repairs or drains.
- **X-rays:** Serial X-rays might be repeated to monitor the progression or resolution of certain conditions like pneumothorax, fracture alignment, and the status of any surgical hardware.

TARGETED IMAGING APPROACHES FOR SPECIFIC TRAUMA SCENARIOS

Following the primary survey, imaging strategies are typically customized based on the specific regions involved and the nature of the injuries. Except in cases of polytrauma or when patients remain hemodynamically unstable, targeted imaging is employed to scrutinize affected areas more precisely.

Head Trauma

In the evaluation of head trauma, imaging plays a critical role from the emergency setting to detailed follow-up assessments. The choice of imaging modalities is strategic, tailored to reveal various types of injuries and to guide subsequent treatment decisions.

Baseline and Advanced Imaging Modalities

- **Computed tomography (CT)** is the cornerstone of initial trauma assessment due to its rapid acquisition and high sensitivity for detecting acute hemorrhages, fractures, and other traumatic brain injuries. The volume rendering technique (VRT) from 3D CT data sets provides detailed visualizations of complex fractures and cranial sutures, which are invaluable for surgical planning and assessment of injury severity **(Fig. 33.3)**.
- **Magnetic resonance imaging (MRI):** MRI is more sensitive than CT for detecting parenchymal brain lesions and is used when CT results are inconclusive or when the clinical condition of a patient does not align with CT findings. It's particularly advantageous for evaluating diffuse axonal injury, small vessel damage, and subtle parenchymal injuries that CT might miss.
- **CT angiography (CTA)** is recommended when vascular injuries are suspected, which could be due

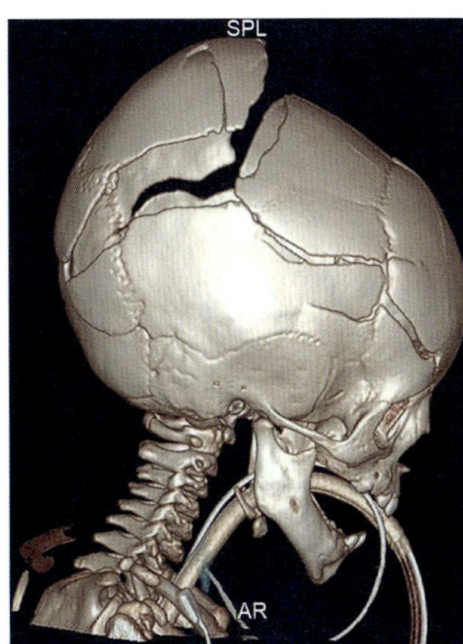

Fig. 33.3: Volume rendering technique (VRT), obtained from a 3D CT-scan data set, reveals multiple skull fractures and displaced bone fragments.

to mechanisms like high-energy impacts or penetrating traumas. This modality is critical for identifying vascular dissections or occlusions that might require immediate intervention.

Specific Traumatic Injuries and Imaging Approaches

Scalp Lesions and Skull Fractures

Scalp lesions, often evident as lacerations or hematomas, generally serve as indicators of possible underlying skull fractures. While these are usually minor, their identification can direct more focused imaging evaluations. Skull fractures, particularly those involving the base of the skull or crossing suture lines, require detailed CT imaging to assess for potential complications such as cranial nerve injury or vascular damage.

Intracranial Hemorrhages

Acute management of head trauma frequently involves identifying various types of intracranial hemorrhages:

- **Epidural hematomas (EDH)** and **subdural hematomas (SDH)** are best diagnosed with CT, which can delineate their extent, and any associated midline shift or mass effect.
- **Subarachnoid hemorrhage (SAH)**: While CT is effective for initial detection, MRI, particularly FLAIR sequences, is better at evaluating the extent and resolving subtle or chronic stages **(Table 33.3)**.

Table 33.3: Comparative radiological characteristics of intracranial hemorrhages on CT and MRI.

Feature	*Epidural hematoma*	*Subdural hematoma*	*Subarachnoid hemorrhage*
Shape on CT	Biconvex (lens-shaped)	Crescent-shaped	Diffuse or layered blood, often along contours of the brain
Crossing sutures	Does not cross sutures	Can cross sutures	Does not apply; fills subarachnoid space around the brain
Typical density on CT	Hyperdense due to arterial origin	Varies from hyperdense to isodense depending on age of hematoma	Often hyperdense, particularly acute bleeding
Location on CT	Located between the skull bone and dura mater	Between dura and arachnoid (subdural space)	Between arachnoid membrane and pia mater (subarachnoid space)
Effect on adjacent structures on CT	May cause local mass effect with midline shift	Typically causes smoother mass effect with possible midline shift	May cause minimal direct mass effect but significant secondary effects like hydrocephalus
Blood accumulation pattern on CT	Usually localized to site of impact	Spreads over the surface of the brain following contour of the brain	Fills the subarachnoid space, often visible in the basins of the sulci and cisterns
MRI appearance	Isointense or hypointense on T1, hyperintense on T2 depending on the age of the blood	Isointense or hypointense on T1, hyperintense on T2 depending on the age of the blood	Blood in subarachnoid space shows up hyperintense on FLAIR, especially in acute phase
MRI sensitivity	Useful for detecting associated soft tissue and vascular injuries	More sensitive than CT in detecting chronic or isodense hematomas	Superior for evaluating secondary effects like hydrocephalus and complications like vasospasm

Cerebral Contusions and Diffuse Axonal Injury

Cerebral contusions might be initially detected by CT but are further delineated by MRI, which can differentiate between hemorrhagic and nonhemorrhagic contusions and reveal associated edema. Diffuse axonal injury, a severe form of brain injury that results from strong rotational forces, is not always apparent on CT scans. MRI, especially with diffusion tensor imaging (DTI), is crucial for its detection and assessment.

Vascular Injuries

Vascular injuries suspected from mechanisms of injury or initial CT findings warrant further investigation with CT angiography or MR angiography. These modalities provide detailed views of blood vessel integrity and help identify dissections, occlusions, or aneurysms that require urgent intervention.

Imaging in Chest Trauma

Chest trauma, encompassing both blunt and penetrating injuries, necessitates prompt and precise imaging to diagnose potentially life-threatening conditions and guide appropriate management strategies. The complexity of chest injuries, which may involve the lungs, heart, major blood vessels, and the bony thorax, requires a systematic imaging approach to ensure no significant injury is missed.

Radiological Techniques and their Applications

- **Chest X-ray:** The chest X-ray serves as the first line of imaging in chest trauma due to its rapid availability. It effectively identifies pneumothorax, hemothorax, rib fractures, and mediastinal shifts. While essential for initial assessment, chest X-rays may miss less obvious injuries such as small pneumothoraces, pulmonary contusions, or cardiac injuries.
- **Computed tomography (CT) scan:** CT scans provide a more detailed assessment and are superior for evaluating complex injuries, including those to the lungs and mediastinum. CT angiography is particularly valuable for visualizing vascular injuries.
- **Ultrasound:** Point-of-care ultrasound (POCUS), including echocardiography, is advantageous due to its portability and real-time imaging capabilities. It is particularly useful for evaluating the heart and detecting pericardial effusions in the setting of trauma.
- **Magnetic resonance imaging (MRI):** MRI is generally reserved for specific indications in chest trauma due to its longer acquisition times. It is particularly useful for assessing vascular injuries and cardiac contusions when CT is contraindicated.

Clinical Relevance of Imaging Findings

Rapid imaging is crucial for identifying life-threatening injuries such as tension pneumothorax, which require immediate decompression. Further, decisions between surgical intervention and conservative management of chest injuries often hinge on the detailed insights provided by CT imaging. Imaging also plays a vital role in the follow-up of chest trauma, helping to monitor the healing of injuries and guiding further treatment and rehabilitation.

Polytrauma

Polytrauma, characterized by multiple concurrent injuries that may affect various body regions or systems, demands a structured and rapid imaging response to accurately diagnose and manage life-threatening conditions. The advancement in radiological technologies and the establishment of comprehensive protocols have significantly enhanced the role of imaging in managing such complex clinical scenarios.

Core Imaging Strategies

- **Ultrasound and extended fast (EFAST):** Ultrasound, including the EFAST protocol, is the first line imaging tool for quick bedside assessments to detect free fluid in the abdominal, pericardial, or thoracic cavities. It's particularly valuable in unstable patients where immediate decisions about surgical intervention are necessary.
- **Whole body computed tomography (WBCT):** WBCT is pivotal for immediate and comprehensive assessment in polytrauma due to its ability to simultaneously visualize multiple body areas. It is particularly effective for identifying occult injuries that may not be clinically apparent.
- **Focused imaging protocols:** Depending on the patient's stability and the suspected injury locations, more focused imaging assessments like targeted CT scans or MRIs might be conducted. This tailored approach helps in detailed evaluation of suspected areas without unnecessary exposure to radiation.

OPERATIONAL AND CLINICAL CONSIDERATIONS

- **Integration within trauma centers:** The physical location of imaging facilities relative to the emergency department is crucial. Moving CT scanners closer to or within the emergency departments or portable CT has shown to reduce delays significantly, which is vital for improving survival outcomes.
- **Interventional radiology (IR):**
  - *Immediate availability:* Rapid access to interventional radiology can be lifesaving, especially for managing vascular injuries and controlling internal bleeding in hemodynamically unstable patients.
  - *Communication and coordination:* Efficient communication between radiologists and trauma teams is essential for quick interpretation and application of imaging results in best clinical decision-making. All the imaging modalities should be integrated with PACS.

LAST MINUTE REVISION

- FAST scan is a critical part of the primary assessment in trauma care. Extended FAST (E-FAST) includes thoracic examination, allowing for the assessment of pneumothorax in addition to abdominal and pericardial evaluations.
- CT scans are typically performed during the secondary survey.
- MRI is used selectively in the tertiary survey.
- Whole Body CT (WBCT) is recommended for comprehensive assessment in polytrauma cases.

REVIEW QUESTIONS

Multiple Choice Questions (MCQs)

1. **What is the primary goal of the FAST scan in trauma assessment?**
   a. To evaluate bone fractures
   b. To detect free fluid in the peritoneal, pericardial, or pleural spaces
   c. To assess soft tissue damage
   d. To confirm the presence of pneumothorax

2. **Which imaging modality is considered most appropriate for assessing vascular injuries in chest trauma?**
   a. Ultrasound
   b. X-ray
   c. MRI
   d. CT angiography
3. **During which survey is whole body CT (WBCT) typically used in the management of polytrauma patients?**
   a. Primary survey
   b. Secondary survey
   c. Tertiary survey
   d. It is not used in trauma surveys
4. **MRI is particularly useful for evaluating which type of injury in trauma patients?**
   a. Bone fractures
   b. Lung contusions
   c. Diffuse axonal injury
   d. Abdominal free fluid
5. **Which statement is true regarding the use of X-rays in trauma imaging?**
   a. They are primarily used for detailed vascular assessments.
   b. They are not useful for detecting pneumothorax.
   c. They provide a quick and effective method for identifying major bony injuries and chest trauma.
   d. They are the best choice for evaluating soft tissue damage.

Answer Key

1. b   2. d   3. b   4. c   5. c

SUGGESTED READING

1. Lomoschitz FM, Eisenhuber E, Linnau KF, Peloschek P, Schoder M, Bankier AA. Imaging of chest trauma: radiological patterns of injury and diagnostic algorithms. Eur J Radiol. 2003;48(1):61-70.
2. Thippeswamy PB, Rajasekaran RB. Imaging in polytrauma—Principles and current concepts. J Clin Orthop Trauma. 2020;16:106-13.

CHAPTER

34 Radiology in Intensive Care Unit

"In the ICU, every scan is a lifeline—radiologists provide answers when time and certainty matter most."

INTRODUCTION

The intensive care unit (ICU) is a high-stakes environment where timely and accurate diagnosis is essential for patient management. Radiology plays a pivotal role in the ICU by providing critical imaging information that influences clinical decisions. This chapter aims to elucidate the various radiological techniques used in the ICU, their applications, advantages, and limitations, with a focus on portable chest radiography and computed tomography (CT).

PORTABLE CHEST RADIOGRAPHY (FIG. 34.1)

Portable chest radiography is the most commonly requested radiographic examination in the ICU. It is favored for its availability and cost-effectiveness. However, it is often hampered by technical limitations, such as variable image quality due to differences in film exposure and scattered radiation as commonly done CXR in ICU is AP view but for better lung imaging the most preferable view is chest PA. The implementation of wide-latitude screen film systems and digital radiography has significantly improved image quality.

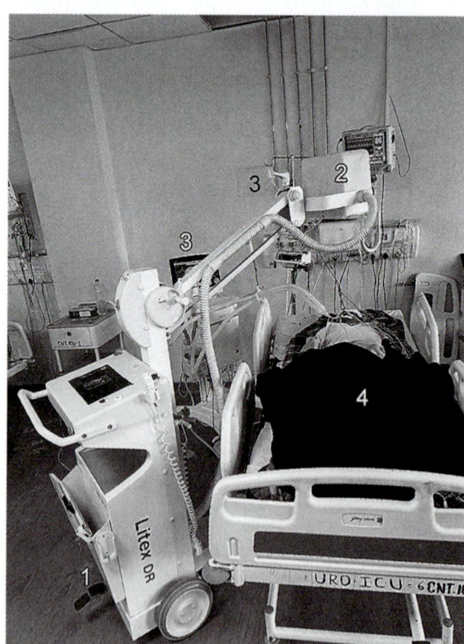

Fig. 34.1: ICU setup showing portable digital x-ray machine (1) with its tube end (2) above the patient (3) on patient right side (4) lying supine on ICU bed with ventilator apparatus.

Portable chest radiography is routinely performed in the ICU as a complement to the physical examination. Despite its advantages, portable radiography can have technical and diagnostic limitations. Variations in film exposure and scattered radiation often lead to inferior image quality, frustrating both clinicians and radiologists. However, recent advancements in digital radiography, including features like exposure compensation and image processing, have consistently produced diagnostic quality radiographs.

PACS IN THE ICU (FIG. 34.2)

The introduction of PACS has enhanced the management of ICU patients by allowing rapid acquisition, distribution, and review of radiographic images. PACS integrates digital radiography, image processing, and network transmission, facilitating simultaneous observation by ICU clinicians as well as radiologists. The ability to manipulate images at viewing stations enhances diagnostic accuracy and clinician confidence in interpretation. The user interface emphasizes speed and simplicity, with a variety of viewing tools.

PACS networks consist of image acquisition devices, network display devices, image servers or archives, and storage devices. Radiographs can be acquired directly by a digital radiographic device or digitized from conventional radiographs. These images are then transmitted via a computer network for display at workstations in multiple locations within minutes of their acquisition, allowing simultaneous and prompt viewing by both the clinician in the ICU and the radiologist. The soft-copy images read from a high-quality display are as accurate as screen film bedside chest radiographs.

Although PACS has significantly improved the quality of images and their accessibility, the actual impact on patient care is still being evaluated. Hospital-wide, the introduction of PACS has increased viewing of images by clinicians and generated increased utilization of imaging services. However, this trend has not been observed in the ICU, where the frequency of images assessed was similar between film and filmless operations. For nonroutine ICU radiographs, prompt clinical actions were initiated more quickly once image findings were known, compared to the pre-PACS era.

Accuracy and Efficacy

Despite the widespread use of portable chest radiographs, their accuracy in diagnosing pulmonary conditions in ICU patients varies. Studies indicate that up to 65% of daily radiographs reveal

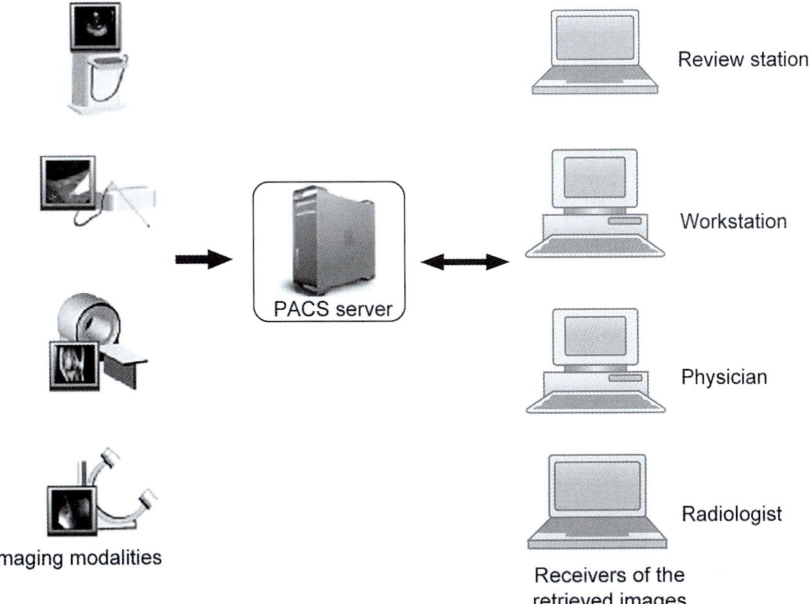

Fig. 34.2: Shows working of PACS integrating all modalities with radiologist.

(RIS: Radiology information system) and other clinicians; (HIS: Hospital information system) through hardware (server) as well as various softwares/network.

significant abnormalities affecting patient management. However, routine radiographs often yield fewer clinically significant findings compared to those taken after a change in clinical status.

COMMON RADIOGRAPHIC APPEARANCES OF SUPPORT DEVICES (FIGS. 34.3 TO 34.5)

Endotracheal and Tracheostomy Tubes

Radiographs frequently guide the repositioning of endotracheal (ET) tubes. The ideal position for an ET tube is mid-trachea **(Fig. 34.3)**. Misplacement can lead to complications such as right main stem intubation.

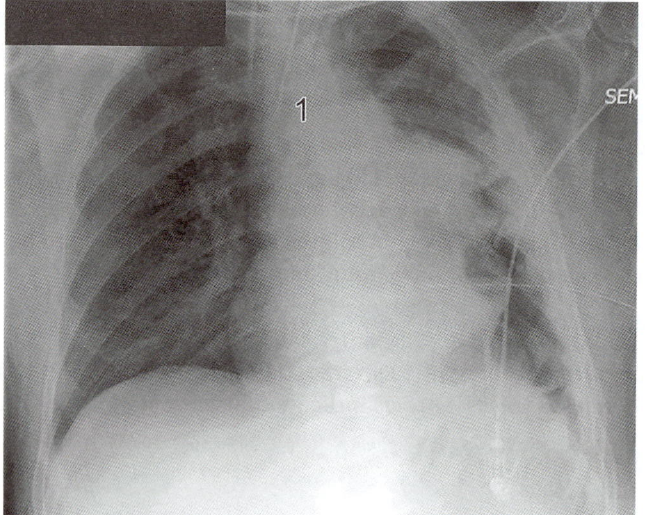

Fig. 34.3: Chest X-ray AP in ICU setup shows endotracheal tube (1) in situ.

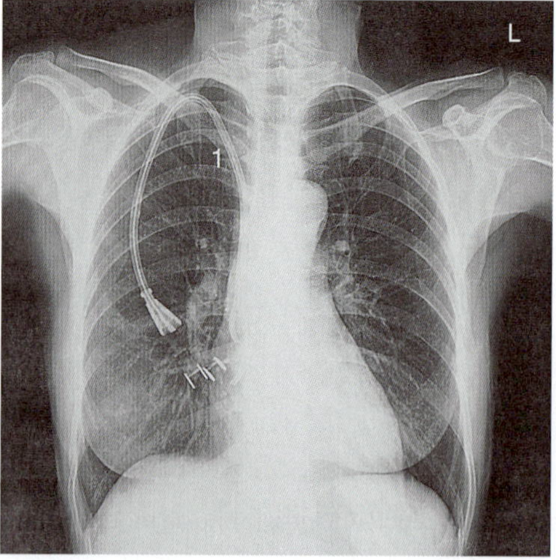

Fig. 34.4: Chest X-ray shows SVC catheter in situ.

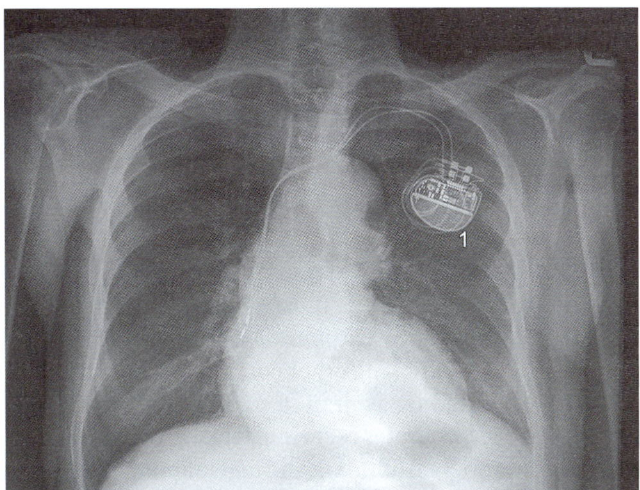

Fig. 34.5: Shows chest x-ray with pacemaker in situ.

The ideal position for the ET tube, with the head in the neutral position, is in the mid-trachea. Head flexion and extension are associated with a tube excursion of 2 cm; with the chin "down," the tip is "down" at the lowest point. Too low positioning results in right main stem intubation, whereas too high placement is associated with a theoretical risk of inadvertent extubation and vocal cord injury. Following intubation, physical examination identified tube malposition in only 2–5% of patients, whereas radiographs revealed suboptimal positioning in 10–25%.

Tracheotomy tubes are rarely malpositioned, and the role of the radiograph is to exclude postsurgical complications of hemorrhage or abnormal air collections. Tracheal stenosis is a late complication, usually occurring at the stoma or tube tip.

Enteric Tubes

Proper placement of nasogastric and feeding tubes is critical to prevent complications like aspiration. Malpositioning is more frequent with small-bore feeding tubes and can be reliably detected via chest radiography.

Malpositioning occurs in 1% of cases and is more frequent with small-bore feeding tubes than nasogastric tubes. It is important to ensure that the distal side holes of the nasogastric tube lie in the stomach to prevent aspiration. Following insertion of a feeding tube, a chest radiograph is mandatory to confirm correct positioning. Feeding tubes may inadvertently be placed in the major bronchi or pleural space.

Pulmonary Artery Catheters

Pulmonary artery catheter placement complications include malposition, vascular trauma, and thromboembolic events. Radiographs ensure proper positioning and identify complications such as pulmonary artery pseudoaneurysms and thromboembolic phenomena.

The ideal location for the pulmonary artery catheter tip is central, lying within 2 cm of the hilar point. The catheter tip on balloon deflation should not extend beyond the proximal interlobar arteries. Distal placement is associated with an increased risk of vascular trauma and thromboembolic events. Nonfatal asymptomatic ruptures are manifest as the sudden appearance of localized air space opacification around the catheter tip, representing focal hemorrhage.

Thromboembolic complications are increasingly recognized, with a reported incidence between 1 and 11%. Thrombus formation may occur from persistent wedging of the catheter in small arteries, leading to stagnant flow, or it may originate at the site of catheter insertion, or a mural thrombus may arise from catheter contact with the vessel wall. Subsequent pulmonary embolism and pulmonary infarction is a significant risk.

COMMON PULMONARY COMPLICATIONS IN THE ICU

Nosocomial Pneumonia

Ventilator-associated pneumonia (VAP) is the most common nosocomial infection in the ICU. Radiographic signs include new or progressive pulmonary opacities, but diagnosis is challenging, due to nonspecific findings often mimicking other conditions like pulmonary edema or ARDS.

Most episodes of VAP are caused by aspiration of oropharyngeal contents into the distal airways. Endotracheal intubation promotes recurrent leakage of bacteria-laden oropharyngeal and gastric secretions despite proper positioning and cuff inflation. These secretions pool above the cuff and can be radiographically observed. Oropharyngeal colonization by Gram-negative bacteria occurs rapidly in critically ill patients, often within 24 hours of admission to the ICU, and up to 40% of patients will be colonized by 5 days.

Establishing the diagnosis of VAP is difficult. Clinical criteria to define pneumonia include fever, leukocytosis, purulent tracheobronchial secretions, and the radiographic appearance of a new or progressive pulmonary opacity. However, in mechanically ventilated patients, these parameters are less reliable. Studies have shown that fever, leukocytosis or leukopenia, and bacterial pathogens in sputum are often present in the absence of pneumonia. The majority of air space opacities in critically ill patients therefore do not represent pneumonia.

Studies comparing the accuracy of chest radiography in diagnosing pneumonia to the gold standards of autopsy examination or protected brush catheter specimens reveal a radiographic specificity of 27–35%.

Atelectasis

Atelectasis, particularly postsurgical, is common in ICU patients. Radiographs show linear bands of opacification or lobar opacification. Differentiating atelectasis from pneumonia can be challenging but is aided by observing the resolution of opacities over time.

Atelectasis occurs most frequently in the left lower lobe (66%) compared to the right lower lobe (22%) and the right upper lobe (11%). Radiographically, atelectasis may be manifest as linear bands of opacification, patchy opacities mimicking pneumonia, or complete lobar opacification. If the opacity fluctuates or resolves within minutes or hours, the air space opacification is likely due to atelectasis.

The portable radiograph is relatively insensitive to the detection of air space opacities in the lung bases. When a basal opacity is identified on the chest radiograph, the extent of the abnormality is frequently underestimated. Studies comparing postoperative supine radiographs with CT studies reported a sensitivity of only 74%.

Pulmonary Edema

Radiographs are sensitive for detecting pulmonary edema but less so in differentiating its causes. Features like cardiomegaly, septal thickening, and pleural effusions are common, and CT scans can provide additional clarity, especially in distinguishing cardiogenic from noncardiogenic edema.

Additional CT findings of congestive cardiac failure include dilated arteries and veins with the nondependent vessels enlarged disproportionately (cephalization). The airspace opacification tends to be central with a ventral dorsal distribution of increasing density. The distribution of pulmonary edema may be altered by patient positioning due to the effects of gravity and by underlying lung disease. These features are usually absent in noncardiogenic pulmonary edema.

Aspiration Pneumonia

Aspiration is prevalent in ICU patients due to various factors such as anesthesia and enteral feeding. Radiographic signs include bilateral nodular opacities and asymmetric distribution, often requiring CT for detailed evaluation.

Aspiration is a significant risk for patients receiving enteral nutrition. The method of feeding (nasal, gastric, or jejunal) does not increase the frequency of aspiration. The clinical manifestations of aspiration include the development of chemical pneumonitis, pleuropulmonary infection, and acute airway obstruction. The extent and severity of lung injury depend on the volume of aspirated material, its acidity, and the amount of particulate matter in the aspirate. Aspiration occurs more commonly on the right and in the supine position, involving the posterior aspects of the lungs.

Following aspiration of sterile gastric contents, the majority of patients have an uncomplicated recovery. Radiographic findings are nonspecific but include bilateral nodular or confluent opacities with central and lower zone predominance with an asymmetric distribution. Typically, radiographic resolution is rapid, with some improvement seen as early as the first 24 hours. In a minority of patients, acute respiratory failure develops or following an initial period of clinical and radiographic stability, bacterial pneumonia and the development of ARDS supervenes.

Complications of aspiration pneumonia include lung abscess formation, pleural effusions, and bronchopleural fistula. Most lung abscesses resolve with antibiotic therapy and postural drainage. Medically refractory abscesses should be considered for percutaneous image-guided drainage. Percutaneous drainage is effective and has a low incidence of complications. CT provides the best depiction of the size and location of the abscess.

Acute airway obstruction may occur following aspiration of solid material from the oropharynx or stomach. The clinical outcome and radiographic manifestations of airway obstruction depend on the level and degree of obstruction. Obstruction of a central bronchus may lead to complete lung collapse, whereas obstruction of a major bronchus may lead to lobar collapse. The chest radiograph may reveal atelectasis or demonstrate features of air trapping with unilateral hyperinflation and mediastinal shift.

COMPUTED TOMOGRAPHY (CT) IN THE ICU

CT scans offer detailed imaging of thoracic structures and are increasingly used for diagnosing conditions like pulmonary embolism, sepsis, and postsurgical complications. Multislice CT scanners enable rapid imaging, even in dyspneic patients, providing invaluable information for therapeutic procedures and image-guided interventions.

CT has a high sensitivity and specificity for detecting pulmonary embolism, with CT pulmonary angiography becoming the gold standard for evaluation. CT also provides superior imaging for diagnosing sepsis of unknown etiology, postsurgical complications, and for guiding interventional procedures. The ability to perform multiplanar reconstructions and 3D imaging further enhances the diagnostic utility of CT in the ICU.

Pleural complications such as effusions, pneumothorax, and hemothorax are common in ICU patients and are often challenging to diagnose with portable radiographs alone due to suboptimal position of patient. CT provides detailed imaging of pleural abnormalities, helping to differentiate between various causes and guiding therapeutic interventions like thoracentesis and chest tube placement.

CONCLUSION

Radiology is an indispensable tool in the ICU, enhancing the diagnosis and management of critically ill patients. Portable chest radiography remains a cornerstone of routine evaluation, while CT offers detailed imaging for complex conditions. The integration of PACS has further streamlined radiological services, improving image accessibility and diagnostic efficiency. Continuous dialogue between clinicians and radiologists is essential for optimizing patient care and interpreting imaging findings effectively.

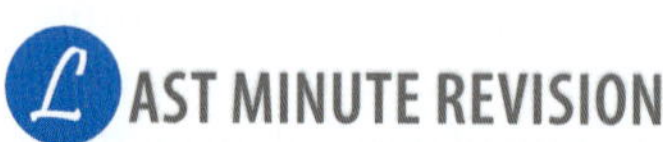

- Portable chest radiography is the most commonly used imaging modality in the ICU due to its availability and cost-effectiveness.
- Picture archiving and communication system (PACS) significantly enhances image accessibility and diagnostic efficiency in ICU settings.
- Portable X-rays can detect up to 65% of significant pathologies in ICU patients.
- CT scans provide detailed imaging for diagnosing pulmonary embolism, sepsis, and surgical complications.
- Atelectasis frequently occurs in the left lower lobe and can present as linear opacities or complete lobar collapse.

REVIEW QUESTIONS

Multiple Choice Questions (MCQs)

1. **What is the primary imaging modality used in the ICU for routine evaluation of patients?**
   a. MRI
   b. CT scan
   c. Portable chest radiography
   d. Ultrasound
2. **Which system has revolutionized the accessibility and efficiency of radiological services in the ICU?**
   a. Digital radiography (DR)
   b. Computed radiography (CR)
   c. Picture archiving and communication system (PACS)
   d. Fluoroscopy
3. **Which of the following is NOT a common complication of pulmonary artery catheter placement?**
   a. Malposition
   b. Vascular trauma
   c. Pleural effusion
   d. Thromboembolic events
4. **What is the most specific radiographic sign for differentiating increased permeability edema from hydrostatic pulmonary edema?**
   a. Cardiomegaly
   b. Septal thickening
   c. Patchy airspace opacification
   d. Pleural effusion

5. What is the typical radiographic feature of aspiration pneumonia in ICU patients?

a. Unilateral hyperinflation
b. Bilateral nodular opacities with asymmetric distribution
c. Cardiomegaly
d. Hilar lymphadenopathy

Answer Key

1. c 2. c 3. c 4. c 5. b

SUGGESTED READING

1. Hall JB, White SR, Karrison T. Efficacy of daily routine chest radiographs in intubated, mechanically ventilated patients. Crit Care Med. 1991;19(5):689-93.
2. Wunderink RG, Woldenberg LS, Zeiss J, et al. The radiologic diagnosis of autopsy-proven ventilator-associated pneumonia. Chest. 1992;101:458-63.

UNIT 7

Advanced Techniques and Professional Practice

Unit Outline

CHAPTER

35 Nuclear Medicine in Radiology

"With targeted isotopes and intelligent imaging, nuclear medicine brings radiology to the molecular frontier."

INTRODUCTION

Nuclear medicine is a branch of medicine which utilizes various radiopharmaceuticals (radiotracers) for diagnosis and treatment of various human diseases. After administration of radiopharmaceutical, patient becomes radioactive source (internal radiation source). It differs from conventional radiology and radiotherapy techniques, where source of radiation lies external to the patient. Nuclear medicine studies provide functional (physiological) information whereas conventional radiology studies provide morphological (anatomical) information. Nuclear medicine has become quite widespread since its inception in the 1950s.

TYPES OF RADIATION

Gamma (γ) ray emission and positron emission are two main types of radiation used for Nuclear medicine imaging. Gamma photons are detected with a gamma camera as either planar (2D) images or tomographic (3D) images using single photon emission computed tomography (SPECT). The annihilation photons from positron emission are detected using a positron emission tomography (PET) camera. Hybrid/fusion imaging is the combination of SPECT or PET cameras with CT/MRI scanners in a single imaging device. SPECT-CT, PET-CT and PET-MRI are examples of hybrid imaging techniques which provides both physiological and anatomical information with higher sensitivity and specificity.

Radiopharmaceutical comprises of two words—radionuclide and pharmaceutical. Radionuclide emits radiation and pharmaceutical helps in localization within the body. Thus, utilization of biodistribution of the radiopharmaceutical within the body is the basis of diagnosis and treatment in Nuclear medicine.

Nuclear fission or neutron activation (nuclear reactor), charged-particle bombardment in a particle accelerator (cyclotron) and decay of a radioactive parent to radioactive daughter (generator) are various methods of radionuclide production.

99mTechnetium (6 hours half-life) and 18F-Fluorodeoxyglucose (FDG, 110 minutes half-life) are workhorses of SPECT and PET imaging respectively. Increased glucose metabolism of cancer cells forms the fundamental basis of FDG PET/CT tumor imaging. It is characterized by increased expression of GLUT1 and GLUT3 glucose transporters and upregulation of hexokinase enzyme activity of malignant cells.

Commonly used radionuclides for diagnostic applications includes: Technetium-99m (Tc-99m), Iodine-131 (I-131), Thallium-201 (Tl-201), etc., in SPECT while, Fluorine-18 (F-18), Carbon-11 (C-11) and Oxygen-15 (O-15) in PET imaging **(Tables 35.1 and 35.2)**. Beside diagnosis, radionuclides are also used for therapeutic applications, e.g., Iodine-131 sodium iodide used in hyperthyroidism and thyroid cancer.

Table 35.1: Technetium-99m labeled radiopharmaceuticals.

Radiopharmaceutical	*Clinical applications*
Tc-99m methylene diphosphonate (MDP)	Skeletal scintigraphy **(Fig. 35.1)**
Tc-99m diethylenetriaminepentaacetic acid (DTPA)	Renal dynamic scintigraphy, lung ventilation scintigraphy, glomerular filtration rate estimation **(Fig. 35.2)**
Tc-99m mercaptoacetyltriglycine (MAG3)	Renal dynamic scintigraphy
Tc-99m dimercaptosuccinic acid (DMSA-V)	Renal cortical scintigraphy
Tc-99m sestamibi	Myocardial perfusion scintigraphy, parathyroid scintigraphy
Tc-99m sodium pertechnetate	Meckel's diverticulum detection, salivary and thyroid gland scintigraphy
Tc-99m sulfur colloid	Lymphoscintigraphy, liver/spleen scintigraphy, bone marrow scintigraphy, gastroesophageal reflux (GER), gastric emptying study
Tc-99m iminodiacetic acid (HIDA)/Tc-99m mebrofenin	Hepatobiliary scintigraphy **(Fig. 35.3)**
Tc-99m Technegas	Lung ventilation scintigraphy

Table 35.2: Common PET radiopharmaceuticals (Fig. 35.4).

Radiopharmaceutical	*Clinical applications*
F-18 fluorodeoxyglucose (FDG)	Tumor imaging Infection/inflammation imaging Myocardial viability, sarcoid diagnosis Brain: Dementia, interictal seizure
Ga-68 DOTATATE	Somatostatin-positive neuroendocrine tumor (NET)

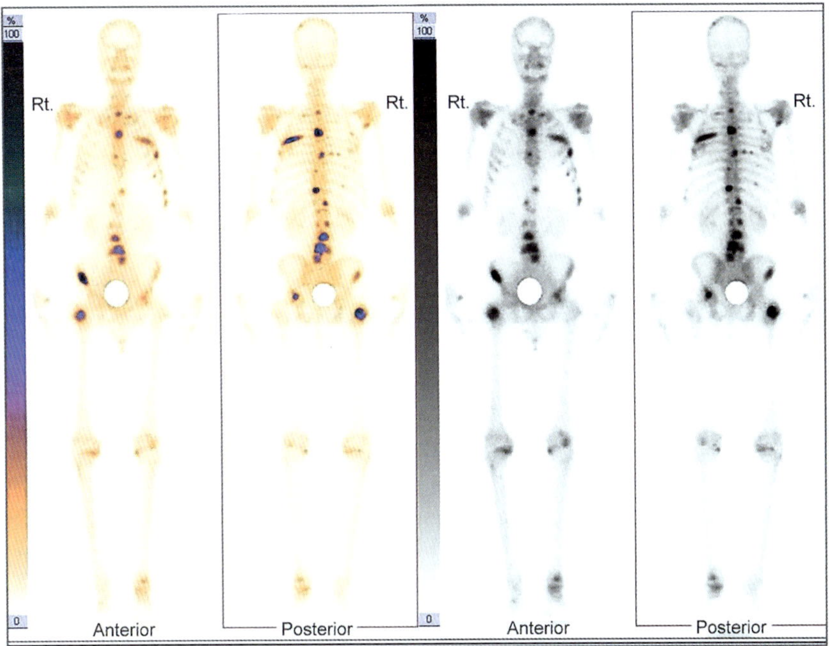

Fig. 35.1: Tc-99m MDP whole-body bone scan shows extensive bone metastases in a patient of prostate cancer.

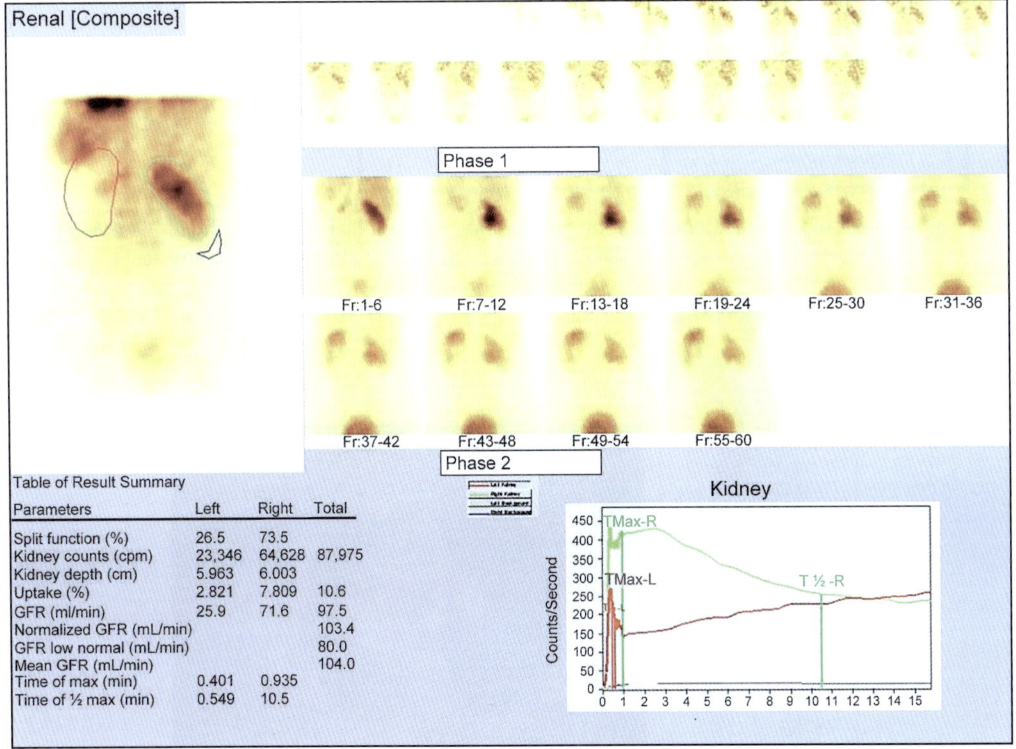

Fig. 35.2: Diuretic renal dynamic scintigraphy using Tc-99m DTPA showing progressive filling of left dilated PCS.

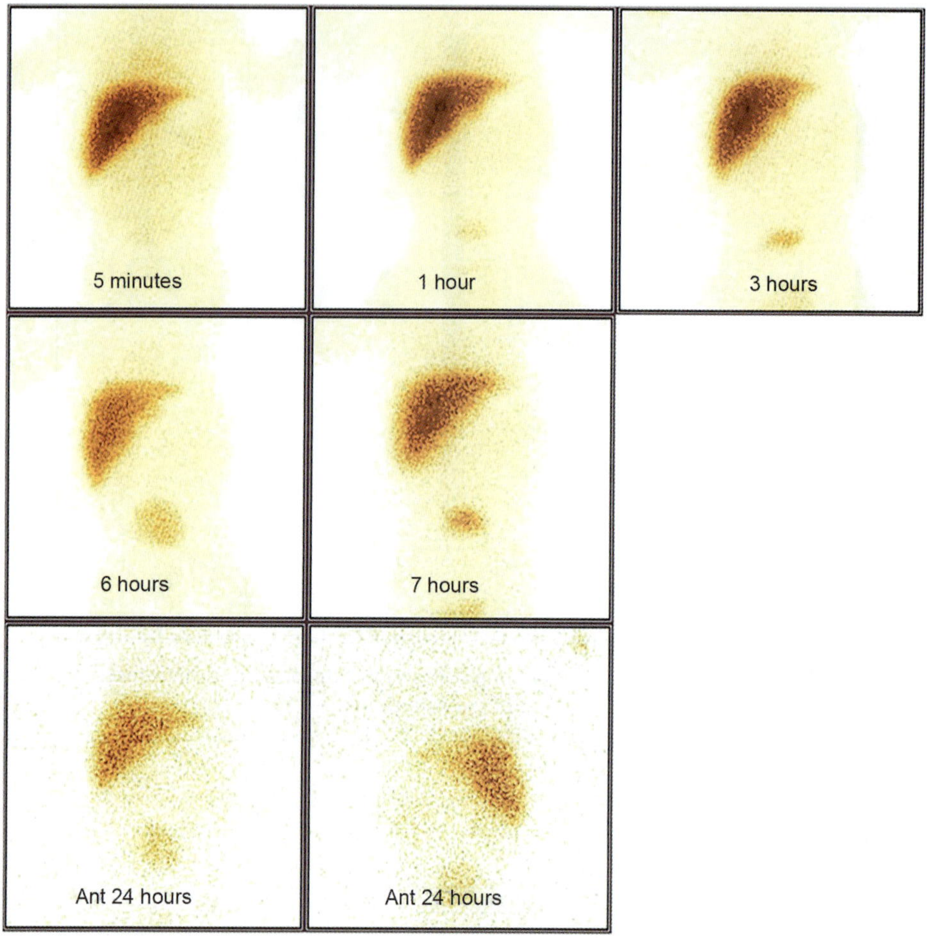

5 minutes
1 hour
3 hours
6 hours
7 hours
Ant 24 hours
Ant 24 hours

Fig. 35.3: 16 weeks old child under evaluation for jaundice. Hepatobiliary scintigraphy Tc-99m Mebrofenin shows no biliary excretion over 24 hours suggests possibility of biliary atresia.

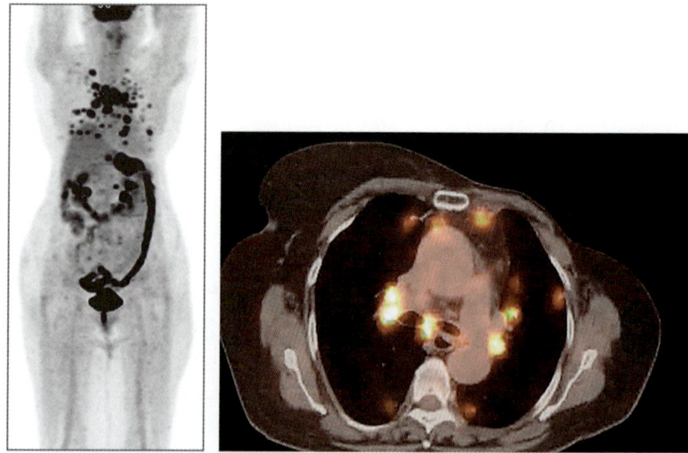

Fig. 35.4: Whole-body F-18 FDG PET/CT scintigraphy in an operated case of breast carcinoma showing bilateral lung and mediastinal lymphnode metastases.

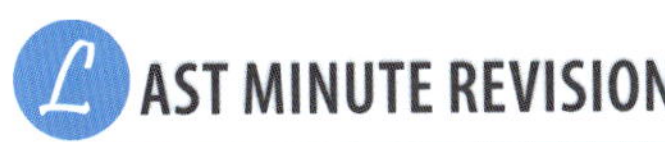

LAST MINUTE REVISION

- Nuclear medicine is a medical specialty that involves the use of various radiopharmaceuticals for diagnostic and therapeutic clinical applications, virtually in all organs of the body.
- SPECT, PET, SPECT-CT, PET-CT and PET-MRI are various diagnostic imaging modalities in nuclear medicine.
- The most commonly used radionuclides for diagnostic purposes are Tc-99m and F-18, and for therapeutic applications is Iodine-131.
- Most recently clinical applications of PET-MRI and alpha emitters radionuclide therapy are having many futuristic promising clinical applications.

REVIEW QUESTIONS

Multiple Choice Questions (MCQs)

1. **Which of the following SPECT radiopharmaceutical is used for myocardial perfusion imaging?**
   a. N-13 ammonia
   b. Tc-99m sestamibi
   c. Rb-82 chloride
   d. O-15 water
2. **What is the half-life of the most commonly used SPECT radionuclide in diagnostic nuclear medicine?**
   a. 110 minutes
   b. 8 days
   c. 6 hours
   d. 68 minutes
3. **Which of the following is an example of hybrid imaging?**
   a. PET-MRI
   b. PET
   c. SPECT
   d. MRI
4. **Which of the following radiopharmaceutical is used for renal cortical scintigraphy?**
   a. Tc99m-MAG3
   b. Tc99m-DTPA
   c. Tc99m-EC
   d. Tc-99m DMSA
5. **Which of the following Iodine radioisotope is used for treatment of well-differentiated thyroid cancer?**
   a. Iodine-127
   b. Iodine-123
   c. Iodine-131
   d. Iodine-125

Answer Key

1. b 2. c 3. a 4. d 5. c

SUGGESTED READING

1. Crişan G, Moldovean-Cioroianu NS, Timaru DG, Andrieş G, Căinap C, Chiş V. Radiopharmaceuticals for PET and SPECT Imaging: A Literature Review over the Last Decade. Int J Mol Sci. 2022;23(9):5023. doi: 10.3390/ijms23095023. PMID: 35563414; PMCID: PMC9103893.
2. Lee WW. K-SPECT Group. Clinical Applications of Technetium-99m Quantitative Single-Photon Emission Computed Tomography/Computed Tomography. Nucl Med Mol Imaging. 2019;53(3):172-181. doi: 10.1007/s13139-019-00588-9. Epub 2019 Mar 15. PMID: 31231437; PMCID: PMC6554391.

CHAPTER

36 Imaging in Transplantation

"In transplant imaging, radiologists safeguard second chances—ensuring compatibility, function, and follow-up with precision."

INTRODUCTION

Transplantation is a medical procedure in which an organ, tissue, or cells are transferred from one location to another within the same person's body or from one individual to another to replace damaged or absent parts. This can include organs like the heart, kidneys, liver, lungs, and pancreas, tissues such as skin and corneas, or cells such as stem cells and bone marrow. The most common type of transplantation worldwide is the transplantation of blood components, specifically red blood cell transfusions. These are routinely performed in medical settings ranging from emergency trauma care to management of conditions like severe anemia or during surgery. After that abdominal organ transplantation has witnessed remarkable success in treating end -stage organ diseases over the past few decades. With advancements in surgical techniques, immunosuppressive therapies and post-transplant care, kidney and liver transplants, in particular, have become highly effective in prolonging and improving the quality of life for patients with end-stage organ disease. Radiologists play a crucial role in evaluating donor and recipient before, during and after transplantation. Radiologist awareness about various surgical techniques of transplantation, complications and associated imaging features that may occur at varying time points following transplantation is essential to effectively guide clinical management and to facilitate intervention in time that saves graft organs and lives. This chapter endeavors to provide insights into the radiological aspects of liver and kidney transplantation.

RENAL TRANSPLANTATION

Compared to grafts from deceased donors, allografts from living donors offer significant advantages in terms of both graft and patient survival. Living donor transplantation provides the benefit of prearranged scheduling, which helps to minimize any unnecessary delays and enables the possibility of pre-emptive transplantation.

Radiological Evaluation of Potential Renal Donor

- The potential donor must be evaluated in detail to ensure adequate kidneys for both donor and recipient, for preventing donor complications and assuring good recipient graft function.
- Ultrasound (US) is the primary imaging tool for pre donation screening—in identifying incidental conditions like unilateral agenesis, horseshoe shaped kidney, cortical atrophy, polycystic disease that are absolute contraindication for donation.

Also useful for assessing kidney size, the presence of any solid or cystic mass, and nephrolithiasis, which are not absolute contraindications for donation but require thorough assessment.

- Following this, 99mTc-DTPA (diethylene-triamine-pentaacetate) scan is used to determine relative contribution of each of two kidneys. If there is asymmetry in the renal function the kidney with better function should remain with the donor and donating kidney should be adequate.
- Computed tomography (CT) angiography and intravenous urography (IVU) serve as the final step in the imaging process to provide information on renal vasculature including number of renal arteries and veins, their course, early branching pattern, renal parenchyma, and collecting system.

Radiological Evaluation of Potential Renal Recipient

The following is standard protocol:

- **Chest x-ray:** To evaluate pulmonary manifestation of chronic kidney disease.
- **Ultrasound of abdomen:** To determine the potential need for nephrectomy, particularly in cases of infection or polycystic kidney disease.
- **Doppler of iliac vessels:** For presence and severity of atherosclerotic changes that may cause difficulty in anastomosis.
- Sometimes, CT may be needed to reinforce the findings of x-ray and/or Sonography/Doppler

Important Surgical Technique

- The transplanted kidney is usually placed extraperitoneally in the patient's right iliac fossa (less commonly in left iliac fossa), with end-to-side anastomosis of renal vessels to the external iliac vasculature **(Fig. 36.1)**. Less commonly an end-to-end anastomosis of renal artery to the recipient internal iliac artery is performed.
- Deceased donor kidneys are commonly procured with an intact main renal artery and an attached portion of the aorta (Carrel patch).
- If the harvested kidney has more than one renal artery, they can be anastomosed with each other in a side-to-side fashion (pantaloons) during bench surgery or there could be separate anastomoses.

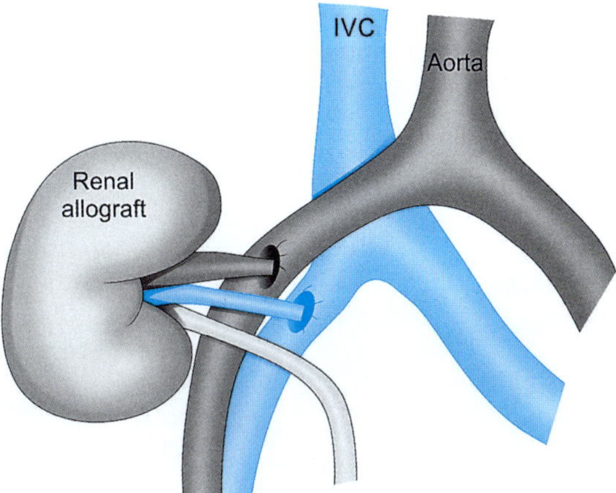

Fig. 36.1: Diagrammatic representation of anatomical layout and end-to-side anastomosis in renal transplantation.

- In cases of multiple renal veins, usually the larger vein is anastomosed, and the smaller veins are ligated.
- Currently ureteroneocystostomy is a method of choice for restoring urinary drainage in which the ureter is implanted directly into the dome of the bladder. In some cases, ureteroureterostomy or pyeloureterostomy may also be performed.

Postrenal Transplant Evaluation

Ultrasound and Doppler

Doppler ultrasonography plays a pivotal role in monitoring renal transplant during the postoperative period. It is a method of choice due to easy availability, portability (can be done bedside) nonionizing, noninvasive, can be repeated frequently and without need of contrast media.

A baseline Doppler evaluation is usually performed in the first 24–48 hours after transplantation. Before commencing, it is useful to review the operative notes to get a clear idea of the number of arteries anastomosed and the type of anastomosis. Grayscale ultrasound should be used to see for renal size, echogenicity, corticomedullary differentiations, and dilatation of collecting system or ureter and for evaluation of postoperative collections. Color Doppler is used to see the intrarenal perfusion. Visualizing interlobar, segmental, arcuate arteries, corresponding veins, renal artery and veins at the hilum, along their entire length and at the anastomosis is crucial. Resistive index (RI) and peak systolic velocity (PSV) should be measured. RI up to 0.75 and PSV up to 300 cm/s at anastomosis in early post-transplant period is considered normal **(Figs. 36.2A and B)**. Iliac vessels should be evaluated for possible signs of thrombosis, stenosis or occlusion. There should be normal triphasic waveform in iliac artery.

Ultrasound is also useful in guiding renal biopsies and for percutaneous drainage of collection if any.

Cross-sectional imaging is used only when ultrasound/Doppler findings are equivocal or when vascular intervention to be carried out.

CT Scan

CT provides excellent vascular anatomy but has disadvantage of ionizing radiation and iodinated contrast media. Sometimes in presence of postoperative collection CT is used to see for exact volume and the extent of the collection.

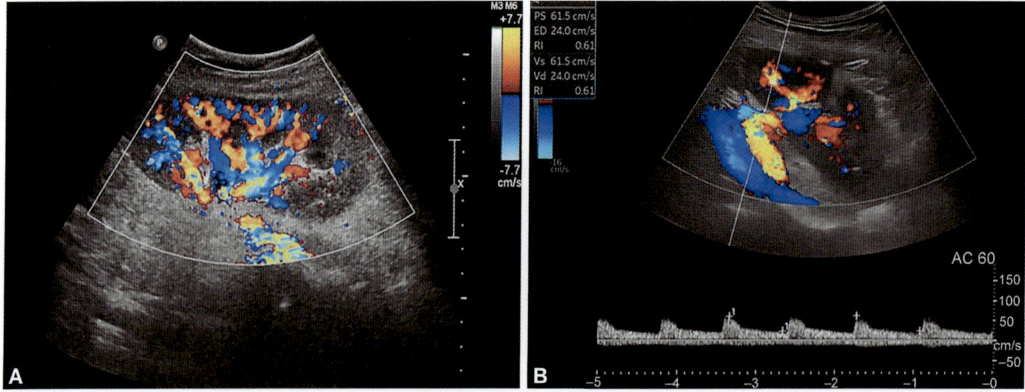

Figs. 36.2A and B: (A) Normal Color Doppler image of transplanted kidney and (B) Spectral Doppler of intrarenal arterial branch showing normal biphasic flow pattern, end-diastolic flow being approximately one-third or greater of the amplitude of peak systolic velocity.

Magnetic Resonance Imaging (MRI)

MRI is an excellent alternative tool in terms of contrast and radiation risk. The disadvantages are expensive, accessibility, time-consuming and contraindicated in patients with a cardiac implantable electronic device, metallic intraocular foreign body, implantable neurostimulation system, cochlear implant etc.

Postrenal Transplant Complications (Table 36.1)

Postrenal transplant complications are classified into four primary categories:

Table 36.1: Postrenal transplant complications.

Type of complication	*Conditions*	*Diagnostic features*
1. Vascular complications	Renal artery thrombosis	Enlarged and hypoechoic kidney on grayscale ultrasound, devoid of arterial and venous flow
(Selective angiography is gold standard but is reserved for patient needed intervention, due to availability of CTA/MRA)	Renal artery stenosis (RAS)	Focal aliasing at stenotic segments on Doppler ultrasound, peak systolic velocity >300 cm/s, PSV of renal artery/external iliac artery >/= 1.8, high resistive index >0.7, acceleration time >0.07s, index <3 and intrarenal tardus-parvus; CT or MR angiography for detailed assessment
	Renal vein thrombosis (RVT)	Swollen, hypoechoic graft on ultrasound; absence of venous flow, reversal or absence of diastolic flow in renal artery on Doppler
	Kinking of artery	• Common in right renal allograft due to longer length of renal artery • Tardus-parvus pattern on Doppler ultrasound; CT/MR angiography for detailed evaluation
	Torsion of graft	Shift in kidney axis, diminished or absent perfusion. CT and MRI can reveal vascular pedicle kinking
	Extraparenchymal pseudoaneurysm **(Fig. 36.3)**	Common at anastomosis site. Cystic lesion with color flow, to-and-fro spectral pattern on Doppler; CT or MR angiography needed for detailed evaluation
2. Urological complications	Ureteric leak	Common site is distal ureter, notably at ureteroneo-cystostomy. Anechoic fluid collection without septa on ultrasound commonly at lower pole; CT for precise relation of fluid collection to kidney; Tc-99m MAG3 scan and antegrade pyelography for confirmation
	Urinary obstruction	Common at site of anastomosis into bladder (lower third ureter due to lack of blood supply). Hydronephrosis with dilated ureter up to the level of obstruction on ultrasound or cross-sectional imaging
3. Peritransplant fluid collections	Urinoma	Rapidly enlarging anechoic fluid collection without septations near lower pole of kidney on ultrasound
	Hematoma	Complex and echogenic appearance initially on ultrasound, decreasing echogenicity over time
	Lymphocele	Anechoic appearance with or without internal septa on ultrasound, may compress adjacent structures
	Peritransplant abscess	Low-level echoes and thick irregular wall on ultrasound; presence of air may indicate an abscess

Contd...

Contd...

Type of complication	*Conditions*	*Diagnostic features*
4. Renal parenchymal diseases	Acute tubular necrosis (ATN)	Normal appearance in mild cases, or enlarged, edematous, and echo-poor kidney with elevated resistive index on Doppler in severe cases
	Hyperacute rejection	Imaging plays no role; Doppler may show absence of perfusion
	Acute rejection	Enlarged graft, reduced cortical echogenicity, loss of cortico-medullary differentiation, echogenic sinus fat, focal hypoechoic areas on ultrasound; elevated resistive index, possibly absent or reversed diastolic flow on Doppler
	Chronic rejection	Hyperechogenic kidney, cortical thinning, reduced intrarenal perfusion, mild hydronephrosis on ultrasound; resistive index measurements are unreliable
	Infection and abscesses	Imaging findings similar to those in native kidneys; specific characteristics depend on the type of infection or abscess

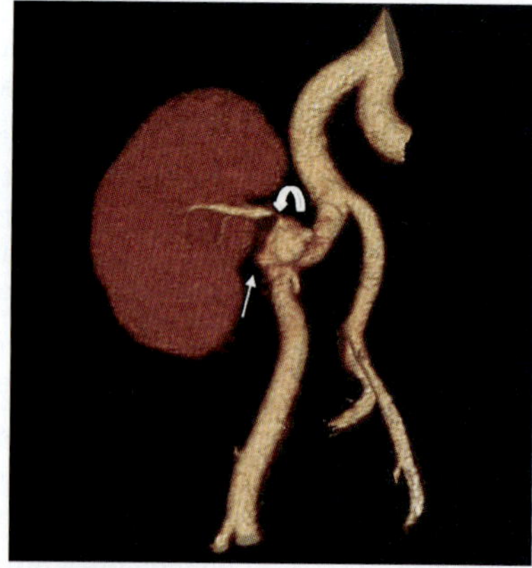

Fig. 36.3: 3D volume rendered image (VRT) image of CT angiography showing stenosis in graft renal artery (curved arrow) and contrast filled outpouching (straight arrow) at anastomosis suggest pseudoaneurysm.

Post-transplant Extrarenal Complication

- Increased chances of malignancy due to use of immunosuppressive drugs - like Kaposi's sarcoma, post-transplant lymphoproliferative disorder (associated with Epstein-Barr virus infection) and skin cancer.
- Osteonecrosis related to long steroid use
- Long-term renal transplant recipients may see disease recurrence with conditions like diabetes, amyloidosis, cystinosis, active vasculitis, and oxalosis. Graft loss may result from primary glomerulonephritis and inherited metabolic diseases.

Newer Imaging Techniques in Renal Transplantation

Contrast-enhanced Ultrasound (CEUS)

CEUS is increasingly recognized as a valuable adjunct to color Doppler in renal transplantation. The key advantages include rapidity of execution, real time acquisition and use of non-nephrotoxic contrast agent. CEUS enables the assessment of both macro- and microcirculation, facilitating the detection of parenchymal abnormalities associated with rejection, acute tubular necrosis (ATN), impaired perfusion, and focal lesions. It offers comparable diagnostic value to a (99m) Tc-DTPA scan in perfusion abnormality.

Elastography

Shear wave elastography (SWE) is the most effective noninvasive technique for assessing renal fibrosis after transplantation and assessing tissue velocity in response to a low-frequency pulse, a low velocity being indicative of tissue stiffness.

LIVER TRANSPLANTATION

There continues to be a wide disparity between the demand and supply of livers for transplantation, in spite of relatively well-developed deceased donor organ donation program. Living donor transplantation, an alternative that was first started for pediatric recipients and later expanded to adults, can alleviate this shortfall and decrease the number of deaths of patients on waiting lists.

Living donor surgery is not without risk and potential donors must be carefully assessed for their suitability. Radiology and imaging play a significant role in this process. Unlike kidney, liver is transplanted into right hypochondrium following native hepatectomy. The liver has an extraordinary ability to regenerate up to 75–95% of its original mass and fully restore its functions within a span of 8–15 days following surgery.

Radiological Evaluation of Potential Liver Donor

Assessment of Liver Parenchyma for Fatty Infiltration

- After initial screening by ultrasound abdomen, noncontrast CT should be done for hepatic fat estimation. Liver attenuation index (LAI) should be calculated; that is the difference between mean hepatic and splenic attenuation. LAI >5 HU suggest absence of significant macrovesicular steatosis. LAI values of -10 to 5 HU suggest of mild to moderate steatosis (6–30%) and should be further evaluated. LAI values of less than -10 HU suggest moderate to severe hepatic steatosis (i.e., ≥30% fat) and donor is unacceptable for donation.
- MR imaging is another sensitive modality for noninvasive assessment of fatty liver. It mainly utilize MR spectroscopy or chemical shift imaging. Sometimes biopsy may be necessary to quantify steatosis.

Depiction of Arterial, Portal Venous, Hepatic Venous and Biliary Anatomy; and Identification of Important Vascular Variants

- Triphasic CT of upper abdomen should be performed for arterial, portal and hepatic venous anatomy which is crucial for surgical planning to mitigate the risk of graft ischemia.
- MRCP is used to delineate biliary anatomy.

Accurate Measurement of Total and Segmental Liver Volume

- Accurate assessment of graft and whole liver volumes is essential for evaluating potential donor candidates. This ensures that both the graft and remnant liver possess adequate volume for liver regeneration and functional sustenance during the immediate postoperative phase.
- Volume is measured in CT images either by manual method or by automated software.
- When the graft volume is inadequate, there is a risk of "small-for-size" syndrome—where grafts are susceptible to dysfunction due to inadequate liver volume and potential injury from excessive portal perfusion.

- When graft exceeds the ideal size, it may causes vascular compression and challenges with abdominal closure. Therefore, accurate noninvasive liver volumetry is necessary for planning of liver transplant.

Radiological Evaluation of Potential Liver Recipient

- Pretransplant imaging plays a key role in identification of cirrhosis and sequel to portal hypertension, varices, for staging of hepatocellular carcinoma (HCC), for assessment of vascular patency and anatomical variant that may influence surgical planning. It's also useful for identification of contraindication to transplantation like complete thrombosis of entire portal vein and superior mesenteric vein; extrahepatic malignancy, and diffuse hepatic tumor invasion.
- Ultrasound and Doppler used as primary screening modality. However cross-sectional imaging (CT/MRI) is necessary to see for exact location of tumor and extent of vascular involvement if any.
- CT thorax and PET scan should be done if clinically indicated.

Surgical Technique

In adult live donor liver transplant, the prevailing technique involves right hemihepatectomy, where segments V-VIII are harvested, preserving the middle hepatic vein (MHV) with the donor liver.

Sound knowledge of Couinaud anatomy of liver segmentation which divides liver into eight segments is essential to understand radiology of liver transplantation.

Intraoperative Evaluation

Here, Probes are directly positioned on the graft and its vasculature for real-time assessment. It serves as a valuable tool for evaluating patency and detecting early complications before the conclusion of the operative procedure, thereby enabling prompt intervention.

Post-transplant Evaluation

Ultrasound and Doppler

Ultrasound and Doppler is the primary imaging modality for evaluating post-liver transplant (LT) patients offering bedside accessibility and swift evaluation of hepatic parenchyma, perihepatic area, biliary tree, and vasculature.

Post-transplant Doppler examinations are usually conducted for five consecutive days, commencing within the first 24 hours after surgery. The initial postoperative Doppler establishes a baseline, and any deterioration in the hepatic arterial waveform during subsequent evaluations consistently indicates an arterial complication.

CT

CT is commonly utilized as a secondary imaging method, primarily to corroborate or dismiss clinical suspicions and/or ultrasound findings.

MRI

It is preferred noninvasive modality for evaluation of biliary complications.

Post-liver Transplant Complications

Post-transplant complications can be divided into medical and surgical complications.

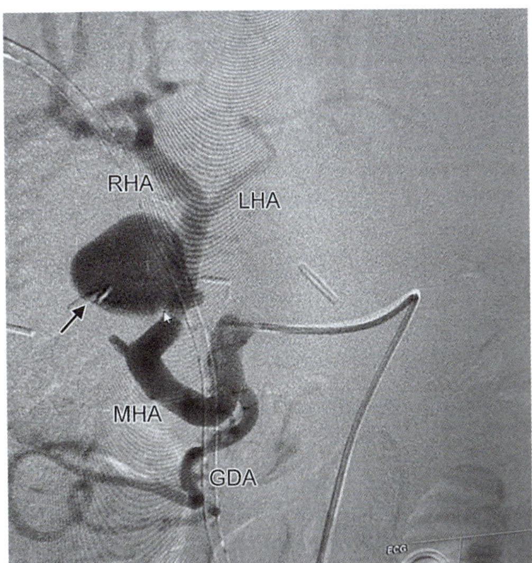

Fig. 36.4: Selective arteriography image showing contrast filled pseudoaneurysm (arrow) at anastomosis of hepatic artery (MHA – main hepatic artery, GDA- gastroduodenal artery, RHA-right hepatic artery, LHA-left hepatic artery).

Medical complication include rejection and primary graft dysfunction. Nonspecific findings, such as liver parenchymal inhomogeneity and periportal hypodensity due to edema, are seen.

Post-liver transplant surgical complications includes: Hepatic artery complications (thrombosis, stenosis, pseudoaneurysm formation **(Fig. 36.4)**. Portal venous complications (stenosis, thrombosis), hepatic venous/IVC complications and biliary complications.

Other Complications

Other complication includes hematoma, seroma, abscess, infarction, recurrence of hepatocellular carcinoma and post-transplant lymphoproliferative disorders.

Summary

Radiologists must possess a comprehensive understanding of anatomy, pathophysiology, and imaging characteristics to distinguish normal transplants from complications. Ultrasonography and Doppler examination are invaluable tools for accurately depicting and characterizing many potential transplant complications. They enable prompt and precise diagnosis, guiding appropriate treatment interventions.

LAST MINUTE REVISION

- **For kidney transplantation**, ultrasound (US), CT angiography, and 99mTc-DTPA scans are essential for evaluating renal function, vascular anatomy, and detecting contraindications.
- **For liver transplantation**, non-contrast CT for fatty liver assessment, triphasic CT for vascular anatomy, and MRCP for bile duct evaluation are critical.
- **In kidney transplantation** the kidney is usually placed in the right iliac fossa with anastomosis to external iliac vessels.
- **In liver transplantation** of adults, the right hemi-liver is commonly used, whereas in pediatric cases, the left lateral segment is preferred.

REVIEW QUESTIONS

Multiple Choice Questions (MCQs)

1. **A 14-year-old boy who underwent living donor renal transplantation presented with hematuria on 3rd postoperative day. Which is the first investigation of choice?**
   a. CT scan
   b. MRI
   c. USG and Doppler
   d. All of above
2. **The liver has how many segments?**
   a. 5
   b. 6
   c. 8
   d. 10
3. **Which of following is contraindication for kidney donation?**
   a. Polycystic kidney
   b. Horseshoe kidney
   c. Both A and B
   d. None of above
4. **A 50-year-old male who underwent live donor liver transplantation, found to have elevated liver enzymes on 2nd-month follow-up. Ultrasound and Doppler show normal appearance of hepatic artery, portal vein and outflow tract but reveals mildly dilated central IHBR; which is the next choice of investigation?**
   a. MRCP
   b. Triphasic CT scan
   c. ERCP
   d. All of above
5. **Which radionuclide study useful to determine split renal function?**
   a. 99mTc-DTPA scan
   b. Tc-99m MAG3 scan
   c. DMSA scan
   d. All of above

Answer Key

1. c 2. c 3. c 4. a 5. a

SUGGESTED READING

1. Chong WK, Beland JC, Weeks SM. Sonographic evaluation of venous obstruction in liver transplants. AJR Am J Roentgenol. 2007;188(6):W515–W21.
2. García-Criado A, Gilabert R, Nicolau C, Real I, Arguis P, Bianchi L, et al. Early detection of hepatic artery thrombosis after liver transplantation by Doppler ultrasonography: prognostic implications. J Ultrasound Med. 2001;20:51-58.
3. Järv L, Kull I, Riispere Z, et al. Ultrasound elastography correlations between anthropometrical parameters in kidney transplant recipients. J Investig Med. 2019;67:1137-41.
4. Limanond P, Raman SS, Lassman C, Sayre J, Ghobrial RM, Busuttil RW, et al. Macrovesicular hepatic steatosis in living related liver donors: correlation between CT and histologic findings. Radiology. 2004;230:276-80.
5. Sugi MD, Joshi G, Maddu KK, Dahiya N, Menias CO. Imaging of Renal Transplant Complications throughout the Life of the Allograft: Comprehensive Multimodality Review. Radiographics. 2019;39:1327-55.

CHAPTER 37

Medicolegal Aspects in Radiology

"In the medicolegal world, your image is your word—accuracy, clarity, and integrity define the radiologist's shield."

INTRODUCTION

Radiology, a pivotal branch of medical science, involves the use of imaging techniques to diagnose and treat diseases. Given the critical nature of these activities, radiology is heavily intertwined with medicolegal considerations. Though radiology is the most demanding and interesting branch, due to its high expenses in latest machine installation and management as well as medicolegal part, many of good radiologist don't get best working environment of which they really deserve. That's why understanding of these aspects is essential for radiologists to practice ethically in best setup, avoid legal pitfalls, and provide the best care for patients.

Radiologist should be well aware of medicolegal duties at various levels.

At the Level of Patient

- **Standard of care**: It should be maintained like spacious clean area, drinking water and toilet should be provided.
- **Documentation**: Emphasize thorough and accurate documentation of all investigation and communications with patients and other healthcare providers so any patient related information can't be missed before initiation of doing scan of that patent.

At Level of Doctor

- **Negligence**: We should know which terminology should be avoided in reporting format or in other documents so can not become part of negligence or failure to diagnose or misdiagnosis, and delayed diagnosis.
- **Informed consent**: Always take informed consent before procedures, detailing the risks, benefits, and alternatives.
- **Privacy laws**: Patient report and all documents should be kept confidential.
- **Defensive medicine**: Learn the concept of defensive medicine, by which additional tests or procedures may be advised primarily to protect against potential lawsuits or diagnostic errors.
- Every doctor set its own working protocol for making work easier.
- **Continuing education**: Continuing medical education program should be attended to stay in touch with evolving standards and regulations.
- Resident are well trained to above all these aspects while their residency under guidance of experienced senior radiologist so they deal properly with patients, help to maintain documents as well as by promoting various academic activities like case presentation, tutorials etc.

At Level of Machines

Licensing and accreditation: All machine should be registered by their respective board and authorities. For example, AERB provide certificate for X-ray related machines and USG machine are governed by PC-PNDT laws.

Various machines are checked yearly or renewal of certificate done at specific duration. Some rules related to various machines are described below:

Computed Tomography (CT)

- **Regulatory compliance**: Ensure CT scanners meet standards set by bodies like ACR, FDA, etc. **(Table 37.1)**.
- **Radiation safety**: Implement protocols for dose optimization and radiation protection.
- **Quality control**: Regular calibration and maintenance of equipment. Participate in accreditation programs.
- **Patient communication**: Obtain informed consent, explain procedures, and discuss potential risks.

Magnetic Resonance Imaging (MRI)

- **Regulatory compliance**: Adhere to guidelines from ACR, MHRA, and Health Canada for MRI safety and performance.

Table 37.1: Common regulatory boards related with radiology machines and its working.

Regulatory body/ act	*Jurisdiction*	*Key regulations/acts*	*Radiology modality*	*Management by radiologists*
American College of Radiology (ACR)	USA	ACR accreditation program	All modalities (CT, MRI, ultrasound, mammography, nuclear medicine)	Ensure accreditation and adherence to ACR standards for equipment, staff qualifications, and quality control. Participate in ACR's quality improvement programs
Food and Drug Administration (FDA)	USA	Mammography Quality Standards Act (MQSA), Medical device amendments	Mammography, medical devices	Comply with MQSA for mammography, including annual inspections and personnel qualifications. Ensure FDA-approved devices are used correctly
Health Insurance Portability and Accountability Act (HIPAA)	USA	HIPAA privacy rule	All modalities	Implement and maintain policies to protect patient privacy and secure medical records. Regular staff training on HIPAA compliance
Nuclear Regulatory Commission (NRC)	USA	10 CFR Part 20 - Standards for protection against radiation	Nuclear medicine, PET	Obtain necessary licenses for handling radioactive materials. Follow NRC regulations for radiation protection and safety

- **Safety protocols**: Screen patients for contraindications (e.g., metallic implants), ensure safe use of contrast agents.
- **Quality assurance**: Regularly update and calibrate MRI machines. Engage in continuous professional education.
- **Patient interaction**: Explain the procedure, manage claustrophobia, and ensure patient comfort.

Ultrasound

- **Regulatory compliance**: Follow standards set by the PC-PNDT act.
- **Equipment management**: Ensure ultrasound machines are properly maintained and calibrated.
- **Clinical guidelines**: Adhere to clinical protocols for specific examinations (e.g., obstetric, vascular).
- **Documentation**: Accurate reporting of findings and maintaining thorough patient records, especially in obstetric patients.

Mammography

- **Regulatory compliance**: Comply with MQSA and ACR guidelines for mammography.
- **Quality control**: Regular inspections, equipment maintenance, and quality assurance tests.
- **Radiation safety**: Minimize radiation exposure while maintaining image quality.
- **Patient care**: Obtain informed consent, explain the process, and provide appropriate follow-up.

Nuclear Medicine and PET

- **Regulatory compliance**: Obtain necessary licenses from NRC or equivalent bodies.
- **Radiation safety**: Implement strict protocols for handling and disposing of radioactive materials.
- **Quality assurance**: Regular equipment checks and adherence to safety standards.
- **Patient communication**: Explain the procedure, potential risks, and post-procedure precautions.

General Radiography (X-ray)

- **Regulatory compliance**: Adhere to guidelines from regulatory bodies like AERB, MCI, etc. (**Table 37.2**).
- **Radiation protection**: Use appropriate shielding and dose reduction techniques.
- **Equipment maintenance**: Regular calibration and maintenance of X-ray machines.
- **Patient interaction**: Explain the procedure, ensure safety, manage patient positioning as well as report.

Note: Duplicate report with all documents should be stored in all medicolegal cases like trauma and age determination, etc. Separate system or register is maintained in government institutions for this tedious task.

THE PRECONCEPTION AND PRENATAL DIAGNOSTIC TECHNIQUES (PCPNDT) ACT AND RULES

Introduction

The Preconception and Prenatal Diagnostic Techniques (Prohibition of Sex Selection) Act, commonly referred to as the PCPNDT Act, was enacted in 1994 to address the alarming issue of sex-selective abortions in India. The primary aim of this legislation is to prohibit the use of prenatal diagnostic techniques for determining the sex of the fetus and to prevent female feticide. This chapter provides an in-depth overview of the PCPNDT Act, its rules, its historical context, and its implications for medical practitioners and patients. Total 8 chapters are there.

Table 37.2: Regulatory boards and acts affecting radiology practices in India.

Regulatory body/ act	*Jurisdiction*	*Key regulations/ acts*	*Radiology modality*	*Management by radiologists*
Medical Council of India (MCI)	India	Indian Medical Council (Professional conduct, Etiquette, and Ethics) Regulations, 2002	All modalities	Adhere to MCI guidelines for ethical practice, maintaining professional competence, and patient communication. Engage in continuous medical education (CME)
Atomic Energy Regulatory Board (AERB)	India	Atomic Energy (Radiation Protection) Rules, 2004	Modalities using ionizing radiation (X-ray, CT, Nuclear Medicine)	Obtain necessary licenses for equipment. Implement radiation protection protocols and regular safety checks. Ensure staff training in radiation safety
Bureau of Indian Standards (BIS)	India	BIS Standards for Medical Devices	All modalities	Ensure medical devices comply with BIS standards. Conduct regular maintenance and quality assurance checks
Health Ministry	India	Clinical Establishments (Registration and Regulation) Act, 2010	All modalities	Register radiology facilities and comply with standards for infrastructure, equipment, and staffing. Ensure quality and safety protocols are in place
Drugs and Cosmetics Act	India	Regulation of diagnostic imaging contrast agents	Modalities using contrast agents (CT, MRI)	Ensure use of approved contrast agents. Monitor for adverse reactions and report as required
National Accreditation Board for Hospitals and Healthcare Providers (NABL)	India	NABL Standards for diagnostic center	All modalities	Adhere to NABL standards for patient safety, equipment maintenance, and quality control. Participate in accreditation processes
Indian Radiological and Imaging Association (IRIA)	India	IRIA Guidelines	All modalities	Follow IRIA guidelines for best practices in radiology, ethical conduct, and continuous professional development
Preconception and Prenatal Diagnostic Techniques (PCPNDT) Act	India	Regulation of the use of prenatal diagnostic techniques	Ultrasound	Ensure compliance with PCPNDT Act, including proper documentation, record-keeping, and reporting. Prevent misuse of diagnostic techniques for sex determination
National Health Mission (NHM)	India	Various health initiatives and standards like 6 months USG training and doing USG in less amount in private set up under Pradhan Mantri Yojana	All modalities	Participate in NHM initiatives for improving healthcare access and quality. Implement relevant health programs and protocols

Historical Background

The PCPNDT Act has evolved significantly since its inception, with several amendments aimed at strengthening its provisions and enforcement mechanisms.

Key Milestones

- **1978**: The act was first implemented in Maharashtra as a state initiative to combat sex-selective abortions.
- **September 20, 1994**: The Prenatal Diagnostic Techniques (Regulation and Prevention of Misuse) Act was enacted.
- **January 1, 1996**: The act came into force nationwide.
- **2003**: The act was amended to the Preconception and Prenatal Diagnostic Techniques (Prohibition of Sex Selection) Act, 2002, which expanded its scope to include preconception techniques.
- **2014**: The PCPNDT (6 months training rules) were introduced.

Key Provisions of the PCPNDT Act

The PCPNDT Act includes several crucial provisions designed to regulate the use of diagnostic techniques and prevent their misuse:

1. **Prohibition of sex selection**: The act strictly prohibits sex selection, both before and after conception.
2. **Regulation of diagnostic techniques**: It regulates the use of prenatal diagnostic techniques like ultrasound, amniocentesis, and chorionic villus sampling.
3. **Registration of clinics**: All genetic counseling centers, genetic laboratories, and genetic clinics must be registered under the act.
4. **Maintenance of records**: Clinics and laboratories are required to maintain detailed records of all diagnostic procedures conducted.
5. **Regulation of advertisements**: The act prohibits any form of advertisement related to pre-conception and prenatal sex determination.
6. **Penalties**: It prescribes severe penalties for violations, including imprisonment and fines.

Detailed Provisions (Table 37.3)

Prohibition of Sex Selection

The cornerstone of the PCPNDT Act is the prohibition of sex selection. This includes any procedures or techniques used before or after conception that are intended to determine the sex of the fetus. The act emphasizes that the use of diagnostic techniques should be strictly for medical purposes, such as detecting genetic abnormalities or assessing the health of the fetus, and not for revealing its sex.

Table 37.3: Key provisions of the PCPNDT Act.

Provision	*Description*
Prohibition of sex selection	Strict prohibition of sex selection before and after conception
Regulation of diagnostic techniques	Regulation of ultrasound, amniocentesis, and other prenatal diagnostic techniques
Registration of clinics	Mandatory registration of genetic counseling centers, laboratories, and clinics
Maintenance of records	Requirement to maintain detailed records of all diagnostic procedures
Regulation of advertisements	Prohibition of advertisements related to sex determination and selection
Penalties	Imprisonment and fines for violations

Table 37.4: Steps for registration of clinics.

Step	Description
1.	Submission of application form along with necessary documents
2.	Inspection of premises by the appropriate authority
3.	Verification of qualifications of medical practitioners
4.	Issuance of registration certificate upon meeting all criteria
5.	Regular audits and inspections to ensure ongoing compliance

Regulation of Diagnostic Techniques

The act specifies that only registered medical practitioners with appropriate qualifications and certifications can conduct prenatal diagnostic procedures. These procedures must be carried out in registered institutes, ensuring that only authorized personnel handle sensitive diagnostic equipment. The act outlines the circumstances under which these procedures can be performed, emphasizing that they should only be done for valid medical reasons.

Registration of Clinics (Table 37.4)

To ensure accountability and transparency, the PCPNDT Act mandates the registration of all genetic counseling centers, genetic laboratories, and clinics that offer prenatal diagnostic services. The registration process involves a thorough inspection of the facilities, verification of the qualifications of the medical staff, and adherence to the standards set by the act. Registered clinics are required to display their registration certificates prominently, at working place along with its photo and their registered NMC certificate.

Note: Registration initiates with application in Form A, with fees within 60 days (fresh registration) while 30 days in case of renewal prior to date of expiry. It has to be renewed every 5 years.

Maintenance of Records

One of the critical requirements of the PCPNDT Act is the maintenance of detailed records of all prenatal diagnostic procedures. This includes information about the patient, the referring doctor, the reasons for the procedure, and the results. The records must be meticulously kept and made available for inspection by authorized personnel (at least for 2 years). The purpose of maintaining these records is to ensure that the procedures are not misused for sex determination.

Regulation of Advertisements

The act prohibits any form of advertisement that promotes preconception or prenatal sex determination. This includes advertisements in newspapers, magazines, online platforms, and other media. The prohibition aims to eliminate the commercial exploitation of sex determination technologies and to discourage the societal preference for male children.

Penalties (Table 37.5)

The PCPNDT Act prescribes stringent penalties for violations. These include imprisonment, fines, and the suspension or cancellation of the medical practitioner's license. The severity of

Table 37.5: Penalties under the PCPNDT Act.

Offense	Penalty
Conducting sex selection	Imprisonment up to 3 years and fine up to ₹ 50,000
Advertising sex selection	Imprisonment up to 3 years and fine up to ₹ 50,000
Non-registration of clinics	Imprisonment up to 5 years and fine up to ₹ 1,00,000
Failure to maintain records	Imprisonment up to 3 years and fine up to ₹ 10,000
Repeat offenses	Imprisonment up to 5 years and increased fines

the penalties reflects the seriousness with which the government views the misuse of diagnostic techniques for sex selection. Repeat offenders face even harsher consequences to deter habitual violations.

Implementation and Enforcement

The implementation of the PCPNDT Act is overseen by both central and state authorities. The central supervisory board and state supervisory boards are responsible for monitoring and ensuring compliance with the act. They conduct regular inspections and audits of registered clinics and laboratories.

Central and State Supervisory Boards

The central supervisory board is responsible for advising the government on policy matters related to the implementation of the PCPNDT Act. It also monitors the functioning of state supervisory boards, ensuring that they comply with the act's provisions. The state supervisory boards oversee the implementation of the act within their respective states, conducting inspections, reviewing records, and taking action against violators.

Inspections and Audits

Regular inspections and audits are a crucial part of the enforcement mechanism. Authorized officers visit registered clinics and laboratories to verify that they comply with the act's provisions. This includes checking the records, inspecting the facilities, and ensuring that the procedures are conducted by qualified personnel. Any discrepancies or violations found during these inspections can result in penalties, including the suspension or cancellation of the facility's registration.

Legal and Administrative Actions

The PCPNDT Act empowers the authorities to take legal and administrative actions against violators. This includes filing criminal cases, imposing fines, and suspending or canceling the licenses of medical practitioners and clinics. The act also provides for the establishment of advisory committees at the district level to assist in the implementation and enforcement of the act.

Essential Record Keeping

Form F is a critical component of the PCPNDT Act, used to maintain records of all prenatal diagnostic procedures. Proper filling and maintenance of Form F (it should be filled in two hard copies which has to be updated on same day in pyaribitiya.com by opening login id of registered center) are mandatory to ensure transparency and accountability. The form includes detailed information about the patient, and her children details, the referring doctor, the procedure performed with it's indication, and the results. Below is an example of Form F:

FORM F (TO BE FILLED IN TWO COPIES ONE GIVEN TO PATIENT AND OTHER KEPT AT CENTRES AS RECORD)

[Refer Proviso to Section 4(3) Rules 9(4) and 10(1A)]

FORM FOR MAINTENANCE OF RECORDS IN CASE OF PRENATAL DIAGNOSTIC TEST/PROCEDURE BY GENETIC CLINIC/ULTRASOUND CLINIC/IMAGING CENTRE

Section A: To be Filled in for All Diagnostic Procedure Tests

1. Name and complete address of the genetic clinic/ultrasound clinic/imaging centre:

   ____

2. Registration no. (Under PC & PNDT Act, 1994)

   ____

3. Patient's name

4. Total number of living children

   ____

   A. Number of living sons with age of each living son (in years or months)

   ____

   B. Number of living daughter with age of each living daughter (in year months)

5. Husband's/wife/father's/mother' name

   ____

6. Full postal address of the patient with contact number, if any

   ____

7a. Referred by (Full name and addresses of doctor (s)/genetic counseling centre

   ____

   (Referral slips to be preserved carefully with form F)

b. Self-referral by Gynecologist/Radiologist/Registered Medical Practitioner conducting the diagnostic procedure:

   ____

   (Referral note with indications and case papers of the patient to be preserved with form F) **(Self-referral does not mean a client coming to a clinic and requesting for the test or the relative/s requesting for the test of a pregnant woman)**

8. Last menstrual period or weeks of pregnancy:

   ____

Section B: To be Filled In for Performing Noninvasive Diagnostic Procedures/Tests Only

9. Name of the doctor performing the procedure/s:

   ____

10. Indication/s for diagnosis procedures ______________________________ (specify with reference to the request made in the referral slip or in a self-referral note)
    Ultrasonography prenatal diagnosis during pregnancy should only be performed when indicated. The following is the representative list of indications for ultrasound during pregnancy. (Put "Tick" against the appropriate indication/s for ultrasound).
    i. To diagnose intrauterine and/or ectopic pregnancy and confirm viability
    ii. Estimation of gestational age (dating)
    iii. Detection of number of fetuses and their chorionicity
    iv. Suspected pregnancy with IUCD in-situ or suspected pregnancy following contraceptive failure/MTP failure.
    v. Vaginal bleeding/leaking.
    vi. Follow-up of cases of abortion
    vii. Assessment of cervical canal and diameter of internal os.
    viii. Discrepancy between uterine size and period of amenorrhea
    ix. Any suspected adnexal or uterine pathology/abnormality
    x. Detection of chromosomal abnormalities, fetal structural defects and other abnormalities and their follow-up
    xi. To evaluated fetal presentation and position
    xii. Assessment of liquor amnii
    xiii. Preterm labor/preterm premature rupture of membranes
    xiv. Evaluation of placental position, thickness, grading and abnormalities (placenta previa, retro placental hemorrhage, abnormal adherence, etc.)
    xv. Evaluation of umbilical cord-presentation, insertion, nuchal encirclement, number of vessels and presence of true knot
    xvi. Evaluation of previous caesarean Section scars
    xvii. Evaluation of fetal growth parameters, fetal weight and fetal well-being
    xviii. Color flow mapping and duplex Doppler studies
    xix. Ultrasound guided procedures such as medical termination of pregnancy, external cephalic version, etc. and their follow-up
    xx. Adjunct diagnostic and therapeutic invasive interventions such as chorionic villus sampling (CVS), amniocentesis, fetal blood sampling, fetal skin biopsy, amnioinfusion, intrauterine infusion, placement of shunts, etc.
    xxi. Observation of intra-partum events
    xxii. Medical/surgical condition complicating pregnancy
    xxiii. Research/scientists studies in recognized institutions
11. Procedure carried out (noninvasive) put a "Tick" on the appropriate procedures)
    i. Ultrasound
    (Important note: Ultrasound is not indicated/advised/performed to determine the sex of fetus except for diagnosis of sex-linked diseases such as Duchene Muscular Dystrophy, Hemophilia A&B etc.)
    ii. Any other (specify)
12. Date on which declaration of pregnant women/person was obtained:
    ____
13. Date on which procedure carried out:
    ____

14. Result of the noninvasive procedure carried out (report in brief of the test)

    ____

15. The result of prenatal diagnostic procedures was conveyed to ____________. On ____________

16. Any indication for MTP as per the abnormality detected in the diagnostic procedures/test

    ____

Date: __________

Place: ____________________

Name, signature and registration numbers with seal of the
Gynecologist/Radiologist/Registered Medical Practitioner
performing diagnostic procedure/s

Section C: To be Filled for Performing Invasive Procedure/Test Only

17. Name of the doctor/s performing the procedure/s:

    ____

18. History of genetic/medical disease in the family (specify)

    ____

    a. Clinical
    b. Biochemical
    c. Cytogenetic
    d. Other (e.g., radiological, ultrasonography etc. Specify)

19. Indication for the diagnosis procedure ("Tick" on appropriate indication)
    A. Previous child/children with:
    i. Chromosomal disorders
    ii. Metabolic disorders
    iii. Congenital anomaly
    iv. Mental disability
    v. Hemoglobinopathy
    vi. Sex-linked disorders

vii. Single gene disorder

viii. Any other (specify)

B. Advanced maternal age (35)

C. Mother/Father/sibling has genetic (specify)

D. Other (specify)

20. Date on which consent of pregnant woman/person was obtained if Form G prescribed in PC & PNDT Act, 1994:

____

21. Invasive procedure carried out ("Tick" on appropriate indication/s)
    i. Chromosomal studies
    ii. Biochemical studies
    iii. Molecular studies
    iv. Preimplantation gender diagnosis
    v. Any other (specify)
22. Any complication/s of invasive procedure (specify)

____

23. Additional test recommended (please mention if applicable)
    i. Chromosomal studies
    ii. Biochemical studies
    iii. Molecular studies
    iv. Preimplantation gender diagnosis
    v. Any other (specify)
24. Result of the procedures/test carried out (report in brief of the invasive)
25. Date on which procedure carried out:

____

26. The result of prenatal diagnosis procedure was conveyed to ______________________
27. Any indication for MTP as per the abnormality detected in the diagnostic procedures tests

____

Date: ________________

Place: ______________________________

Name, Signature and registration number with seal of the Gynecologist/ Radiologist/ Registered Medical Practitioner performing diagnostic procedure/s

Section D: Declaration

Declaration of the person undergoing prenatal diagnostic test/procedure
I, Mrs/Mr ____ declare that by undergoing ________________________ prenatal diagnostic test/procedure, I do not want to know the sex of my fetus.

Date: ____________

Signature/Thumb impression of the person undergoing the prenatal diagnostic test/procedure

In case of thumb impression

Identified by (Name): _______________ Age: _______ Sex: ___________

Relation (if any): ____________________ Address and contact no: ________________

____

Signature of person attesting thumb impression _________________ Date: _________

Declaration of Doctor/Person Conducting Prenatal Diagnostic Procedure/Test

I, ____ (name of the person conducting ultrasonography/image scanning) declare that while conducting ultrasonography/image scanning on M/s/ Mr ______________________________ (name of the pregnant woman or the person undergoing prenatal diagnostic procedure/test), I have neither detected nor disclosed the sex of her fetus to anybody in any manner.

Signature: ________________

Date: _______________

Name in capitals, Registration number with seal of the Gynecologist/Radiologist/Registered Medical Practitioner conducting diagnostic procedure

Case Studies and Real-World Applications

The PCPNDT Act has had significant implications for medical practitioners, patients, and society as a whole. Several case studies highlight the impact of the act and the challenges faced in its implementation.

Case Study 1: Successful Prosecution of Violators

In a landmark case, a clinic in a major city was found to be conducting sex determination tests in violation of the PCPNDT Act. Following an investigation by the state supervisory board, the clinic's records revealed numerous instances of unauthorized sex determination procedures. The clinic's license was suspended, and the medical practitioners involved were prosecuted and sentenced to imprisonment. This case served as a deterrent to other clinics and reinforced the importance of adhering to the act's provisions.

Case Study 2: Challenges in Rural Areas

Implementing the PCPNDT Act in rural areas poses unique challenges. Limited access to medical facilities, lack of awareness about the act, and sociocultural factors contribute to the persistence of sex-selective practices. In one rural district, a series of awareness campaigns and training programs for medical practitioners were conducted to address these challenges. The district saw a gradual improvement in compliance with the act and a reduction in sex-selective practices.

Ethical and Legal Implications

The PCPNDT Act has significant ethical and legal implications for healthcare providers. It emphasizes the importance of ethical practices and the responsibility of medical professionals to adhere to the law. Violations not only lead to legal consequences but also damage the trust between healthcare providers and patients.

Ethical Considerations

The PCPNDT Act raises important ethical questions about the use of medical technology and the responsibilities of healthcare providers. Medical practitioners are entrusted with sensitive diagnostic tools that can be misused for unethical purposes. The act underscores the need for medical professionals to prioritize the well-being of their patients and to use their skills and knowledge responsibly. It also highlights the ethical obligation to promote gender equality and to prevent practices that devalue the lives of female children.

Legal Responsibilities

The legal responsibilities under the PCPNDT Act are stringent. Medical practitioners must ensure that they comply with all provisions of the act, including maintaining accurate records, conducting procedures only for valid medical reasons, and avoiding any involvement in sex determination. Failure to comply with the act can result in severe legal consequences, including imprisonment, fines, and the suspension or cancellation of medical licenses. These legal responsibilities serve as a powerful deterrent to unethical practices and help to uphold the integrity of the medical profession.

Challenges and Future Directions

Despite the significant progress made through the PCPNDT Act, several challenges remain. Addressing these challenges requires a multifaceted approach involving legal reforms, increased awareness, and stronger enforcement mechanisms.

Ongoing Challenges

- **Awareness and education**: Many people, especially in rural areas, remain unaware of the PCPNDT Act and its provisions. Continuous efforts are needed to educate both the public and healthcare providers about the importance of the act.
- **Sociocultural factors**: Deep-rooted sociocultural preferences for male children continue to drive the demand for sex determination and sex-selective abortions. Changing these attitudes requires long-term social and cultural interventions.
- **Enforcement**: Ensuring strict enforcement of the PCPNDT Act is a constant challenge. Limited resources, bureaucratic hurdles, and corruption can undermine enforcement efforts. Strengthening the infrastructure and capacity of regulatory bodies is crucial.

Future Directions

- **Technological innovations**: Leveraging technology can enhance the implementation and enforcement of the PCPNDT Act. For example, digital record-keeping systems can improve transparency and accountability.
- **Policy reforms**: Periodic reviews and updates to the PCPNDT Act can address emerging challenges and incorporate best practices. Involving stakeholders in the policy-making process can ensure that the act remains relevant and effective.
- **Community engagement**: Engaging communities in the fight against sex-selective practices is essential. Grassroots initiatives, led by local leaders and community organizations, can drive cultural change and promote gender equality.

Conclusion

The PCPNDT Act is a vital legislative measure aimed at curbing the practice of sex-selective abortions and promoting gender equality. For medical practitioners, understanding and complying with this act is essential to ensure ethical practice and avoid severe legal repercussions. By following the provisions and maintaining proper records, healthcare providers contribute to the larger goal of balancing the sex ratio and upholding the dignity of human life. As we move forward, continuous efforts are needed to address the challenges and to ensure that the act's objectives are fully realized, creating a more equitable and healthy society for all.

LAST MINUTE REVISION

- Radiology facilities must maintain a **clean and safe environment**, provide essential amenities (e.g., drinking water, toilets), and ensure proper documentation of all investigations to avoid missing critical patient information.
- Radiologists must be cautious in their **reporting terminology** to avoid misinterpretation, misdiagnosis, or failure to diagnose. **Informed consent** must be obtained before procedures, detailing risks, benefits, and alternatives.
- Radiologists must **safeguard patient records and reports**, ensuring confidentiality under laws like HIPAA (internationally) and the **PCPNDT Act (India)**, which regulates ultrasound use to prevent illegal sex determination.
- Radiology machines (e.g., X-ray, CT, MRI) must be **registered and maintained** per regulatory standards like **AERB (India) and FDA (USA)**, ensuring adherence to radiation safety protocols, licensing, and periodic audits.
- Radiologists should understand **defensive medicine**, where additional tests may be performed to **avoid litigation risks**. They must also participate in **continuing medical education (CME)** to stay updated on evolving medicolegal regulations.

REVIEW QUESTIONS

Multiple Choice Questions (MCQs)

1. **Which of the following is NOT a primary responsibility of a radiologist in maintaining patient care standards?**
   a. Ensuring informed consent is obtained before procedures
   b. Maintaining accurate and thorough documentation
   c. Disclosing patient information without consent
   d. Participating in continuing medical education programs
2. **What is the purpose of defensive medicine in radiology?**
   a. To avoid unnecessary tests and procedures
   b. To protect against potential lawsuits or diagnostic errors
   c. To increase patient wait times for scans
   d. To reduce the cost of medical care
3. **The PCPNDT Act was enacted in which year to address the issue of sex-selective abortions in India?**
   a. 1984 b. 1994
   c. 2004 d. 2014
4. **Which of the following is a key provision of the PCPNDT Act?**
   a. Permitting sex selection under specific conditions
   b. Prohibition of sex selection before and after conception
   c. Encouraging sex determination for cultural reasons
   d. Allowing unregistered clinics to perform prenatal diagnostic procedures
5. **Which regulatory body in India is responsible for ensuring radiation protection in radiology practices?**
   a. Medical Council of India (MCI)
   b. Bureau of Indian Standards (BIS)
   c. Atomic Energy Regulatory Board (AERB)
   d. Health Ministry

Answer Key

1. c 2. b 3. b 4. b 5. c

SUGGESTED READING

1. Bhaktwani A. The PC-PNDT Act in a nutshell. Indian J Radiol Imaging. 2012;22(2):133-4. doi: 10.4103/0971-3026.101114. PMID: 23162258; PMCID: PMC3498638.
2. Mohapatra D. Role of independent research at AERB for ensuring safety of nuclear facilities in India. Radiat Prot Dosimetry. 2024;200(11-12):973-78. doi: 10.1093/rpd/ncad280. PMID: 39016507.

Annexure

INDICATIONS FOR AND INTERPRET THE REPORT OF USG KUB

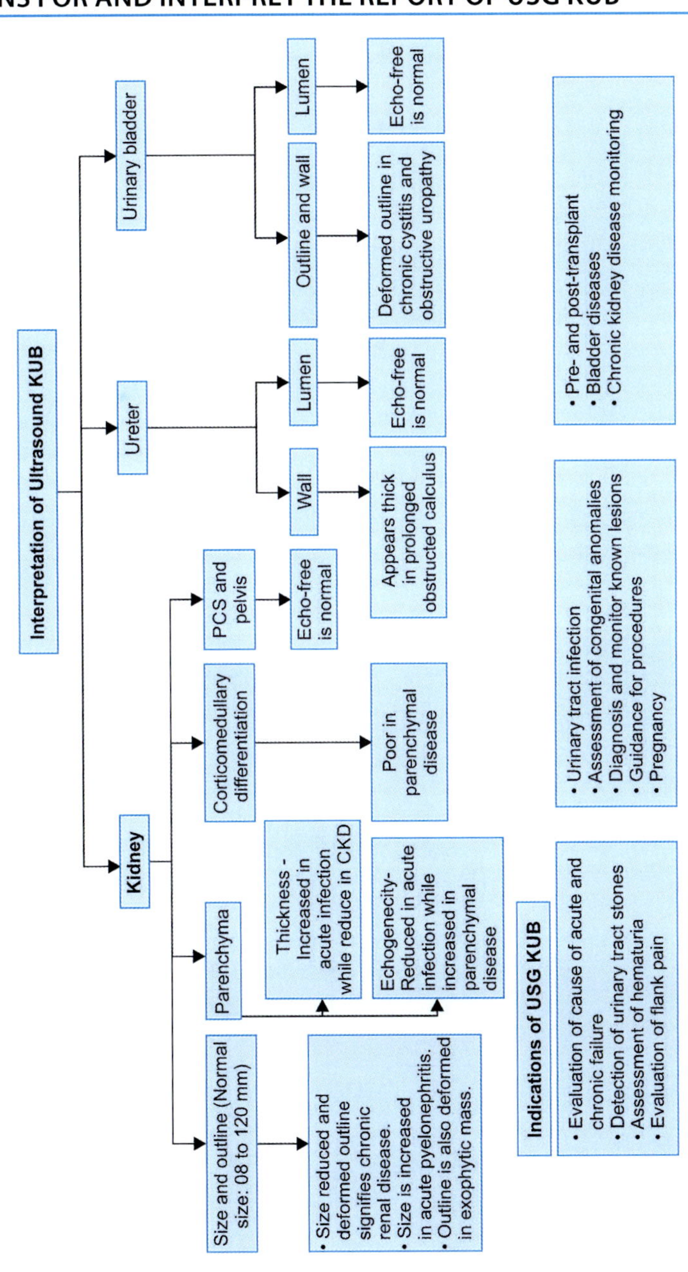

CHEST X-RAY IN FOREIGN BODY ASPIRATION AND ITS INTERPRETATION

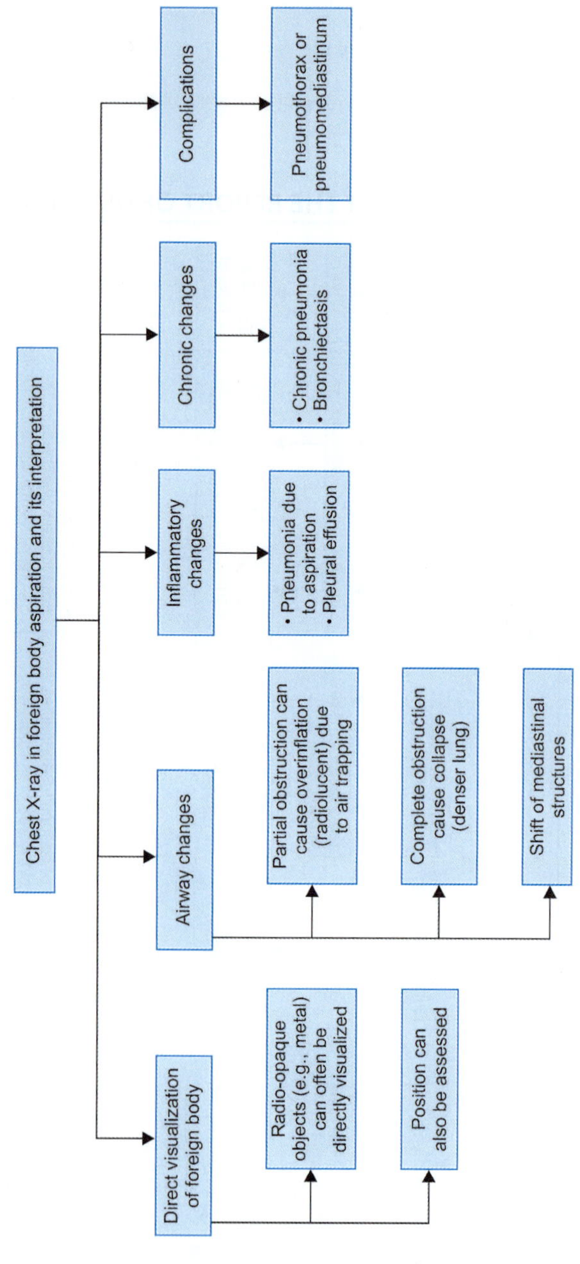

INTERPRETATION OF CHEST X-RAY IN LOWER RESPIRATORY TRACT INFECTION

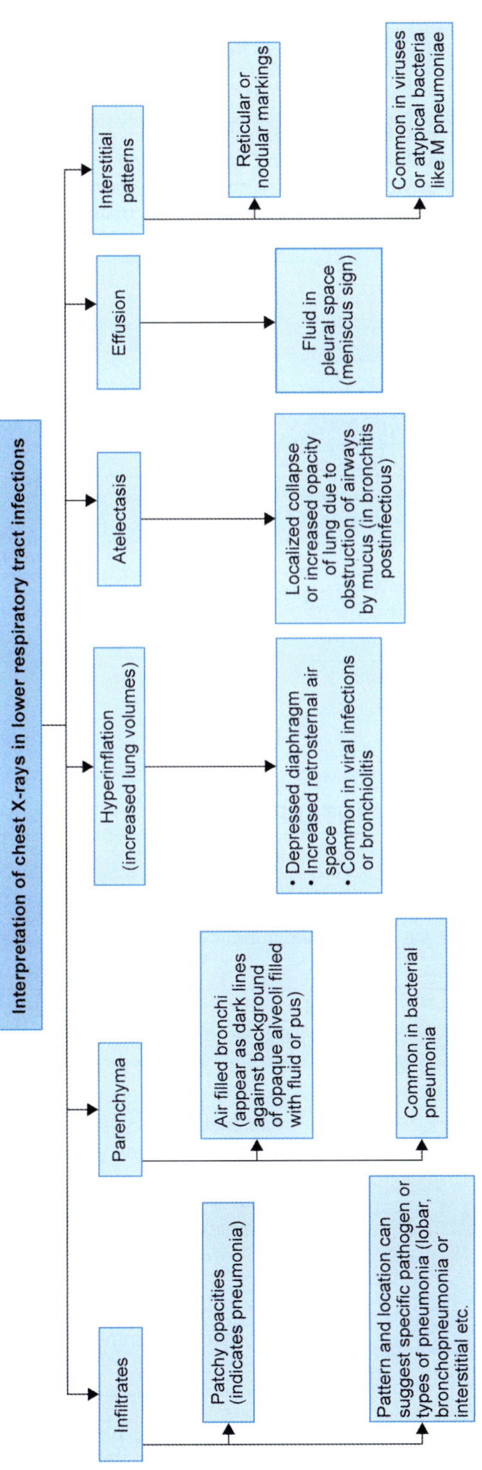

THYMIC SHADOW IN PEDIATRIC CHEST X-RAY

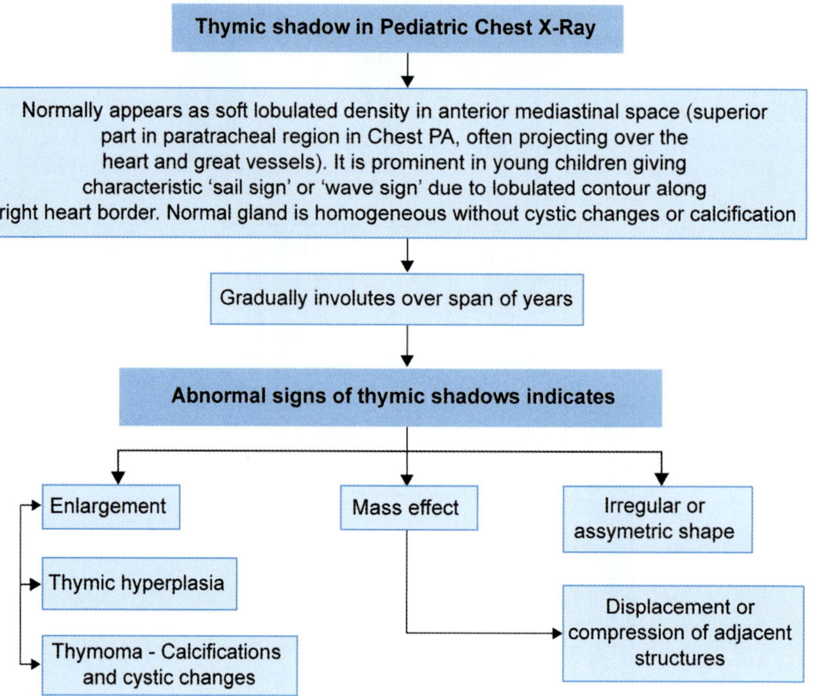

ELECTROENCEPHALOGRAM INTERPRETATION

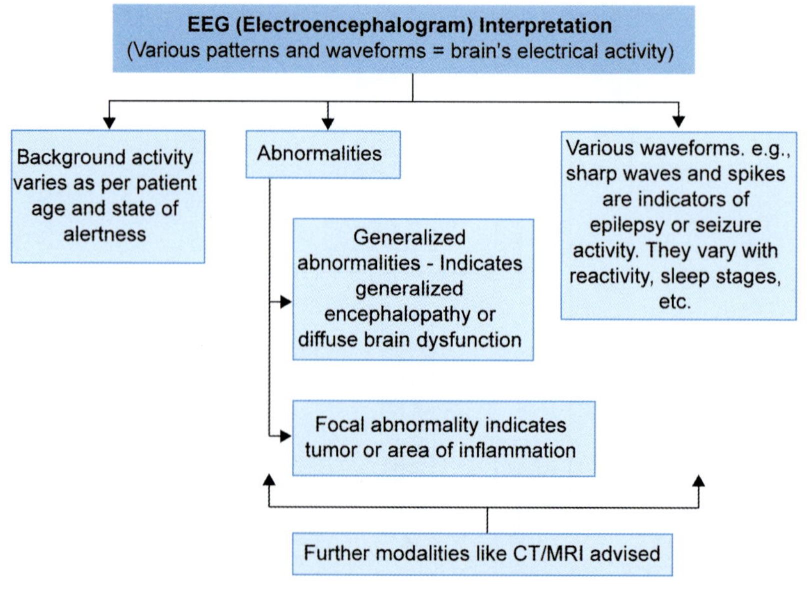

INTERPRETATION OF X-RAY KUB

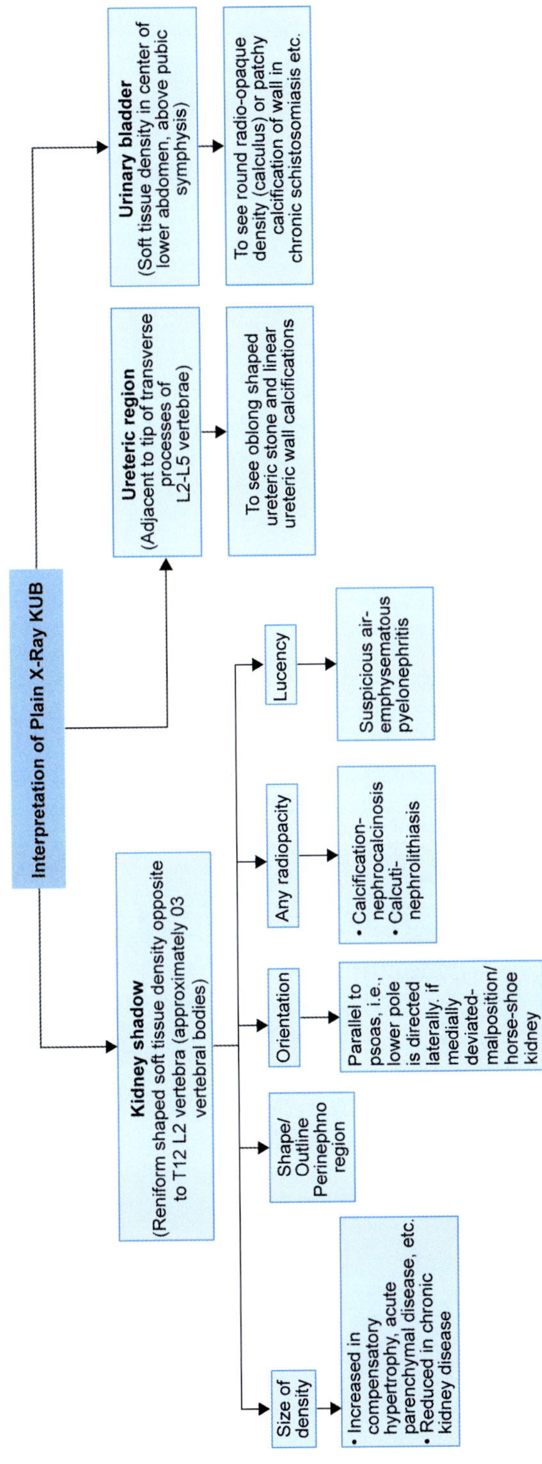

ORDER AND INTERPRET DIAGNOSTIC TESTS BASED ON VARIOUS CLINICAL PRESENTATION

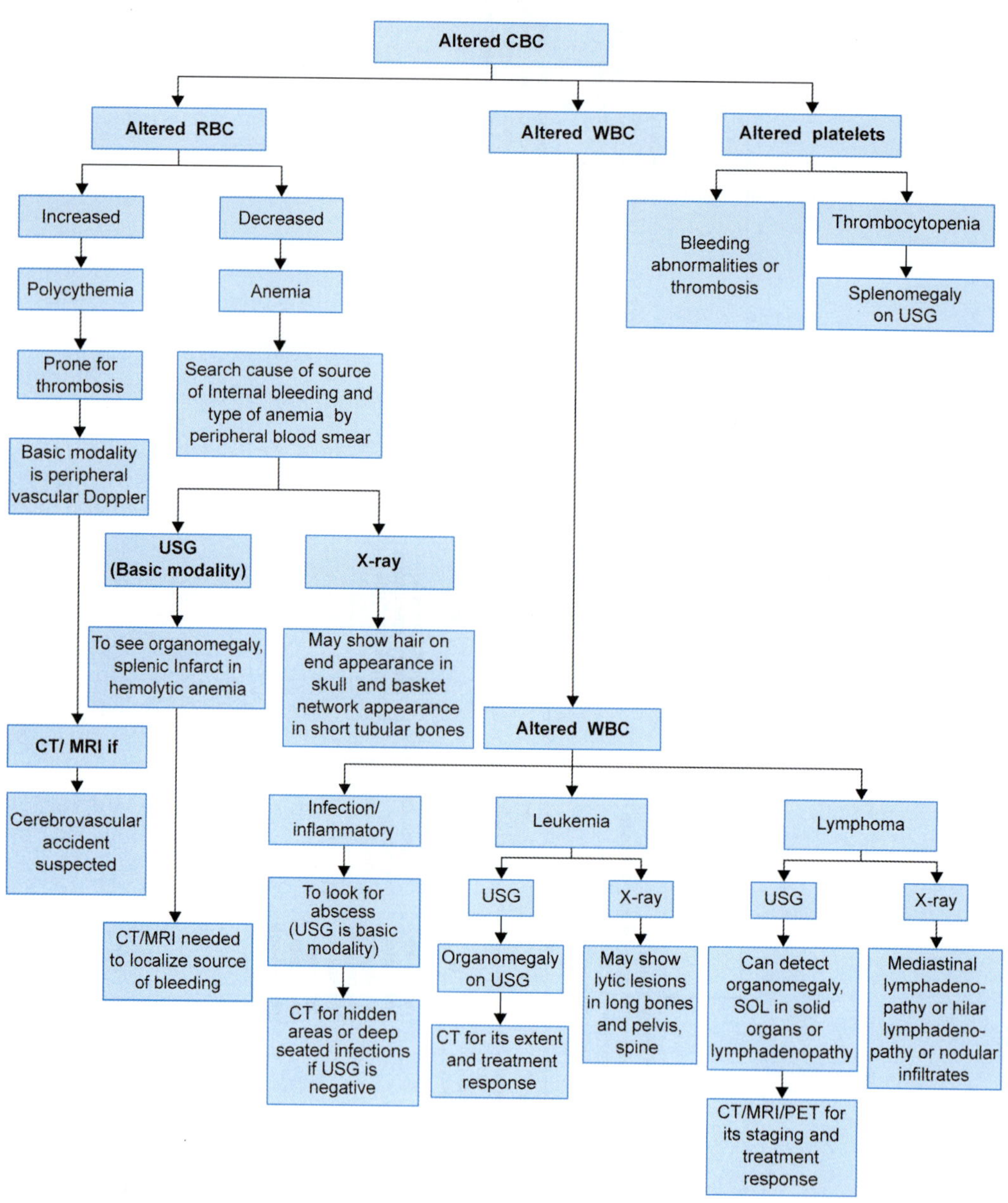

ORDER AND INTERPRET DIAGNOSTIC TESTS BASED ON VARIOUS CLINICAL PRESENTATION

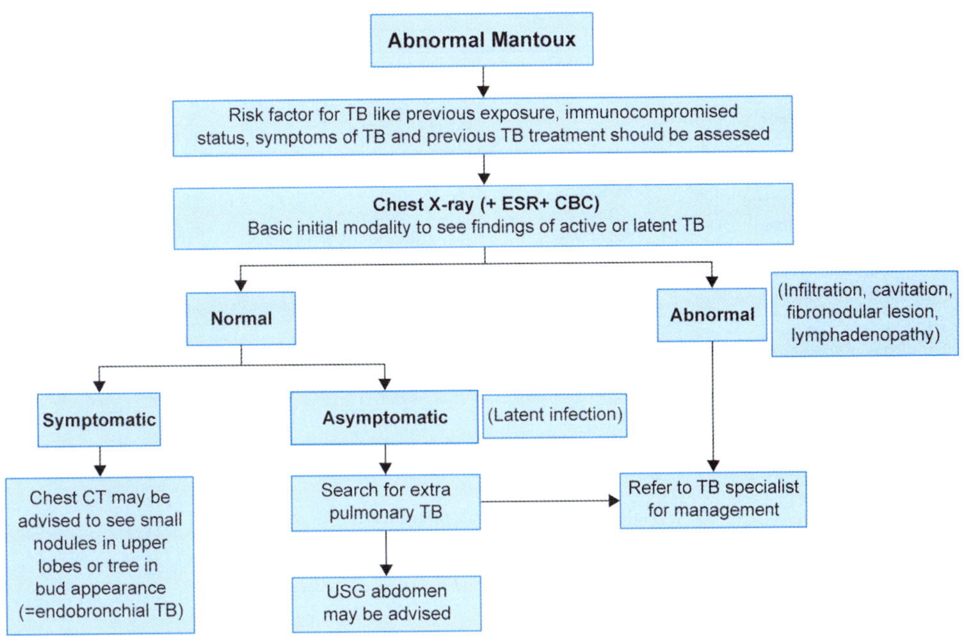

ORDER AND INTERPRET DIAGNOSTIC TESTS BASED ON VARIOUS CLINICAL PRESENTATION

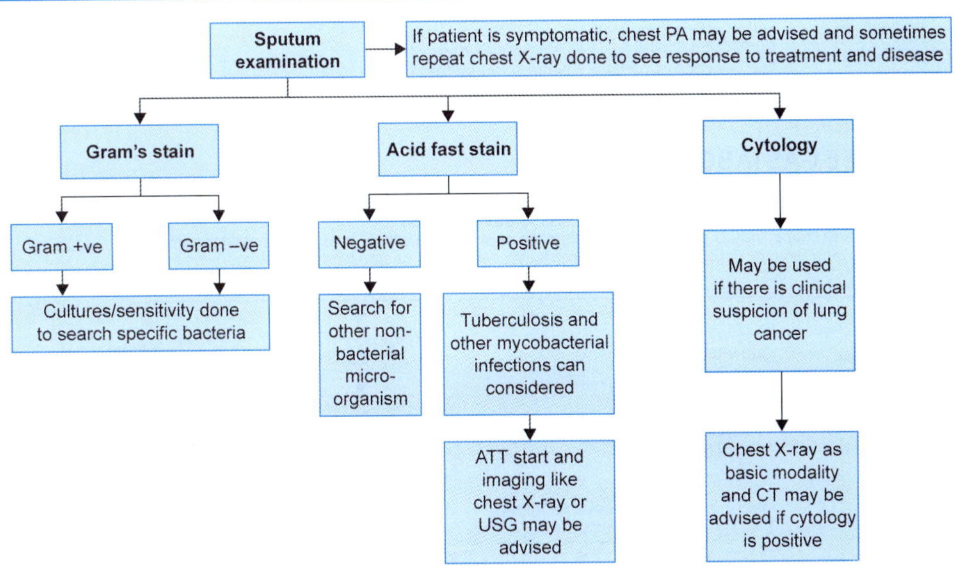

ORDER AND INTERPRET DIAGNOSTIC TESTS BASED ON VARIOUS CLINICAL PRESENTATION

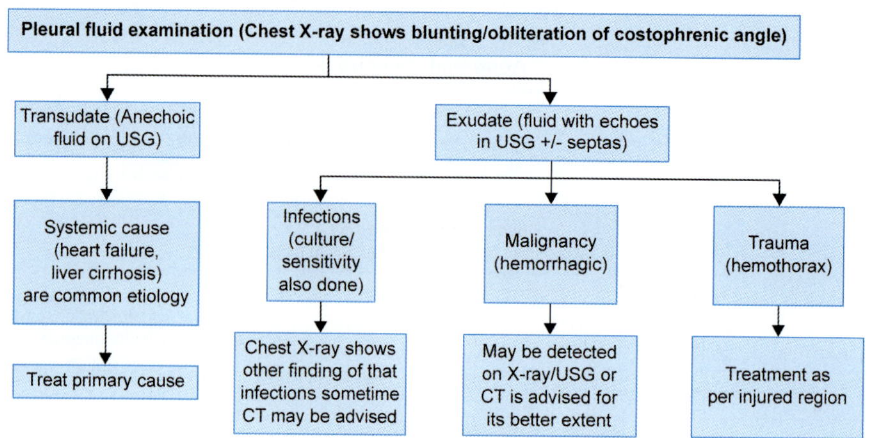

HIV

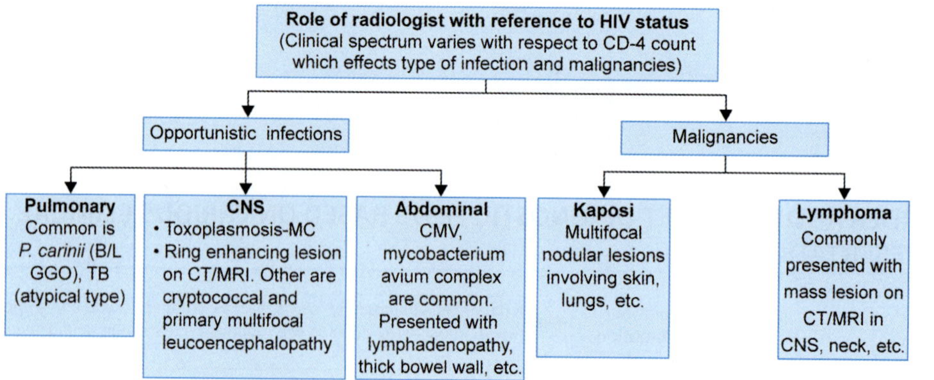

ACID-BASE GAS (ABG) ANALYSIS

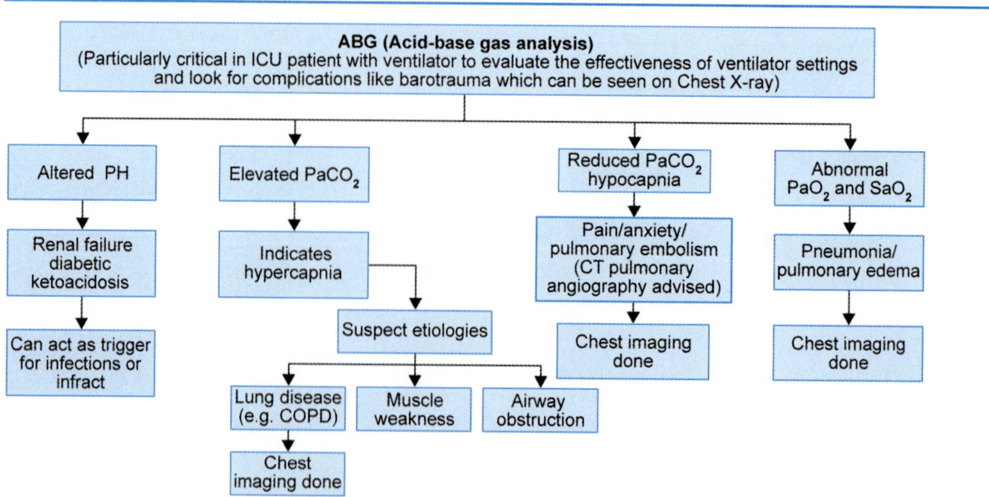

VIRAL CULTURE

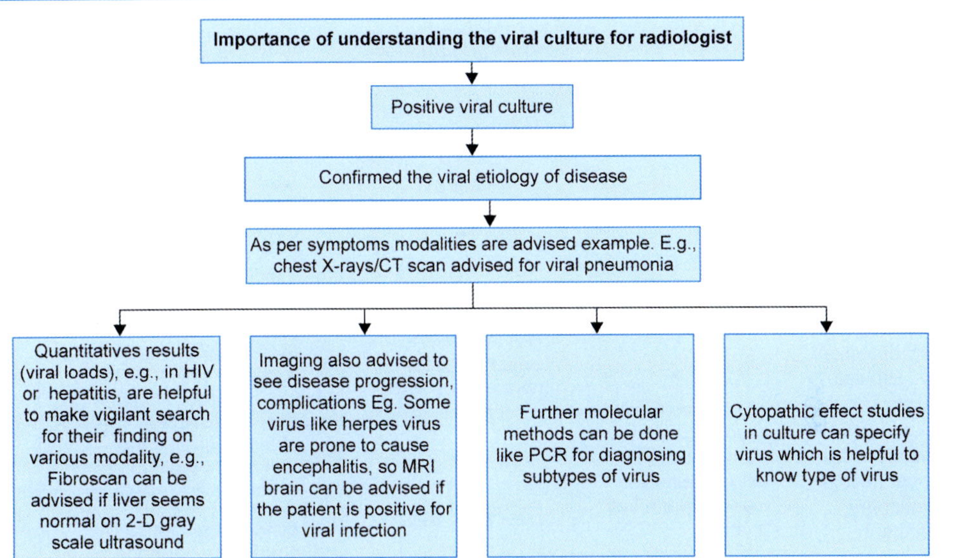

SKIN AND TISSUE BIOPSIES

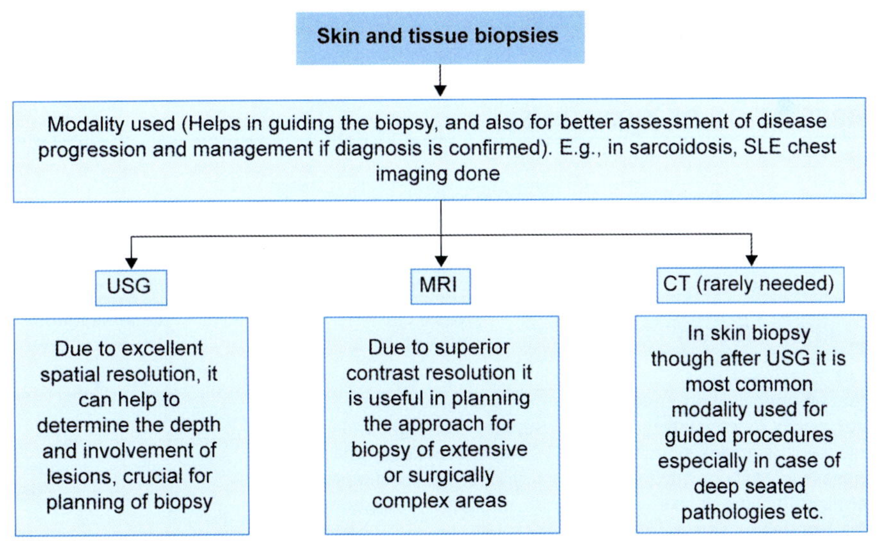

TUMOR MARKERS

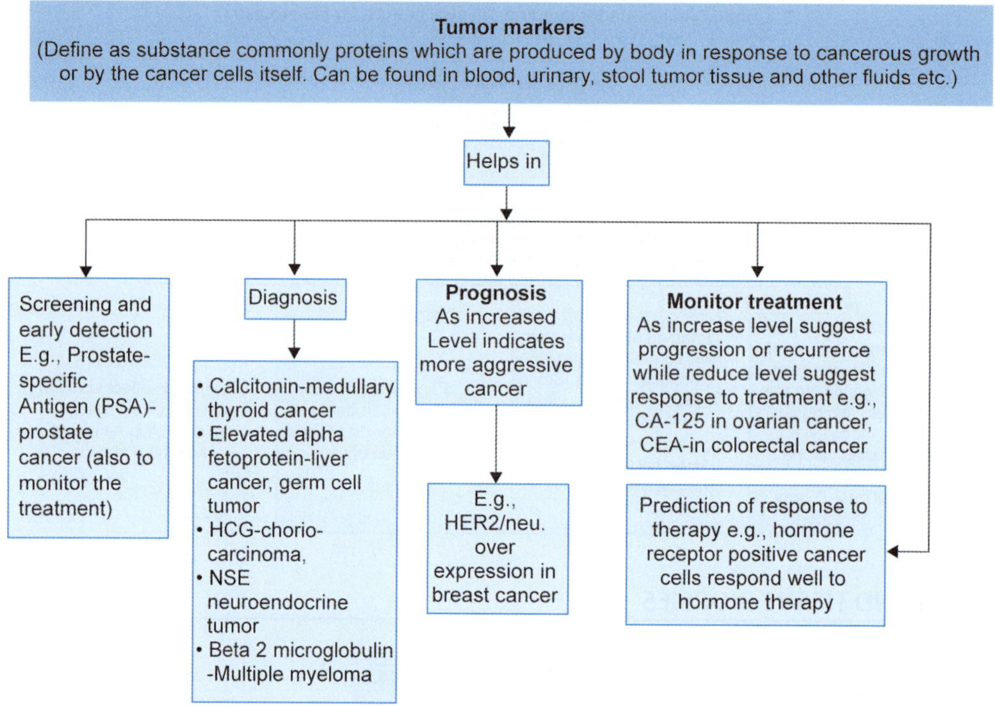

INTERPRETATION OF X-RAY (PNS)

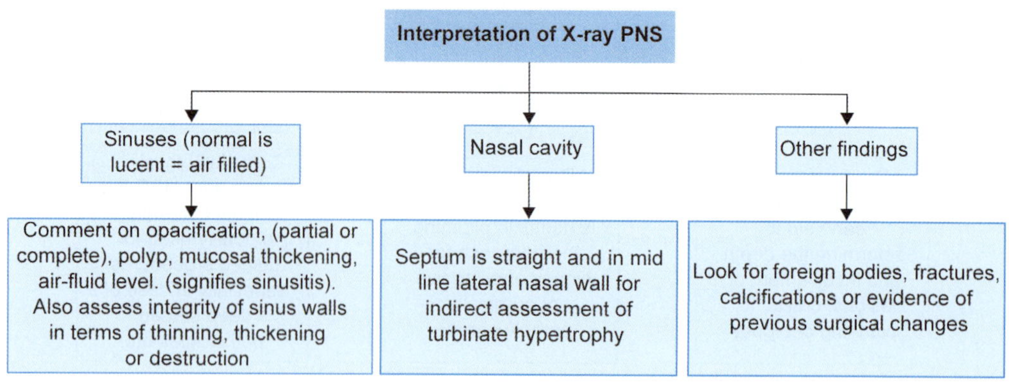

INTERPRETATION OF X-RAY MASTOID

Interpretation of X-ray mastoid

↓

Normally air cells are well aerated-honeycomb radiolucent structure with intact intervening wall

↓

- Opacification = mastoiditis
- Bone destruction or sclerosis - chronic infection
- Look for soft tissue mass
- Always compare from opposite side
- Advise CT if needed

APPROACH TO HEART FAILURE

Aspect	*Acute heart failure*	*Congestive heart failure*
Onset	Rapid onset, often within hours to days	Gradual onset, typically over weeks to months
Primary cause	Often triggered by an acute event (e.g., myocardial infarction, severe hypertension, arrhythmias)	Chronic conditions like hypertension, coronary artery disease, valvular heart disease
Symptoms	Severe dyspnea, orthopnea, chest pain, rapid edema development	Progressive dyspnea, fatigue, chronic peripheral edema, weight gain
Imaging findings	Pulmonary congestion, cardiomegaly on chest X-ray, possible pleural effusion	Cardiomegaly, pulmonary edema, pleural effusion, ascites on imaging
Hemodynamic features	Elevated filling pressures, reduced cardiac output, pulmonary edema	Chronic volume overload, elevated venous pressures, possible right heart failure
Treatment approach	Immediate intervention required, use of diuretics, vasodilators, inotropes	Long-term management, lifestyle modification, use of ACE inhibitors, beta-blockers, diuretics
Prognosis	Depends on underlying cause, can be life-threatening if not treated promptly	Chronic condition with variable prognosis, often managed over years

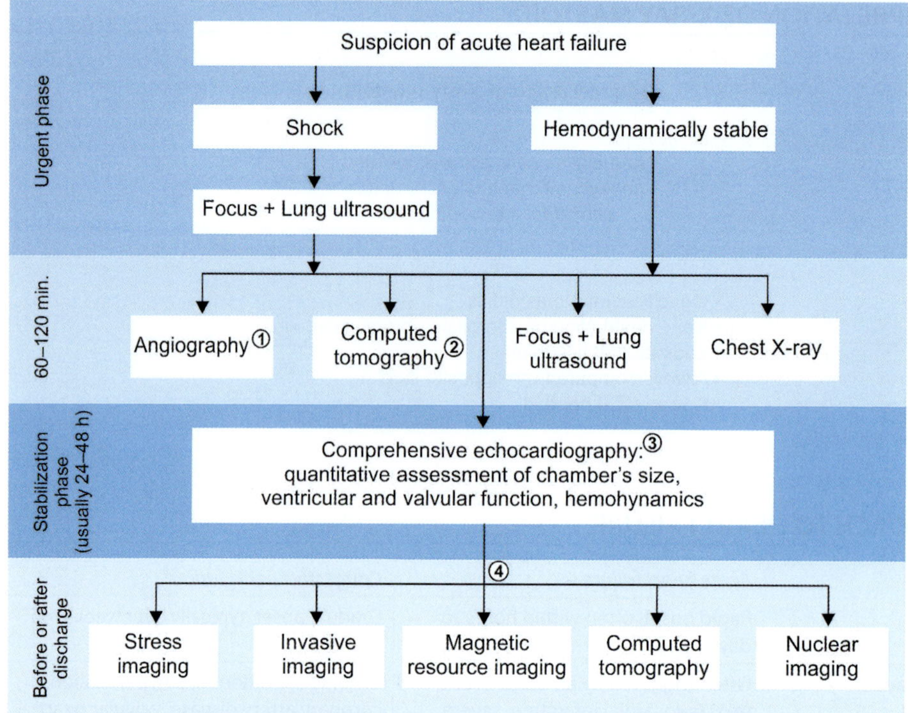

① In suspicion of acute coronary syndrome

② In suspicion of pulmonary embolism, aortic dissection; triple rule out Computed tomography may be used if available

③ Magnetic resonance imaging may be used as replacement of echocardiography in case of bad image quality

④ For etiology and decision making

Clinicoradiological Approach to Acute Heart Failure

Step 1: Patient Presentation

- **Symptoms:** Dyspnea, orthopnea, fatigue, chest pain
- **Signs:** Elevated jugular venous pressure, pulmonary crackles, peripheral edema

Step 2: Initial Assessment

- **Clinical history and physical examination:** Assess for cardiovascular risk factors, past history of heart disease, and signs of systemic congestion
- **Laboratory Tests:**
  - BNP or NT-proBNP levels
  - Troponins for myocardial injury

Step 3: Initial Imaging

Chest X-ray: Evaluate for pulmonary congestion, cardiomegaly, and pleural effusion

Step 4: Echocardiography

- Assess left ventricular ejection fraction (LVEF)
- Identify any structural abnormalities, valvular heart disease, or regional wall motion abnormalities

Step 5: Advanced Imaging (If Needed)

- **Cardiac MRI:** Assess for myocardial viability, fibrosis, or infiltrative diseases
- **CT coronary angiography:** Rule out coronary artery disease

Step 6: Hemodynamic Assessment

Right heart catheterization if needed to measure pulmonary capillary wedge pressure, cardiac output, etc.

Step 7: Management and Follow-Up

Based on findings, initiate treatment for acute heart failure (diuretics, vasodilators, inotropes) and monitor response.

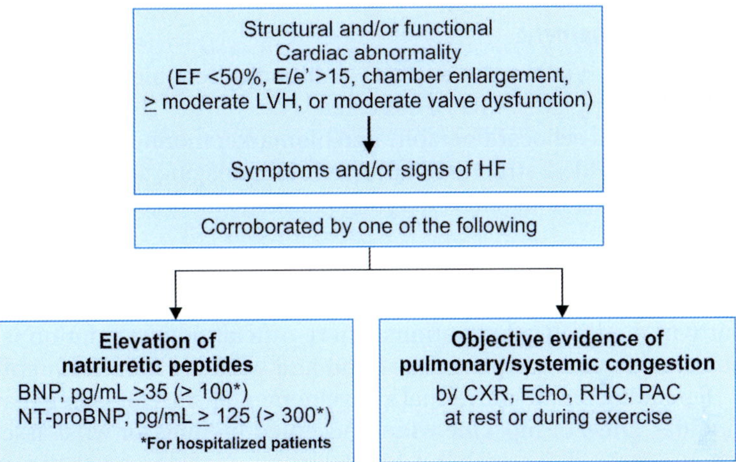

Fig. 1: Universal definition of heart failure according to the recent guideline.

(EF: ejection fraction; LVH: left ventricular hypertrophy; HF: heart failure; BNP: brain natriuretic peptide; CXR: chest x-ray; echo: echocardiography; RHC: right heart catheterization; PAC: pulmonary artery catheter).

Clinicoradiological Approach to Congestive Heart Failure

Step 1: Patient Presentation

- **Symptoms:** Progressive dyspnea, orthopnea, fatigue, exercise intolerance
- **Signs:** Peripheral edema, ascites, elevated jugular venous pressure

Step 2: Initial Assessment

- **Clinical history and physical examination:** Review history of hypertension, diabetes, coronary artery disease, and prior heart failure episodes
- **Laboratory tests:**
  - BNP or NT-proBNP levels
  - Electrolytes, renal function, and liver function tests

Step 3: Initial Imaging

- **Chest X-ray:** Assess for cardiomegaly, pulmonary edema, pleural effusion

Step 4: Echocardiography

- Evaluate LVEF to classify heart failure (HFrEF, HFmrEF, HFpEF)
- Assess diastolic function, chamber size, valvular abnormalities

Step 5: Advanced Imaging (If Needed)

- **Cardiac MRI:** Detailed assessment of myocardial structure, fibrosis, and scar tissue
- **Nuclear imaging (SPECT or PET):** Evaluate myocardial perfusion and viability

Step 6: Multidimensional Assessment

Combine imaging results with biomarkers (e.g., troponin, sST2, galectin-3) for comprehensive evaluation

Step 7: Long-term Management

- Initiate and adjust heart failure therapy (ACE inhibitors, beta-blockers, diuretics)
- Consider device therapy (ICD, CRT) if indicated
- Regular follow-up with echocardiography and biomarker monitoring

These flowcharts provide a structured approach to managing acute and congestive heart failure, integrating clinical evaluation with radiological and laboratory assessments.

Radiographic Standards for Age Determination

Radiographic imaging, alongside dental evaluations, plays a crucial role in determining age, particularly in medicolegal situations where official documentation is unavailable. Among various options, radiographs of the hand and wrist are most frequently utilized for this purpose. Depending on the individual's developmental stage, imaging may also involve the elbow, shoulder, knee, or hip. One widely accepted method for wrist assessment is the Tanner-Whitehouse technique, which involves assigning developmental stages to individual bones, calculating a composite score, and converting it into an estimated bone age. Accurate interpretation across multiple anatomical sites is essential to reduce errors and accurately assign age categories.

Radiographic Indicators of Age: Sequence of Bone Development and Fusion

Approx. age (males)	*Approx. age (females)*	*Bones visible in wrist x-ray*	*Additional skeletal changes*
3 months	3 months	Capitate, hamate	Distal femoral epiphysis, talus, calcaneus
15–18 months	1 year	Epiphyses of 2nd, 3rd, and 4th proximal phalanges; Metacarpal heads; Distal radius	Closure of anterior fontanelle and metopic suture
2 years	18 months	Epiphyses of 2nd, 3rd, and 4th middle phalanges	Occipital condyles fuse with squamous part
2.5 years	2 years	Triquetral bone	Number of visible carpal bones approximates chronological age
3 years	2.5 years	Lunate appears	—
4 years	3 years	Epiphysis of 5th middle phalanx becomes visible	—

Contd...

Contd...

Approx. age (males)	*Approx. age (females)*	*Bones visible in wrist x-ray*	*Additional skeletal changes*
5–6 years	4–5 years	Scaphoid, trapezium, trapezoid	Appearance of medial humeral epicondyle; Fusion of occipital condyle with basiocciput
6 years	4–6 years	Distal epiphysis of ulna	—
7–8 years	6–7 years	—	Union of pubic and ischial rami begins
8–10 years	7–9 years	—	Olecranon becomes radiographically evident
In Later Childhood and Adolescence			
Wrist and hand findings			*Additional skeletal features*
Up to 11 years	Up to 9 years	Epiphyses of phalanges are slightly smaller than the growth plates (physes)	—
11–12 years	10–12 years	Phalangeal epiphyses become marginally broader than physes but remain thin; Pisiform bone begins to appear	—
13 years	11–12 years	Hook of hamate becomes visible	Fusion of lateral humeral epicondyle with the trochlea and capitulum
14 years	13 years	Metacarpal head ossification becomes apparent	Appearance of iliac crest ossification
15 years	14 years	Epiphysis of the proximal phalanx seen	Coracoid process fuses with the scapula; Olecranon joins with ulna
16 years	15 years	Middle phalanx epiphysis becomes evident	—
Adolescence to Early Adulthood			
Epiphyseal fusion in long bones			*Other radiographic milestones*
17–18 years	13–14 years	Fusion of distal ends of the ulna and radius (full maturation)	Epiphysis appears at ischial tuberosity; All components of the elbow joint (except the medial epicondyle) fuse with their shafts; Femoral head and distal tibial epiphysis unite with the shaft
18–20 years	15–18 years	—	Complete fusion of all wrist and knee epiphyses; Clavicular lateral end joins the shaft; Acromion fuses with the scapula
20–22 years	19–21 years	—	Ischial tuberosity fuses with the pelvis
23–25 years	22–24 years	—	Central four sacral vertebrae fuse; Completion of epiphyseal fusion throughout the body

Mnemonic: Up to 11 years: Age determination done by wrist with hand and usually number of ossification center of carpal bones correspond to age in years, up to 7 years except appearance of pisiform at 11 years.

Flowchart 1: Depicting systematic age estimation from radiographs for children below 5 years.

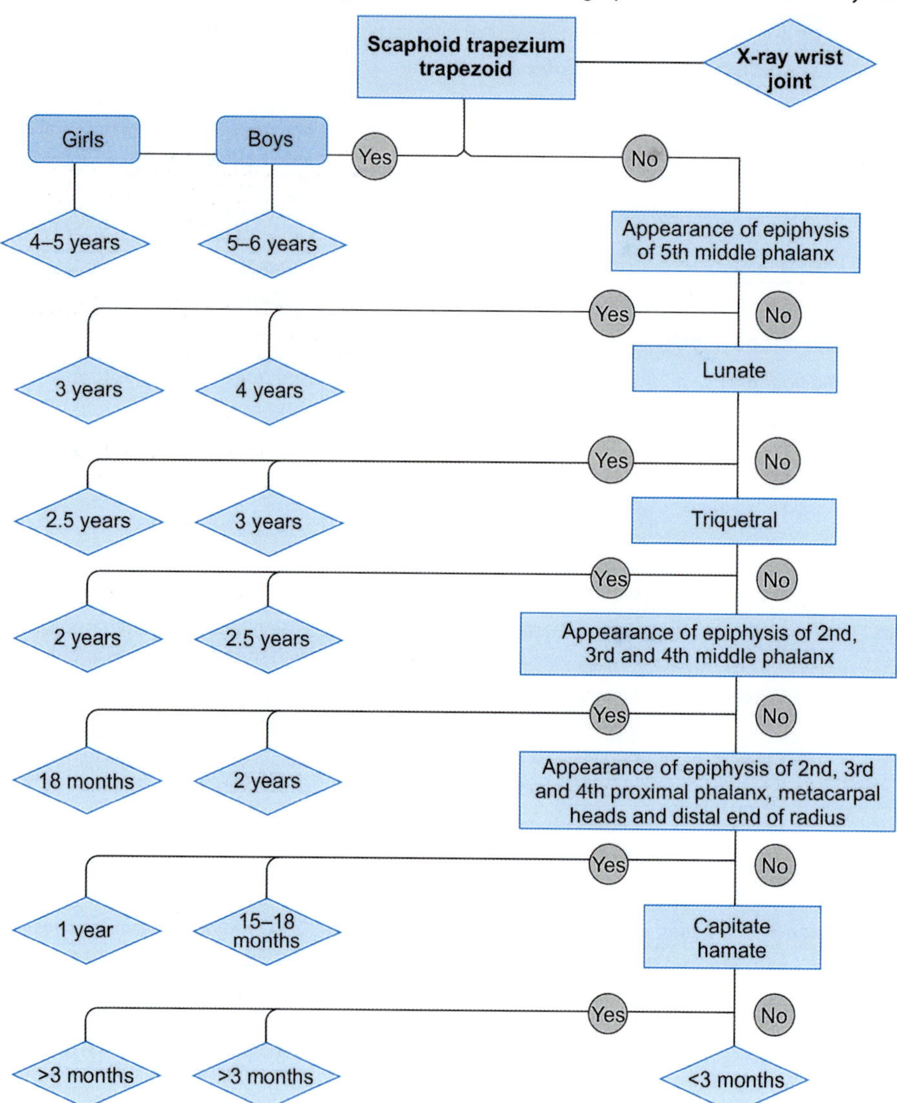

Flowchart 2: Depicting systematic age estimation from radiographs for 5 to 16 years of age.

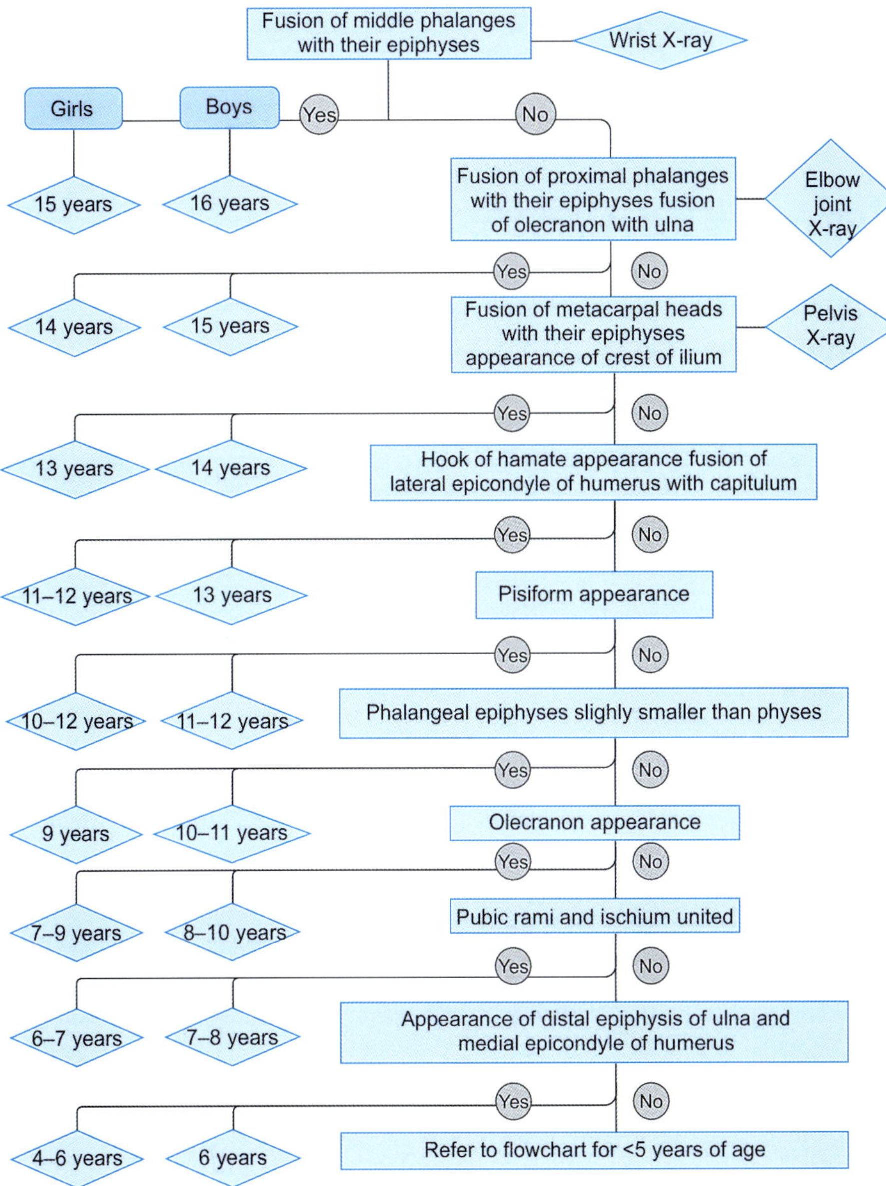

Glossary

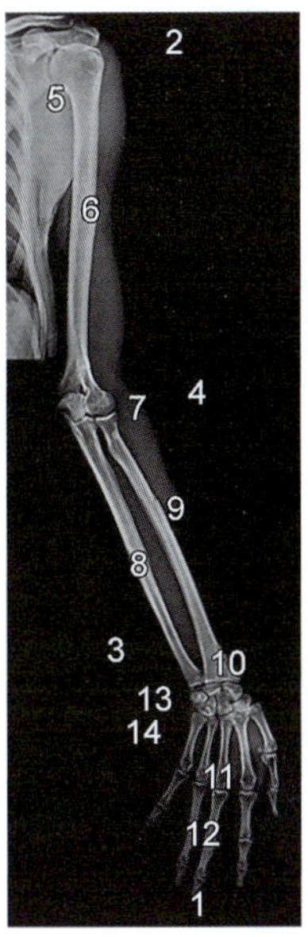

Fig. 1: Complete stitched AP X-ray film of upper limb: 1, 2, 3 and 4. distal, proximal, medially and lateral aspect respectively; 5. Shoulder joint (glenohumeral joint); 6. Humerus (arm); 7. Elbow joint; 8. Ulna; 9. Radius;10. Wrist joint (radiocarpal joint); 11. Metacarpophalangeal joint; 12. Interphalangeal joint;13. Carpal bones;14. Metacarpals.

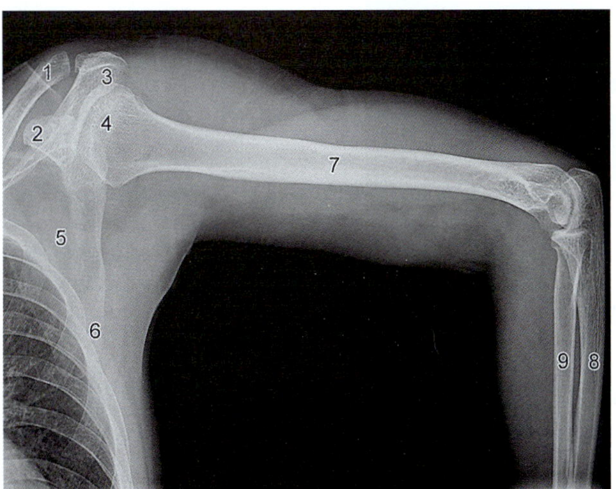

Fig. 2: X-ray arm with shoulder and elbow joint lateral view: 1. Clavicle; 2. Coracoid process; 3. Acromion process; 4. Head of humerus; 5. Body of scapula; 6. Inferior pole of scapula; 7. Shaft of humerus; 8. Radius; 9. Ulna.

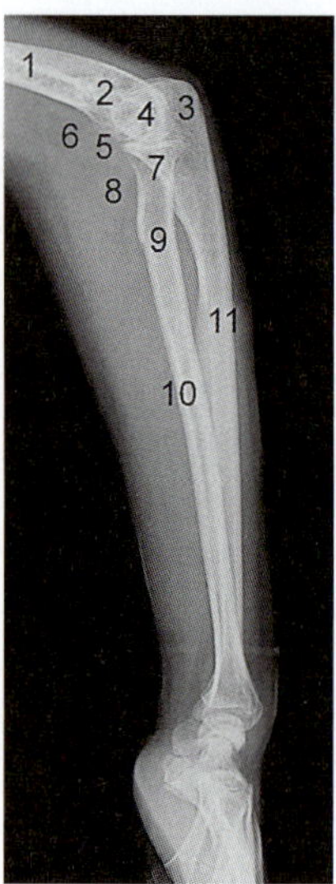

Fig. 3: X-ray elbow with forearm with wrist joint (lateral view): 1. Humerus; 2. Supracondylar ridge; 3. Olecranon process; 4. Trochlear notch; 5. Coronoid process; 6. Capitulum; 7. Head of radius; 8. Neck of radius; 9. Tuberosity of radius; 10. Radius shaft; 11. Ulna shaft.

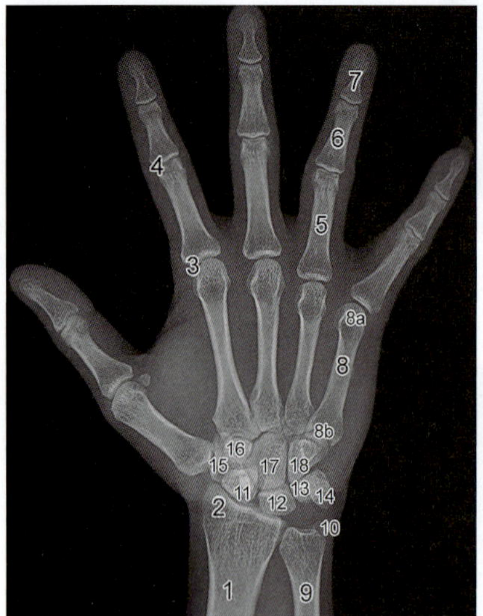

Fig. 4: X-ray wrist joint with hand (AP view): 1. Radius; 2. Styloid process of radius; 3. Metacarpophalangeal joint; 4. Interphalangeal joint; 5. Proximal phalanx; 6. Middle phalanx; 7. Distal phalanx; 8. Metacarpal; 8a. Base of metacarpal; 8b. Head of metacarpal; 9. Ulna; 10. Styloid process of ulna; 11. Scaphoid; 12. Lunate; 13. Triquetrum; 14. Pisiform; 15. Trapezium; 16. Trapezoid; 17. Capitate; 18. Hamate.

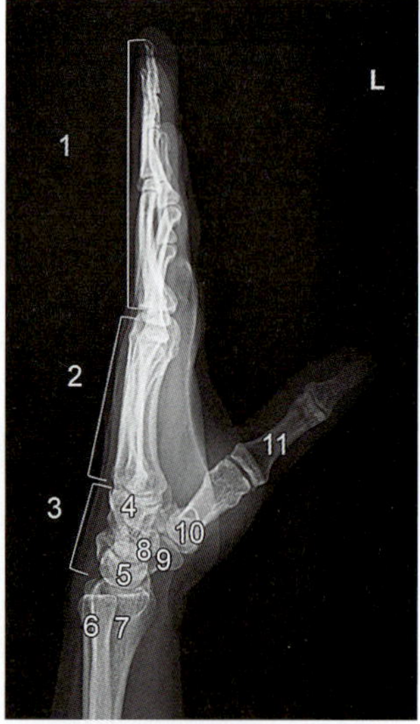

Fig. 5: X-ray wrist joint with hand (lateral view): 1. Phalanges; 2. 2nd and 4th metacarpals; 3. Carpals; 4. Capitate; 5. Lunate; 6. Ulna; 7. Radius; 8. Pisiform; 9. Scaphoid; 10. Trapezium; 11. Metacarpal.

Fig. 6: Complete stitched AP X-ray film of Lower Limb: 1. Pelvic bone (medially); 2. Hip joint; 3. Femur; 4. Knee joint; 5. Tibia; 6. Fibula; 7. Ankle joint; 8. Patella.

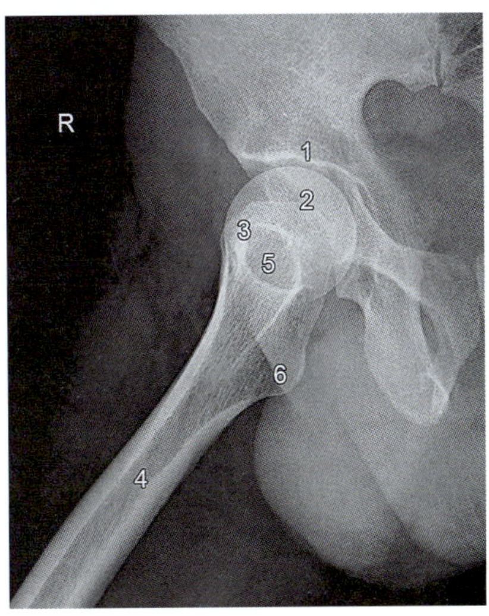

Fig. 7: X-ray right hip joint lateral view (with leg abduction): 1. Acetabulum; 2. Femoral head; 3. Femoral neck; 4. Femur shaft; 5. Greater trochanter; 6. Lesser trochanter.

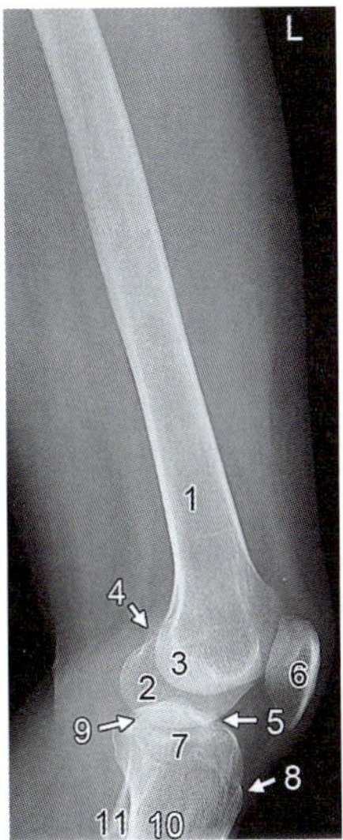

Fig. 8: X-ray thigh with knee joint (lateral view): 1. Femur; 2. Medial condyle; 3. Lateral condyle; 4. Adductor tubercle; 5. Intercondylar tubercle (protruded part); 6. Patella; 7. Tibial condyles; 8. Tibial tuberosity; 9. Tibial plateau; 10. Tibia; 11. Fibula.

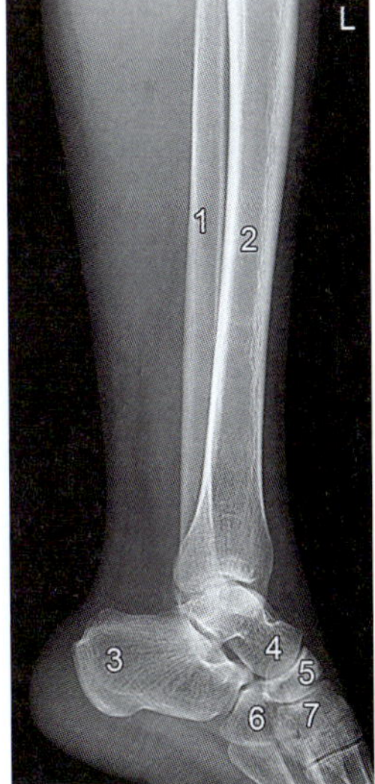

Fig. 9: X-ray leg with ankle (lateral view): 1. Fibula; 2. Tibia; 3. Calcaneum; 4. Talus; 5. Navicular; 6. Cuboid; 7. Cuneiform.

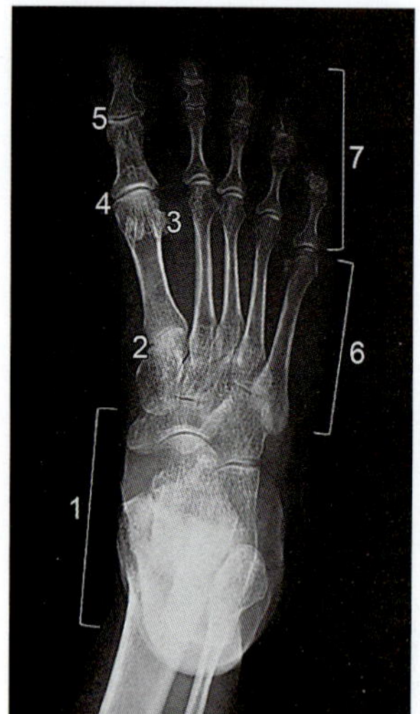

Fig. 10: X-ray foot with ankle (AP view): 1. Tarsals; 2. Tarsometatarsal joint; 3. Sesamoid bone; 4. Metatarsophalangeal joint; 5. Interphalangeal joint; 6. Metatarsals; 7. Phalanges.

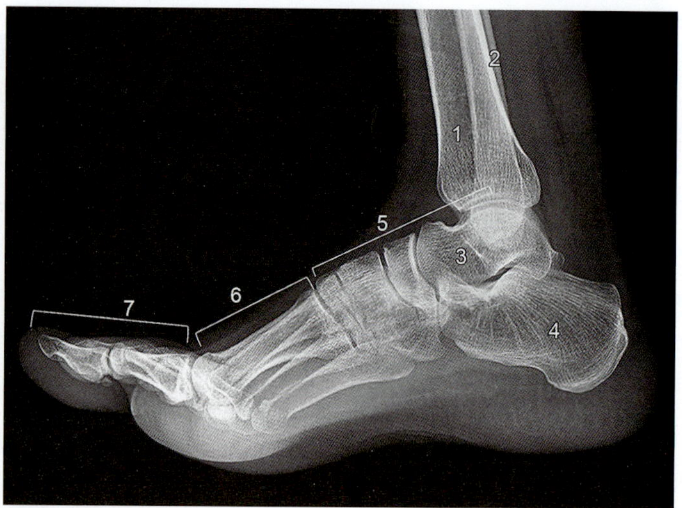

Fig. 11: X-ray foot with ankle (lateral view): 1. Tibia; 2. Fibula; 3. Talus; 4. Calcaneum; 5. Tarsals; 6. Metatarsals; 7. Phalanges.

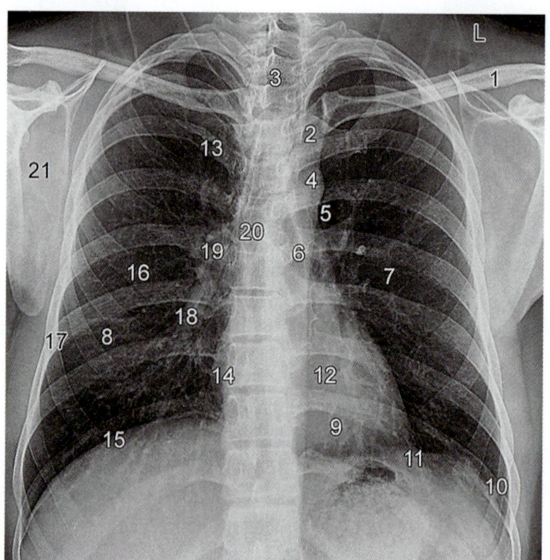

Fig. 12: X-ray chest PA view: 1. Clavicle; 2. Manubrium; 3. Trachea; 4. Aortic knuckle; 5. Pulmonary conus; 6. Left main bronchus; 7. Vascular markings; 8. Lung parenchyma; 9. Left ventricle; 10. Costophrenic angle; 11. Cardiophrenic angle; 12. Heart; 13. Posterior end of rib; 14. Right atrium; 15. Diaphragm; 16. Anterior end of rib; 17. Rib; 18. Descending pulmonary artery; 19. Hilar shadows; 20. Right main bronchus; 21. Scapula.

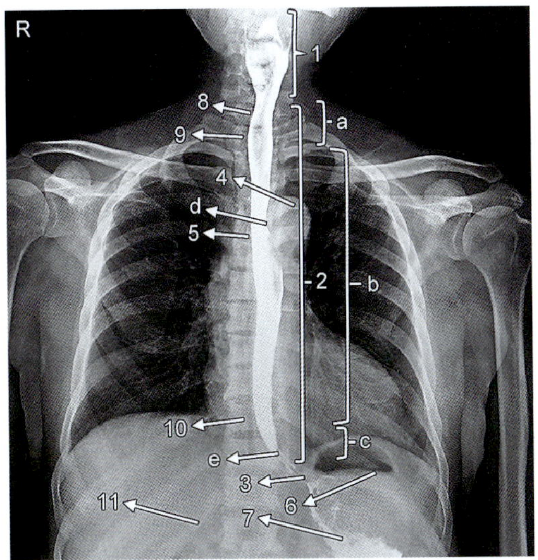

Fig. 13: AP view of barium swallow: 1. Pharynogram; 2. Esophagogram (a) Cervical esophagus, (b) Thoracic esophagus, (c) Intra-abdominal esophagus, (d) Knuckle constriction, (e) Diaphragmatic constriction; 3. Gastroesophageal junction; 4. Aortic knuckle; 5. Tracheal lucency; 6. Air-fluid level of stomach; 7. Barium contrast in stomach; 8. Seventh cervical vertebrae; 9. First thoracic vertebrae; 10. Tenth thoracic vertebrae; 11. Twelfth rib.

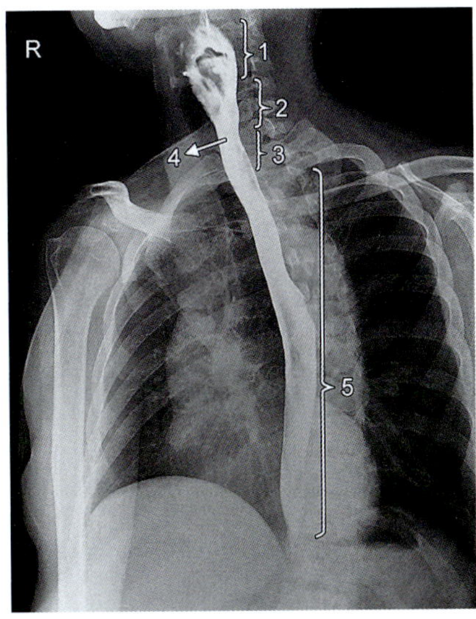

Fig. 14: Oblique view: 1. Oropharynx; 2. Hypopharynx; 3. Cervical esophagus; 4. Cervical constrictions (cricopharynx level); 5. Thoracic esophagus.

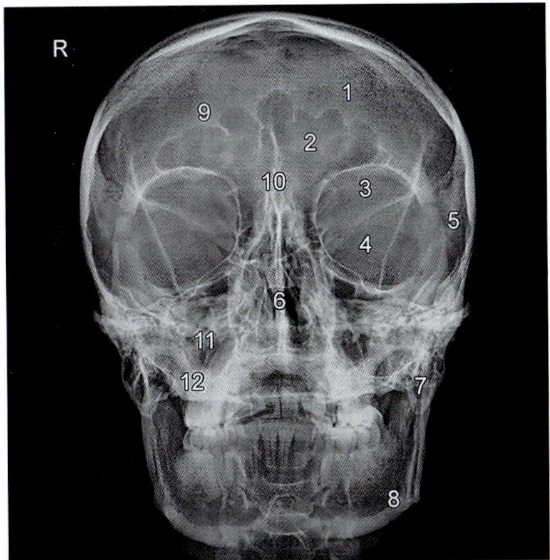

Fig. 15: X-ray skull (AP view): 1. Frontal bone; 2. Frontal sinus; 3. Sphenoid bone—lesser wing; 4. Orbit; 5. Sphenoid bone—greater wing; 6. Nasal septum; 7. Mastoid process; 8. Angle of mandible; 9. Lambdoid suture; 10. Crista galli; 11. Maxillary sinus; 12. Occipital bone.

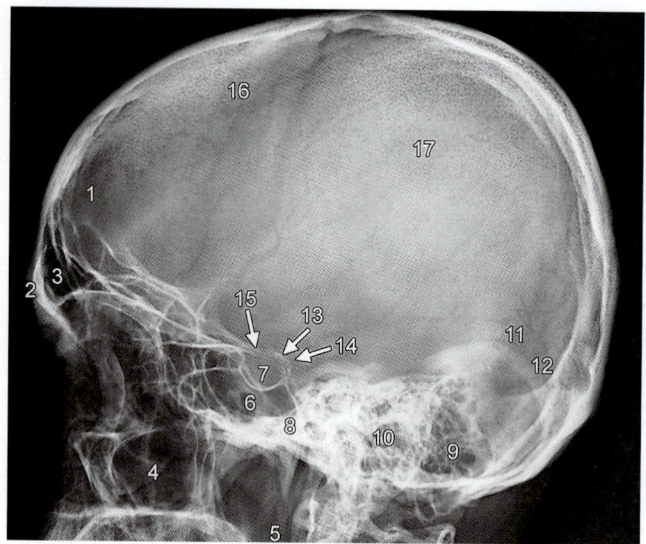

Fig. 16: X-ray skull (lateral view): 1. Frontal bone; 2. Glabella; 3. Frontal sinus; 4. Maxillary sinus; 5. Mandible; 6. Sphenoid sinus; 7. Pituitary fossa; 8. Clivus; 9. Mastoid region; 10. External acoustic meatus; 11. Lambdoid suture; 12. Occipital bone; 13. Dorsum sella; 14. Posterior clinoid process; 15. Anterior clinoid process; 16. Coronal suture; 17. Parietal bone.

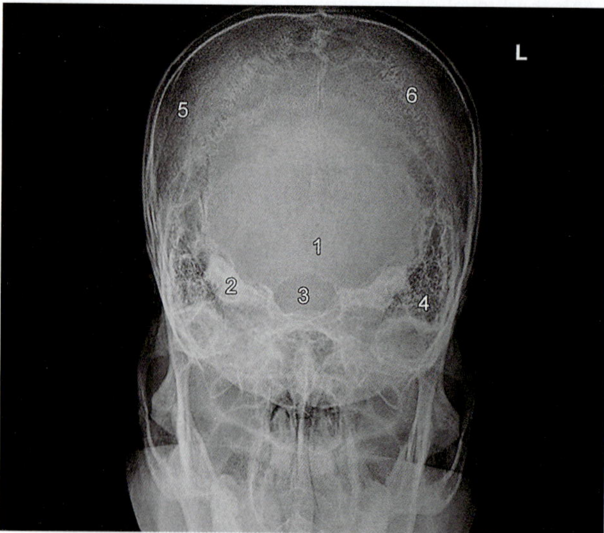

Fig. 17: X-ray mastoid (Towne's view): 1. Occipital bone; 2. Petrous ridge; 3. Foramen magnum; 4. Mastoid with air cells; 5. Parietal bone; 6. Lambdoid suture.

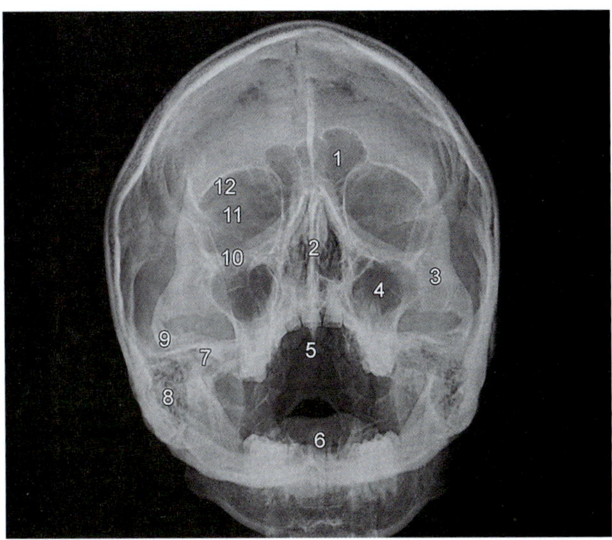

Fig. 18: X-ray paranasal sinus (Water's view): 1. Frontal sinus; 2. Nasal septum; 3. Zygomatic bone; 4. Maxillary sinus; 5. Sphenoid sinus; 6. Odontoid process; 7. Petrous ridge; 8. Mastoid air cells; 9. Zygomatic arch; 10. Inferior orbital rim; 11. Orbit; 12. Retro-orbital fat.

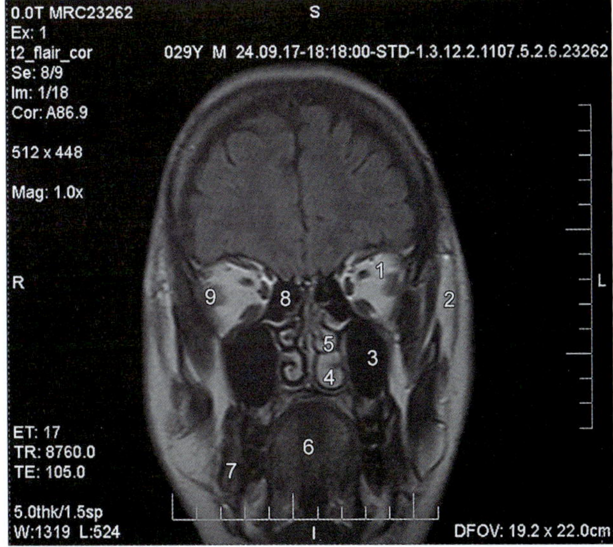

Fig. 19: MRI paranasal sinus (coronal section): 1. Orbital fat; 2. Subcutaneous fat; 3. Maxillary sinus; 4. Inferior turbinate; 5. Middle turbinate; 6. Tongue; 7. Mandible; 8. Ethmoid sinus; 9. Lateral rectus muscle.

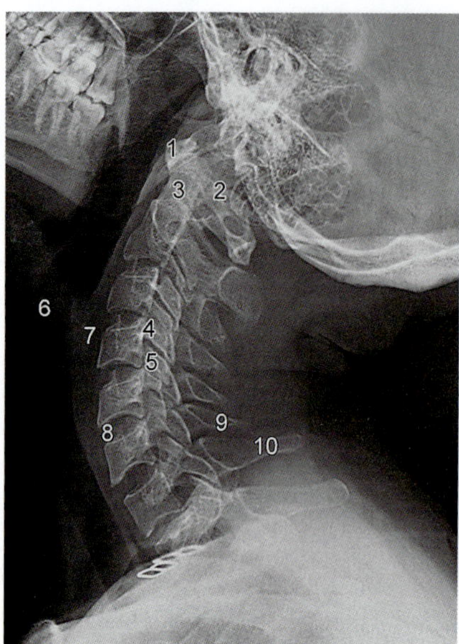

Fig. 20: X-ray cervical spine (lateral view): 1. Anterior arch of atlas; 2. Posterior arch of atlas; 3. Dens of C2 vertebra; 4. Superior articular process; 5. Inferior articular process; 6. Trachea; 7. Pre-vertebral soft tissue; 8. Intervertebral disc space; 9. Spinous process; 10. Vertebrae prominence.

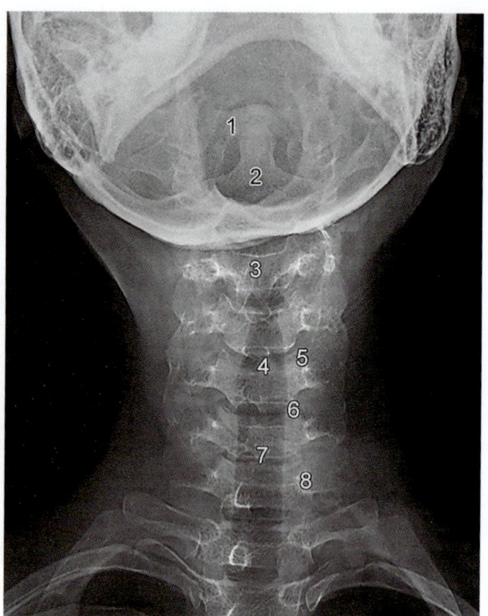

Fig. 21: X-ray cervical spine (AP view): 1. C1 – atlas vertebra; 2. C2 – axis vertebra; 3. C3 – vertebra; 4. Trachea; 5. Superior articular process; 6. Intervertebral disc space; 7. Spinous process; 8. Pedicle.

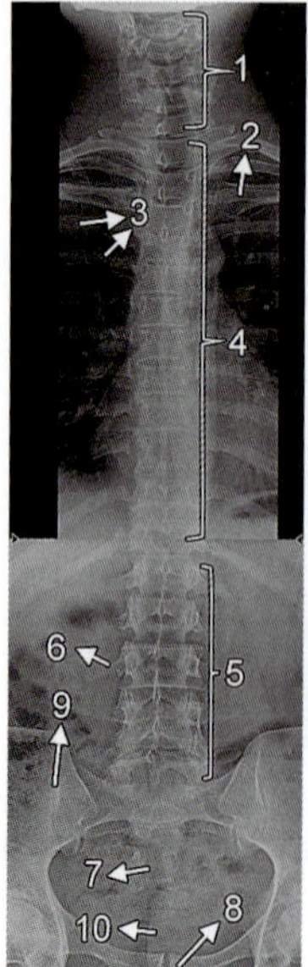

Fig. 22: Stitch spine (AP view): 1. Cervical vertebrae; 2. Clavicle; 3. Ribs; 4. Thoracic vertebrae; 5. Lumbar vertebrae; 6. Transverse process of lumbar vertebra; 7. Sacrum; 8. Pubis; 9. Sacroiliac joint; 10. Coccyx.

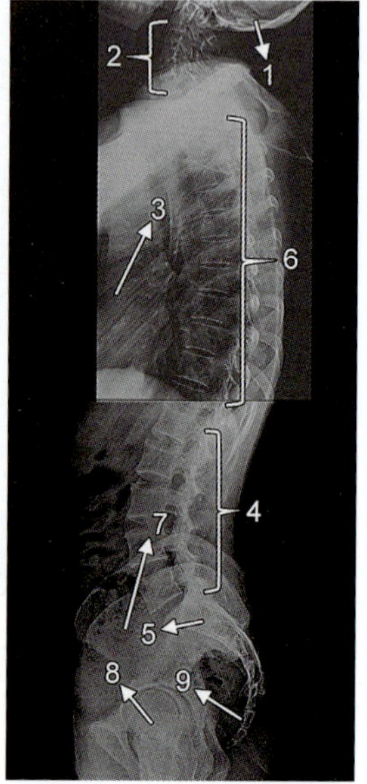

Fig. 23: Stitch spine (lateral view): 1. Occipital bone; 2. Cervical vertebrae; 3. Ribs; 4. Lumbar vertebrae; 5. Sacrum; 6. Thoracic vertebrae; 7. Ilium; 8. Femur; 9. Coccyx.

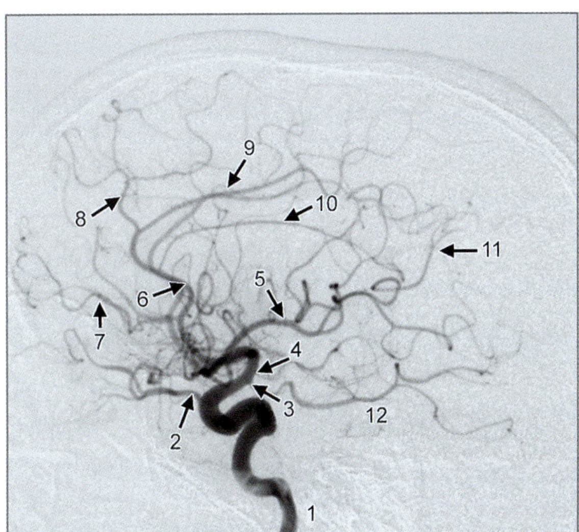

Fig. 24: ICA lateral angiogram: 1. Internal cerebral artery; 2. Ophthalmic artery; 3. Posterior communicating artery; 4. Anterior choroidal artery; 5. Middle cerebral artery; 6. Anterior cerebral artery; 7. Frontopolar branch; 8. Prefrontal branch; 9. Callosomarginal artery; 10. Pericallosal artery; 11. Temporo-occipital branch; 12. Posterior cerebral artery.

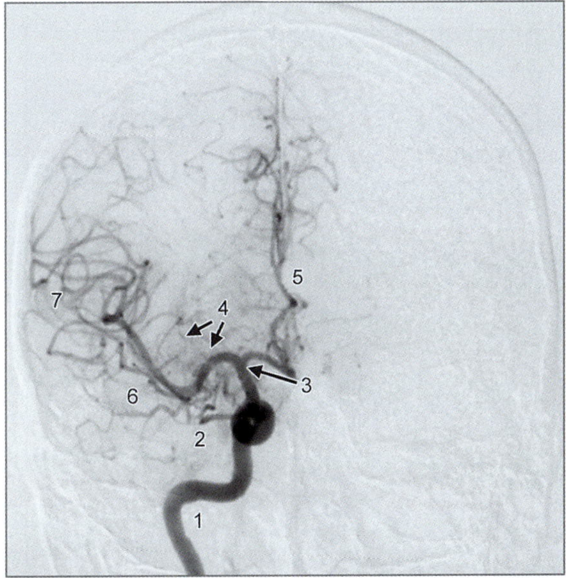

Fig. 25: ICA AP projection: 1. Internal cerebral artery; 2. Ophthalmic artery; 3. ICA bifurcation into ACA and MCA; 4. Lenticulostriate branches; 5. Anterior cerebral artery; 6. Middle cerebral artery; 7. Insular branches of MCA.

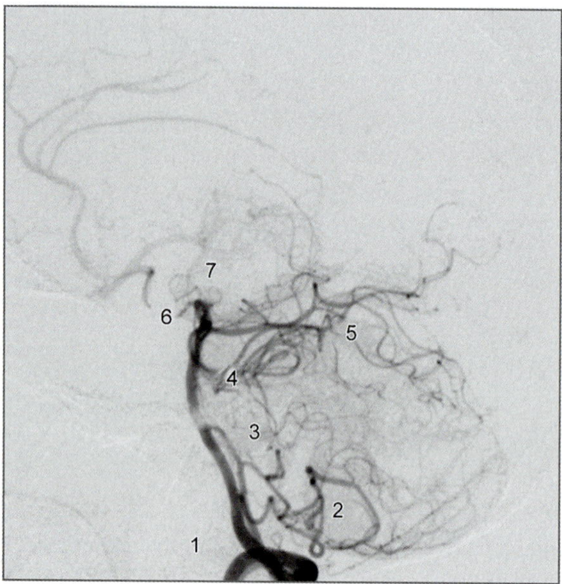

Fig. 26: Vertebral lateral angiogram: 1. Vertebral artery; 2. Posterior inferior cerebellar artery; 3. Anterior inferior cerebellar artery; 4. Superior cerebellar artery; 5. Posterior cerebral artery; 6. Posterior communicating artery; 7. Thalamoperforators.

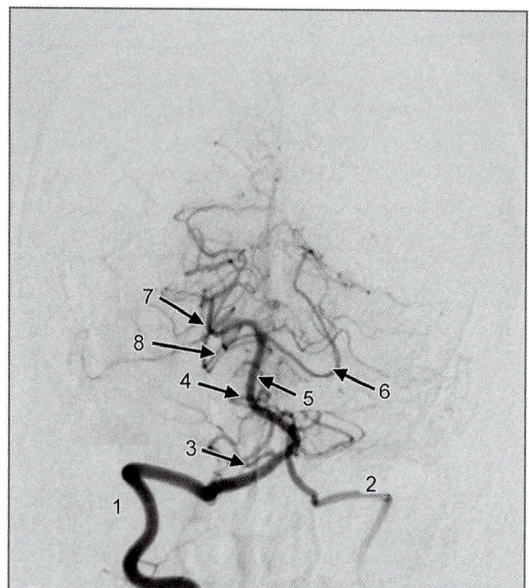

Fig. 27: Vertebral angiogram AP Townes projection: 1. Right vertebral artery; 2. Left vertebral artery; 3. Right posterior inferior cerebellar artery; 4. Right anterior inferior cerebellar artery; 5. Basilar artery; 6. Left superior cerebellar artery; 7. Right posterior cerebral artery; 8. Right duplicated superior cerebellar artery.

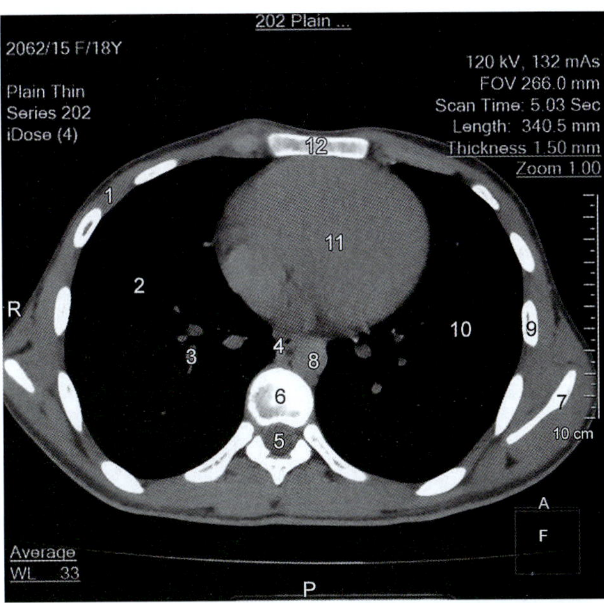

Fig. 28: NCCT chest at T8 level (axial section): 1. Chest wall; 2. Right lung; 3. Bronchial vessels; 4. Esophagus; 5. Spinal canal; 6. T8 vertebral body; 7. Scapula; 8. Descending thoracic aorta; 9. Rib; 10. Left lung; 11. Heart; 12. Sternum.

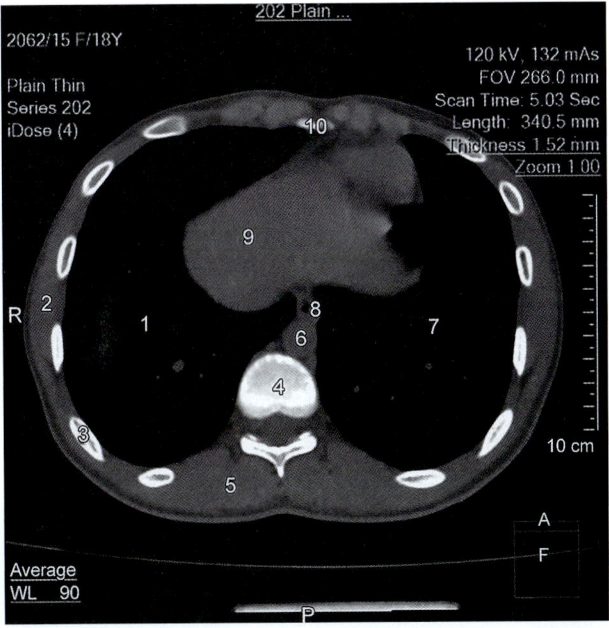

Fig. 29: NCCT chest at T10 level (axial section): 1. Right lung; 2. Chest wall; 3. Rib; 4. T10 vertebral body; 5. Paraspinal muscles; 6. Descending thoracic aorta; 7. Left lung; 8. Esophagus; 9. Liver; 10. Sternum.

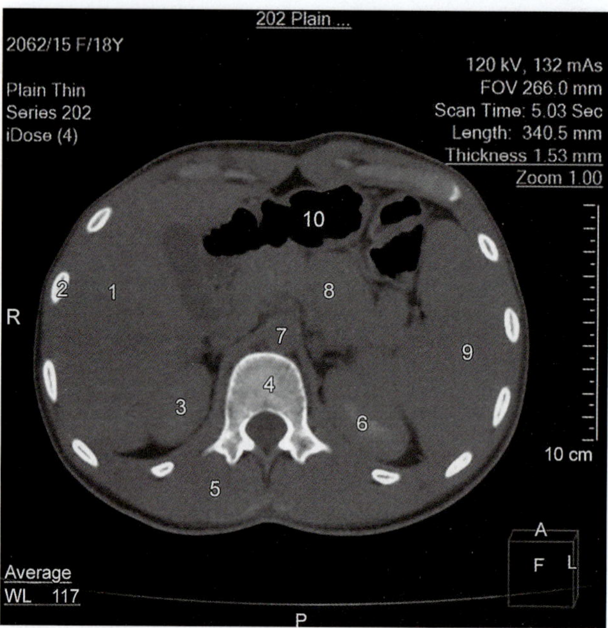

Fig. 30: NCCT abdomen at L1 level (axial section): 1. Liver; 2. Rib; 3. Right kidney; 4. L1 vertebral body; 5. Paraspinal muscles; 6. Left kidney; 7. Descending abdominal aorta; 8. Pancreas; 9. Spleen; 10. Large bowel.

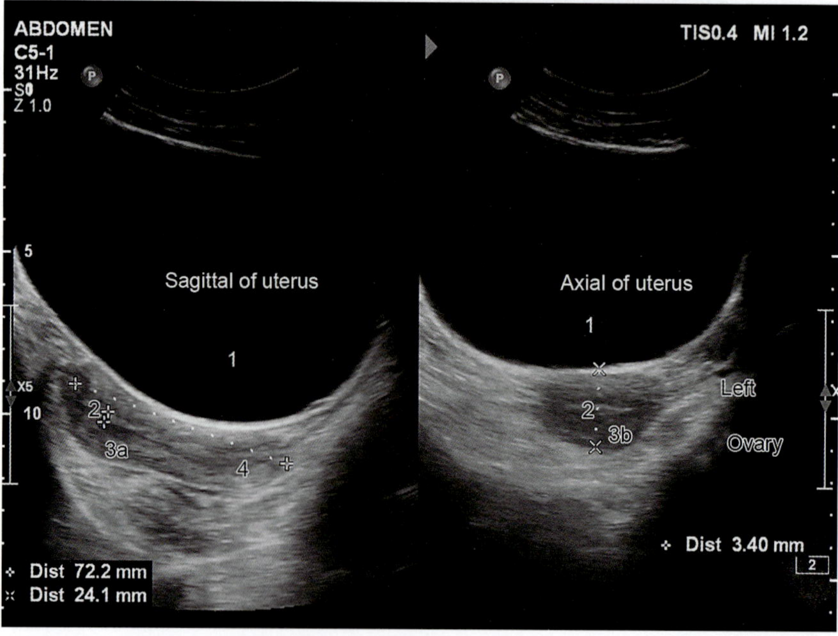

Fig. 31: USG female pelvis (sagittal and axial view): 1. Urinary bladder; 2. Endometrium; 3a. Uterus (sagittal); 3b. Uterus (axial); 4. Cervix.

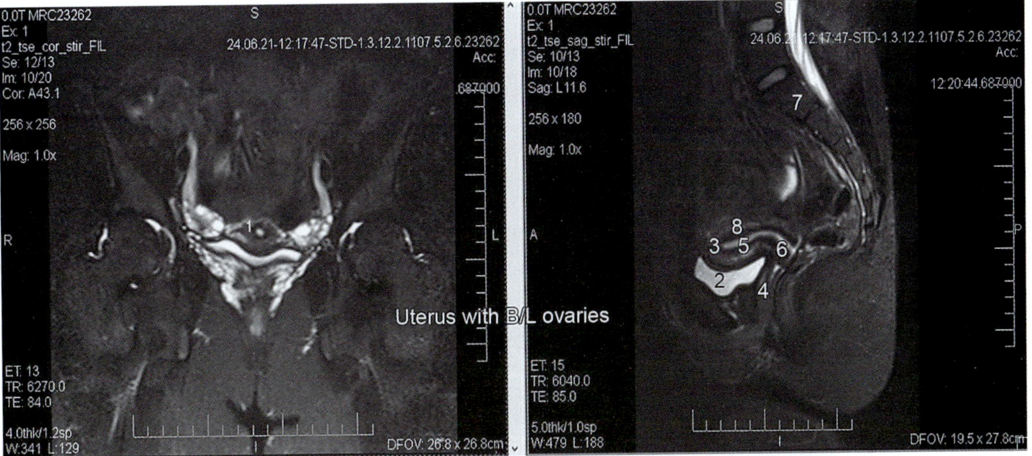

Fig. 32: MRI female pelvis (coronal and sagittal section): 1. Axial uterus; 2. Urinary bladder; 3. Sagittal uterus; 4. Vagina; 5. Endometrial lining; 6. Cervix; 7. Sacrum; 8. Myometrium.

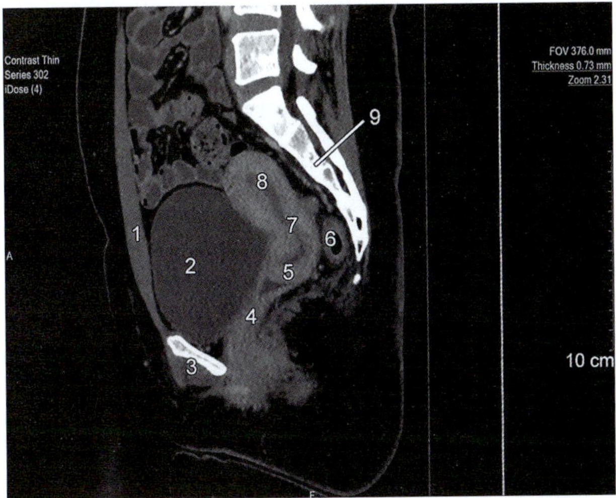

Fig. 33: CECT female pelvis (sagittal section): 1. Rectus muscle; 2. Urinary bladder; 3. Pubic symphysis; 4. Vagina; 5. Cervix; 6. Rectum; 7. Uterus; 8. Endometrium; 9. Sacrum.

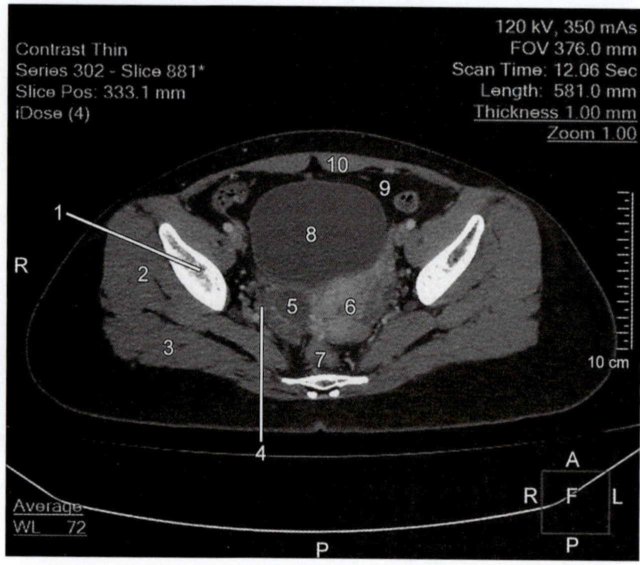

Fig. 34: CECT female pelvis (axial section): 1. Ilium; 2. Gluteus medius; 3. Gluteus maximus; 4. Ovary; 5. Follicle; 6. Uterus (transverse); 7. Rectum; 8. Urinary bladder; 9. Mesenteric fat; 10. Rectus muscle.

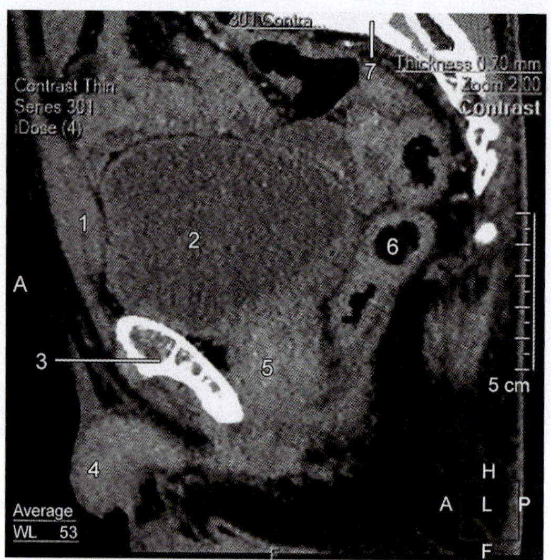

Fig. 35: CECT male pelvis (sagittal section): 1. Rectus; 2. Urinary bladder; 3. Pubic symphysis; 4. Penis; 5. Prostate; 6. Rectum; 7. Sacrum

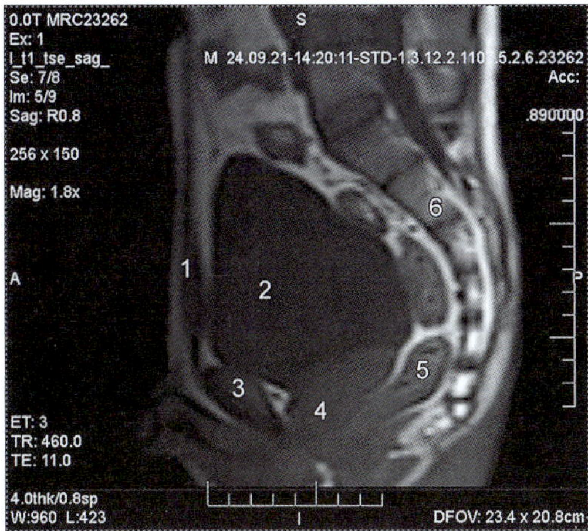

Fig. 36: MRI male pelvis (sagittal section): 1. Rectus; 2. Urinary bladder; 3. Pubic symphysis; 4. Prostate; 5. Rectum; 6. Sacrum

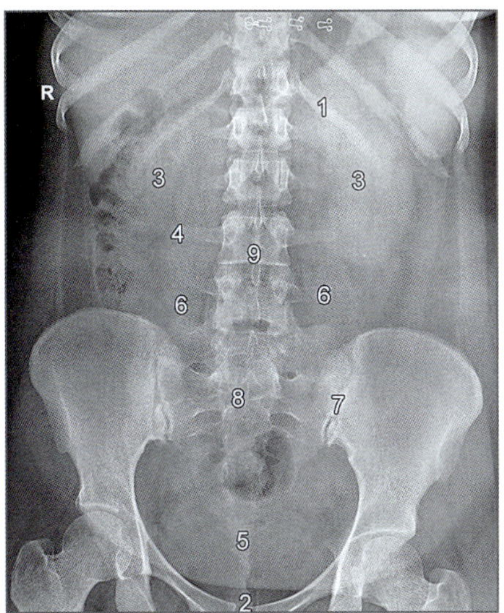

Fig. 37: Plain X-ray abdomen KUB region: 1. 12th Rib; 2. Pubic symphysis; 3. Kidney position showing bean-shaped density; 4. Tip of transverse process of lumbar vertebra (ureteric position); 5. Bladder density; 6. Psoas shadow; 7. Sacroiliac joint; 8. Sacrum; 9. Lumbar vertebra.

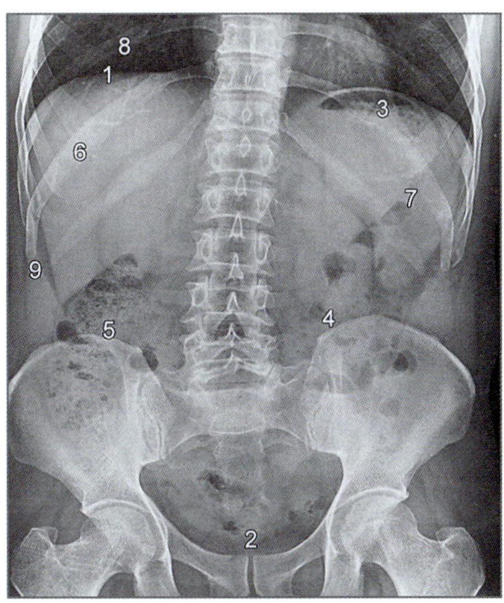

Fig. 38: Plain X-ray abdomen erect: 1. Dome of diaphragm(radio-opaque); 2. Pelvis (bowel gas); 3. Gastric bubble; 4. Bowel gas (small bowel); 5. Bowel gas (ascending colon); 6. Liver shadow/ density; 7. Splenic shadow; 8. Lower zone of chest (lung air); 9. Pro-peritoneal fat.

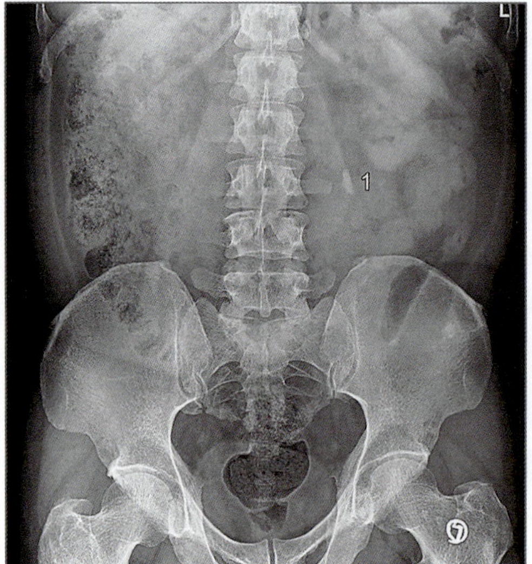

Fig. 39: Plain X-ray abdomen KUB region: 1. Left ureteric calculus/stone (oblong density adjacent to transverse process).

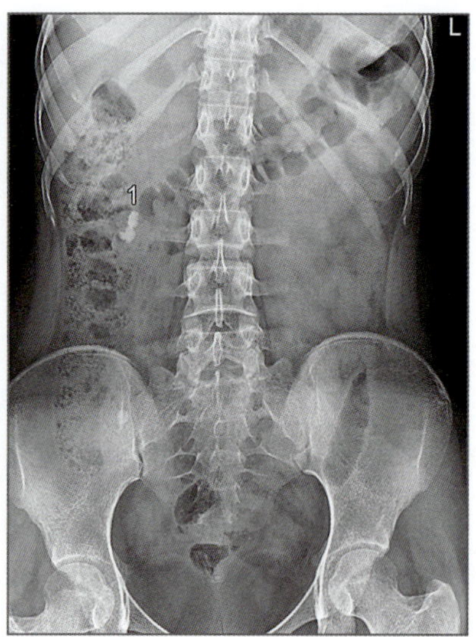

Fig. 40: Plain X-ray abdomen KUB region: 1. Right renal calculi/Stone (density of calyceal shape, along renal region).

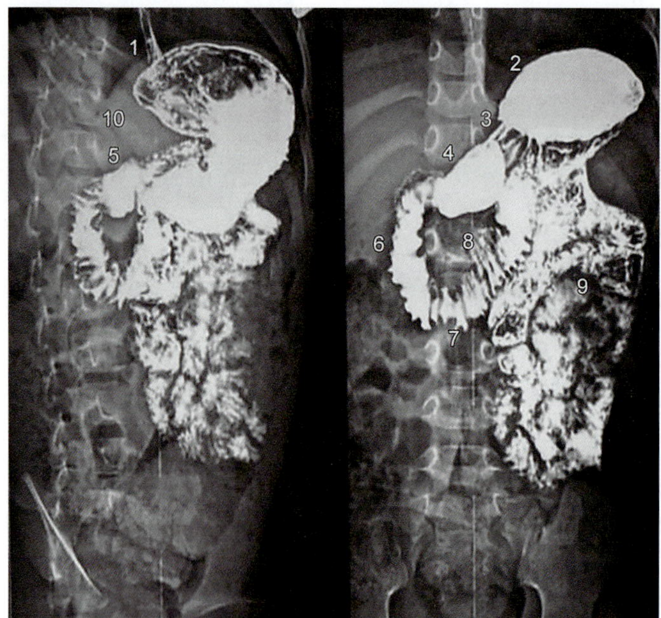

Fig. 41: Oblique and AP of Barium Meal: 1. Gastroesophageal junction; 2. Cardia of stomach; 3. Body; 4. Pylorus; 5. Duodenal cap (D1); 6. Second part of duodenum; 7. Third part of duodenum; 8. Fourth part of duodenum; 9. Jejunum (left upper abdomen); 10. Fundus of stomach.

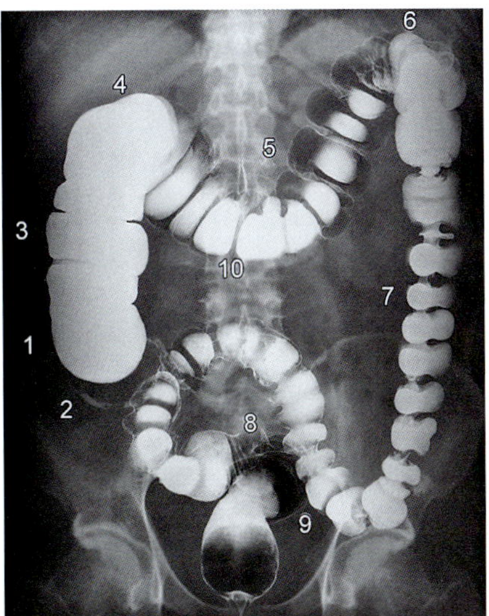

Fig. 42: Barium enema: 1. Cecum; 2. Appendix; 3. Ascending colon; 4. Hepatic flexure; 5. Transverse colon; 6. Splenic flexure; 7. Descending colon; 8. Pelvic colon; 9. Rectum;10. Haustral folds.

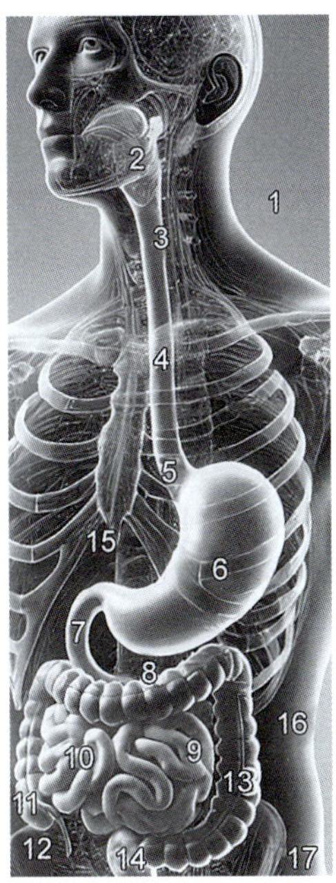

Fig. 43: Diagrammatic representation of barium studies: 1. Depicts part of GIT studied in swallow; 2. Oropharynx; 3. Hypopharynx; 4. Esophagus; 5. Gastroesophageal junction; 6. Stomach; 7. Duodenum; 8. Duodeno-jejunal junction; 9. Jejunum; 10. Ileum; 11. Cecum; 12. Ileocecal junction; 13. Colon; 14. Distal to pelvic colon (rectum and ano-rectal region); 15. Depicts part of GIT studied in Barium meal; 16. Depicts part of GIT studied in BMFT; 17. Depicts part of GIT studied in Barium enema.

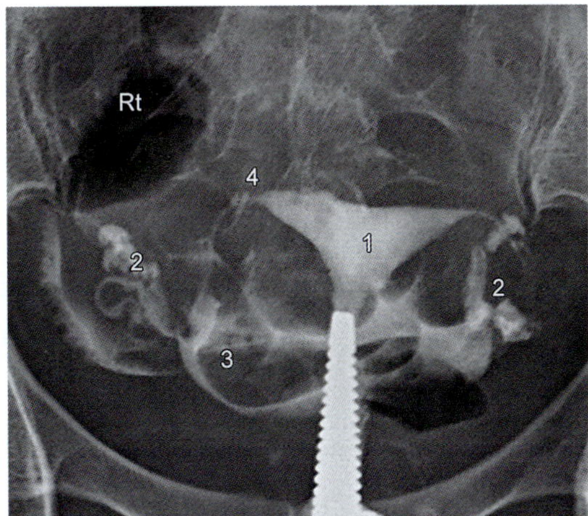

Fig. 44: Contrast study showing normal hysterosalpingogram: 1. Uterine cavity; 2. Bilateral fallopian tube with normal caliber; 3. Free peritoneal spillage; 4. Cornual end.

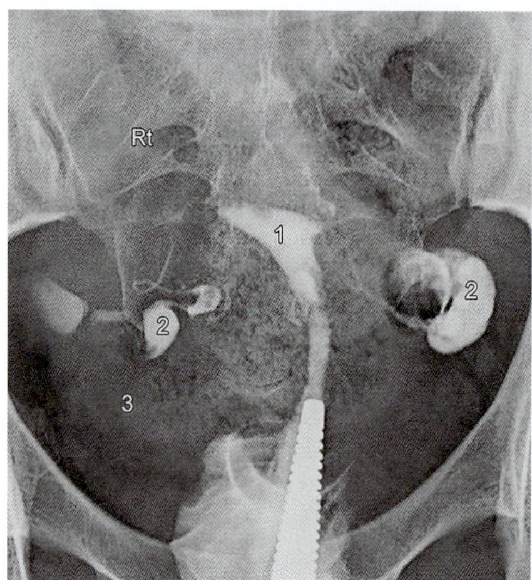

Fig. 45: Contrast study showing hysterosalpingogram: 1. Uterine cavity; 2. Bilateral dilated fallopian tube (hydrosalpinx); 3. No peritoneal spillage (=blocked tube at fimbrial end).

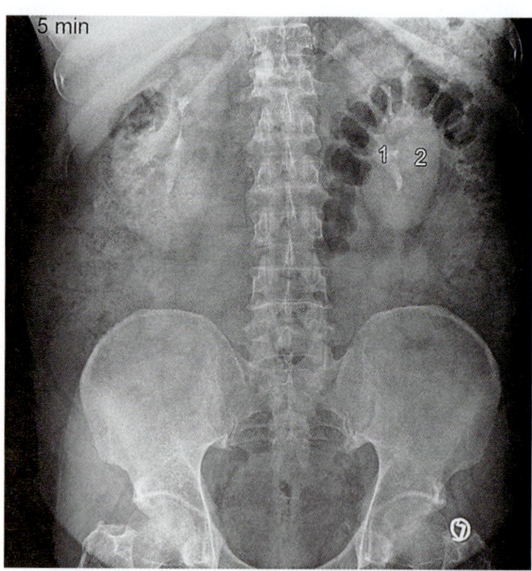

Fig. 46: Intravenous pyelogram 5 minutes post-contrast (AP): 1. Pelvicalyceal system; 2. Nephrogram.

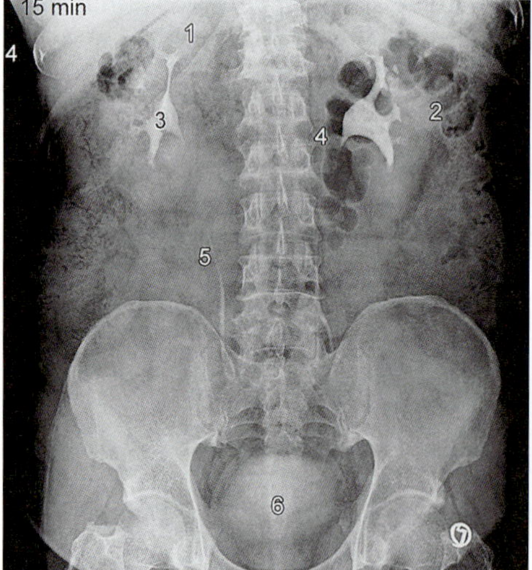

Fig. 47: Intravenous pyelogram 15 minutes post-contrast (AP): 1. Minor calyx; 2. Major calyx; 3. Renal pelvis; 4. Pelvi-ureteric junction; 5. Ureter; 6. Urinary bladder.

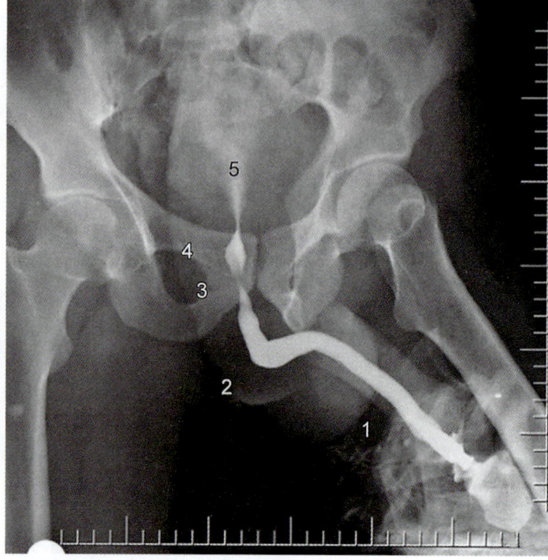

Fig. 48: Retrograde urethrogram (RGU): 1. Penile urethra; 2. Bulbous urethra; 3. Membranous urethra; 4. Prostatic urethra; 5. Contrast in urinary bladder.

Index

Page numbers followed by *f* refer to figure and *t* refer to table.

C

D

G

H

M

N

O

P

Q

R

S

T

U